Controlled Drug Delivery Systems

Controlled Drug Delivery Systems

Edited by
Emmanuel Opara

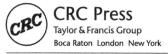

CRC Press
Taylor & Francis Group
Boca Raton London New York

CRC Press is an imprint of the
Taylor & Francis Group, an **informa** business

CRC Press
Taylor & Francis Group
6000 Broken Sound Parkway NW, Suite 300
Boca Raton, FL 33487-2742

First issued in paperback 2023

© 2020 by Taylor & Francis Group, LLC
CRC Press is an imprint of Taylor & Francis Group, an Informa business

No claim to original U.S. Government works

ISBN 13: 978-0-367-18717-0 (hbk)
ISBN 13: 978-1-03-265392-1 (pbk)
ISBN 13: 978-0-429-19783-3 (ebk)

DOI: 10.1201/9780429197833

Visit the Taylor & Francis Web site at
http://www.taylorandfrancis.com

and the CRC Press Web site at
http://www.crcpress.com

Contents

Foreword

Pharmaceutical agents, or drugs, are chemical substances that are applied to the body where they are metabolized and have, or are expected to have, a beneficial effect in treating, mitigating, or preventing disease or discomfort, facilitating repair of injury or otherwise beneficially altering human physiological performance. Drugs have been the mainstay of many branches of medicine for centuries and have a powerful impact on both health status and health economics around the world.

The ability of a drug to achieve its desired effect efficiently and safely depends on many factors, primarily including the ease with which it is administered to, and absorbed by, the body, its mechanism of action in the body, and the way in which the body responds to the presence of the drug, taking into account the characteristics of distribution and metabolic fate. As drugs have become more complex, and their potential to do harm as well as good becomes more evident, attention has been increasingly drawn to the need for greater selectivity with respect to exactly where the drug is targeted in the body, to the preciseness with which the drug molecule attaches to the required site, and the relationship between the level of a drug in the body and time.

Traditionally and most easily, drugs are delivered to a patient by mouth, as in swallowing a tablet, or by inhalation as with an asthma nebulizer. If the drug is not easily absorbed by either of these routes, then alternatives such as intramuscular injection or intravenous infusion may be used, albeit with much lower levels of convenience. There is an inherent problem with conventional delivery regimes since the whole body experiences a peak load of the medication, which then decreases substantially as the drug is metabolized and cleared from the body, until the next dose. At times the level in the patient is likely to be higher than is strictly necessary, and at times it may well be lower than the threshold at which it has an effect. More importantly, the whole body and not just the relevant part experiences these levels. This is hardly a well-controlled delivery process, although it is often quite effective and is usually very convenient as far as the patient is concerned.

The process of achieving greater selectivity in drug delivery may be referred to as controlled drug delivery, controlled drug release, or targeted drug delivery. It may be that the delivery mechanism is quite different, as with an implantable micropump to deliver morphine or insulin, or with transdermal or transmucosal patches. More often we find that the best results are obtained when the drug is combined with a suitable biomaterial. This could involve a physical dispersion of a drug in a biodegradable polymer, which is injected or implanted into the patient, where the drug is released by combinations of diffusion, erosion, osmotic, and degradation processes. In addition, many new drugs do not have the required solubility in the body and biomaterials may assist in this process. It could also involve the chemical coupling of a drug to a soluble polymer, where the linkage between the two is broken under specific *in vivo* conditions.

The technology of the controlled delivery and targeting of active molecules to the body is of immense importance; this book attempts to cover the most relevant aspects. It is necessary to emphasize here that the development of these technologies has taken place since the 1950s, with varying periods of rapid growth in our understanding of mechanisms but of far less growth in their translation into clinical practice. A vast amount of experimental work and preclinical studies have been undertaken. So far, relatively few products have reached full regulatory approval for widespread clinical use; it is very opportune, therefore, to reflect at this time just what are the hopes for the future and the challenges that we face. Thus the contents of the book include discussions of mechanisms of delivery of drugs from materials and devices (such as with thermosensitive hydrogels), the nature of drug delivery biomaterials and their modification (including biopolymers, synthetic polymers, and liposomes), site-specific issues with, for example, transdermal delivery, therapeutic-specific issues such as with cell-secreted products, probiotics and insulin, and with clinical targets such as vaccination and regenerative medicine.

In view of these wide-ranging technological areas, and the up-to-date discussions of opportunities and challenges associated with these applications, the book should provide readers from technology, materials science, pharmacology, and clinical disciplines with very valuable information.

David Williams
Professor, Wake Forest Institute of Regenerative Medicine

Preface

Controlled drug delivery technologies have emerged as an offshoot of Biomaterials Science, a discipline that actually began as early as 3000 BC with the earliest report of a surgical suture in ancient Egypt. By 1829, HS Levert had performed studies to assess the responses to implanted metals in living dogs. Over the years Biomaterials Science has grown tremendously, and today a biomaterial can be defined as a natural or synthetic material (such as a metal or polymer) that is suitable for introduction into living tissue especially as part of a medical device. The device or construct loaded with therapeutic agents can be fabricated to enable a sustained release of a drug over an extended period in the body. The biomaterial used in the construct could be designed to be responsive to different stimuli for the release of a given therapeutic agent. Such a release system would generally result in enhanced therapeutic efficacy achieved with lower doses of drugs that reduce or eliminate unwanted side effects and promote better patient compliance.

The purpose of this book is to provide a unique forum to review the promise of various controlled release systems for which different stimuli, that include pH- and heat-sensitivities, trigger drug release. The book highlights different mechanisms by which tunable polymeric materials can be used in the design of controlled release systems for various purposes, particularly in the emerging field of regenerative medicine. Of particular note in this book is the description of the potential role of engineered polymeric materials for delivery of proteins and targeted delivery of other therapeutic biologics such as probiotics and vaccines.

Controlled Drug Delivery Systems is intended to be a reference handbook for researchers, engineers, clinicians, and other healthcare professionals, and patients, who will find in the book, detailed descriptions of methods of designing biomedical devices suitable for controlled delivery of therapeutic agents. The book also includes elaborate descriptions of methods to engineer polymeric materials for different biomedical applications. Furthermore, individuals or family members of individuals afflicted with certain diseases for which innovative systems of controlled delivery of therapeutic agents are required will find the book to be a good informative resource as they research new therapeutic options in drug delivery for improved efficacy. In addition, entrepreneurs/investors and scientists who work with them in pharmaceutical and biotechnology industries will find this book to be a great reference for assessment of the promise of different models of controlled drug delivery to enable them make informed decisions about where to make rewarding investments that would move the field forward for the benefit of patients.

I would like to express my sincere gratitude to certain individuals with whom I have interacted personally since I have been working in the area of controlled drug delivery. First, I would like to thank Mark E Welker, PhD, professor and immediate past chair of the Department of Chemistry at Wake Forest University in Winston-Salem, North Carolina, whose expertise and collaboration with me have opened new horizons for drug delivery in my laboratory. I am also grateful to my long-term collaborators Eric M. Brey, PhD, professor and chair of the Department of Biomedical Engineering at the University of Texas at San Antonio, Texas, and Justin M. Saul, PhD, professor of chemical and biomedical engineering at Miami University of Ohio, Oxford, Ohio, whose collaborations with me have significantly enriched my knowledge in this area. I also acknowledge the contribution of some postdoctoral fellows and students who have worked with me in developing controlled delivery systems, including Sittadjody Sivanandane, PhD, Surya Banks, PhD, Kevin Enck, PhD, and Brittany Kleszynski Muhlstadt, DVM, for their dedication and productivity in my research in this area. In addition, I would like to acknowledge the great patience, personal sacrifice, and unqualified support of my lovely wife, Clarice, and our children, Ogechi, Chiedu, Chucky, and Ike and his wife, Erin.

Finally, I would like to dedicate this book to the memory of my late beloved uncle, Sir Livinus O. Opara, who taught me the virtues of perseverance, hard work, and fairness, which have guided my career.

Emmanuel Opara
*Wake Forest Institute for Regenerative Medicine, Wake Forest School of Medicine
and
Virginia Tech-Wake Forest School of Biomedical Engineering & Sciences (SBES)
Wake Forest School of Medicine, Winston-Salem, North Carolina*

Editor

Professor Emmanuel Opara earned his PhD in medical sciences from the University of London, England. He came to the USA in 1984 as a World Health Organization (WHO) Fellow in Endocrinology/Metabolism at the Mayo Clinic in Rochester, Minnesota. He later moved to the National Institute of Diabetes, Digestive and Kidney diseases (NIDDK) of the National Institutes of Health in Bethesda, Maryland, where he served as a Visiting Fellow from 1986 to 1988 prior to accepting a faculty position in the Department of Surgery at Duke University Medical Center, Durham, North Carolina. In 2003, after 15 years at Duke, he was appointed a research professor at the Pritzker Institute of Biomedical Science and Engineering at the Illinois Institute of Technology (IIT), Chicago, while serving as a senior investigator in the Human Islet Transplant Program at the Pritzker School of Medicine of the University of Chicago. He currently serves as a professor of regenerative medicine and biomedical engineering at the Wake Forest School of Medicine and the graduate program director at the Wake Forest University Campus of the Joint Virginia Tech-Wake Forest School of Biomedical Engineering and Sciences (SBES).

Contributors

Mmesoma Anike
Wake Forest School of Medicine
Winston-Salem, North Carolina
and
Wake Forest Institute for Regenerative
    Medicine, Wake Forest School of Medicine
Winston-Salem, North Carolina

Mohammad Reza Askari
Department of Chemical and Biological
    Engineering
Illinois Institute of Technology
Chicago, Illinois

Anthony Atala
Wake Forest Institute for Regenerative
    Medicine, Wake Forest School of Medicine
Winston-Salem, North Carolina

Gunjan Vasant Bonde
Department of Pharmaceutical Engineering &
    Technology
Indian Institute of Technology (Banaras Hindu
    University)
Varanasi, India
School of Health Sciences, University
    of Petroleum and Energy Studies,
    Dehradun India

Rachel Brandt
Department of Biomedical Engineering
Illinois Institute of Technology
Chicago, Illinois

Eric M. Brey
Department of Biomedical Engineering and
    Chemical Engineering
The University of Texas at San Antonio
San Antonio, Texas

Jacob Brown
Department of Biomedical Engineering and
    Chemical Engineering
The University of Texas at San Antonio
San Antonio, Texas

Zishuai Chou
Wake Forest Institute for
    Regenerative Medicine, Wake Forest
    School of Medicine
Winston-Salem, North Carolina

Ali Cinar
Department of Chemical and Biological
    Engineering
Illinois Institute of Technology
Chicago, Illinois
and
Department of Biomedical Engineering
Illinois Institute of Technology
Chicago, Illinois

Fernando Freitas de Lima
Department of Biochemistry and Tissue
    Biology, Institute of Biology
University of Campinas-UNICAMP
Campinas, Brazil

Lígia Nunes de Morais Ribeiro
Department of Biochemistry and Tissue
    Biology, Institute of Biology
University of Campinas-UNICAMP
Campinas, Brazil
and
School of Veterinary Medicine
Federal University of Uberlândia
Uberlândia, Brazil

Thomas DePalma
Department of Biomedical Engineering
The Ohio State University
Columbus, Ohio

Eneida de Paula
Department of Biochemistry and Tissue
    Biology, Institute of Biology
University of Campinas-UNICAMP
Campinas, Brazil

Kevin Enck
Virginia Tech-Wake Forest School of
    Biomedical Engineering and Sciences
    (SBES)
Wake Forest Institute for Regenerative
    Medicine, Wake Forest School of Medicine
Winston-Salem, North Carolina

Elham Ghadiri
Wake Forest Institute for Regenerative
    Medicine, Wake Forest School of Medicine
Winston-Salem, North Carolina
and
Department of Chemistry
Wake Forest University
Winston-Salem, North Carolina

Jian Guan
School of Pharmacy
Shenyang Pharmaceutical University
Shenyang, China

Iman Hajizadeh
Department of Chemical and Biological
    Engineering
Illinois Institute of Technology
Chicago, Illinois

Nicole Hobbs
Department of Biomedical Engineering
Illinois Institute of Technology
Chicago, Illinois

Katie Hogan
Department of Bioengineering
Rice University
Houston, Texas

Adam Jorgensen
Wake Forest Institute for Regenerative
    Medicine, Wake Forest School of Medicine
Winston-Salem, North Carolina

Alec Jost
Wake Forest School of Medicine
Winston-Salem, North Carolina
and
Wake Forest Institute for Regenerative
    Medicine, Wake Forest School of Medicine
Winston-Salem, North Carolina

Jareer Kassis
Wake Forest Institute for Regenerative
    Medicine, Wake Forest School of Medicine
Winston-Salem, North Carolina

W.F. Kendall Jr
Department of Surgery,
University of Florida
Gainesville, Florida

Shirui Mao
School of Pharmacy
Shenyang Pharmaceutical University
Shenyang, China

Kevin J. McHugh
Department of Bioengineering
Rice University
Houston, Texas

Antonios G. Mikos
Department of Bioengineering
Rice University
Houston, Texas

Brahmeshwar Mishra
Department of Pharmaceutical Engineering &
    Technology
Indian Institute of Technology (BHU)
Varanasi, India

Sean Murphy
Wake Forest Institute for
    Regenerative Medicine, Wake Forest
    School of Medicine
Winston-Salem, North Carolina

Kylie G. Nairon
Department of Biomedical Engineering
The Ohio State University
Columbus, Ohio

Juliana Damasceno Oliveira
Department of Biochemistry and Tissue
    Biology, Institute of Biology
University of Campinas-UNICAMP
Campinas, Brazil

Emmanuel Opara
Wake Forest School of Medicine
Winston-Salem, North Carolina
and
Wake Forest Institute for Regenerative
    Medicine, Wake Forest School of Medicine
Winston-Salem, North Carolina
and
Virginia Tech-Wake Forest School of
    Biomedical Engineering & Sciences, Wake
    Forest School of Medicine
Winston-Salem, North Carolina

Victor Hugo Pérez-Luna
Department of Chemical and Biological
    Engineering
Illinois Institute of Technology
Chicago, Illinois

Mudassir Rashid
Department of Chemical and Biological
    Engineering
Illinois Institute of Technology
Chicago, Illinois

Sediqeh Samadi
Department of Chemical and Biological
    Engineering
Illinois Institute of Technology
Chicago, Illinois

Justin M. Saul
Chemical, Paper and Biomedical Engineering
Miami University
Oxford, Ohio

Mert Sevil
Department of Biomedical Engineering
Illinois Institute of Technology
Chicago, Illinois

Ashkan Shafiee
Wake Forest Institute for Regenerative
    Medicine
Wake Forest School of Medicine
Winston-Salem, North Carolina

Binita Shrestha
Department of Biomedical Engineering and
    Chemical Engineering
The University of Texas at San Antonio
San Antonio, Texas

Sivanandane Sittadjody
Wake Forest Institute for Regenerative
    Medicine, Wake Forest University School of
    Medicine
Winston-Salem, North Carolina

Hemamylammal Sivakumar
Department of Biomedical Engineering
The Ohio State University
Columbus, Ohio

Aleksander Skardal
Department of Biomedical Engineering
The Ohio State University
Columbus, Ohio
and
The Ohio State University Wexner Medical
    Center
Columbus, Ohio
and
The Ohio State University Comprehensive
    Cancer Center
Columbus, Ohio

Mark E. Welker
Department of Chemistry
Wake Forest University
Winston-Salem, North Carolina

Xin Zhang
School of Pharmacy
Shenyang Pharmaceutical University
Shenyang, China

1 Introduction – Approaches to Controlled Drug Delivery

Katie Hogan and Antonios G. Mikos
Rice University

Professor Emmanuel Opara is a leading researcher in drug delivery technologies. This textbook, *Controlled Drug Delivery Systems*, stems from this expertise and seeks to enlighten readers on topics and techniques of interest within the field of drug delivery. The goal of controlled drug delivery systems is to provide a means for predictable *in vivo* release of therapeutics over a desired timeframe. This design objective allows for more targeted therapeutic responses that reduce the need for high dosing frequency and large systemic doses. As may be seen throughout this book, the specific criteria for controlled drug delivery vary widely based on the drug of interest and its intended target, and these requirements have led to the development of diverse types of drug delivery systems. Here, the role of biomaterials in drug delivery for a variety of applications (direct therapeutic response, tissue regeneration, etc.) will be discussed as well as delivery systems designed to interact with specific tissues.

The first portion of this book describes the formulation and modification of hydrogel systems for drug delivery. In Chapter 2 the use of alginates and their chemical modification via covalent bond-forming reactions for drug delivery and regenerative medicine applications are detailed. These modifications are explored via the type of modifying reaction used and the intended function of the resulting alginate material. Chapter 3 looks into the tunability of hydrogel systems for specific applications involving the long-term release of cell-secreted products with therapeutic potential. Chapter 4 similarly deals with potential methods for hydrogel modification, looking specifically at thermoresponsive hydrogels such as those based on N-isopropylacrylamide. Methods using glutathione to address one of the key disadvantages of hydrogels composed of linear polymer chains, poor *in vivo* degradation, are discussed in detail.

Subsequent chapters discuss specific applications of controlled drug delivery systems and unique challenges encountered with tissue- and organ-specific targeting. In Chapter 5, for instance, the use of biodegradable particles as single-injection vaccine systems is discussed as an alternative to traditional multidose vaccine regimens. The authors describe the many factors that must be considered for controlled-release vaccine development, including device formulation strategies and large-scale clinical distribution considerations.

Tissue engineering and regenerative medicine is a key application for controlled drug delivery systems. Thus, the next several chapters describe general and specific applications of drug delivery systems for tissue engineering. Endocrine pathways are far-reaching and often have systemic side effects which are not immediately obvious. Chapter 6 discusses general hormone delivery and controlled release methods, introducing the concept of hormone pellet implants. Chapter 7 describes an application of hormone delivery and targeting that clearly demonstrates this concept – delivery of ovarian hormones for the preservation of bone health. The challenges and benefits of this strategy are explored within the context of tissue engineering and regenerative medicine approaches that seek to harness cellular production and delivery of these hormones. In Chapter 8, the use of controlled molecular delivery for tissue engineering and biofabrication is more generally discussed. Growth factors and other bioactive molecules are frequently introduced into tissue engineered constructs to induce processes such as cellular differentiation and angiogenesis. Here, the authors discuss methods of delivery and release of these molecules alongside current techniques used in tissue regeneration. Looking deeper at a specific integral component of engineering tissue, Chapter 9 delves into the importance and intricacies of stim-ulating vasculogenesis via the delivery of angiogenic proteins. Vascularization is an important compo-nent in the solution to issues with tissue engineered construct scalability, survival, and integration with native tissue. Within this chapter, strategies including polymer delivery systems are discussed, which seek to produce closely controlled and timely release of growth factors to provide greater therapeutic efficacy and angiogenesis compared with single growth factor administration. Chapter 10 describes advances in tissue engineering for wound healing and the role of drug delivery in skin regeneration technologies. Specifically, the importance of hydrogel-based biomaterials is examined as a vehicle for biological elements such as stem cells and cytokines as well as essential proteins for skin regeneration like collagen. The chapter discusses patient successes in skin regeneration and the use of technologies like 3D printing to improve cell and growth factor delivery for improved therapeutic effects.

The next three chapters explore the development of different approaches to controlled drug deliv-ery for a single application: insulin regulation. Diabetic patients often need exogenous insulin to regulate glucose levels. However, the need for multiple daily injections often leads to inconsistent patient compliance. Chapter 11 explores how an adaptive model predictive control algorithm may be used in conjunction with a multivariable artificial pancreas to characterize glucose concentration dynamics. This information may then be used to calculate exogenous insulin dosing from an insulin pump in simulated case studies. Focusing on an alternative strategy, Chapter 12 reviews research related to the development of an oral insulin formulation. Specifically, this survey reveals advances in addressing key challenges related to an oral formulation, namely enzymatic degradation of and mucosal transport of polypeptide insulin, and discusses challenges that must be mitigated before clinical translation. Next, Chapter 13 offers yet another prospective solution for insulin delivery which harnesses tissue engineering strategies for the creation of a bioartificial pancreas. It details limitations of previously developed artificial pancreas strategies, including pancreatic tissue trans-plantation, and describes strategies for biomaterial-based devices that provide structural support for cell-based systems and employ selective permeability.

The next section of this book explores additional routes of controlled drug delivery in greater depth. For instance, Chapter 14 offers a description of transdermal delivery systems. The chapter addresses unique advantages that make this technique desirable for local or systemic drug delivery as well as challenges. Additionally, basic components of transdermal delivery systems, common architectures, material evaluation, and novel formulation strategies are discussed. In Chapter 15, oral drug delivery systems are once again examined, this time regarding specific new technologies which seek to address inherent issues with this delivery route. This chapter investigates in depth the mucoadhesive properties of chitosan and the application of its derivatives to create nanoparticle delivery systems for oral drug delivery. Similarly, Chapter 16 describes liposomes as a means of tar-geted therapy delivery for applications including pain management, treating infections, and cancer therapeutics. The various materials which can be used to create liposomes and increase their tissue specificity and the unique systems which may be generated using these concepts are described in detail. Further, focusing on the clinical translatability of these technologies, those liposomal formu-lations which have been tested in clinical trials or reached market and their clinical applications are discussed. Finally, in Chapter 17, emerging technologies are reviewed which allow for oral delivery of probiotics with increased efficacy. Therapeutic bacteria operate via a symbiotic relationship with gut bacteria, and this chapter illustrates ways in which cell encapsulation strategies have provided orally delivered cells from acidic destruction and demonstrates how engineered polymers have pro-vided new routes for targeted bacterial delivery to the intestine.

Taken together, this textbook provides a comprehensive overview of topics relevant to controlled drug delivery systems in a wide array of formulations and applications. We hope that readers enjoy the excellent tour of systems for targeted therapeutic release provided by Professor Opara's textbook and are inspired to create new solutions to clinical challenges in drug delivery.

2 Chemical Modifications of Alginates for Use in Drug Delivery and Regenerative Medicine Applications

Mark E. Welker
Wake Forest University

CONTENTS

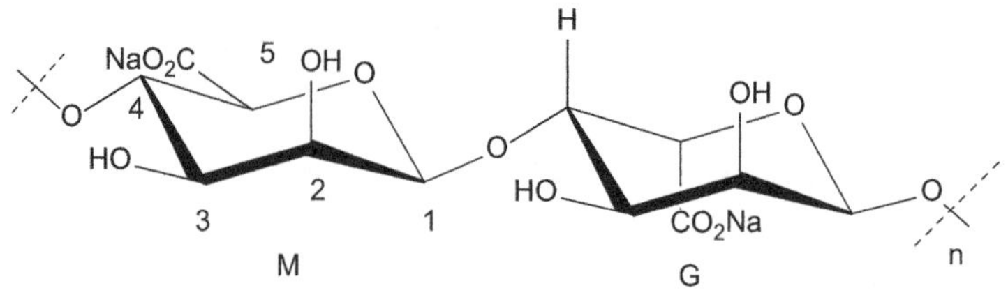

FIGURE 2.1 Alginate structure.

2.1 INTRODUCTION

This chapter covers covalent bond forming chemical modification of alginates that are subsequently used for drug delivery and regenerative medicine applications. Many mixtures of alginates with other polysaccharides and other additives have been used in drug delivery and regenerative medicine, but that work will not be covered here since that type of work does not involve planned covalent bond modification of alginates. A book chapter that has good coverage of the structures of alginates and a chronological history of chemical modifications of its hydroxyl and carboxylic acid functional groups appeared in 2017 [1]. Review articles on the chemical modifications of alginates for use in biomedical applications have appeared in 2010–2014, so this chapter will largely cover this topic for the last 5 years (2014–2018) [2–7]. The articles reviewed here came from one of the three topical searches within the Science Citation Index. A search using keywords alginate and regenerative medicine yielded 285 references which were subsequently checked for reported organic chemistry. A second search using keywords alginate and drug delivery yielded 2,191 references with 146 of them within the subtopic of organic chemistry and those were also checked for reported chemical functionalization of alginates. Last, a search using keywords alginate derivative yielded 267 references with 40 of them within the subtopic of organic chemistry which were also checked for chemical modification of alginates and had possible uses in drug delivery or regenerative medicine. Two nice reviews of chemical functionalization of polysaccharides for uses in biomedical science with some references to alginates appeared in 2018 [8,9]. There are many recent reviews that focus on biomedical and clinical applications of polysaccharides, where all or part of the review content focuses on alginates [10–26].

Alginates are composed of linked β-D-mannuronic acid (M) and α-L-guluronic acid (G) monosaccharides. The M/G ratio of the polysaccharide depends on the source and can contain M-blocks, G-blocks, and M-G blocks interspersed with M-G disaccharide linkages. Alginates isolated from algae are typically polydisperse with molecular weights of 100,000–1,000,000 g/mol, so 500–5,000 residues per chain. M and G are C-5 epimers, and most of the covalent bond forming organic chemistry of alginates occurs at the C-5 carboxylic acid functional group or at the C-2/C-3 hydroxyl functional groups (Figure 2.1).

2.2 COMMON CHEMICAL REACTIONS OF ALGINATES

Before we embark on a review of alginate chemical modification work from the last 5 years, it may be helpful for the reader to see generic examples of the most common alginate modification reactions.

2.2.1 SIMPLE MONOSACCHARIDE MODIFICATION REACTIONS

2.2.1.1 Hydroxyl Modification

Acetylation, phosphorylation, and sulfation of the C-2/C-3 hydroxyl groups are well-known reactions, and it is generally difficult to control whether M or G hydroxyls are functionalized in those reactions. Ester formation off the C-2/C-3 hydroxyls can be effected by treating alginates with acid chlorides (Figure 2.2).

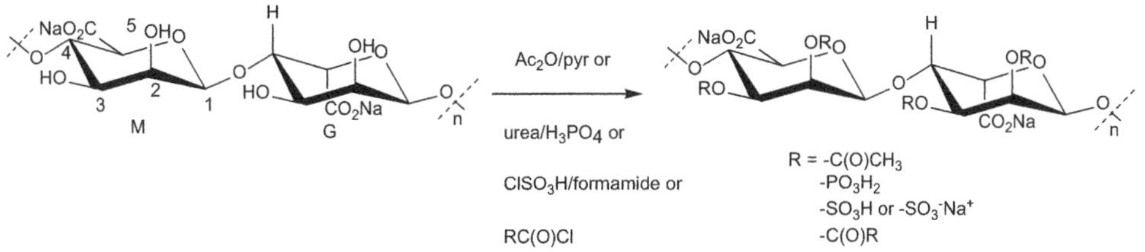

FIGURE 2.2   Common alginate hydroxyl group modifications.

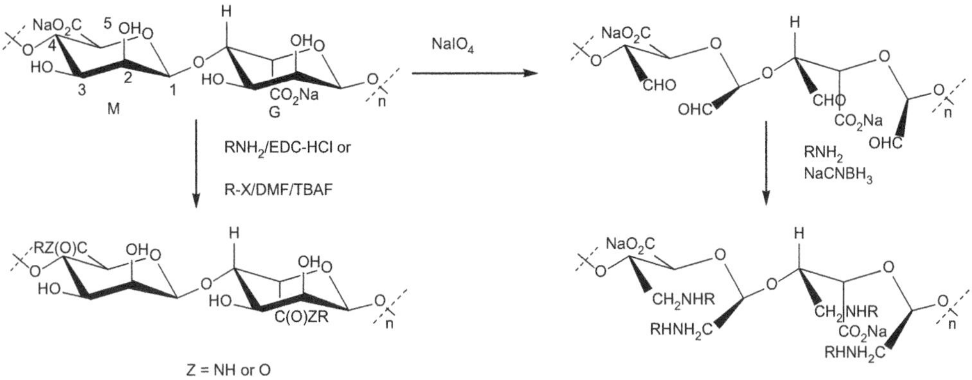

FIGURE 2.3   Reductive amination of partially oxidized alginates and amide/ester formation from carboxylates.

Likewise, periodate oxidative cleavage of the C–C bond between the C-2/C-3 hydroxyls is well known and in many cases is followed by reductive amination (Figure 2.3).

2.2.1.2   Carboxylic Acid Modification

The most common organic reaction of the carboxylic acid functional group is carbodiimide mediated coupling with an amine to form an amide. Ester rather than amide formation at the carboxylate can be accomplished by treating the carboxylate anions with a primary alkyl halide (Figure 2.3).

2.2.2   CHEMICAL MODIFICATIONS FOR *IN SITU* COVALENTLY CROSSLINKING ALGINATES

Three different synthetic methods are most commonly used for covalently linking alginate polymer chains *in situ* to one another: (i) ether linkages generated from alginate hydroxyl group reactions with epichlorhydrin, (ii) ether linkages generated from alginate hydroxyl group reactions with glutaraldehyde, and (iii) amide linkages generated from diamine reactions with alginate carboxylic acids (Figure 2.4).

2.2.3   CHEMICAL MODIFICATIONS THAT ARE SUBSEQUENTLY USED FOR CROSSLINKING

2.2.3.1   Modifications That Are Followed by Photochemical Crosslinking

Two different synthetic methods are most commonly used for photochemically linking alginate polymer chains *in situ* to one another: (i) photochemical coupling of acrylates and (ii) photochemical thiol–alkene click reactions (Figure 2.5).

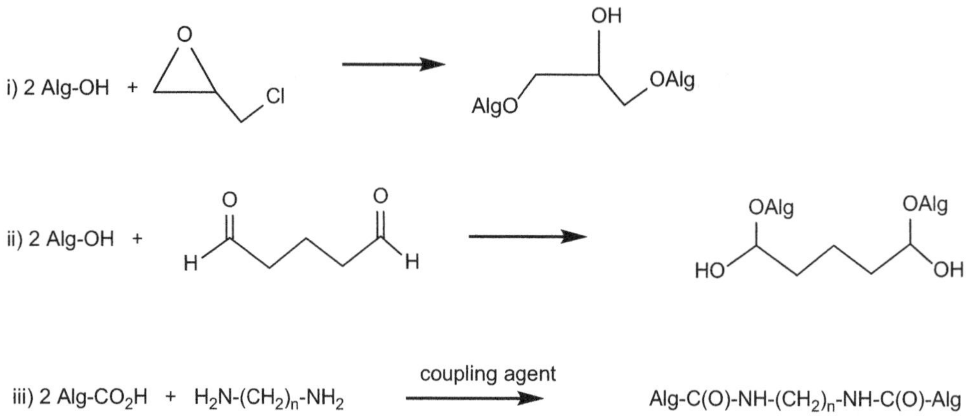

FIGURE 2.4 Common methods for *in situ* covalent crosslinking of alginate chains.

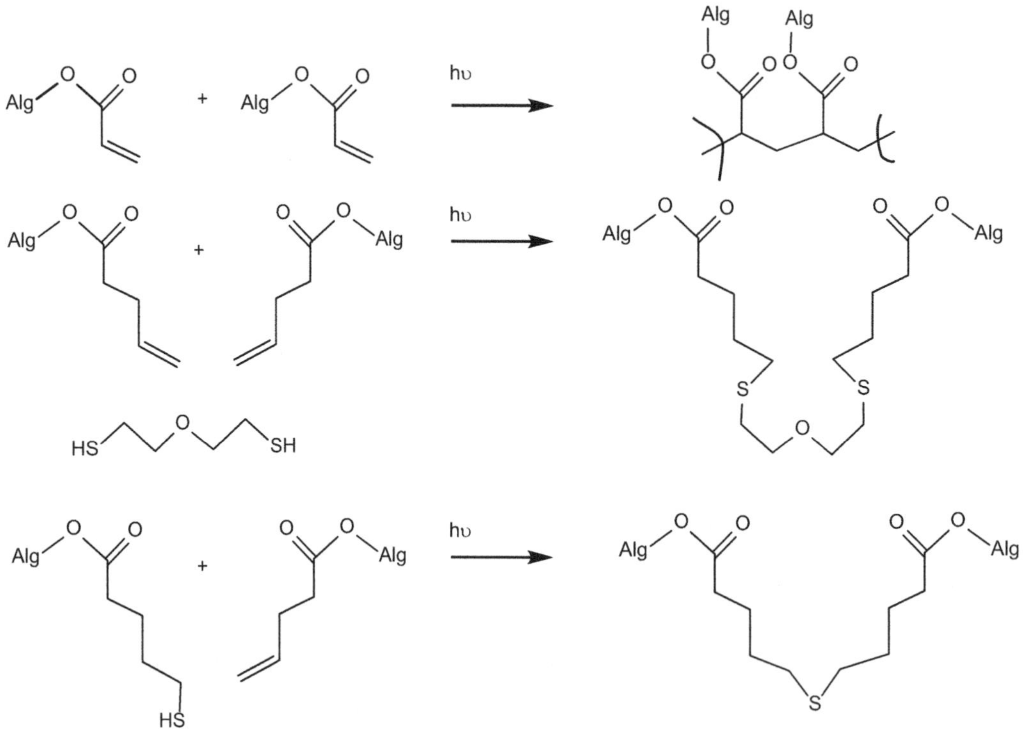

FIGURE 2.5 Chemical modifications of alginates that are followed by photochemical crosslinking.

2.2.3.2 Modifications That Are Followed by Nucleophile–Electrophile or Cycloaddition Reaction Crosslinking

A number of chemical reactions fit into this category and generally involve bond formation between a modified alginate which can be classified as an electron acceptor and an electron donor. Examples of acceptors are strained ring alkynes, aldehydes or ketones, and α,β-unsaturated carbonyl compounds or sulfones. Examples of electron donors are azides, amides, hydrazines, hydrazones, and thiols (Figure 2.6).

Alg-acceptor + Alg-donor ⟶ Alg-acceptor-donor-Alg

FIGURE 2.6 Nucleophile–electrophile reactions between modified alginate chains.

2.2.4 CHEMICAL MODIFICATIONS TO ADD LIGANDS TO THE POLYSACCHARIDE

Ligand addition reactions are most commonly amidation or esterification reactions of the carboxylic acids or reductive amination reactions of the partially oxidized polysaccharides, many times used to add drugs which can be ligated while still attached to the polysaccharide or released via hydrolysis.

2.2.5 CHEMICAL MODIFICATIONS THAT ADD BOTH CROSSLINKING CAPABILITY AND LIGANDS

Combinations of the reactions are discussed under Sections 2.2.1–2.2.3 above.

2.3 REVIEW OF RECENT ALGINATE COVALENT BOND FORMING REACTION CHEMISTRY

Most of the reaction chemistry reported in the last 5 years starts with either alginate periodate oxidation or alginate amidation as the first chemical bond forming step, so we will break this discussion along those two categories initially and then finish the discussion with alginate modifications that begin with something other than these two types of reactions.

2.3.1 MODIFICATIONS THAT BEGIN WITH PERIODATE OXIDATION

2.3.1.1 Modifications That Begin with Periodate Oxidation Where the Alginate Application Is Cell Growth or Survival

In 2014, the groups of Yan, Chen, Cui, and Yin and their co-workers reported that hydrazide modified poly (L-glutamic acid) (PLGA-ADH) could be reacted with periodate oxidized alginate (ALG-CHO) to make an imine crosslinked two-polymer component hydrogel (Figure 2.7) [27]. This hydrogel showed injectability, rapid *in vivo* gel formation, mechanical stability, rabbit chondrocyte ingrowth, and ectopic cartilage formation, indicating that this hydrogel has attractive properties for cartilage tissue engineering.

In 2015, Bernkop-Schnurch and co-workers reported preparation and characterization of a novel S-protected thiolated alginate [28]. Partially oxidized alginate was treated with cysteine and NaCNBH$_3$ to effect reductive amination. Properties of this thiol-modified alginate were determined, and it was also incorporated into a disulfide using 2-mercaptonicotinic acid (Figure 2.8). The thiol

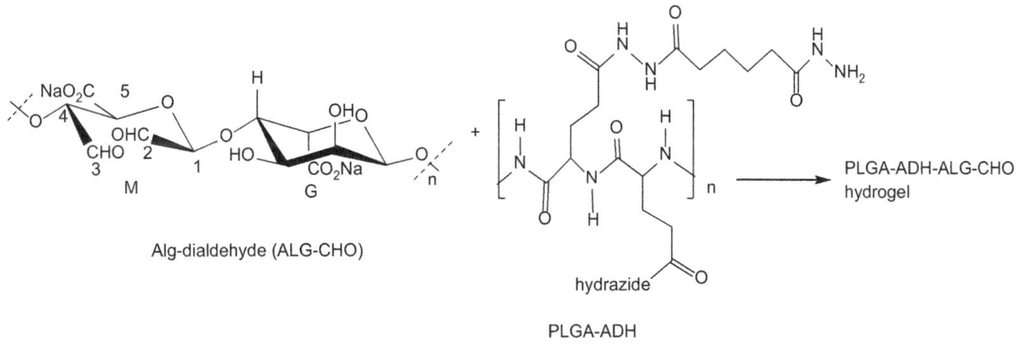

FIGURE 2.7 Oxidized alginate–hydrazide modified polyglutamic acid hydrogel.

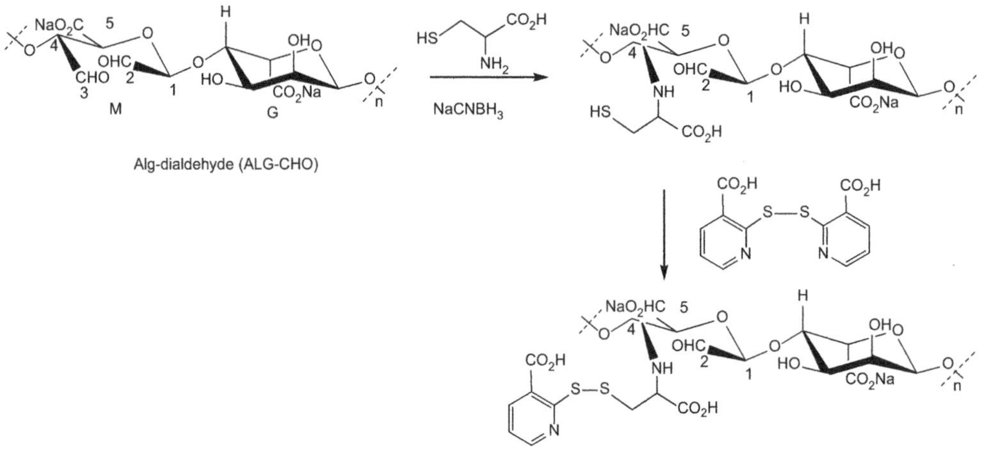

FIGURE 2.8 Oxidized and disulfide modified alginate.

protected material showed increased viscosity relative to unmodified alginate and also behaved similarly after treatment with H_2O_2 to effect disulfide formation. Mucoadhesive properties of both thiolated and disulfide-containing alginate were significantly better than unmodified alginate, and these modified alginates were not cytotoxic toward Caco-2 cell lines.

In 2016, Du and co-workers reported crosslinking alginate dialdehyde with carboxymethylchitosan (Figure 2.9) with and without the addition of polyethylene oxide (PEO) to each of the polysaccharide solutions [29]. Presumably with PEO present there is more chain-to-chain crosslinking in addition to the imine bonds formed between chitosan NH_2 groups and aldehydes. The nanofibers produced using PEO promoted the adhesion, proliferation, and alkaline phosphatase activity of mouse bone marrow stromal cells making them candidates for bone regeneration applications.

Also that year, Christensen and co-workers used reductive amination to functionalize alginate with three different bioactive peptides (Figure 2.10) [30]. Three different peptide sequences (GRGDYP, GRGDSP, and KHIFSDDSSE) were coupled to 8% oxidized alginate with degrees of substitution ranging between 4% and 7%. The alginate with covalently attached GRGDSP was found to excel in binding mouse skeletal myoblasts and human dental stem cells.

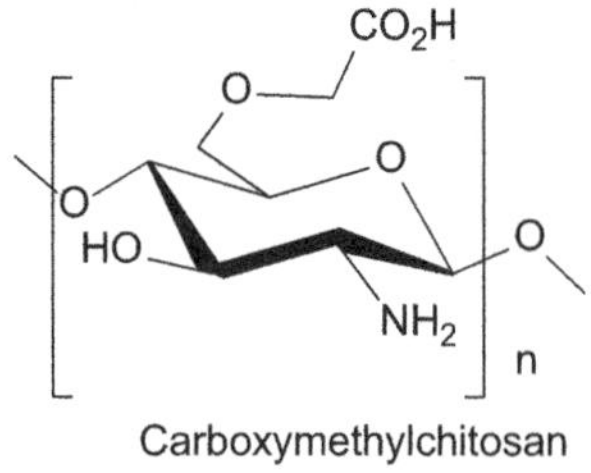

FIGURE 2.9 Carboxymethylchitosan.

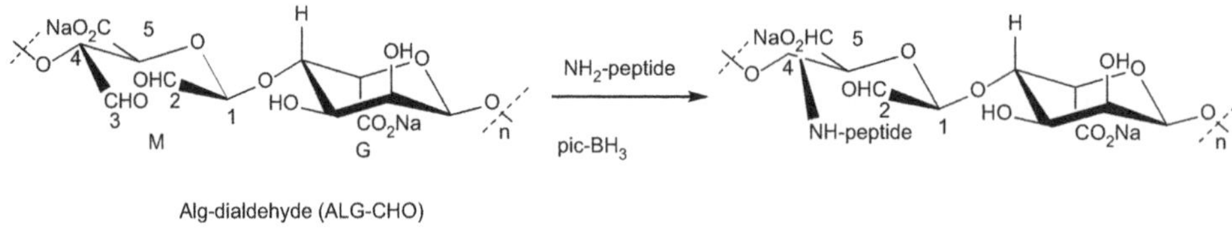

FIGURE 2.10 Peptide reductive amination of oxidized alginate.

In 2017, Mo and co-workers reported the preparation of alginate which had been modified first by periodate oxidation and then by amidation with 2-aminoethyl methacrylate [31]. Separately gelatin was treated with ethyl-(N,N′-dimethylamino)propylcarbodiimide hydrochloride (EDC) and ethylene diamine to form a primary amine containing gelatin. The amino gelatin and the dialdehyde alginate were then first mixed to effect imine formation and alginate chain to gelatin chain cross-linking, and this was followed by photolysis to form alginate chain to alginate chain crosslinks via the photochemical dimerization of acrylates (Figure 2.11). These dual crosslinked hydrogels were then shown to have better mechanical properties and slower degradation than the corresponding singly crosslinked gels. These dual crosslinked gels also had lower cytotoxicity and proved to be suitable environments for the growth of L929 mouse fibroblast cells.

In 2018, Karvinen and co-workers reported a modified alginate-modified polyvinylalcohol (PVA) hydrogel that could be used as a supportive biomaterial for neuronal cell cultures [32]. The PVA was first converted to a carbamate by treatment with carbonyl diimidazole (CDI) and glycine ethyl ester. That carbamate was then treated with hydrazine to make a hydrazide modified PVA (Figure 2.12). The modified PVA was then mixed with partially oxidized alginate in a 10% sucrose solution to produce hydrogels presumably crosslinked via imine bond formation. These alginate–PVA hydrogels were shown to be supportive of growth of human pluripotent stem cell derived neuronal cells.

In late 2018, Nan, Li, and co-workers reported injectable gelatin, oxidized sodium alginate (Na-Alg), and adipic acid dihydrazide (ADH) (Figure 2.13) hydrogels which remained in liquid form and flowed easily for several minutes after initial mixing at room temperature but gelled rapidly at 37°C [33]. Gelation time could be regulated by varying ratios of the three components, and gelation presumably comes from a mixture of imine formation between oxidized alginate and gelatin and acylhydrazone formation between oxidized alginate and ADH. Both L929 and NIH 3T3 cells proliferated on these hydrogels, so the authors believe they would be safe injectable self-healing hydrogels for both tissue engineering and drug delivery purposes.

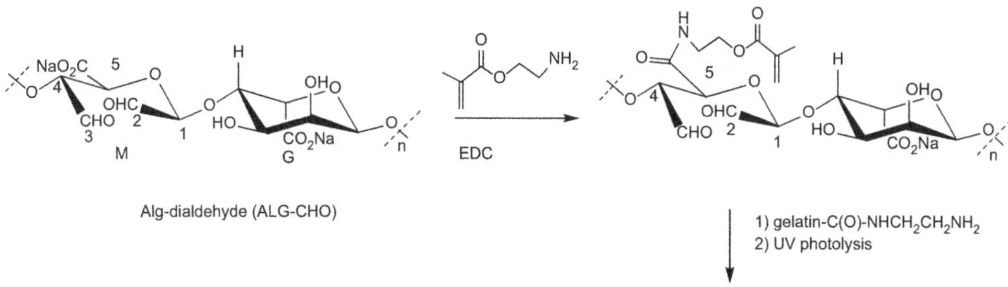

FIGURE 2.11 Oxidized and acrylate modified alginate crosslinked with gelatin.

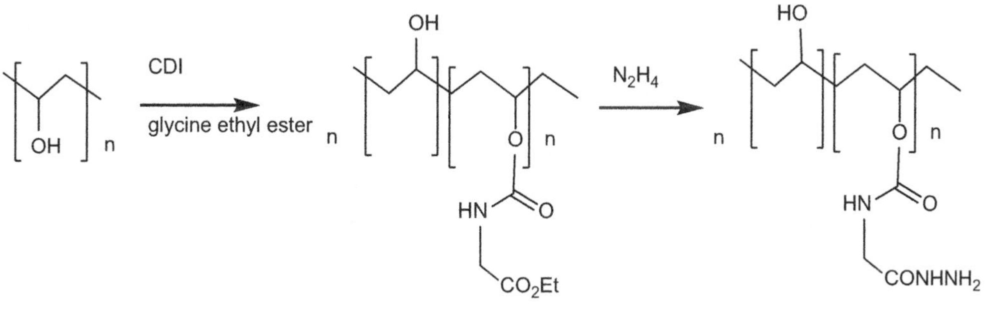

FIGURE 2.12 Modified polyvinyl alcohol prior to oxidized alginate addition.

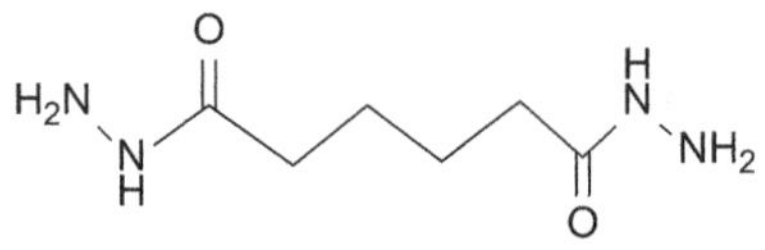

FIGURE 2.13   Adipic acid dihydrazide.

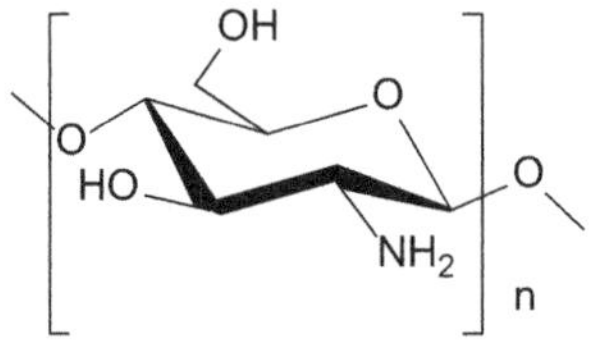

Chitosan

FIGURE 2.14   Chitosan.

2.3.1.2   Modifications That Begin with Periodate Oxidation Where the Alginate Application Is Drug Delivery

In 2015, Grondahl and co-workers partially oxidized alginate to the dialdehyde and then treated it with chitosan (Figure 2.14) in acetic acid [34]. Some chitosan-alginate crosslinking occurred through imine formation between chitosan amine groups and aldehydes. The oxidized alginate-chitosan conjugate was then assembled onto silica and alginate in a layer-by-layer approach, and the swelling that occurred was studied as a precursor to using this layer-by-layer approach to control drug diffusion from such gels.

Similarly, in 2015, James and co-workers treated partially oxidized alginate with gelatin and sodium borate to form gelatin–alginate conjugates via imine linkages [35]. The gels thus formed were shown not to cause significant hemolysis of whole blood and were not cytotoxic to MCF-7 cancer cell lines indicating that these gels were candidates for drug delivery applications.

In 2018, Liu and co-workers reported some folate and rhodamine modified oxidized alginates which are intended for cancer treatment [36]. Partially oxidized alginate was first treated with a 1:1 mixture of folate terminated poly(ethylene glycol) amine (FA-PEG-NH$_2$) (Figure 2.15) and rhodamine B-terminated poly(ethylene glycol) amine (RhB-PEG-NH$_2$) (Figure 2.15) along with N-hydroxysuccinimide (NHS) and EDC to effect amidation. That modified alginate was then treated with the diamine, cystamine [NH$_2$(CH$_2$)$_2$S-]$_2$, along with NHS and EDC to effect alginate chain crosslinking. Finally, the crosslinked gel was treated with doxorubicin (Figure 2.15) under basic conditions to attach the drug to the oxidized alginate via an imine linkage. These hydrogels were used for pH-specific doxorubicin release for cancer chemotherapy using HepG2 cells.

Lastly in 2018, there were two reports of reactions of oxidized alginates with hydrazides where the modified alginates prepared were tested for drug delivery. In early 2018, Yang and co-workers prepared a hydrazide terminated poly(ethylene glycol) (PEG-DTP) via the reaction of PEG-diacid with 3,3′-dithiobis (propionohydrazide) (Figure 2.16) [37]. The PEG-DTP thus prepared and oxidized Na-Alg were then used to prepare hydrogels where the gelation seen presumably occurs via acylhydrazone bond formation. The hydrogels thus produced showed reduced hydrophobicity relative to unmodified oxidized alginate and enhanced mechanical performance. These hydrogels were also shown to have low cytotoxicity as A549 cells showed good viability (>90%) after incubation with these gels for 24 hours. These gels were then used to encapsulate and release rhodamine B as a model drug. Rhodamine B release from the gels was affected by treatment with the reducing agent dithithreitol (DTT) which cleaves disulfide bonds.

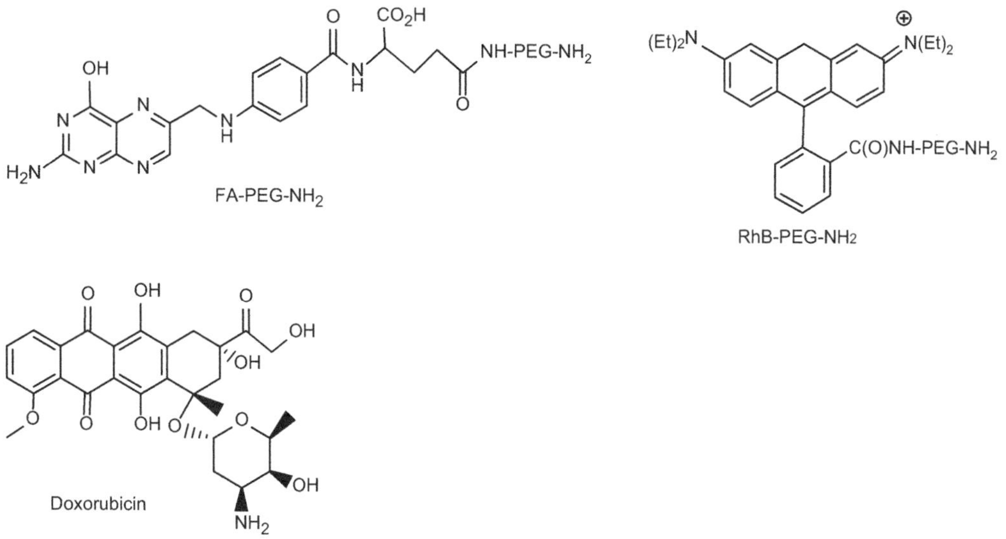

FIGURE 2.15   Modified folate, modified rhodamine, and doxorubicin structures.

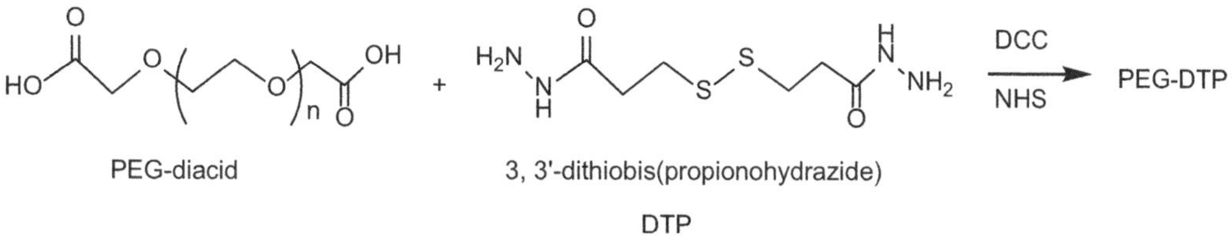

FIGURE 2.16   Reaction of PEG-diacid and DTP.

Jang and Cha reported the preparation of polyaspartamides containing hydrazides or primary amines which were conjugated to partially oxidized alginate via acyl hydrazone/imine linkages [38]. In this work, polysuccinimide (PSI) was first treated with ADH and 2-aminoethanol or diethylene triamine and 2-aminoethanol in order to prepare polyaspartamides which contained hydrazide or primary amine functional groups (Figure 2.17). These polyaspartamides were then treated with partially oxidized alginate to make imine crosslinked hydrogels. The mechanical properties of these hydrogels could be controlled over a wide range, and they were used for a drug release model study using bovine serum albumin (BSA) as a control protein drug.

2.3.2   MODIFICATIONS THAT BEGIN WITH AMIDATION

2.3.2.1   Modifications That Begin with Amidation and Any Crosslinking Is Nucleophile–Electrophile or Cycloaddition Chemistry Where the Alginate Application Is Enhanced Cell Growth or Survival

In 2015, Strand and co-workers reported a chemoenzymatic protocol for preparing peptide modified alginates which were used for cell encapsulation [39]. In this work, mannuronan was first coupled at low levels (0.1%–0.2%) to the peptide GRGDSP using N-hydroxysulfosuccinimide (sulfo-NHS) and EDC. This peptide modified alginate was then treated with epimerases to produce low (30%–50%) and high (60%–80%) G content alginates (Figure 2.18). These alginates were then used to encapsulate olfactory ensheathing cells (OECs) and myoblasts, and while cell attachment and improved cell

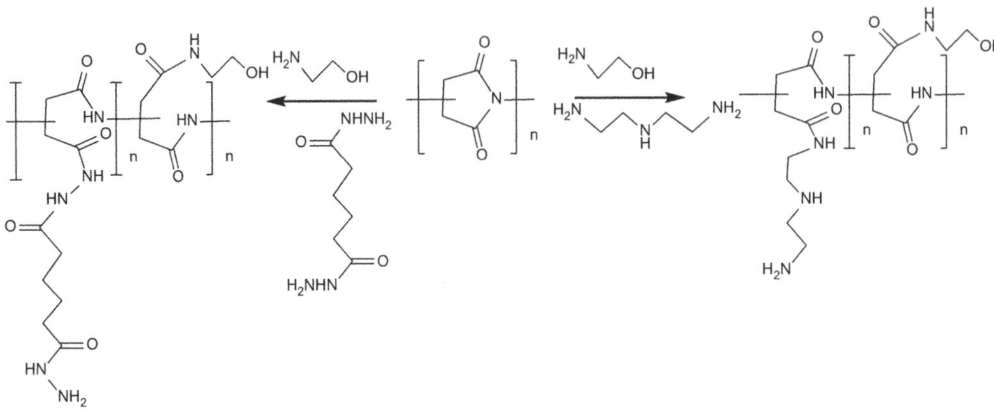

FIGURE 2.17 Reactions of PSI with dihydrazides and triamines.

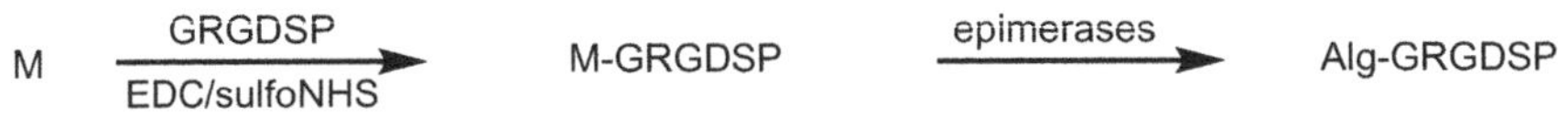

FIGURE 2.18 Preparation and epimerization of mannuronan–peptide conjugates.

viability was noted on some 2D surfaces, these studies did not show enhanced cell survival *in vitro* as a result of this peptide coupling onto alginates.

In 2016, Kirsching, Drager, and co-workers reported a sequential click strategy for modifying alginates [40]. The first step of this sequence involved amidation of alginate with an amino-functionalized ring-strained oxanorbornadiene. After this initial modification of alginate, two sequential click approaches were used to (i) add a ligand to alginate and (ii) crosslink alginate chains (Figure 2.19). In one sequence, alginate was first treated with an azide containing peptide. That alginate was then oxidatively cleaved with periodate and crosslinked via hydrazine to imine formation to a second alginate containing acyl hydrazine functional groups. Conversely, alginate was also oxidatively cleaved first and then treated with the azide containing peptide and the hydrazine containing alginate. The gels thus formed were found to be noncytotoxic to human fibroblast cell cultures indicating that in principle they would have applications in tissue engineering.

In 2017, Mano and co-workers reported a layer-by-layer deposition and amidation of chitosan and alginate in order to tune the cell adhesive properties of polysaccharides [41]. In this work, chitosan and alginate were deposited in alternating layers on polystyrene for five deposition cycles. Human plasma fibronectin or murine LM-1 proteins were then covalently bonded to the alginate using treatment with EDC and sulfo-NHS. Successful tests with human umbilical vein endothelial cells were used to show the potential of these films to alter cell adhesion, spreading, and proliferation.

Also in 2017, Hu, Mao and co-workers reported the synthesis of some additional modified alginates which could be crosslinked by click chemistry [42]. In this work NHS/EDC catalyzed amidation reactions between alginate and benzylaminotetrazine, norbornene methanamine or *trans*-cyclooctenamine were first performed (Figure 2.20). Additionally, biotin-PEG$_3$-amine was also used to modify alginate via amide bond formation.

They then used these modified alginates to form two different types of what they called binding pair molecule (BPM) self-assembling hydrogels and compared the properties of those hydrogels. One BPM gel type was formed via a click reaction between benzylaminotetrazine modified alginate and either norbornene or *trans*-cyclooctene modified alginate. The second gel type was formed via soluble streptavidin protein binding to biotin modified alginate. The click reaction gels and the

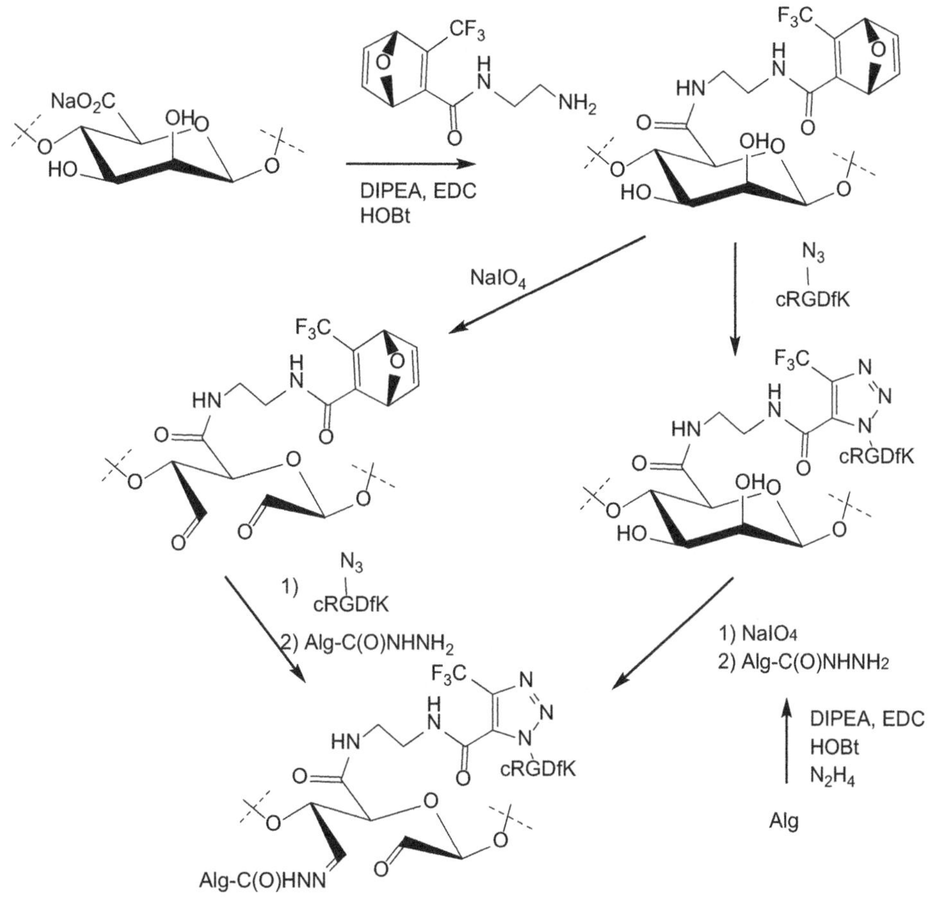

FIGURE 2.19 Preparation and click modification of alginates containing strained rings.

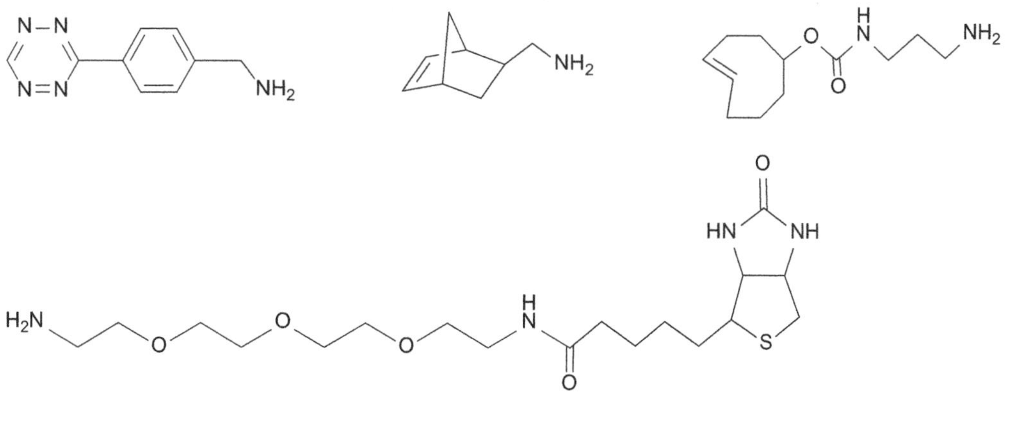

FIGURE 2.20 Clickable amines and biotin-PEG$_3$-amine.

biotin gel were found to have similar physical properties as long as sufficient time was allowed for completion of the click reaction for gel assembly. All gels were found to be capable of viably encapsulating murine mesenchymal stem cells without losing their assembly properties indicating they were viable models for future cell infusion therapies.

Also in 2017, Skardal, Zhang, and co-workers reported conjugating gelatin and heparin to alginate via amidation chemistry and then the use of hydrogels made from those modified alginates for promotion of myogenic differentiation of human muscle progenitor cells [43]. In this work, alginate was first treated with base and chloroacetic acid to carboxymethylate-free hydroxyl groups and to increase the number of carboxylic acids on the polysaccharide chain. This carboxymethylated alginate was then treated with EDC and gelatin, followed by treatment with 2kDa PEG-diamine/EDC, and lastly with heparin/EDC (Figure 2.21). This alginate–gelatin–heparin material was then converted into a hydrogel using $CaCl_2$. This modified material, combined with an extracellular matrix (ECM) solution, prepared from skeletal muscle proved superior for skeletal muscle progenitor cell maintenance and differentiation. The gelatin promotes cell adherence and the heparin supports sequestration of heparin binding cytokines, thus providing a material that could be used as a treatment for muscular injuries.

In 2018, Paul and co-workers reported treating alginate with a type A gelatin (collagen) mixture and three different amounts of NHS/EDC in order to prepare hydrogel coatings that could be used on ceramic scaffolds for bone repair [44]. The modified ceramic coatings survived compression, and their cytocompatibility was assessed by testing the proliferation and osteogenic differentiation of human adipose stem cells (hASCs). Stem cells seeded on the coated ceramic scaffolds also had higher expression of alkaline phosphatase activity making them valid candidates for bone tissue engineering applications.

This same year, Zhao and co-workers reported using EDC/NHS to couple bone forming peptide-1 (BFP-1) to alginate [45]. This peptide decorated alginate (Figure 2.22) was then used to promote osteodifferentiation of human mesenchymal stem cells (hMSCs).

Lee and co-workers reported that hyaluronate-alginate hybrid (HAH) hydrogels could be coupled via amidation reactions to arginine–glycine–aspartate (RGD) and/or histidine–alanine–valine (HAV) [46]. They showed that the viability and growth of mouse chondrocytes increased significantly when cultured on RGD modified HAH hydrogels. Cell aggregates formed on HAV modified HAH resulted in enhanced chondrogenic differentiation via enhanced cell–cell interactions.

Lastly in 2018, Zimmermann and co-workers reported the preparation of some poly(amidoamine)-alginate hydrogels using EDC/NHS amidation reaction conditions and then used these hydrogels to prepare differently charged surfaces via the amount of poly(amidoamine) that was conjugated (Figure 2.23) [47]. They monitored how surface charge impacted protein absorption and noted that mesenchymal stem cells showed enhanced attachment to increasingly positively charged surfaces and that charge had an effect on differentiation toward bone and fat cells.

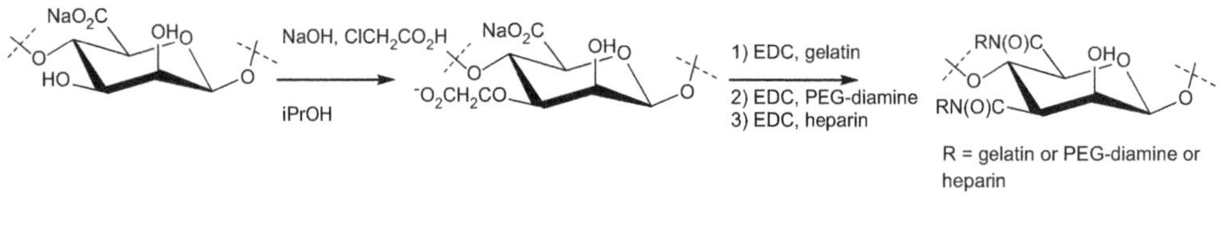

FIGURE 2.21   Amidation reactions of carboxymethylated alginate.

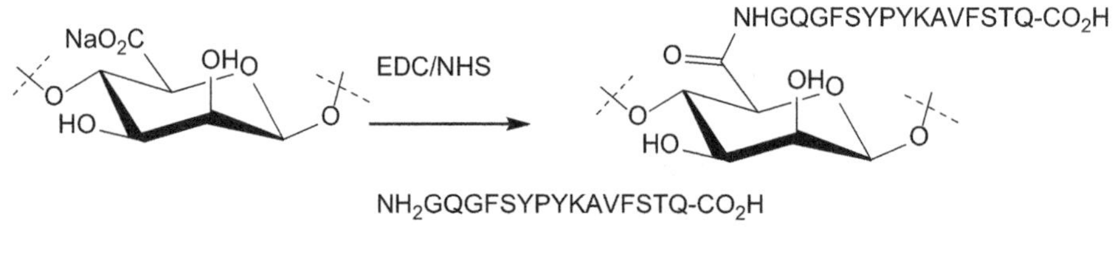

FIGURE 2.22   Conjugation of bone forming peptide to alginate.

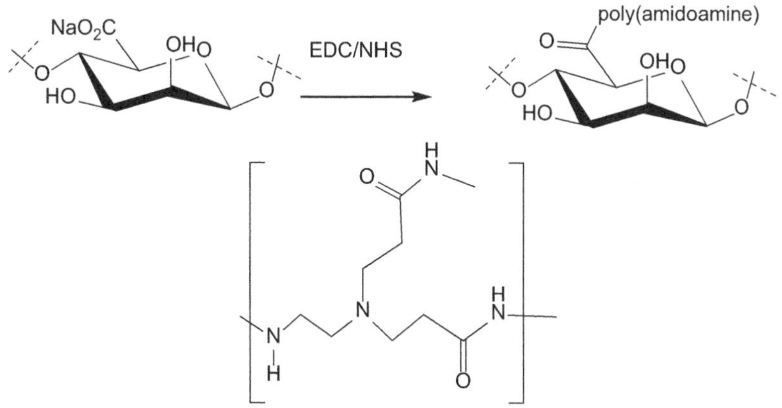

FIGURE 2.23   Preparation of poly(amidoamine) alginates.

2.3.2.2   Modifications That Begin with Amidation and Any Crosslinking Is Nucleophile–Electrophile or Cycloaddition Chemistry Where the Alginate Application Is Drug Delivery

In 2015 Chiang and Chu reported preparation of an alginate–cyclodextrin conjugate [48]. Na-Alg was treated with 6-amino-β-cyclodextrin (CD) and EDC/NHS to prepare an alginate-CD hybrid. The CD was used as a coordination host for diazobenzene terminated polyethylene glycol (Az$_2$-PEG) (Figure 2.24). The original trans diazobenzene isomer encapsulated in the CD dissociates when photolyzed and converts to the cis isomer. This irreversible dissociation leaves comb-like cavities in the gel and released entrapped dye molecules, hence this material may have phototriggered drug release applications.

In 2016, Lee and co-workers reported preparation of a heparin modified alginate that was used to entrap and release transforming growth factor beta 1 (TGF-β1) [49]. To prepare the alginate, Na-Alg was first treated with ethylene diamine and EDC/sulfo-NHS to form amide linkages off the alginate that would be terminated with primary amine groups. That modified alginate was then conjugated to heparin also using EDC/sulfo-NHS. This heparin modified alginate was crosslinked with iron oxide nanoparticles using CaCl$_2$ in the presence of TGF-β1 in order to entrap it. Application of a magnetic field to these ferrogels regulated TGF-β1 release, which was demonstrated by monitoring growth of ATDC5 cells used as a model chondrogenic cell line.

In 2017 and 2018, Bitton and Ochbaum used standard EDC/NHS amidation chemistry to link three different peptides (G$_6$KRGDY, A$_6$KRGDY, and V$_6$KRGDY) to alginate [50,51].

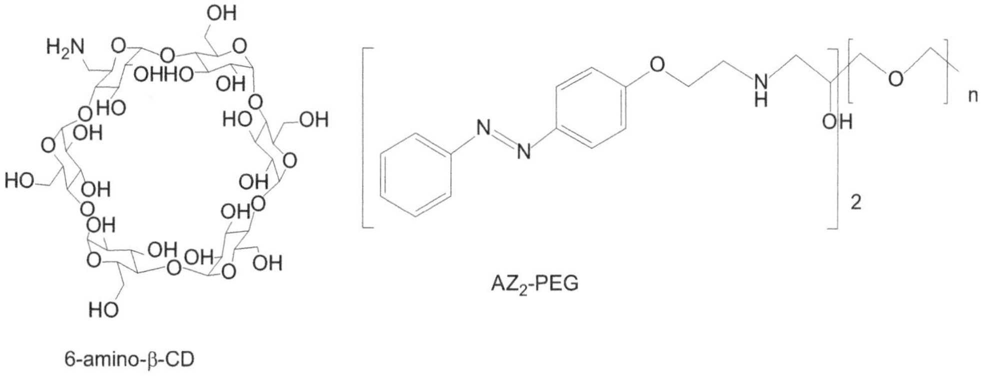

6-amino-β-CD

AZ$_2$-PEG

FIGURE 2.24   Aminocyclodextrin and diazobenzene terminated PEG.

This conjugation chemistry was followed by a study of their self-assembly. Alg-A_6 and Alg-V_6 had a higher viscosity and denser network than native alginate in water, and this change in properties was attributed to peptide hydrogen bonding and noted as a modified alginate property which should be measured and considered prior to drug encapsulation.

Also in 2017, Peled and co-workers reported preparation and testing of an alginate modified with maleimide terminated PEG as a drug carrier [52]. In this work, Na-Alg was first treated with EDC and cysteine to produce a cysteine substituted alginate (Alg-SH). This material was then treated with PEG dimaleimide (PEGDM) (Figure 2.25). This dimaleimide probably serves as a chain cross-linker, but nuclear magnetic resonance evidence also showed that there were unreacted maleimide groups in the product. The aim was to have unreacted maleimide groups present, which could react via Michael addition reactions with mucin glycoproteins and thus function as a mucoadhesive agent. Sustained drug release from these mucin modified alginate mixtures was also demonstrated using ibuprofen as a model drug.

There were many reports of amidation of alginates in 2018 where the alginates thus produced were used for drug delivery. Fort and co-workers used 4-(4,6-dimethoxy-1,3,5-triazin-2-yl)-4-methylmorpholinium chloride (DMTMM) to amidate Na-Alg with amino acids and aminomonosaccharides (Figure 2.26) [53]. The amine grafted alginates they produced showed increased resistance to degradation by alginate lyases, and the carbohydrate amidated alginates were efficient inhibitors of concanavalin A lectin indicating they may have applications as new anti-infection agents.

Siqueira Petri and co-workers reported conjugation of the diamine containing antibiotic gentamicin sulfate (GS) to Na-Alg using carbodiimide chemistry [54]. Materials with different Alg:GS ratios were prepared and tested for antibiotic activity against Pseudomonas and Staphylococcus strains and Alg-GS (1:2) showed the highest microbicidal activity (Figure 2.27).

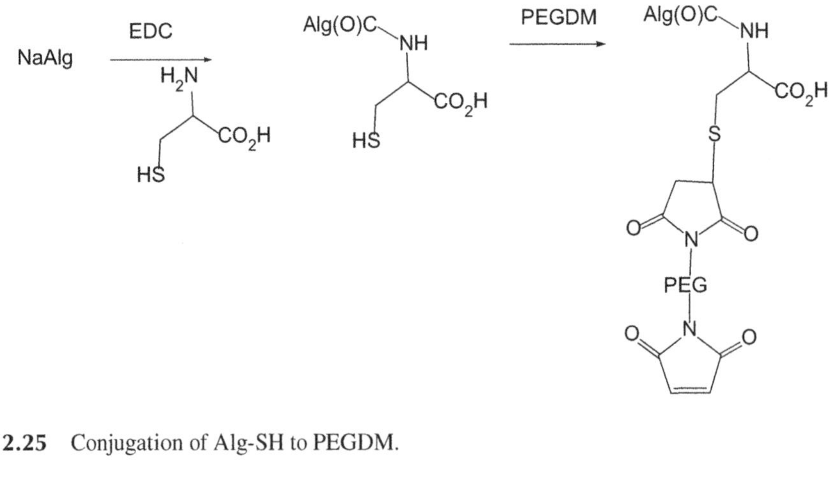

FIGURE 2.25 Conjugation of Alg-SH to PEGDM.

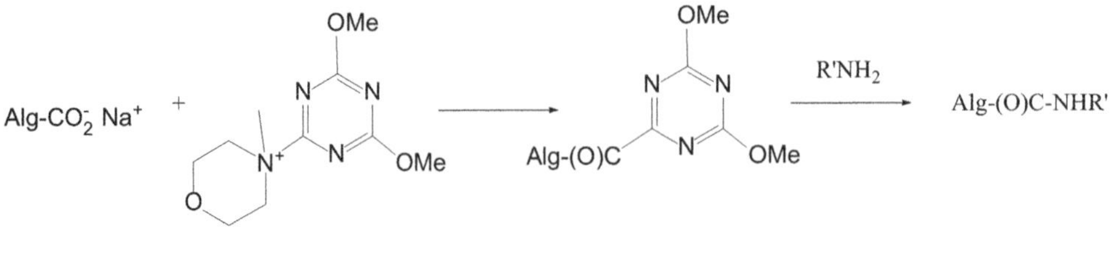

FIGURE 2.26 Amidation of alginate using DMTMM.

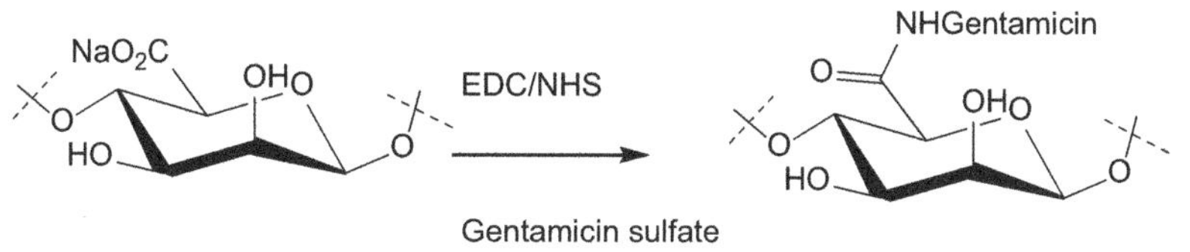

FIGURE 2.27 Conjugation of GS to alginate.

Staikos and co-workers reported an alginate grafted with an acrylamide (AA) polymer and its thermoresponsive behavior [55]. NH_2 terminated poly(N-isopropylacrylamide) (PNIPAM) of three different molecular weight ranges was prepared by polymerizing N-isopropylacrylamide with potassium persulfate in the presence of 2-aminoethanthiol. These PNIPAM-NH_2 chains were then grafted onto Na-Alg using standard amidation chemistry (EDC/N-hydroxybenzotriazole (HOBt). Thermothickening behavior of these graft copolymers was then studied in water and 0.1N NaCl and found to depend on both the degree of PNIPAM grafting and the length of those chains. The authors speculate that these materials may have applications in drug delivery but reported no tests of this.

Two groups independently reported amidation of alginate with furfurylamine in 2018 and then used that furan group in alginate crosslinking Diels-Alder reactions. Averous and co-workers reported some furfurylamine modified alginates that were converted into click crosslinked hydrogels for model compound delivery [56]. Alginate was first coupled to furfurylamine using EDC. This modified alginate was then treated with PEG bis maleimide as a Diels-Alder active crosslinking agent (Figure 2.28). The hydrogels thus formed were used in vanillin release studies as models for drug delivery applications.

Ghanian, Mirzadeh, and Baharvand independently also reported amidation of alginate with furfurylamine using EDC/NHS [57]. This group separately prepared a four-arm poly(ethylene glycol) (4-arm-PEG) which was then tosylated and converted to an amine terminated 4-arm PEG-NH_2 by treatment with ammonia. This 4-arm-PEG-NH_2 was conjugated to 3-(maleimido)propionic acid NHS ester to yield a maleimide functionalized 4-arm-PEG. The furan substituted alginate (FAlg) and this 4-arm-PEG-maleimide were used to form hydrogels via a click furan-maleimide Diels-Alder reaction at 37°C (Figure 2.29). The hydrogels thus produced were used to encapsulate human

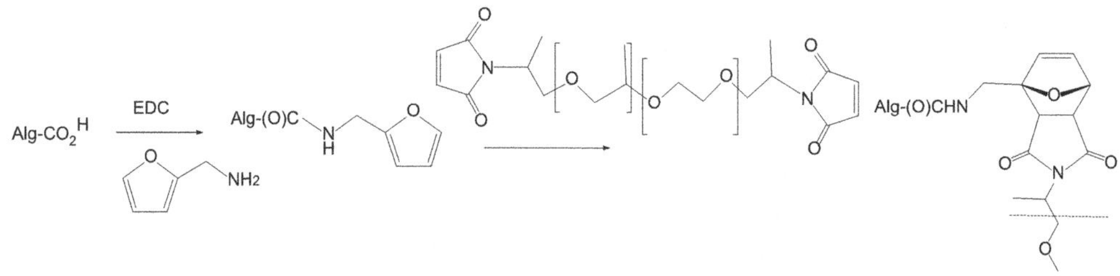

FIGURE 2.28 Reaction of furfurylamine modified alginate with bismaleimides.

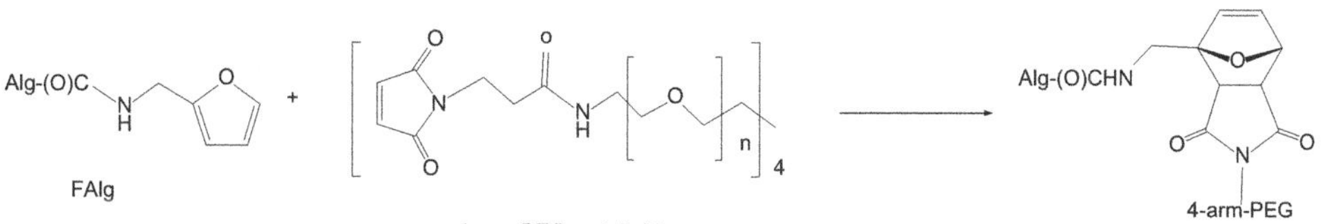

FIGURE 2.29 Reaction of furfurylamine modified alginate with 4-arm-PEG.

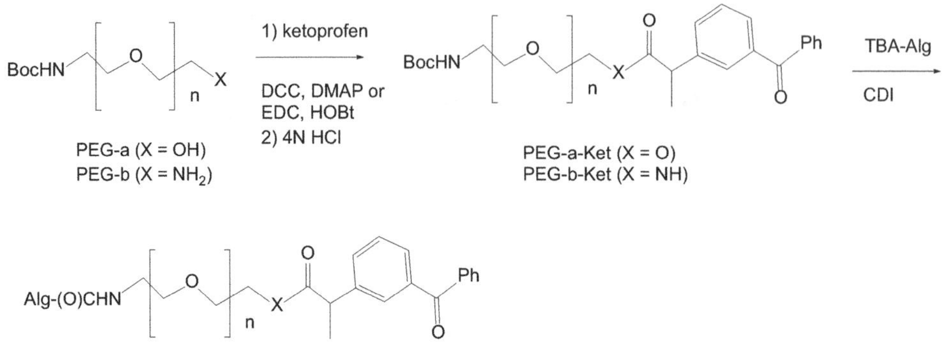

FIGURE 2.30 Preparation of ketoprofen grafted alginate.

cardiac progenitor cells which showed a high viability rate (>90%) after 7 days under physiological conditions. Additionally, unreacted maleimide groups in the 4-arm-PEG were shown to react with a thiol bearing model drug, thiolated fluorescein (FITC-SH).

Lastly in 2018, Gerber-Lamaire and co-workers reported the preparation of ketoprofen-grafted alginate and its use to deliver higher concentrations of this anti-inflammatory drug to aid in transplantation of insulin producing cells [58]. In this work, semi Boc NH protected PEG with both OH and NH$_2$ unprotected termini were first conjugated to ketoprofen using dicyclohexylcarbodiimide/dimethylaminopyridine to form ester linkages and EDC/HOBt to form amide linkages to the drug. These PEGylated ketoprofen derivatives were then grafted onto tetrabutylammonium alginate (TBA-alg) using carbodiimidazole chemistry to produce alginate with grafting degrees of 7% and 20% (Figure 2.30). Microspheres of these alginates and insulin producing MIN6 cells containing these microspheres were evaluated for their ability to do controlled release of the ketoprofen. The covalent conjugation of ketoprofen through an ester linkage resulted in regular and sustained drug release up to 14 days, whereas the amide linkage only released a trace amount of the drug. Quantification of collagen deposition on microspheres transplanted under the kidney capsule in immune competent mice indicated that the conjugation of ketoprofen through an ester linkage can strongly reduce pericapsular fibrotic overgrowth while maintaining the insulin secretion capacity of the microencapsulated cells.

2.3.3 Modifications That Involve Radical Chemistry

In 2014, Ray and Samanta reported a radical initiated coupling of alginate and polyacrylamide to form a hydrogel that was then used for controlled release of acetaminophen [59]. In this work, Na-Alg was mixed with AA and N,N′-methylene bisacrylamide (MBA) (Figure 2.31) and treated with ammonium persulfate/sodium metabisulfite to form alkoxy radicals on the alginate which would then induce polymerization/crosslinking of AAs. Hydrogels thus formed with differing ratios of AA to MBA to Na-Alg were tested for swelling characteristics as well as their ability to entrap and release acetaminophen at pH 7.5.

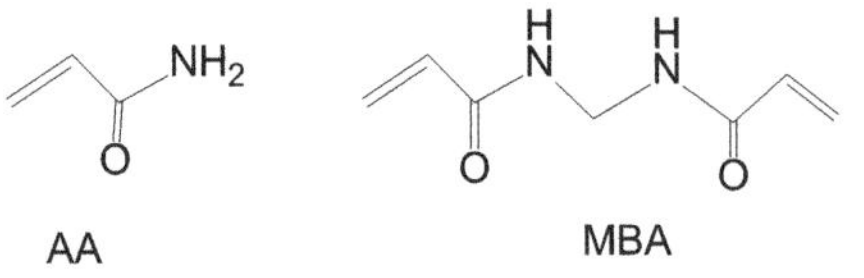

FIGURE 2.31 Structures of AA and N,N′-MBA.

Similarly, Yang and co-workers reported making hydrogels in 2014 via persulfate treatment of alginate, itaconic acid (Figure 2.32), and AA [60]. Na-Alg was treated with potassium persulfate to generate alginate radicals, and this was done in the presence of AA, itaconic acid, and N,N′- MBA as radical acceptors and propagators. This modified and crosslinked alginate was then mixed with the silicate, sodium rectorite, in the presence of MBA. This final mixture was then used to encapsulate salicyclic acid and compared to Na-Alg alone for drug release, and this modified alginate showed a slower and more continuous release than Na-Alg.

Ma and co-workers prepared a methacrylated alginate (AlgMA) followed by persulfate initiated polymerization crosslinking with an AA and used this material for both controlled drug and protein release [61]. The secondary alcohol groups of Na-Alg were first methacrylated with methacryloyl anhydride under basic conditions. This AlgMA was then copolymerized/crosslinked with PEG-methacrylate and N-isopropyl AA using ammonium persulfate as radical initiator. The hydrogels thus formed were used to encapsulate the drug diclofenac sodium (DCS) as well as the protein BSA. DCS release was shown to be slow at pH 2.1 and rapid at 7.4. BSA release could be controlled over 13 days showing this hydrogel was also a candidate for controlled protein release.

In 2015 Ostrowski and co-workers reported some iron(III)-alginate hydrogels that were used for phototriggered drug release [62]. The authors prepared Fe(III) coordinated alginates of different M/G ratios and irradiated them with visible light (Figure 2.33). Presumably irradiation initiates electron transfer mediated decarboxylation, and the carbon centered radicals thus formed dimerize or otherwise crosslink alginate chains to some extent. They also reported Fe(III) alginate beads that contained chloramphenicol and folic acid and studied their phototriggered release from the alginates.

Jayabalan and Finosh reported what they called bimodal hydrogels consisting of polyesters copolymerized with alginates and then crosslinked with diacrylates under radical initiated crosslinking [63]. In this work, sebacic acid, D-mannitol, and maleic anhydride were first heated to form a polyester of undefined chemical connectivity. This polyester was then heated with alginate in conc. H_2SO_4 to presumably esterify free carboxylic acid groups in alginate. This alginate was then treated with poly(ethylene glycol)diacrylate (PEGDA) and diethylene glycol dimethacrylate (DEGDMA) (Figure 2.34) along with ammonium persulfate to effect radical catalyzed crosslinking of alginate chains. The materials reported here were only characterized by FT-IR spectroscopy, so relatively little is known about their chemical composition. These materials supported the co-culture of fibroblasts and cardiomyoblasts so they may be candidates for cardiac tissue engineering.

Also in 2015 Cunningham, Neufeld, and co-workers prepared polymethylmethacrylate (PMMA)-alginate micelles using a living radical polymerization approach [64]. In this work, low molecular weight alginic acid was prepared and converted to its TBA salt. This salt was then treated with the acyl imidazole of α-bromoisobutyric acid in order to esterify some of the secondary OH groups with

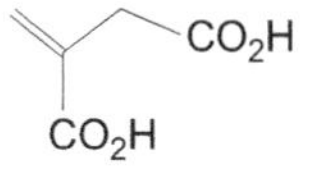

FIGURE 2.32   Itaconic acid.

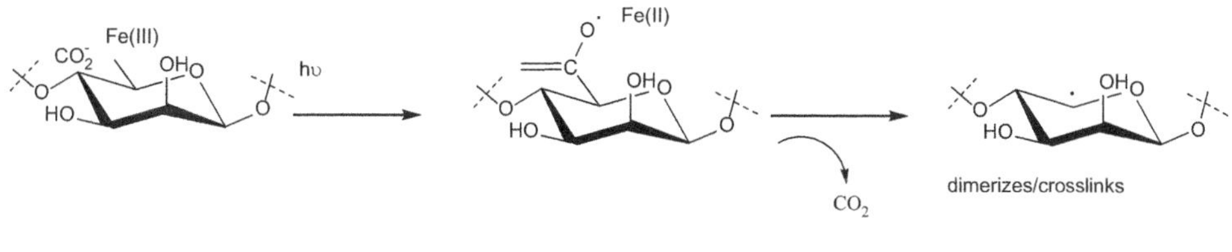

FIGURE 2.33   Irradiation of iron-alginate hydrogels.

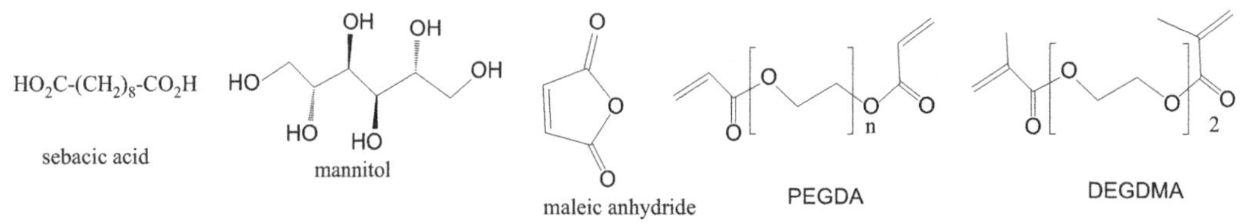

FIGURE 2.34 Components of bimodal alginate hydrogels.

a bromide that could then be used to initiate copper catalyzed radical polymerization with methylmethacrylate (Figure 2.35). The PMMA thus formed produced a micelle with an alginate shell. The hope is that these alginate graft copolymers will have applications in the area of drug delivery.

In 2017, Ahmad and co-workers reported work aimed at radical induced coupling of PVA and alginates [65]. A mixture of Na-Alg (Na-Alg) and PVA was first treated with 2-acrylamido-2-methylpropanesulfonic acid (AMPS) and ammonium peroxydisulfate (APS) and sodium hydrogen sulfite (SHS) with the hope that the AMPS would predominantly couple to secondary alcohols in Na-Alg and PVA. To this solution, ethylene glycol dimethacrylate (EGDMA) (Figure 2.36) was then added with the expectation that this would predominantly crosslink the Na-Alg carboxylates to the PVA secondary alcohols. In reality, a lot of different crosslinking and addition chemistry is possible under these reaction conditions, but the authors took the products of reaction conditions using different amounts of reagents and tested them as polymer networks for tramadol release, where they showed pH-independent drug release.

In 2018, Sakai and co-workers reported the preparation of an alginate derivative that could be used for a light induced radical gelation reaction [66]. In this work Na-Alg was first treated with tyramine under amidation reaction conditions (EDC/NHS), and then this tyramine modified alginate was irradiated with visible light in the presence of $[Ru(bpy)_3]^{2+}$ and sodium persulfate (Figure 2.37). The resultant hydrogel presumably has biphenyl crosslinking and phenyl ether crosslinking from the radicals being formed from the tyramine phenol group. This gel was used to encapsulate mouse fibroblast cells that maintained more than 90% viability for 1 week.

In 2018 Li and Yang and co-workers reported a polyacrylamide/graphene oxide/gelatin/alginate hydrogel that might prove to be useful for nerve cell regeneration [67]. In this work, polyacrylamide mixed with graphene oxide was then treated with Na-Alg and ammonium persulfate as a

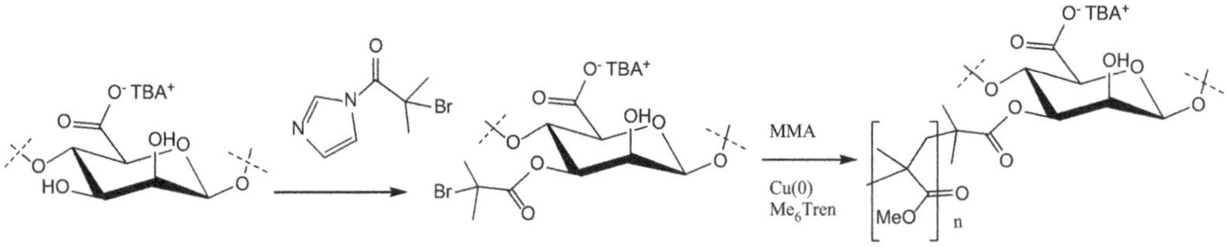

FIGURE 2.35 Preparation of alginate graft PMMA copolymers.

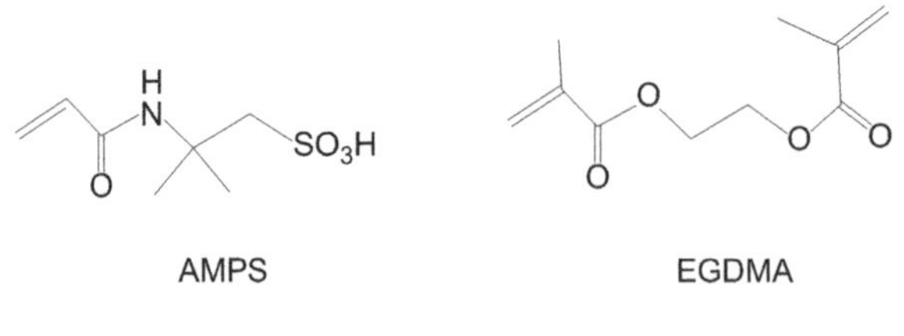

FIGURE 2.36 Structures of AMPS and EGDMA.

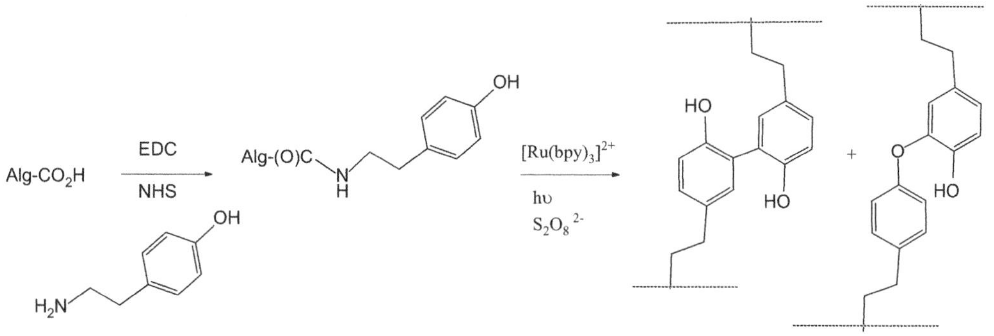

FIGURE 2.37 Preparation and irradiation of tyramine modified alginate.

radical initiator. The persulfate radical anion presumably forms AA radicals, graphene radicals, and alginate radicals in this system so there is no real way to chemically characterize the hydrogel formed by this protocol other than to say radical crosslinking of the alginate is presumably occurring. This hydrogel was used to support attachment and proliferation of Schwann cells so it may have nerve tissue engineering applications.

In 2018, Paul and colleagues reported a gelatin–alginate–polydopamine hydrogel system used to modulate osteogenic differentiation of adipose-derived stem cells [68]. To prepare the hydrogel gelatin, methacrylamide was first photolyzed with alginate, which presumably causes both alginate to AA and AA to AA radical crosslinking. This gel was then treated with calcium and followed by a dexamethasone–polydopamine complex. This gel showed enhanced osteoinductive drug dexamethasone adsorption and retention over 21 days compared to the gel with no polydopamine.

2.3.4 MODIFICATIONS THAT BEGIN WITH REACTIONS OTHER THAN PERIODATE OXIDATION, AMIDATION, OR RADICAL CHEMISTRY

Two examples of modification of alginates via esterification reactions have occurred recently. Sreenivasan and Dey reported that conjugation of curcumin onto alginate via an ester linkage enhanced both aqueous solubility and stability of curcumin [69]. Na-Alg was treated with DCC and DMAP followed by curcumin in order to produce an alginate–curcumin conjugate via esterification (Figure 2.38). The hypothesis was that the Alg-curcumin could be used as a curcumin delivery vehicle, and this was tested and shown to be true via cytotoxicity studies using L-929 mouse fibroblast cells.

In 2017 Dewards-Levy, Bliard, and co-workers reported preparation of several new alginate esters which were used to encapsulate human serum albumin (HSA) [70]. In this work TBA salts of alginic acid were treated with bromoethane, bromopropane, 2-bromoethanol, or 3-bromopropanol under basic conditions with differing degrees of esterification (Figure 2.39). The alginate esters formed were then used to microencapsulate HSA and the hydroxyalkyl alginates with high degrees of esterification (>50%) performed best.

In 2014, Cohen, Brik, and co-workers reported an end group modified alginate that formed a hydrogel which was significantly more stable than the gels formed from unmodified alginate [71].

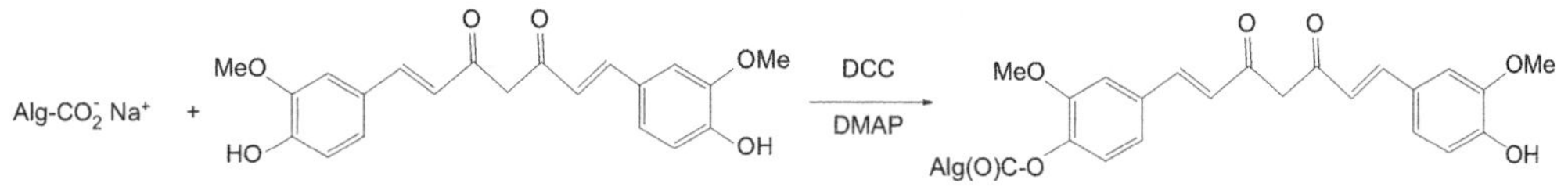

FIGURE 2.38 Conjugation of curcumin onto alginate.

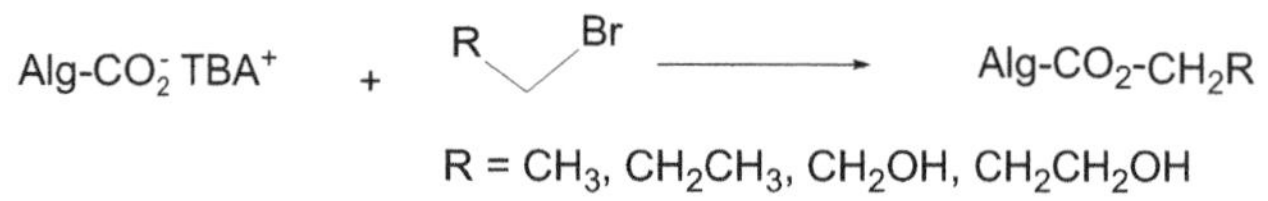

Alg-CO$_2^-$ TBA$^+$ +   R⌄Br   ———————→   Alg-CO$_2$-CH$_2$R

R = CH$_3$, CH$_2$CH$_3$, CH$_2$OH, CH$_2$CH$_2$OH

FIGURE 2.39   Alginate carboxylate esterification.

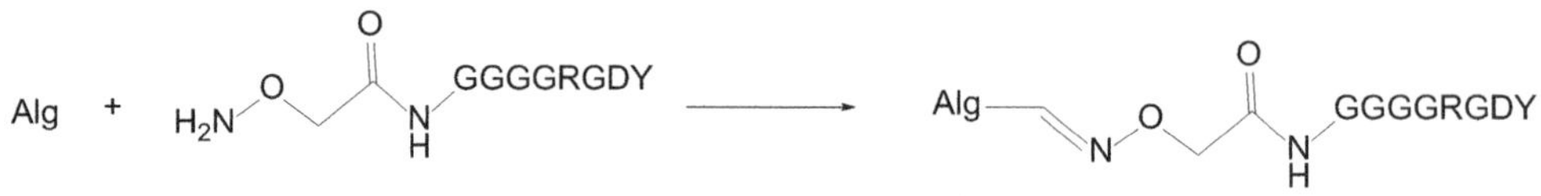

Alg   +   H$_2$N⌄O⌄(C=O)⌄N(H)⌄GGGGRGDY   ———————→   Alg⌄N⌄O⌄(C=O)⌄N(H)⌄GGGGRGDY

FIGURE 2.40   Preparation of peptide oxime terminated alginate.

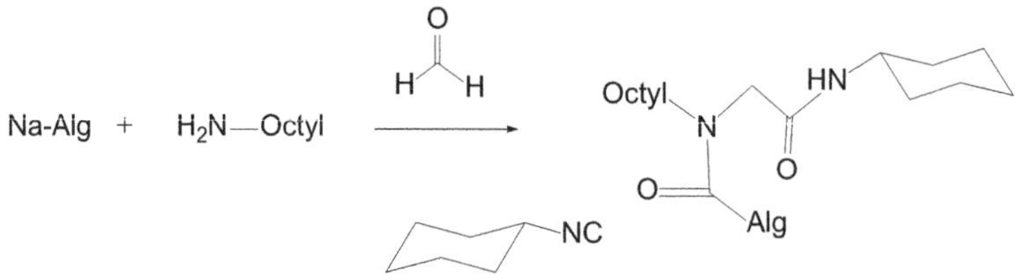

Na-Alg   +   H$_2$N—Octyl   ———————→

FIGURE 2.41   Alginate Ugi reaction using octylamine.

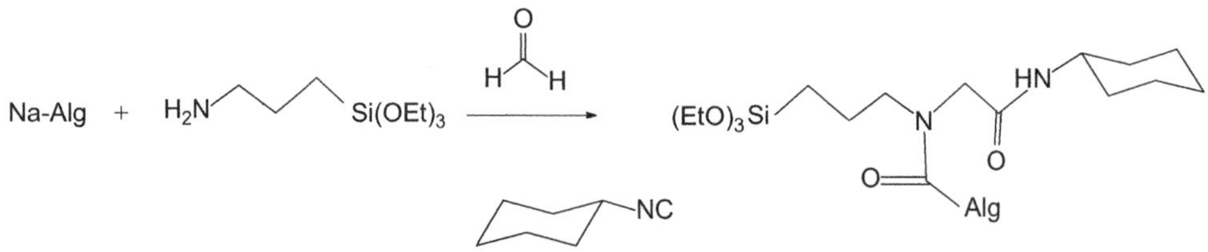

Na-Alg   +   H$_2$N⌄⌄Si(OEt)$_3$ ———————→

FIGURE 2.42   Alginate Ugi reaction with APTES.

In this work, they reported reaction conditions for selectively modifying the reducing end of alginate by forming an oxime from an aminooxyacetic acid (Aoa) terminated peptide (Figure 2.40). Alginate hydrogels formed from this modified material were more stable and had better adhesive properties than hydrogels formed from alginates that had been randomly modified with this same protein via amide linkages.

Two different examples of modification of alginates via Ugi reactions appeared in 2016 and 2017. Lin and co-workers reported an Ugi reaction of formaldehyde, octylamine, and cyclohexyl isocyanide with Na-Alg (Figure 2.41) [72]. This modified alginate was shown to form stable self-aggregated micelles in aqueous media, which the authors took as an indicator that this material would have applications in both drug delivery and tissue engineering.

In 2017, Li, Feng, and co-workers reported use of an Ugi reaction to graft alginate to silica, and they used this alginate modified silica for controlled release of λ-cyhalothrin [73]. In this work, silica, which had been surface modified with aminopropyltriethoxysilane (APTES) treatment was reacted with Na-Alg, formaldehyde, and cyclohexylisocyanide to effect an Ugi reaction to link the modified silica to the alginate (Figure 2.42). Emulsions of these silica–alginate aggregates were used to encapsulate λ-cyhalothrin. A sustained release assay over a pH range of 3 to 8 showed that the emulsion can function as a pH triggered drug delivery system.

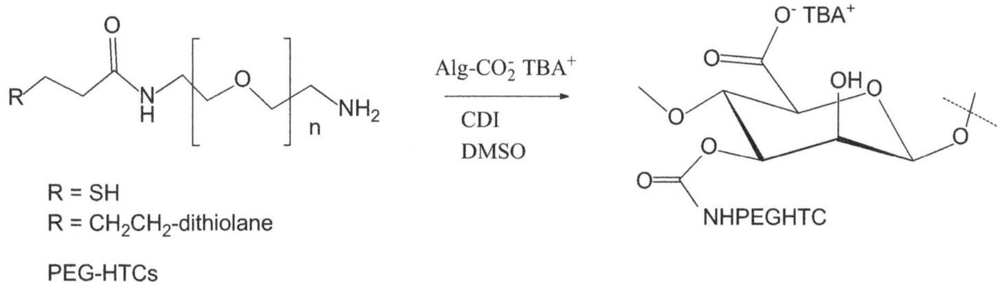

R = SH
R = CH_2CH_2-dithiolane

PEG-HTCs

FIGURE 2.43   Attachment of PEG amines to alginates via carbamate linkages.

In 2017 Aghdam and co-workers reported making an injectable conducting hydrogel from polypyrrole, alginate, and collagen [74]. In this work pyrrole was polymerized with $FeCl_3$ in the presence of alginate but there is no real way to know the extent or type of covalent bond formation that may have occurred between alginate and polypyrrole. The product of this reaction was washed and dried and then mixed with differing amounts of collagen. Physical properties of these hydrogels were measured including conductivity, and its cytotoxicity was measured against human bone marrow mesenchymal stem cells. The good levels of syringeability and cell viability attained led the authors to postulate that this material could be useful for myocardial regeneration.

Gerber-Lemaine and co-workers reported the preparation of heterotelechelic PEG derivatives (PEG-HTC) with amino (NH_2) groups at one PEG terminus and thiol or dithiolane groups at the other terminus [75]. These modified PEG derivatives were then linked to the hydroxyl groups of Na-Alg via carbamate linkages using CDI) (Figure 2.43). The resulting hydrogels were then used to encapsulate a mouse insulinoma cell line, MIN6 cells. Cell viability after encapsulation averaged 70% after both 3 and 15 days which the authors suggested showed potential for cell transplantation applications.

In 2017, Li, Zhang, and co-workers reported preparation of low molecular weight polymannuronates (PM) and polyguluronates (PG) that contained phosphate, phosphonate, and sulfate groups on the alginate monosaccharide units [76]. These modified polysaccharides were tested for their heparin-like activities and the sulfated polysaccharides proved superior in this regard and the sulfated PG was superior to the sulfated PM.

Strand and co-workers reported a number of properties of mixed alginate/cellulose hydrogels [77]. In this work, alginate–cellulose composite hydrogels of differing compositions were prepared and their physical properties were compared. One of the cellulose samples used was from chemically oxidized cellulose, but there was no attempt made by the authors to characterize any covalent bonds that might have been formed between alginate and oxidized cellulose. However, since rupture strength, compressibility, and rigidity as well as saline stability of these hydrogels could be controlled the authors believed they would be useful for tissue engineering.

2.4   CONCLUSIONS

The last 5 years have seen a host of reports of oxidation, amidation, and radical chemistry of alginates and alginate mixtures. Reports of the use of organic chemistry to both control the properties of alginates as well as add ligands or drugs to the alginates continues to grow and can be expected to continue to do so. Alginates will always present tough problems for finely controlled organic chemistry due to the presence of many carboxylic acid and secondary alcohol functional groups. Perhaps over time, reagents will be developed that can better distinguish between axial and equatorial functional groups in the monosaccharides and even more controllable organic chemistry will become possible.

REFERENCES

1. J. Venkatesan, S. Anil, S.-K. Kim, Seaweed Polysaccharides -1st Edition, (2017). www.elsevier.com/books/seaweed-polysaccharides/venkatesan/978-0-12-809816-5 (accessed October 10, 2018). Elsevier.
2. N. Chopin, X. Guillory, P. Weiss, J.L. Bideau, S. Colliec-Jouault, Design polysaccharides of marine origin: Chemical modifications to reach advanced versatile compounds, *Current Organic Chemistry.* 18 (2014) 867–895. www.eurekaselect.com/122191/article (accessed October 4, 2018).
3. J. Sun, H. Tan, J. Sun, H. Tan, Alginate-based biomaterials for regenerative medicine applications, *Materials.* 6 (2013) 1285–1309. doi:10.3390/ma6041285.
4. S.N. Pawar, K.J. Edgar, Alginate derivatization: A review of chemistry, properties and applications, *Biomaterials.* 33 (2012) 3279–3305. doi:10.1016/j.biomaterials.2012.01.007.
5. K.Y. Lee, D.J. Mooney, Alginate: Properties and biomedical applications, *Progress in Polymer Science.* 37 (2012) 106–126. doi:10.1016/j.progpolymsci.2011.06.003.
6. J.-S. Yang, Y.-J. Xie, W. He, Research progress on chemical modification of alginate: A review, *Carbohydrate Polymers.* 84 (2011) 33–39. doi:10.1016/j.carbpol.2010.11.048.
7. M.D. Cathell, J.C. Szewczyk, C.L. Schauer, Organic modification of the polysaccharide alginate, *Mini-Reviews in Organic Chemistry.* 7 (2010) 61–67. www.eurekaselect.com/85554/article (accessed October 4, 2018).
8. A. Kirschning, N. Dibbert, G. Dräger, Chemical functionalization of polysaccharides—towards biocompatible hydrogels for biomedical applications, *Chemistry – A European Journal.* 24 (2018) 1231–1240. doi:10.1002/chem.201701906.
9. R. Afshari, A. Shaabani, Materials functionalization with multicomponent reactions: State of the art, *ACS Combinatorial Science.* 20 (2018) 499–528. doi:10.1021/acscombsci.8b00072.
10. G. Sun, Y.-I. Shen, J.W. Harmon, Engineering pro-regenerative hydrogels for scarless wound healing, *Advanced Healthcare Materials.* 7 (2018) 1800016. doi:10.1002/adhm.201800016.
11. E. Ruvinov, S. Cohen, Alginate biomaterial for the treatment of myocardial infarction: Progress, translational strategies, and clinical outlook: From ocean algae to patient bedside, *Advanced Drug Delivery Reviews.* 96 (2016) 54–76. doi:10.1016/j.addr.2015.04.021.
12. E. Axpe, M. Oyen, E. Axpe, M.L. Oyen, Applications of alginate-based bioinks in 3D bioprinting, *International Journal of Molecular Sciences.* 17 (2016) 1976. doi:10.3390/ijms17121976.
13. R. Zafar, K.M. Zia, S. Tabasum, F. Jabeen, A. Noreen, M. Zuber, Polysaccharide based bionanocomposites, properties and applications: A review, *International Journal of Biological Macromolecules.* 92 (2016) 1012–1024. doi:10.1016/j.ijbiomac.2016.07.102.
14. M. Cardoso, R. Costa, J. Mano, M.J. Cardoso, R.R. Costa, J.F. Mano, Marine origin polysaccharides in drug delivery systems, *Marine Drugs.* 14 (2016) 34. doi:10.3390/md14020034.
15. S. Ahadian, R.B. Sadeghian, S. Salehi, S. Ostrovidov, H. Bae, M. Ramalingam, A. Khademhosseini, Bioconjugated hydrogels for tissue engineering and regenerative medicine, *Bioconjugate Chemistry.* 26 (2015) 1984–2001. doi:10.1021/acs.bioconjchem.5b00360.
16. M. de Jesus Raposo, A. de Morais, R. de Morais, M.F. de Jesus Raposo, A.M.B. de Morais, R.M.S.C. de Morais, Marine polysaccharides from algae with potential biomedical applications, *Marine Drugs.* 13 (2015) 2967–3028. doi:10.3390/md13052967.
17. E. Rodríguez-Velázquez, M. Alatorre-Meda, J.F. Mano, Polysaccharide-based nanobiomaterials as controlled release systems for tissue engineering applications, *Current Pharmaceutical Design.* 21 (2015) 4837–4850. www.eurekaselect.com/134146/article (accessed October 23, 2018).
18. W.L. Stoppel, C.E. Ghezzi, S.L. McNamara, L.D. Black III, D.L. Kaplan, Clinical applications of naturally derived biopolymer-based scaffolds for regenerative medicine, *Annals of Biomedical Engineering.* 43 (2015) 657–680. doi:10.1007/s10439-014-1206-2.
19. E.S. Dragan, Advances in interpenetrating polymer network hydrogels and their applications, *Pure and Applied Chemistry.* 86 (2014) 1707–1721. doi:10.1515/pac-2014-0713.
20. K.B. Fonseca, P.L. Granja, C.C. Barrias, Engineering proteolytically-degradable artificial extracellular matrices, *Progress in Polymer Science.* 39 (2014) 2010–2029. doi:10.1016/j.progpolymsci.2014.07.003.
21. G.D. Mogoşanu, A.M. Grumezescu, Natural and synthetic polymers for wounds and burns dressing, *International Journal of Pharmaceutics.* 463 (2014) 127–136. doi:10.1016/j.ijpharm.2013.12.015.
22. N.B. Shelke, R. James, C.T. Laurencin, S.G. Kumbar, Polysaccharide biomaterials for drug delivery and regenerative engineering, *Polymers for Advanced Technologies.* 25 (2014) 448–460. doi:10.1002/pat.3266.
23. L. Gasperini, J.F. Mano, R.L. Reis, Natural polymers for the microencapsulation of cells, *Journal of The Royal Society Interface.* 11 (2014) 20140817. doi:10.1098/rsif.2014.0817.

24. D.P. Pacheco, E. Marcello, N. Bloise, A. Sacchetti, E. Brenna, L. Visai, P. Petrini, Design of multi-functional polysaccharides for biomedical applications: A critical review, *Current Organic Chemistry.* 22 (2018) 1222–1236. doi:10.2174/1385272822666171212153320.

25. D. Merli, A. Profumo, P. Quadrelli, C.R. Arciola, L. Visai, Drug delivery systems for chemothera-peutics through selected polysaccharidic vehicles, *Current Organic Chemistry.* 22 (2018) 1157–1192. doi:10.2174/1385272822666180122161444.

26. K.M. Park, K.D. Park, In situ cross-linkable hydrogels as a dynamic matrix for tissue regenerative medi-cine, *Tissue Engineering and Regenerative Medicine.* 15 (2018) 547–557. doi:10.1007/s13770-018-0155-5.

27. S. Yan, T. Wang, L. Feng, J. Zhu, K. Zhang, X. Chen, L. Cui, J. Yin, Injectable in situ self-cross-linking hydrogels based on poly(L-glutamic acid) and alginate for cartilage tissue engineering, *Biomacromolecules.* 15 (2014) 4495–4508. doi:10.1021/bm501313t.

28. S. Hauptstein, S. Dezorzi, F. Prüfert, B. Matuszczak, A. Bernkop-Schnürch, Synthesis and in vitro characterization of a novel S-protected thiolated alginate, *Carbohydrate Polymers.* 124 (2015) 1–7. doi:10.1016/j.carbpol.2015.01.049.

29. X. Zhao, S. Chen, Z. Lin, C. Du, Reactive electrospinning of composite nanofibers of carboxymethyl chitosan cross-linked by alginate dialdehyde with the aid of polyethylene oxide, *Carbohydrate Polymers.* 148 (2016) 98–106. doi:10.1016/j.carbpol.2016.04.051.

30. M.Ø. Dalheim, J. Vanacker, M.A. Najmi, F.L. Aachmann, B.L. Strand, B.E. Christensen, Efficient functionalization of alginate biomaterials, *Biomaterials.* 80 (2016) 146–156. doi:10.1016/j.biomaterials.2015.11.043.

31. L. Yuan, Y. Wu, Q. Gu, H. El-Hamshary, M. El-Newehy, X. Mo, Injectable photo crosslinked enhanced double-network hydrogels from modified sodium alginate and gelatin, *International Journal of Biological Macromolecules.* 96 (2017) 569–577. doi:10.1016/j.ijbiomac.2016.12.058.

32. J. Karvinen, T. Joki, L. Ylä-Outinen, J.T. Koivisto, S. Narkilahti, M. Kellomäki, Soft hydrazone cross-linked hyaluronan- and alginate-based hydrogels as 3D supportive matrices for human pluripotent stem cell-derived neuronal cells, *Reactive and Functional Polymers.* 124 (2018) 29–39. doi:10.1016/j.reactfunctpolym.2017.12.019.

33. L. Wang, F. Deng, W. Wang, A. Li, C. Lu, H. Chen, G. Wu, K. Nan, L. Li, Construction of injectable self-healing macroporous hydrogels via a template-free method for tissue engineering and drug deliv-ery, *ACS Applied Materials and Interfaces.* 10 (2018) 36721–36732. doi:10.1021/acsami.8b13077.

34. R. Aston, M. Wimalaratne, A. Brock, G. Lawrie, L. Grøndahl, Interactions between chitosan and alginate dialdehyde biopolymers and their layer-by-layer assemblies, *Biomacromolecules.* 16 (2015) 1807–1817. doi:10.1021/acs.biomac.5b00383.

35. P.R. Sarika, P.R. Anil Kumar, D.K. Raj, N.R. James, Nanogels based on alginic aldehyde and gelatin by inverse miniemulsion technique: Synthesis and characterization, *Carbohydrate Polymers.* 119 (2015) 118–125. doi:10.1016/j.carbpol.2014.11.037.

36. M. Pei, X. Jia, X. Zhao, J. Li, P. Liu, Alginate-based cancer-associated, stimuli-driven and turn-on theranostic prodrug nanogel for cancer detection and treatment, *Carbohydrate Polymers.* 183 (2018) 131–139. doi:10.1016/j.carbpol.2017.12.013.

37. L. Wang, W. Zhou, Q. Wang, C. Xu, Q. Tang, H. Yang, An injectable, dual responsive, and self-healing hydrogel based on oxidized sodium alginate and hydrazide-modified poly(ethyleneglycol), *Molecules.* 23 (2018) 546. doi:10.3390/molecules23030546.

38. J. Jang, C. Cha, Multivalent polyaspartamide cross-linker for engineering cell-responsive hydrogels with degradation behavior and tunable physical properties, *Biomacromolecules.* 19 (2018) 691–700. doi:10.1021/acs.biomac.8b00068.

39. I. Sandvig, K. Karstensen, A.M. Rokstad, F.L. Aachmann, K. Formo, A. Sandvig, G. Skjåk-Bræk, B.L. Strand, RGD-peptide modified alginate by a chemoenzymatic strategy for tissue engineering applications, *Journal of Biomedical Materials Research Part A.* 103 (2015) 896–906. doi:10.1002/jbm.a.35230.

40. N. Dibbert, A. Krause, J.-C. Rios-Camacho, I. Gruh, A. Kirschning, G. Dräger, A synthetic toolbox for the in situ formation of functionalized homo- and heteropolysaccharide-based hydrogel libraries, *Chemistry – A European Journal.* 22 (2016) 18777–18786. doi:10.1002/chem.201603748.

41. J.M. Silva, J.R. García, R.L. Reis, A.J. García, J.F. Mano, Tuning cell adhesive properties via layer-by-layer assembly of chitosan and alginate, *Acta Biomaterialia.* 51 (2017) 279–293. doi:10.1016/j.actbio.2017.01.058.

42. Y. Hu, A.S. Mao, R.M. Desai, H. Wang, D.A. Weitz, D.J. Mooney, Controlled self-assembly of algi-nate microgels by rapidly binding molecule pairs, *Lab Chip.* 17 (2017) 2481–2490. doi:10.1039/c7lc00500h.

43. H. Yi, S. Forsythe, Y. He, Q. Liu, G. Xiong, S. Wei, G. Li, A. Atala, A. Skardal, Y. Zhang, Tissue-specific extracellular matrix promotes myogenic differentiation of human muscle progenitor cells on gelatin and heparin conjugated alginate hydrogels, *Acta Biomaterialia.* 62 (2017) 222–233. doi:10.1016/j.actbio.2017.08.022.

44. S. Pacelli, S. Basu, C. Berkland, J. Wang, A. Paul, Design of a Cytocompatible Hydrogel Coating to Modulate Properties of Ceramic-Based Scaffolds for Bone Repair, *Cellular and Molecular Bioengineering.* 11 (2018) 211–217. doi:10.1007/s12195-018-0521-3.

45. Y. Yang, Z. Luo, Y. Zhao, Osteostimulation scaffolds of stem cells: BMP-7-derived peptide-decorated alginate porous scaffolds promote the aggregation and osteo-differentiation of human mesenchymal stem cells, *Biopolymers.* 109 (2018) e23223. doi:10.1002/bip.23223.

46. H. An, J.W. Lee, H.J. Lee, Y. Seo, H. Park, K.Y. Lee, Hyaluronate-alginate hybrid hydrogels modified with biomimetic peptides for controlling the chondrocyte phenotype, *Carbohydrate Polymers.* 197 (2018) 422–430. doi:10.1016/j.carbpol.2018.06.016.

47. A. Schulz, A. Katsen-Globa, E.J. Huber, S.C. Mueller, A. Kreiner, N. Pütz, M.M. Gepp, B. Fischer, F. Stracke, H. von Briesen, J.C. Neubauer, H. Zimmermann, Poly(amidoamine)-alginate hydrogels: Directing the behavior of mesenchymal stem cells with charged hydrogel surfaces, *Journal of Materials Science: Materials in Medicine.* 29 (2018) 105. doi:10.1007/s10856-018-6113-x.

48. C.-Y. Chiang, C.-C. Chu, Synthesis of photoresponsive hybrid alginate hydrogel with photo-controlled release behavior, *Carbohydrate Polymers.* 119 (2015) 18–25. doi:10.1016/j.carbpol.2014.11.043.

49. H. Kim, H. Park, J.W. Lee, K.Y. Lee, Magnetic field-responsive release of transforming growth factor beta 1 from heparin-modified alginate ferrogels, *Carbohydrate Polymers.* 151 (2016) 467–473. doi:10.1016/j.carbpol.2016.05.090.

50. G. Ochbaum, R. Bitton, Effect of peptide self-assembly on the rheological properties of alginate-peptide conjugates solutions, *Polymer.* 108 (2017) 87–96. doi:10.1016/j.polymer.2016.11.048.

51. G. Ochbaum, M. Davidovich-Pinhas, R. Bitton, Tuning the mechanical properties of alginate–peptide hydrogels, *Soft Matter.* 14 (2018) 4364–4373. doi:10.1039/C8SM00059J.

52. Y. Shtenberg, M. Goldfeder, A. Schroeder, H. Bianco-Peled, Alginate modified with maleimide-terminated PEG as drug carriers with enhanced mucoadhesion, *Carbohydrate Polymers.* 175 (2017) 337–346. doi:10.1016/j.carbpol.2017.07.076.

53. F. Labre, S. Mathieu, P. Chaud, P.-Y. Morvan, R. Vallée, W. Helbert, S. Fort, DMTMM-mediated amidation of alginate oligosaccharides aimed at modulating their interaction with proteins, *Carbohydrate Polymers.* 184 (2018) 427–434. doi:10.1016/j.carbpol.2017.12.069.

54. S. Kondaveeti, P.V. de Assis Bueno, A.M. Carmona-Ribeiro, F. Esposito, N. Lincopan, M.R. Sierakowski, D.F.S. Petri, Microbicidal gentamicin-alginate hydrogels, *Carbohydrate Polymers.* 186 (2018) 159–167. doi:10.1016/j.carbpol.2018.01.044.

55. O.-N. Ciocoiu, G. Staikos, C. Vasile, Thermoresponsive behavior of sodium alginate grafted with poly(N-isopropylacrylamide) in aqueous media, *Carbohydrate Polymers.* 184 (2018) 118–126. doi:10.1016/j.carbpol.2017.12.059.

56. C. García-Astrain, L. Avérous, Synthesis and evaluation of functional alginate hydrogels based on click chemistry for drug delivery applications, *Carbohydrate Polymers.* 190 (2018) 271–280. doi:10.1016/j.carbpol.2018.02.086.

57. M.H. Ghanian, H. Mirzadeh, H. Baharvand, In situ forming, cytocompatible, and self-recoverable tough hydrogels based on dual ionic and click cross-linked alginate, *Biomacromolecules.* 19 (2018) 1646–1662. doi:10.1021/acs.biomac.8b00140.

58. F. Noverraz, E. Montanari, J. Pimenta, L. Szabó, D. Ortiz, C. Gonelle-Gispert, L.H. Bühler, S. Gerber-Lemaire, Antifibrotic effect of ketoprofen-grafted alginate microcapsules in the transplantation of insulin producing cells, *Bioconjugate Chemistry.* 29 (2018) 1932–1941. doi:10.1021/acs.bioconjchem.8b00190.

59. H.S. Samanta, S.K. Ray, Synthesis, characterization, swelling and drug release behavior of semi-interpenetrating network hydrogels of sodium alginate and polyacrylamide, *Carbohydrate Polymers.* 99 (2014) 666–678. doi:10.1016/j.carbpol.2013.09.004.

60. L. Yang, X. Ma, N. Guo, Y. Zhang, Preparation and characteristics of sodium alginate/Na+rectorite-g-itaconic acid/acrylamide hydrogel films, *Carbohydrate Polymers.* 105 (2014) 351–358. doi:10.1016/j.carbpol.2014.01.043.

61. J. Zhao, X. Zhao, B. Guo, P.X. Ma, Multifunctional interpenetrating polymer network hydrogels based on methacrylated alginate for the delivery of small molecule drugs and sustained release of protein, *Biomacromolecules.* 15 (2014) 3246–3252. doi:10.1021/bm5006257.

62. G.E. Giammanco, C.T. Sosnofsky, A.D. Ostrowski, Light-responsive iron(III)–polysaccharide coordination hydrogels for controlled delivery, *ACS Applied Materials and Interfaces*. 7 (2015) 3068–3076. doi:10.1021/am506772x.

63. G.T. Finosh, M. Jayabalan, Hybrid amphiphilic bimodal hydrogels having mechanical and biological recognition characteristics for cardiac tissue engineering, *RSC Advances*. 5 (2015) 38183–38201. doi:10.1039/c5ra04448k.

64. V. Kapishon, R.A. Whitney, P. Champagne, M.F. Cunningham, R.J. Neufeld, Polymerization induced self-assembly of alginate based amphiphilic graft copolymers synthesized by single electron transfer living radical polymerization, *Biomacromolecules*. 16 (2015) 2040–2048. doi:10.1021/acs.biomac.5b00470.

65. H. Anwar, M. Ahmad, M.U. Minhas, S. Rehmani, Alginate-polyvinyl alcohol based interpenetrating polymer network for prolonged drug therapy, optimization and in-vitro characterization, *Carbohydrate Polymers*. 166 (2017) 183–194. doi:10.1016/j.carbpol.2017.02.080.

66. S. Sakai, H. Kamei, T. Mori, T. Hotta, H. Ohi, M. Nakahata, M. Taya, Visible light-induced hydrogelation of an alginate derivative and application to stereolithographic bioprinting using a visible light projector and acid red, *Biomacromolecules*. 19 (2018) 672–679. doi:10.1021/acs.biomac.7b01827.

67. Y. Zhao, Y. Wang, C. Niu, L. Zhang, G. Li, Y. Yang, Construction of polyacrylamide/graphene oxide/gelatin/sodium alginate composite hydrogel with bioactivity for promoting Schwann cells growth, *Journal of Biomedical Materials Research Part A*. 106 (2018) 1951–1964. doi:10.1002/jbm.a.36393.

68. S. Pacelli, K. Rampetsreiter, S. Modaresi, S. Subham, A.R. Chakravarti, S. Lohfeld, M.S. Detamore, A. Paul, Fabrication of a double-cross-linked interpenetrating polymeric network (IPN) hydrogel surface modified with polydopamine to modulate the osteogenic differentiation of adipose-derived stem cells, *ACS Applied Materials and Interfaces*. 10 (2018) 24955–24962. doi:10.1021/acsami.8b05200.

69. S. Dey, K. Sreenivasan, Conjugation of curcumin onto alginate enhances aqueous solubility and stability of curcumin, *Carbohydrate Polymers*. 99 (2014) 499–507. doi:10.1016/j.carbpol.2013.08.067.

70. I. Hadef, M. Omri, F. Edwards- Lévy, C. Bliard, Influence of chemically modified alginate esters on the preparation of microparticles by transacylation with protein in W/O emulsions, *Carbohydrate Polymers*. 157 (2017) 275–281. doi:10.1016/j.carbpol.2016.09.090.

71. S. Bondalapati, E. Ruvinov, O. Kryukov, S. Cohen, A. Brik, Rapid end-group modification of polysaccharides for biomaterial applications in regenerative medicine, *Macromolecular Rapid Communications*. 35 (2014) 1754–1762. doi:10.1002/marc.201400354.

72. H. Yan, X. Chen, J. Li, Y. Feng, Z. Shi, X. Wang, Q. Lin, Synthesis of alginate derivative via the Ugi reaction and its characterization, *Carbohydrate Polymers*. 136 (2016) 757–763. doi:10.1016/j.carbpol.2015.09.104.

73. K. Chen, G. Yu, F. He, Q. Zhou, D. Xiao, J. Li, Y. Feng, A pH-responsive emulsion stabilized by alginate-grafted anisotropic silica and its application in the controlled release of λ-cyhalothrin, *Carbohydrate Polymers*. 176 (2017) 203–213. doi:10.1016/j.carbpol.2017.07.046.

74. F. Ketabat, A. Karkhaneh, R.M. Aghdam, S.H.A. Tafti, Injectable conductive collagen/alginate/polypyrrole hydrogels as a biocompatible system for biomedical applications, *Journal of Biomaterials Science, Polymer Edition*. 28 (2017) 794–805. doi:10.1080/09205063.2017.1302314.

75. S. Passemard, L. Szabó, F. Noverraz, E. Montanari, C. Gonelle-Gispert, L.H. Bühler, C. Wandrey, S. Gerber-Lemaire, Synthesis strategies to extend the variety of alginate-based hybrid hydrogels for cell microencapsulation, *Biomacromolecules*. 18 (2017) 2747–2755. doi:10.1021/acs.biomac.7b00665.

76. Q. Li, Y. Zeng, L. Wang, H. Guan, C. Li, L. Zhang, The heparin-like activities of negatively charged derivatives of low-molecular-weight polymannuronate and polyguluronate, *Carbohydrate Polymers*. 155 (2017) 313–320. doi:10.1016/j.carbpol.2016.08.084.

77. O. Aarstad, E.B. Heggset, I.S. Pedersen, S.H. Bjørnøy, K. Syverud, B.L. Strand, Mechanical properties of composite hydrogels of alginate and cellulose nanofibrils, *Polymers*. 9 (2017) 378. doi:10.3390/polym9080378.

3 Tunable Hydrogel Systems for Delivery and Release of Cell-Secreted and Synthetic Therapeutic Products

Kylie G. Nairon, Thomas DePalma, and Hemamylammal Sivakumar
The Ohio State University

Aleksander Skardal
The Ohio State University
The Ohio State University Wexner Medical Center
The Ohio State University Comprehensive Cancer Center

CONTENTS

3.1 INTRODUCTION

Hydrogel biomaterials have been widely explored for applications in regenerative medicine and drug delivery. In particular, due to the ability to customize their crosslinking and swelling characteristics, manipulate available functional moieties such as cell adhesion sites, and load and immobilize a variety of agents such as cytokines and nanoparticles, hydrogels have seen extensive exploration as delivery vehicles and biofabrication materials in which living cells, drugs, and other materials can be incorporated.[1] However, despite countless advances in biomaterial science, until recently, the majority of biomaterials employed in many therapeutic applications remained inadequate, failing either due to difficulties in administration and delivery, biocompatibility, or inefficiency in acting as an optimal delivery vehicle for biologicals such as cells or cytokines. These limitations were largely due to the majority of biomaterials employed by researchers being relatively outdated; many of these materials were developed for completely different biomedical applications, and simply repurposed for regenerative medicine uses. In the past decade or two, we have observed a significant effort in developing novel biomaterials, and in particular hydrogels, that are designed from the ground up with innovative features with specific end applications.[2–4] These developments have helped spur acceleration in technologies such as bioprinting,[5,6] microphysiological systems (e.g. organoids for drug screening),[7,8] cell therapies,[9] and drug delivery methodologies,[10] amongst a host of other applications.

3.2 HYDROGEL OVERVIEW

The term *biomaterials* comprises a wide range of materials that continues to evolve. Biomaterials range widely from soft hydrogels capable of cell encapsulation, to rigid and durable load bearing metal or ceramic implants; from nanoparticles and contrast agents for drug delivery and imaging, to mechanical or electric medical devices such as pacemakers and artificial hearts. As research in materials science continues to expand, so will the number of subclassifications of biomaterial types.[11,12] In the context of regenerative medicine, biomaterials generally are limited to two primary categories. The first category is that of curable polymers that result in mechanically robust and durable materials that provide structure and scaffolding. Many such materials typically require high temperatures or toxic solvents to be processed. The second category of biomaterials is that of soft biomaterials such as hydrogels, generally with a high water content, inside of which cells are capable of residing or that can be loaded with drug compounds, biologicals, and other agents. These can be comprised of synthetic or natural polymers, and do not possess the same levels of mechanical properties as curable support polymers. One of the major problems that the field of regenerative medicine currently faces is the lack of novel biomaterials that are designed specifically for use in delivery applications. In this section, we provide an overview of some of the traditional materials used as hydrogels in regenerative medicine applications (Table 3.1).

TABLE 3.1

Summary of Mathematical Release Kinetic Models

Model	Governing Equation	Description
Zero order	$Q_t = Q_0 + K_0 t$	Constant-rate delivery; IV therapies and some functionalized hydrogels
First order	$\dfrac{dC}{dt} = -KC$	Simple diffusion with no barriers; water-soluble drugs delivered in porous shells
Higuchi	$Q_t = K_H \cdot \sqrt{t}$	Molecule diffusion through a polymer matrix; hydrogels
Hixson-Crowell	$\sqrt[3]{Q_t} = K_{HC} t$	Release governed by dissolution or degradation of carrier; dissolving drug tablets or degradable hydrogels
Korsmeyer-Peppas	$F = \dfrac{M_t}{M} = K_M t^n$	Ratio of Fickian to non-Fickian diffusion; determine contributions of diffusion and degradation to release

3.2.1 CELL-SUPPORTIVE AND BIOCOMPATIBLE HYDROGELS

Here we focus specifically on the category of biomaterials consisting of hydrogels that are bio-compatible and have been employed widely in regenerative medicine applications. To be considered cell-supportive, these hydrogels must not induce toxicity in cells and may provide cell-binding motifs to allow for cell adherence, be they innate to the base materials or through chemical modification steps, for integration with tissue *in vivo*. Hydrogels are composed of polymer or peptide chains, which can be synthetically synthesized in the laboratory or derived from natural sources, such as extracellular matrix from tissue or other natural sources from the environment, which are crosslinked to form a macromolecular network. Typically, the polymers that form hydrogels are hydrophilic, allowing the polymer chain network swell with and hold water, hence the name "hydrogel." With the exception of the stiffest tissue types such as bone and teeth, hydrogels can recapitulate a range of elastic modulus (***E'***) (i.e. stiffness) values through manipulation of chemistry, crosslinking density, and polymer concentration, thus mimicking the elastic moduli of most the soft tissues in the body. However, it should be noted that researchers are pushing the limit of mechanical properties of hydrogels, making the more and more mechanically robust. Chemical and mechanical techniques to generate crosslinking reactions can be designed to be noncytotoxic, allowing 3-D encapsulation of cells within the hydrogel polymer networks at the time of crosslinking and hydrogel formation. This is becoming exceedingly important in regenerative medicine applications as there is an increasing movement from 2-D to 3-D tissue culture both for tissue engineering tissue constructs for use in patients and generation of tissue models for *in vitro* applications such as disease modeling and drug screening. Hydrogels that support encapsulation procedures are significantly more efficient for 3-D uses like 3-D cell culture and drug/cell loading than rigid scaffold seeding approaches of the past. Conceptual illustrations of 3-D hydrogels used in delivery applications are described in Figure 3.1.

Hydrogels generally can be placed into one of the two major categories: synthetic hydrogels, which comprised polymers that are synthesized in the laboratory, or naturally derived hydrogels, which comprised polymers, often polysaccharides, and occasionally peptides or proteins, purified from natural sources and are often further modified chemically in the laboratory. Examples of synthetic hydrogels that are widely employed in laboratories include polyethylene glycol (PEG)-based materials, such as PEG diacrylate (PEGDA), as well as polyacrylamide (PAAm)-based gels. Examples of naturally derived materials that are commonly used in research include collagen, hyaluronic acid (HA), alginate, and fibrin. Typically, with synthetic materials, one has a higher degree of control over molecular weights and molecular weight uniformity, as well as crosslinking densities,

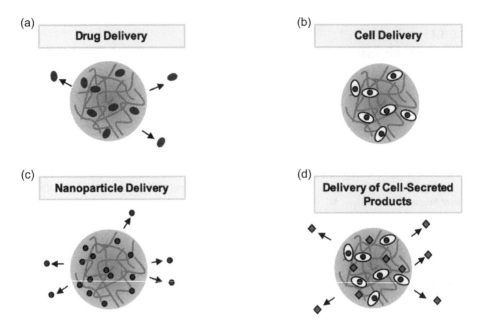

FIGURE 3.1 Uses of hydrogels for delivery applications. Hydrogels can be loaded with a variety of agents for delivery *in vivo*. These include drug compounds (a), nanoparticles (c), local delivery of cells (b), and delivery of cells for the purpose of releasing cell secreted cytokines (d).

facilitating precise control of specific mechanical properties such as elastic modulus E' and pore size. Conversely, the polymers that comprise naturally derived hydrogels are typically more difficult to customize into specific ranges of physical properties, but often have an innate bioactivity through naturally occurring peptide sequences or conformational motifs that cells inherently can identify, aiding with cell and tissue integration and biocompatibility.

3.2.2 Synthetic Polymer Hydrogels

A variety of synthetic materials have been implemented as hydrogels for applications in regenerative medicine. Synthetic polymers are advantageous for one primary reason – as described above, they allow researchers to maintain precise control over chemical and physical properties of the resulting hydrogel. Researchers can chemically modulate molecular weight, functional groups, and hydrophobicity/hydrophilicity at a monomer level. Subsequently, with a reasonable chemistry knowledge base, crosslinking rates and mechanical properties can be customized relatively easily. PEG and PAAm are examples of commonly used synthetic polymers in biomedical applications. PEG, which is a very common synthetic polymer, has been used as medical device coatings for many years to limit host immune responses *in vivo*. It has also been used extensively appended to drug constructs to extend drug half-lives and reduce degradation *in vivo*. It can also be manipulated to form a variety of hydrogels for cell culture and stem cell differentiation. PEG is often chemically modified with acrylate groups to create a photopolymerizable PEGDA in which cells can quickly be encapsulated. The same features that allow such precise control over the chemical and mechanical properties also translate into an inherent drawback. Since synthetic polymer chains typically do not contain natural attachment sites that can interact with cells, all biological activity must be artificially preprogrammed into the material. PEG requires chemical immobilization of cell adhesion motifs in order to support cell adherence. Alternatively, many hydrogels derived from natural polymers and peptides retain some, if not all, of their original biological activity.

3.2.3 COLLAGEN

Collagen is likely the most frequently used protein biomaterial in biomedical research and cell cultures, since it is the most abundant component of the extracellular matrix (ECM) in most types of tissues.[13] Isolation and purification of collagen has been well established for many years, particularly for collagen Type I. Employing collagen as a coating for plastic tissue culture dishes is a common practice in many laboratories. Moreover, generating simple 3-D collagen gels is a straightforward process involving modulation of pH and temperature. Collagen biomaterial matrices are indeed useful and have yielded many important biological advances. However, in normal tissue and ECM, collagen is but one of the many components. The lack of other common ECM components, such as elastin, fibrinogen, laminin, and glycosaminoglycans (GAG), may result in biological signaling that can induce unanticipated cellular changes. Furthermore, collagen fibers and gels primarily contain hydrophobic peptide motifs. As a result, when used as implants or cell delivery agents, collagen gels can exclude water and contract, potentially resulting in decreased diffusion of nutrients and gases. Despite this limitation, there are numerous examples of collagen used as delivery vehicles and carriers for drugs and cells.

3.2.4 GELATIN

Gelatin is derived from collagen that has undergone hydrolytic degradation, resulting in smaller molecular weight peptide sequences that mimic certain properties of collagen. This resulting product can be dissolved in aqueous solutions more easily than collagen, while still maintaining the ability to form simple gels through hydrophobic crosslinking when brought to low temperatures, and supporting cell adhesion through preservation of cell moiety amino acid sequences. The gelation/melt temperature of gelatin solutions/gels lies between 30°C and 35°C, which limits the use of gelatin as a hydrogel in applications that are at or above physiological temperatures, in which case the gelled solutions dissolve. Due to this limitation, gelatin generally requires chemical modification with functional groups, alternative crosslinking techniques, or blending with other polymers or proteins for implementation as 3-D delivery vehicles.

3.2.5 ALGINATE

Alginate is a natural polysaccharide derived from algae or seaweed rather than from extracellular matrix. Because of the simple manner through which alginate can be crosslinked to form a hydrogel, it has been a widely used as a hydrogel in regenerative medicine applications. Crosslinking occurs through a nearly instantaneous sodium–calcium ion exchange reaction. However, it should be noted that barium and magnesium ions can also be employed, but these are accompanied by risk of toxicity to cells. This simple crosslinking reaction – simply mixing or dropping alginate solution with or into a calcium chloride solution – has resulted in alginate being the material of choice for microencapsulation of cells, in which easily available and inexpensive alginic sodium salt, or sodium alginate, which requires no chemical modification, quickly gels into calcium alginate hydrogel microspheres.[14,15] These alginate microcapsules have traditionally been employed for encapsulating liver cells or pancreatic islets inside of a protective capsule.[16]

3.2.6 HYALURONIC ACID

HA, or hyaluronan, is a GAG polysaccharide that is present in the ECM of nearly every tissue type. HA has been harnessed for a wide variety of applications in regenerative medicine.[17,18] Raw HA has been used in the clinic for over four decades,[19] in applications such as treating and lubricating damaged joints.[20,21] While not inert, HA does not inherently have crosslinking capabilities outside of its role in native ECM networks. However, HA has been chemically modified in a number of ways with a variety of functional groups to become a more useful and robust biomaterial that can be crosslinked or loaded with cells or other biomolecules.[22] HA hydrogels can be formed by a variety of crosslinking approaches. Perhaps the most common is photocrosslinking of added methacrylate groups. These groups can undergo free radical polymerization when exposed to ultraviolet light exposure to form soft hydrogels. These photocrosslinkable methacrylated HA (MA-HA) hydrogels have been used in many applications, from cutaneous and corneal wound healing[23] to 3-D extrusion bioprinting.[24] Thiol modification of HA yields another widely used variety of HA that can form hydrogels through direct crosslinking of the thiol groups or through the use of thiol-reactive crosslinkers. Like the MA-HA variety of HA, thiol-modified HA has been implemented in many applications in regenerative medicine such as wound healing,[25] generation of tumor models,[26–29] and bioprinting applications.[30–33]

3.2.7 FIBRIN

Fibrin is another naturally derived material that has been harnessed to generate 3-D hydrogel biomaterials. Fibrin has been employed in tissue culture for various cell and tissues types. Fibrin is a complex that is composed of monomers of fibrinogen that undergo thrombin-mediated cleavage, exposing crosslinking sites, resulting in the cleaved fibrinogen monomers crosslinking to one another. In the human body, fibrin plays a crucial role in blood clotting, injury response, and wound healing. Traditionally, commercial fibrin biomaterials have been prepared in a concentrated glue-like form, which has been used extensively in the clinic as a hemostatic agent, sealant, and surgical glue. This form of fibrin has incredible adhesive properties and can be used as a replacement for stitches and staples after some surgeries. Less concentrated fibrin gels have been used as a tissue engineering scaffold for regenerative medicine applications, including bioprinting and cell delivery due to its fast crosslinking rates.[34,35]

3.3 OVERVIEW OF HYDROGEL RELEASE KINETICS

Hydrogels are hydrophilic, highly porous networks of polymer chains held together by physical entanglement or chemical bonds.[36] This porous structure allows transport and diffusion within the matrix and mimics the high water content of living tissue. For these reasons, hydrogels have attracted study as a method of therapy delivery in biomedical research, as they are capable of both encapsulating cells, drugs, and biomolecules and releasing them to surrounding tissues over a given period of time.[37] This release can occur through diffusion through the hydrogel matrix, degradation of the matrix, or mechanical compression. Additionally, hydrogels form a flexible solid capable of localized insertion into tissue, allowing spatially controlled delivery while retaining the cells, drug, or biomolecule at the desired site. However, to become fully realized as a clinical treatment, hydrogel delivery platforms must have highly characterized total dosage and release profiles to satisfy Food and Drug Administration (FDA) regulations and ensure correct patient treatment. Compared to traditional oral and intravenous (IV) delivery methods, the complex structures and behavior of hydrogel matrices make this rigorous characterization a more difficult task.[38] Cell-based therapies present an even greater challenge, where release kinetics is a function of both gel chemistry and the factor production of living cells.[39]

3.3.1 HYDROGEL LOADING METHODS

The methods by which hydrogels are loaded with drugs and other molecules can be manipulated to improve their release properties.[40] In one method, fully formed gels incubated in solution with a high concentration of drug will absorb molecules into the matrix. While drug stability is unlikely to be impacted, this method also makes it difficult to determine exact loading amounts and is time intensive as the drug takes more time to diffuse into the center of the hydrogel.[41] Distribution throughout the gel is often uneven in diffusion-based loading, which can lead to rapid or unpredictable release profiles. In contrast, the molecules may be incorporated into the uncrosslinked gel prior to solidification. This method is common for encapsulating cells, and the resulting gels have a relatively even distribution and higher quantity of deliverable payload.[42] However, in some few cases, the crosslinking process may interfere with molecular structures or render biomolecules inactive.[40]

3.3.2 MATHEMATICAL MODELING

A number of mathematical models have been employed with loaded hydrogels to describe their release mechanisms and to aid in the design of application-specific systems. Model fitting is influenced by factors including gel geometry, gel chemistry, and loading and release pathways. Classic first-order Fickian diffusion is a commonly used model, governed by the general equation

$$\frac{dC}{dt} = -KC,$$

where C is the drug or biomolecule concentration and K is a rate constant with units of time^{-1}.[43] This release profile describes diffusion through a permeable membrane along a concentration gradient, with an initial "burst" efflux that gradually decreases in rate until maximal release is achieved. Although this model accounts for only the surface barrier of the hydrogel and not its complex internal structure, first-order diffusion models have been commonly used to describe hydrogel behavior in solution. Molecules rapidly diffuse out of the hydrogel directly after implantation into tissue due to the high concentration gradient. As the local tissue concentration increases and hydrogel concentration decreases, release rates taper.

Traditional hydrogels have relatively rapid release, reaching this plateau within 24–48 h.[36] For more sustained release, often necessary in drug and growth factor delivery, gels can be chemically modified. One such modification conjugates heparin, a polymer which binds many cytokines and growth factors, to the hydrogel backbone, allowing the gel to actively retain these molecules for prolonged release.[39,44] With this modification, continuous release has been observed for up to 19 days in poly(ethylene glycol) monomethacrylate (PEGMMA) hydrogels[44] and over a month in heparinized HA hydrogels.[45,46] With increasing modifications and complex molecular interactions, delivery modeling must be adjusted to account for movement through a matrix. The Higuchi model of diffusion, defined by the relation

$$Q_t = K_H \cdot \sqrt{t}$$

where Q_t is the total amount of molecule release at time t, K_H is the Higuchi release constant, and t is the time in days, adjusts standard first-order behavior to account for complex internal polymer networks. In work involving hydrogel delivery of cell-secreted cytokines, the Higuchi model was shown to better fit the experimental release profile than first-order kinetics, suggesting that the internal polymer matrix plays an important role in the delivery timeframe.[39]

Hydrogel structural properties such as pore size can also influence this rate of efflux. In one study, gel precursor concentration was modulated to create gels of varying pore dimensions. Dextrans released from hydrogels with large pores followed the typical rapid "burst" model, while release from nanoporous gels was quasi-linear.[47] This constant rate of release is modeled by zero-order kinetics and represents a system of steady delivery. Clinically, this can be likened to IV infusions and is desirable when maintaining a constant local concentration. Zero-order kinetics avoids the initial burst efflux shown in both the first-order and Higuchi models, which reduces the possibility of overexposure and local toxicity. Although zero-order release kinetics are difficult to achieve with hydrogels, near-zero-order behavior has been reported with heparin-modified alginate–gelatin hydrogels, poly(acrylic acid-g-ethylene glycol) hydrogels, and a G-quadruplex multicomponent hydrogel system.[48–50]

A list of common release kinetic models for hydrogel delivery is outlined in Table 3.1.

3.4 RELEASE METHODS

Delivery pathways from loaded hydrogels into tissues can be categorized into two broad fields: static systems and "smart" stimulus-responsive systems. While static systems rely on the standard diffusion described in the previous section, dynamic systems interact with physiological, environmental, or applied cues to manipulate the hydrogel's state and impact delivery timing. These cues can be classified as internal or external signals, and often induce a change between the hydrogel's swollen and collapsed states. Alternatively, stimuli can induce transition between solid and gel phases or degrade the hydrogel in a controlled manner. This section will discuss the above delivery methods along with their progress and challenges. Figure 3.2 describes several of these approaches conceptually.

3.4.1 STATIC/DIFFUSION-BASED DELIVERY

As discussed previously, systemic treatment via IV or oral routes often results in inadequate concentrations of a drug or molecule at the target site, requiring large total dosages, with the potential to induce off-site toxicity. This is especially true in proposed brain therapies, where <1% of systemically delivered proteins will pass through the blood–brain barrier.[51] Cell therapies generally cannot be administered systemically due to the harsh blood environment and the potential for off-target interactions, and instead require a scaffold or hydrogel capable of maintaining their presence and viability at the desired site. For many such applications, such as wound healing and acute injury treatment, steady-state diffusion is ideal to sustain long-term delivery at a local site.

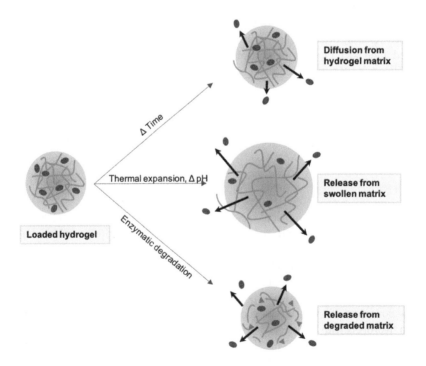

FIGURE 3.2 Examples of hydrogel delivery mechanisms. From a loaded hydrogel, drugs, nanoparticles, or other loaded agents can be released by several methods. Static release is mediated simply by diffusion (top). Several stimuli-sensitive methods of release also exist. Hydrogels can be designed so that changes in temperature or pH cause expansion or contraction of the hydrogel network (middle), thus allowing delivery of the payload. Hydrogels can be designed with enzymatically degradable components, allowing delivery of the payload upon exposure to an environment containing the corresponding enzymes (bottom).

Notably, surface wound therapies can use slow-degrading hydrogels with steady diffusion to maintain local therapy concentrations while minimizing the need for changing dressings, which in turn reduces exposure to contaminants.[52] Further clinical applications such as these will be discussed later in this chapter.

3.4.2 Internal Stimulus-Mediated Delivery

Natural variations in the body's various microenvironments and disease or injury-induced physical and biochemical changes provide stimuli that can be used to guide hydrogel behavior. When designing responsive hydrogels, it is crucial to consider the extent of these physiological variations, as a hydrogel must be capable of substantial structural changes in response to small signal fluctuations. Swelling-induced release and controlled hydrogel degradation are common engineered structural changes to approach this problem. Swelling involves recruiting or expelling water molecules to induce changes in osmotic pressure. As the hydrogel swells, pores widen or crosslinking density decreases, and molecules can more easily diffuse into the surrounding environment. Degradation requires cleaving of the hydrogel structure, and often involves cleavable crosslinkers. Less often, mechanical compression has been targeted as a means of forcing soluble drug out of the hydrogel matrix. In this section, all three methods will be addressed as release pathways.

3.4.2.1 Temperature

Temperature is by far the most studied stimulus for active hydrogel response.[53] Hydrogel thermosensitivity has been used to simplify *in vivo* gel crosslinking without requiring tissue exposure to UV radiation, a common method of initiating the hydrogel gel–sol transitions. Hydrogels with a Lower Critical Solution Temperature (LCST) exist in a solid state above a certain critical temperature and are fluid below this temperature.[54] Inversely, those with an Upper Critical Solution Temperature (UCST) solidify upon cooling.[55] LCST hydrogels synthesized in a cooled state could be injected through a syringe needle into the desired biological site, at which physiological temperatures induce *in situ* solidification and stabilization in the *in vivo* niche.[56] Additionally, in many disease, injury, or infection states, body temperature is elevated or decreased from the standard physiological value of 37°C. To take advantage of this phenomenon, temperature-induced swelling and collapse of polymer networks have been studied as a method of controlled hydrogel degradation and drug release.

3.4.2.2 Local pH

Following thermosensitivity, pH has been an environmental factor that has attracted much research in dynamic hydrogel design. Structurally, pH-sensitive response relies on ionic pendant groups, which develop electrostatic repulsion depending on the pH of the surrounding environment.[57] Swelling can be designed for either low-pH or high-pH release. Anionic hydrogels are ionized above the polymer's pK_a, inducing a rise in osmotic pressure and thus swelling. Cationic hydrogels behave in an opposite fashion, where ionization occurs below the pK_a. Alternatively, crosslinking reactions used during hydrogel synthesis can be designed for pH dependency, where bonds degrade by hydrolysis in a low-pH environment. As these bonds are cleaved, the gel degrades in a tunable manner, providing a temporary scaffold for cell delivery and allowing the molecules to interact with the physiological environment.[58]

3.4.2.3 Biochemical

Disease and injury states are often marked by a local increase in cytokines, enzymes, and other biochemical signals. When designed with enzymatically cleavable motifs, hydrogels can become susceptible to enzymatic degradation specific to the disease state it is intended to treat. This method is especially attractive in cell-based therapies to enable self-remodeling of the hydrogel matrix.[59] Matrix metalloproteinases (MMPs) are a family of enzymes capable of cleaving many ECM components, such as collagen and GAGs, and play a major role in cellular remodeling, and are thus upregulated in environments including cancerous tumors and soft tissue wounds.[60] MMP-cleavable crosslinkers can be customized to the MMPs specific to an injury or disease state, inducing environment-controlled hydrogel degradation.[61]

3.4.2.4 Mechanical

The high degree of flexibility of hydrogels and their close incorporation with the physiological extracellular matrix allow them to transduce mechanical stimuli. Especially in the case of bone, mechanosensitivity and load distribution are crucial to regeneration and healing processes. Additional load-bearing tissues such as cartilage experience greater compression in times of inflammation and thus result in patient pain. Hydrogels subject to cyclical compression patterns have been designed to release free (solubilized) drug during mechanical deformation, which then stimulates an increase in tissue response.[62] The reversible nature of this deformation and recovery allows water molecules to continually penetrate the matrix and further solubilize drug for future release cycles.

3.4.3 EXTERNAL STIMULUS-MEDIATED DELIVERY

An ideal clinical therapy delivers predictable, controlled treatment with minimal side effects. Minimally invasive procedures are a key factor in reducing healing time and patient complications, and thus ways of administering internal therapies from external stimuli are an attractive field for hydrogel applications. Examples of low-risk stimuli capable of soft tissue penetration include near-infrared (NIR) light waves, magnetic fields, and electric fields. Although hydrogel polymer matrices are not often intrinsically responsive to these stimuli at a distance, hydrogel composite structures have been formed with a variety of nanostructures to impart their properties on hydrogel behavior.

3.4.3.1 Photosensitivity

Although light-induced response has long been used for hydrogel formation, it has more recently been pursued as an external trigger for release. The UV and visible spectrum light wavelengths generally applied to initiate hydrogel crosslinking reactions are not viable stimuli due to their quick attenuation when traveling through skin and the negative side effects of UV radiation. NIR wavelengths, however, can overcome both of these challenges, and research has focused on designing hydrogel structures capable of responding to stimulation within this range. Systems have been designed to include NIR-absorbing nanoparticles and nanotubes, which convert the NIR light to thermal energy, causing the gel to contract or degrade and releasing enclosed molecules. Possible nanostructures include carbon nanotubes, gold nanorods, and polydopamine nanoparticles. A second approach converts the NIR to UV light, which is emitted locally and triggers reaction cascades much like standard hydrogel synthesis. To achieve this, upconversion nanoparticles (UCNPs) are incorporated into the polymer matrix, which is crosslinked by photocleavable bonds. When stimulated with NIR light, the UCNPs convert multiple NIR photons into a UV photon, cleaving the crosslinking bonds and degrading the hydrogel.[63]

3.4.3.2 Magnetic Composites

Externally applied magnetic fields have high tissue penetration depths and are commonly used in imaging methods such as magnetic resonance imaging (MRI). Hydrogels with incorporated magnet-sensitive nanostructures can form nanocomposites with a combination hydrogel and nanofiller properties. Upon exposure to an alternating magnetic field, the nanostructures can induce either thermal expansion or mechanical deformation of the hydrogel, which in turn expands or contracts the matrix and flushes solubilized molecules from the hydrogel core. Although less common than magnetic-induced response, conductive nanostructures have been studied for electric field-mediated delivery using similar concepts and release mechanisms.

3.5 APPLICATIONS

3.5.1 Wound Healing

A wound is a disruption in the continuity of the epithelial lining of the skin or mucosa resulting from pathological processes that begin internally or externally.[64,65] Wounds vary in severity, ranging from inconsequential wounds that heal quickly to chronic wounds such as diabetic foot ulcers have been predicted to have a worse 5 years survival rate than cancer.[66] One of the important steps aiding in achieving wound healing is the selection of proper wound dressing.[67] Wound healing is a dynamic interactive process and involves cytokines, growth factors, many cell types, and extracellular matrices.[68] It is a complex series of interrelated processes that begin at the moment of wounding and proceeds in a timely and orderly fashion to restore anatomic and functional integrity to the tissue.[64,65] Tissue regeneration and growth during wound healing progress through four distinct phases: coagulation and hemostasis immediately following injury, an inflammatory phase shortly after the injury followed by the proliferation phase during which new blood vessels and tissue forms, and finally the maturation phase during which the remodeling of the tissue takes place.[68] For effective wound healing to occur, an ideal wound dressing would allow for the various synergistic phases of wound healing to occur unhindered.[69]

3.5.1.1 Characteristics of an Ideal Dressing

An ideal wound dressing has a number of characteristics that help facilitate the healing process. It should maintain wettability and provide a moist environment, thereby promoting epithelial migration and faster reepithelization.[70] It should have the ability to absorb exudate and hydrate the necrotic tissue that increases autolytic debridement.[71] It should allow for gaseous exchange to take place. It should be sterile, nontoxic, biodegradable and a nonirritant. It should serve as a barrier to prevent infection of the wound and thus be impermeable to microorganisms. It should be nonadherent to the wound, thereby promoting easy removal without pain or trauma. It should be able to conform to the wound shape. Lastly, it should be user-friendly and inexpensive to manufacture with a long shelf life.[72]

3.5.1.2 Advantages and Disadvantages of a Hydrogel Wound Dressing

Hydrogels possess most of the qualities of an ideal wound dressing – the most important qualities being able to maintain wettability in the wound zone, the ability to control the lost fluids and liquid from the body, and possessing tissue-like structure and compatibility.[73] It was demonstrated by the work of George Winter that maintaining a moist wound environment is of paramount importance in wound healing and resulted in faster epithelization than under a dry scab.[70] This makes hydrogels a material of choice for burn patients with an added advantage of being able to maintain a cool surface temperature.[74] Hydrogels are advised to be applied to burn wounds if running cold water is unavailable to cool the surface of the wounds and provide pain relief and reduce the damage of the wounds.[75] Hydrogel dressings provide unique advantages such as often being nonadherent, easily removable, promoting wound healing, and reducing inflammatory reaction and pain.[73] Many hydrogels are also relatively inexpensive and easily developed and handled.[73]

Hydrogels are one of the most preferred types of wound dressings in patients requiring debridement, and the only option available to patients who cannot tolerate general anesthesia to undergo surgical debridement of the wound.[71] Hydrogel dressings have been proven to be effective in promoting natural debridement and autolytic debridement, which is particularly useful in healing deeper wounds.[71,73] Hydrogels promote such debridement by rehydrating the necrotic tissue which speeds loosening, and can also absorb the exudates or slough in the wounds.[73,76] Hydrogel wound dressings help in healing of the wound from the base to upward and encourage in rapid granulation and re-epithelialization.[68,73] Some hydrogels in their swollen state have pore sizes which are small enough effectively to prevent bacteria from reaching the wound, while still allowing active biomolecule and gaseous exchange to take place.[77] The bulk of hydrogels is also transparent, which allows for continued monitoring of chronic wounds.[74]

Hydrogels do have the capacity to absorb exudate and maintain wettability in the wound bed, but these dressings lack the ability to absorb more than certain amount of fluid and are not advisable for very wet wounds which could become macerated and infected.[78] In certain types of hydrogels, they lack the mechanical strength which makes them prone to tearing, and it can cause some difficulties in patients handling their dressing on their own.[78,79]

3.5.1.3   Different Types of Hydrogel Dressings

Collagen is the oldest and most frequently used hydrogel wound dressing.[68] Collagen plays an active and vital role in natural healing process, provides mechanical support to the tissue, and facilitates cell migration.[80] Collagen in various forms such as suspensions, foams, membranes, and gels have been employed in wound healing.[73,81] There are a number of collagen-based wound dressings available that incorporate a variety of carriers or combining agents.[82] An example of a commercially available collagen wound dressings is Integra, which is composed of bovine collagen, a silicone protective sheet, and GAGs and has been extensively used in burn patients as well as in soft tissue reconstruction.[83] MatriDerm, another example, is composed of bovine collagen and elastin hydrolysate and has been used in patients for tissue reconstruction and full-thickness wounds.[84]

Poly(vinyl alcohol) (PVA) is the oldest and most frequently used synthetic polymer applied as a wound dressing and for wound management.[73,74] PVA hydrogels are not very elastic and have decreased hydrophilic properties when used on its own.[10] However, PVA has been crosslinked with different materials to counteract the disadvantages of PVA – both natural polymers such as dextran, hydroxyethyl starch, hyaluronan, chitosan, and glucan, as well as synthetic nanoparticle composites such as $AgNO_3$ nanoparticles.

Alginate is a naturally occurring biopolymer that is extracted from a seaweed and is composed of block of (1,4)-linked β-d-mannuronate (M) and α-l-guluronate (G) residues, and the ratio of these residues affects the physical characteristics and behavior of the material.[85] Alginate dressing is manufactured by crosslinking alginate solutions with calcium, magnesium, or barium ions.[86] Examples of some commercial available alginate dressing: Algicell™ (Sodium alginate), AlgiSite M™ (Calcium alginate), and Tromboguard® (Sodium alginate, calcium alginate, chitosan, polyurethane, and silver cations). One disadvantage of alginate is the need to select the correct reagents and initiators that would not result in toxic side effets.[86] Alginate-based hydrogels are widely used in a clinical setting, but more research effort is focused on the development alginate hydrogel wound dressings infused with bioactive agents.[86]

HA is a naturally occurring nonsulfate polysaccharide and is the primary component of the extracellular matrix (ECM) of the connective tissues and has been used in wound dressing because of its physicochemical and biological characteristics.[17,87] HA and gelatin-based hydrogels have been used for the delivery of both cell and tissue-derived cytokines to promote wound healing.[39,88] HYAFF® 11 is a commercially available HA-based wound dressing that is biocompatible and has a safe degradation through a safe metabolic pathway. Hyalomatrix is a double-layered wound contour adapting dermal substitute, which provides immediate wound closure and promotes dermis regeneration.[89]

Amniotic membrane is gaining traction as a wound dressing material because it contains a rich source of biologically active molecules that promote wound healing.[35] HA hydrogel infused with solubilized amniotic membrane has been shown to achieve high rates of wound closure and healing.[88] Human amniotic membrane infused wound dressing have been successfully used in treated infected wound beds.[90] Some of the commercially available amniotic wound dressings are Aminoexcel, Epifix, and Grafix, which have been proven to lead to increased healing in diabetic foot ulcers compared with other available commercial wound dressings. The disadvantages of amniotic membrane dressings are increased processing that it requires and the high cost of manufacturing.[91,92]

3.5.2 HARD AND SOFT TISSUE REGENERATION

3.5.2.1 Hard Tissue Regeneration

Hard tissue regeneration in the human body consists of bone and dental tissues such as tooth enamel, dentin, and cementum. The medical cost related to treating bone trauma, infection, and tumor infiltration, followed by bone regeneration and repair, has continuously increased in the last few years. The need for hard tissue repair and regeneration is on the rise as the world's older population continues to grow at an unprecedented rate.[93] Hydrogels are an exciting alternative to autogenous bone grafts, the current golden standard despite considerable disadvantages such as donor site morbidity.[93–95]

3.5.2.2 Biomaterials for Hard Tissue Regeneration

Biomaterials used as scaffolds for bone regeneration should be osteoinductive, osteoconductive, osteogenic, and osteocompatible to enhance cell adhesion, osteogenic differentiation, and bone formation. The pore size of the scaffold is critical to support the above mentioned functions.[95,96] The scaffolds should be biodegradable but at the same time provide structural stability and guide the incoming progenitor cells and vascular cells until the new bone formation phase.[94] The degradation rate of the biomaterial should be optimal not to risk union failure or graft failure while supporting the new bone formation mechanically and biologically until then.[95,97]

3.5.2.3 Hydrogels in Hard Tissue Regeneration

Hydrogels possess qualities such as being hydrophilic and having a 3-D structure, thereby providing mechanical stability if engineered correctly; ideal when employed as a scaffold for bone regeneration. Hydrogels can mimic the ECM of the bone environment, while aiding in effective transport of nutrient and gaseous exchange. Additionally, when hydrogels are injectable, administration of the materials to a defect in a patient is easier and reduces the pain associated with the administration.[94,98] Hydrogels that have been used or explored for bone regeneration could be either natural polymers such as collagen, chitosan, alginate, HA and fibrin, or synthetic polymers such as polypropylene fumarate (PPF), polylactic acid (PLA), polyglycolic acid (PGA), polycaprolactone (PCL), and PEG.[99–101]

There are several commercially available hydrogel bone graft materials. One example is Collagraft, which is made up of hydroxyapatite, tricalcium phosphate ceramic, and fibrillar collagen, and has been proven to be as functional as an autogenous graft in the cases of acute long bone fractures.[102] cycLOS is a synthetic bone graft substitute composed of sodium hyaluronate and beta-tricalcium phosphate granules. It is used as a bone filler in spinal and craniomaxillofacial defects. It is intraoperatively shaped using a scalpel to fit the bone defect, and the putty is prepared by either adding autologous blood or bone marrow aspirate. The beta-tricalcium phosphate granules in the putty are embedded in a HA carrier.[103] Collagen hydrogels have been formed, subsequently lyophilized into collagen sponges, and then loaded with BMP-2 protein have been used for bone defects successfully, as the collagen sponge could be easily molded to the shape of the defect, and the sponge helps in slow release of the protein.[104] Other hydrogels like chitosan, alginate, and HA have been used as carriers and designed for controlled delivery of BMP-2 protein for bone regeneration as well.[105,106] Alginate hydrogels do not degrade enzymatically but their gelation is due to ionic crosslinking, and these hydrogels disintegrate in a timely fashion in the same timeframe as the bone formation process.[107]

3.5.2.4 Soft Tissue Regeneration

Hydrogels have been explored extensively for soft tissue repair and regeneration of cartilage, neural tissues, vascular tissues, fat and liver tissues by serving as vehicles to deliver cells and cytokines to specific locations *in vivo*. The natural polymers used in hydrogel preparations for soft tissue regeneration are typically collagen, gelatin, fibrin, silk, and polysaccharides such as alginate and HA, while synthetic polymers include poly(lactic-co-glycolic) (PLGA), poly (L-lactic acid) (PLLA), poly(ethylene glycol),), poly(N-isopropylacrylamide) [poly(NIPAAm)], PVA, PPF, and poly(hydroxyethyl methacrylate) (PHEMA).[101]

A hydrogel synthesized with fibrin and alginate; embedded with pancreas specific cells, has been used to form and support large pseudoislet clusters with improved metabolic activity. The pseudoislets constructed with these hydrogels have shown the potential to be employed in diabetic treatment in the future, used to deliver insulin-producing cells.[108] Hyalograft and HYAFF-11 are HA-based polymeric scaffolds loaded with chondrocytes employed with notable success in cartilage engineering.[109] Methacrylated hyaluronic hydrogels match the vocal mucosa with its dynamic viscosity and has been explored as an option in vocal tissue repair.[110] Chitosan–fibrin hydrogels injected on their own have been shown to promote angiogenesis. Hydrogels engineered to release vascular endothelial growth factor (VEGF) and hydrogel scaffolds with endothelial cells in them provide an added advantage in new vessel formation.[111] One such example is a heparinized HA that immobilizes proangiogenic growth factors such as VEGF, fibroblast growth factor (FGF), and platelet-derived growth factor (PDGF), facilitating long-term release for neovascularization and angiogenesis *in vivo*.[45,46,112,113]

3.5.3 DRUG DELIVERY

Over the last decade, there has been a growing interest in the use of hydrogels in drug delivery systems. As Yun et al. outlined in their recent review of emerging drug delivery technologies, research from the 1950s to the 1980s successfully created many clinically by obtaining a strong understanding of the basic release mechanisms.[114] Traditional drug delivery systems often require large and repeated doses in order to achieve the desired therapeutic effect and can often lead to off-target effects due to the systemic nature of the delivery mechanisms.[115] Over the next 30 years, researchers struggled to overcome biological barriers to develop clinically successful drugs in an attempt to create systems that improved long-term release and bioavailability.[114] Attempts to develop therapeutics utilizing proteins, growth factors, RNA, and other unstable therapeutics often break down before reaching the target inside the body.[116,117] Nanoparticles, while effective in treating cancer in small animals, have yet to succeed in human studies, again highlighting the limited success of second-generation drugs.[114,118] It has become evident that there is a need for new modulatory systems that can have controllable physicochemical properties like the first-generation systems and can interact with biological systems in ways that second-generation drugs did not.

Over the last decade, there has been a growing interest in the use of hydrogels in drug delivery systems because of their modulatory chemical and mechanical properties. Hydrogels tend to be biocompatible and highly porous, which means that drugs and other therapeutic molecules can be loaded into the crosslinked network. Precise control over pore size, degradation mechanism, and charge distribution within the crosslinked network make hydrogels great candidates for localized long-term therapeutics applications and delivery of unstable molecules such as peptides and nucleic acids. Hydrogel formulation can also be optimized to improve efficacy of many existing drugs and drugs in development by increasing half-life in the body, decreasing dosage required, and decreasing toxic side effects. In this section, we will outline how we can take advantage of their unique properties to design novel delivery systems and control release kinetics of a variety of molecules.

3.5.3.1 Hydrogel Delivery Systems

As previously described, hydrogels can take many different forms. Macroscopic hydrogels tend to be on the order of millimeters to centimeters, while micro and nanogels tend to be on the order of micrometers and nanometers respectively. Macroscopic hydrogels tend to be useful in regenerative medicine applications and in transepithelial delivery. These larger scale hydrogels are usually implanted into the body or place directly onto the skin or another epithelial layer. One of the most successful clinically approved hydrogel systems is the INFUSE by Medtronic.[10] Collagen gel is loaded with bone morphogenic proteins that are implanted to improve fracture or defect healing in spinal fusions and long bones repair.[119,120] Macroscopic hydrogels have also been used to treat wounds. As previously outlined, hydrogels can be loaded with drug products and applied to wound areas to improve healing and prevent infections.[10] Other systems are being developed with the goal of delivery proteins such as insulin transdermally.

In order to make these implanted hydrogels less invasive, many injectable hydrogel systems are also of great appeal. As described earlier, many hydrogel systems exhibit shear thinning properties. In other words, a viscous material flows like a low-viscosity fluid when a sheer stress is applied but returns to its viscous state when the stress is removed. This allows many hydrogels including HA, PEG, and gelatin to be injected using relatively small gauge needles.[31,121] Currently, injectable hydrogel systems loaded with chemotherapeutic agents are being explored in order to increase the amount of drug delivered to the tumor site and limit off-target effects.[118]

Currently, there are no micro or nanoscale hydrogel formulations that are approved for use in the clinic but continue to be investigated in the lab as intriguing options for drug delivery. For oral and pulmonary delivery, microgels with a diameter around 5 µm. Particles of this size cannot by administered intravenously because they will be rapidly cleared from the blood stream.[10] In one study, orally administered alginate microparticles have been designed to have a pH-dependent release of drug to target the small intestine.[122] Nanohydrogels with a diameter of 10–100 nm can be administered intravenously. These gels are smaller than the microgels so they can carry less payload, but they are small enough to exit the capillary vessels and enter the surrounding tissue on their own.[10] Many nanogels have been designed to deliver DNA therapeutics for long-term gene therapy.[123–125] Other nanogels take advantage of the leaky vasculature in tumors in order to deliver chemotherapeutics directly to the site of the tumor.[126,127] Many are specifically interested in using nanogels to treat glioblastoma because the hydrogel nanoparticles can be modified to increase transport across the blood–brain barrier.[128]

Hydrogels have also proven useful as coatings for implanted medical devices such as orthopedic implants and stents. The use of orthopedic implants to heal fractures and other pathologies comes with an inherent risk of infection, especially in diabetics, smokers, and elderly patients.[129] These patients are also at higher risk if non-unions, or improper healing of the affected site.[129] Thin hydrogel coatings can be applied to the surfaces of implants that release antibiotics into the tissue surrounding the hardware and/or growth factors that will induce healing and remodeling of the bone.[130] Similar technology is being used in stents. Stents can be coated with thin hydrogel coatings containing drugs, including antibiotics, anticoagulation factors, and growth factors such as VEGF to encourage the growth of new vascular cells onto the stent.[131,132]

Hydrogels have also been used in other unique and creative ways to deliver novel therapeutics. One of the most intriguing emerging engineering applications is the use of hydrogels in microneedle delivery systems. Traditionally, vaccines are delivered via bolus subcutaneous injection, but these systems are often limited to use by trained professionals in the clinic and can lead to the spread of blood-borne pathogens, especially in developing countries.[133] Microneedles are fabricated such that they only penetrate the *stratum corneum*, the outermost layer of the skin, and are relatively painless.[133] The array can me molded out of drug-eluting material or it can coat or fill prefabricated needles. Hydrogels have been used to carry and release the vaccine material in a variety of studies. Pearton et al. coated silicon microneedles with thermosensitive PLGA-PEG-PLGA triblock copolymers loaded with plasmid DNA for release into the dermis.[134] In a different study, NIPAAm microgels loaded with drug were imbedded in a PLGA microneedle array, so that when placed in the skin, the hydrogel particles swelled and resulting in successful delivery of the drug.[135]

3.5.3.2 Mechanisms of Controlled Release in Drug Delivery Systems

As outlined previously, there are two broad delivery pathways that can be used to describe the release of molecules from hydrogels: static systems and "smart" stimulus-responsive systems. These mechanisms of release can be engineered to precisely control the delivery of therapeutics to a variety of organs in the body. In the following sections, we will provide some cases where these release mechanisms are used in drug delivery systems. There are limited clinically approved hydrogels for controlled release of therapeutics, so much of the section will focus on systems currently in development.

3.5.3.2.1   Static/Diffusion-Based Delivery

The most hydrogel drug delivery systems, the therapeutic agent, is released from the network via diffusion. By controlling the density of the crosslinked network, the pore size, the charges within the construct, and the size of the drug molecule, the rate of diffusion can be controlled. This is the simplest way to control the rate of drug release, so most, if not all, of the clinically approved hydrogel drug delivery systems are diffusion based. For example, the INFUSE hydrogel mentioned earlier consists of a collagen gel loaded with bone morphogenic protein 2 (BMP2).[10] The hydrogel is injected into the site of a bone defect or fracture where it crosslinks filling the void. Over time, the protein diffuses out of the gel into the surrounding tissue promoting osteocyte infiltration and has been shown to improve bone regrowth in a variety of cases.[119] More recently, hydrogel delivery systems for localized cancer treatment have begun to enter the clinic. Designed to treat prostate cancer, Vantas™ is a hydrogel that is implanted in the upper arm that releases chemotherapies into the body.[136] These clinically successful products have inspired more research into hydrogel delivery of more complex molecules.

Simply changing the pore size of the hydrogel can also change the rate of diffusion of certain molecules from the hydrogel.[137,138] But to create systems that deliver more unstable molecules and therapeutics, we need to modify the hydrogel network to "shield" the payload from the harsh conditions of the body and control the diffusion rate. Heparin conjugated HA hydrogels bind certain growth factors, and by changing the crosslinking density and porosity of the gel, the release rate of the growth factors can be changed.[39] While these hydrogels were specifically studied for use in wound healing applications, the modulatory nature makes them useful in many pharmacological and regenerative medicine applications.[31,39] The interactions of molecules that make up the hydrogel backbone can also impact molecule degradation and diffusion rate. Poly(lactides)s such as PLA are known to form stereocomplexes in solution. Understanding the higher order structures that these molecules create under various conditions, we can change the diffusion rate of molecules from the network.[139]

Static diffusion-based delivery is relatively simple, so it has been applied to a variety of systems. However, the next generation of release systems will be made of smart materials that allow for even more control of release rate and location.

3.5.3.2.2   Temperature

Temperature-sensitive hydrogels have also proven to be very useful in drug delivery systems. The thermoreversible nature of many of these hydrogels means that they are particularly useful as injectables,[56] which means the return to a liquid form after both negatively and positively thermosensitive hydrogels have been studied for use in drug delivery systems.[140] For example, it is known that in breast cancer tumors, the temperature is slightly elevated. Shirakura et al. designed a nanogel that demonstrates increased release of cisplatin, a common chemotherapuertic agent, as temperature increases.[141] These positively thermosensitive nanoparticles could be used in the future to eliminate some of the off-target effects of chemotherary in breast cancer patients. Poly (N-isopropylacrylamide) (pNIPAAm), a negatively thermosenstive hydrogel, is probably the most studied thermoresponsive hydrogel.[140] It has been used in a variety of drug delivery systems including protein delivery and the delivery of vaccines via microneedle arrays.[135,142]

3.5.3.2.3   Local pH

Hydrogels that respond to pH can also be used for "smart" drug delivery. For a long time, researchers have observed that the pH in many tumor types is slightly acidic. Therefore, pH-responsive hydrogels seem to be a logical choice for designing localized chemotherapies. In one particular study, the anticancer drug bortezomib was covalently bound to an alginate-based hydrogel via a pH-sensitive bond, so that the drug is released only when the hydrogel is in the tumor microenviroment.[143] In a similar system, doxorubicin was conjugated to an injectable chitosan–alginate hydrogel using a pH-sensitive bond and was shown to effectively kill breast cancer cells in an animal model.[144] In another recent study, pH-sensitive hydrogel microparticles were designed for oral drug delivery. Alginate was chemically modified such that it was stable at the acidic pH and degraded rapidly in the neutral to basic pH. This means that the material is stable in the stomach but will release the drug once it reaches the intestine, making it a strong candidate for targeted drug delivery to the duodenum.[122]

3.5.3.2.4   Biochemical

The rate of degradation of hydrogels can be controlled by changing the crosslinkers used. In one simple case, Nuttelman et al. functionalized a PEG hydrogel with dexamethasone using lactide bonds. Over time, the ester bonds formed in the crosslinking reaction were hydrolyzed and the drug was released.[145] In other systems, the breaking of the covalent bonds in the hydrogel network requires enzymes. For example, it has been shown that the degradation of silk fibroin hydrogels and the release of bound molecules via protease activity can be controlled by making changes to the processing procedure.[146] There are also specific crosslinkers that can be used to control network degradations. MMP-sensitive sequences are often used for this purpose. In one study, researchers developed a PEG hydrogel with a MMP degradable crosslinker that releases the chemotherapeutic drug cisplatin when exposed to a glioma cell line showing that this system could be used for localized drug delivery to treat aggressive brain tumors.[147] MMP degradable hydrogels have been studied for use in a variety of systems including orally administered treatments.[148] There are also a variety of other enzymatically cleavable crosslinkers that have been explored for use in many other applications.[118,149]

3.5.3.2.5   Mechanical

Mechanical forces can also be applied to hydrogels to induce the release of drugs. Oftentimes hydrogels undergo compression when they are exposed to physiological systems. Therefore, hydrogels can be engineered to release drugs under these conditions.[150] In one case, an alginate hydrogel was designed to release angiogenic factors in response to compressive forces and shear stresses. A diabetic mouse model was used to show that these mechanically responsive hydrogels lead to an increase in blood vessel formation after injury.[62] In a separate study, the release of hydrocortisone from modified alginate hydrogels was shown to increase as mechanical stress increased.[151] Similarly, a mechanoresponsive modified HA-based hydrogel was designed to release the anti-inflammatory dexamethasone in response to mechanical stress.[152] This system could be used to reduce inflammation in wound healing or in mechanically active tissues. Recently, hydrogels that respond to tension have also been developed. In one study, an enzyme was covalently bound to the hydrogel backbone. As the gel was stretched, more of the enzymes were exposed to the outside environment and the enzymatic activity increased.[153]

3.5.3.2.6   External Stimulus-Mediated Delivery

Some hydrogel systems have been designed to release drugs as a result of an external stimulus. The rate and amount of drug released can often be controlled with great precision compared with other mechanisms discussed but there is often risks and limitations associated with the stimuli used. Huebsch et al. used ultrasound to release a burst of drug from an alginate hydrogel.[154] This technique is appealing because ultrasound is already widely used in the clinic, and it provides a high level of control over the release of the drug. Composite hydrogels have also been designed to release the drug when exposed to a magnetic field. In one particular case, a chitosan hydrogel was loaded with iron oxide magnetic nanoparticles along with an anticancer drug and was injected into an animal. The study shows that the drug was released when exposed to a magnetic field and resulted in an improved response compared with the control.[155] Similarly, hydrogels that release chemotherapeutic drugs in response to stimulation with NIR light are being developed.[156,157] These systems are appealing because the light can be focused to a small area of tissue and could be engineered to induce an extremely localized response. However, the penetration may not be as good as ultrasound or magnetic fields. Finally, there are composite hydrogel systems that release drug in response to low energy electric fields.[158,159] While these models are effective *in vitro*, it is not clear whether there would be any negative side effects that would result from exposure to an electric field.

3.6 CONCLUSIONS

Hydrogel biomaterials have often been thought of as tools mostly for tissue engineering, serving as scaffolds for cells to biofabricate tissue constructs. However, these materials are far more versatile with many more applications, including as delivery vehicles. In this chapter we have outlined hydrogel types, hydrogel release kinetics categories, and highlighted applications of hydrogel-based release of cells, cell-derived products, and therapeutics in several biological applications. As the development of more nuanced and novel hydrogel biomaterial technologies continue to advance, we expect that hydrogels will continue to replace more traditional delivery vehicles for clinical applications, and in the end, providing better care for patients in the clinic.

REFERENCES

1. Lee, J. H. Injectable hydrogels delivering therapeutic agents for disease treatment and tissue engineering. *Biomater Res* **22**, 27 (2018). doi: 10.1186/s40824-018-0138-6.
2. Skardal, A. Perspective: "Universal" bioink technology for advancing extrusion bioprinting-based biomanufacturing. *Bioprinting* **10**, e00026 (2018).
3. Wang, H. & Heilshorn, S. C. Adaptable hydrogel networks with reversible linkages for tissue engineering. *Adv Mater* **27**, 3717–3736 (2015). doi: 10.1002/adma.201501558.
4. Li, L., Scheiger, J. M. & Levkin, P. A. Design and applications of photoresponsive hydrogels. *Adv Mater* **31**, e1807333 (2019). doi: 10.1002/adma.201807333.
5. Skardal, A. & Atala, A. Biomaterials for integration with 3-d bioprinting. *Ann Biomed Eng* **43**, 730–746 (2015). doi: 10.1007/s10439-014-1207-1.
6. Datta, P. et al. Essential steps in bioprinting: From pre- to post-bioprinting. *Biotechnol Adv* (2018). doi: 10.1016/j.biotechadv.2018.06.003.
7. Mazzocchi, A. R., Soker, S. & Skardal, A. Biofabrication technologies for developing in vitro tumor models. In *Tumor Organoids*, (eds S. Soker & A. Skardal) pp. 51–70. Springer Nature: Switzerland (2017).
8. Skardal, A., Shupe, T. & Atala, A. Organoid-on-a-chip and body-on-a-chip systems for drug screening and disease modeling. *Drug Discovery Today* **21**, 1399–1411 (2016). doi: 10.1016/j.drudis.2016.07.003.
9. Youngblood, R. L., Truong, N. F., Segura, T. & Shea, L. D. It's all in the delivery: Designing hydrogels for cell and non-viral gene therapies. *Mol Ther* **26**, 2087–2106 (2018). doi: 10.1016/j.ymthe.2018.07.022.
10. Li, J. & Mooney, D. J. Designing hydrogels for controlled drug delivery. *Nat Rev Mater* **1** (2016). doi: 10.1038/natrevmats.2016.71.
11. Williams, D. The continuing evolution of biomaterials. *Biomaterials* **32**, 1–2 (2011). doi: 10.1016/j.biomaterials.2010.09.048.
12. Williams, D. F. On the nature of biomaterials. *Biomaterials* **30**, 5897–5909 (2009). doi: 10.1016/j.biomaterials.2009.07.027.
13. Hesse, E. et al. Collagen type I hydrogel allows migration, proliferation, and osteogenic differentiation of rat bone marrow stromal cells. *J Biomed Mater Res A* **94**, 442–449 (2010). doi: 10.1002/jbm.a.32696.
14. Santos, E., Zarate, J., Orive, G., Hernandez, R. M. & Pedraz, J. L. Biomaterials in cell microencapsulation. *Adv Exp Med Biol* **670**, 5–21 (2010).
15. Sittadjody, S. et al. Encapsulation of mesenchymal stem cells in 3D ovarian cell constructs promotes stable and long-term hormone secretion with improved physiological outcomes in a syngeneic rat model. *Ann Biomed Eng* (2019). doi: 10.1007/s10439-019-02334-w.
16. Opara, E. C., Mirmalek-Sani, S. H., Khanna, O., Moya, M. L. & Brey, E. M. Design of a bioartificial pancreas(+). *J Investig Med* **58**, 831–837 (2010). doi: 10.231/JIM.0b013e3181ed3807.

17. Allison, D. D. & Grande-Allen, K. J. Review. Hyaluronan: A powerful tissue engineering tool. *Tissue Eng* **12**, 2131–2140 (2006). doi: 10.1089/ten.2006.12.2131.

18. Knudson, C. B. & Knudson, W. Cartilage proteoglycans. *Semin Cell Dev Biol* **12**, 69–78 (2001).

19. Kuo, J. W. *Practical Aspects of Hyaluronan Based Medical Products*. CRC/Taylor & Francis: Boca Raton, FL (2006).

20. Galus, R., Antiszko, M. & Wlodarski, P. Clinical applications of hyaluronic acid. *Pol Merkur Lekarski* **20**, 606–608 (2006).

21. Schiavinato, A., Finesso, M., Cortivo, R. & Abatangelo, G. Comparison of the effects of intra-articular injections of Hyaluronan and its chemically cross-linked derivative (Hylan G-F20) in normal rabbit knee joints. *Clin Exp Rheumatol* **20**, 445–454 (2002).

22. Prestwich, G. D. & Kuo, J. W. Chemically-modified HA for therapy and regenerative medicine. *Curr Pharm Biotechnol* **9**, 242–245 (2008).

23. Miki, D. et al. A photopolymerized sealant for corneal lacerations. *Cornea* **21**, 393–399 (2002).

24. Skardal, A. et al. Photocrosslinkable hyaluronan-gelatin hydrogels for two-step bioprinting. *Tissue Eng Part A* **16**, 2675–2685 (2010). doi: 10.1089/ten.TEA.2009.0798.

25. Kirker, K. R., Luo, Y., Morris, S. E., Shelby, J. & Prestwich, G. D. Glycosaminoglycan hydrogels as supplemental wound dressings for donor sites. *J Burn Care Rehabil* **25**, 276–286 (2004).

26. Liu, Y., Shu, X. Z. & Prestwich, G. D. Tumor engineering: Orthotopic cancer models in mice using cell-loaded, injectable, cross-linked hyaluronan-derived hydrogels. *Tissue Eng* **13**, 1091–1101 (2007).

27. Aleman, J. & Skardal, A. A multi-site metastasis-on-a-chip microphysiological system for assessing metastatic preference of cancer cells. *Biotechnol Bioeng* (2018). doi: 10.1002/bit.26871.

28. Mazzocchi, A. R., Rajan, S. A. P., Votanopoulos, K. I., Hall, A. R. & Skardal, A. In vitro patient-derived 3D mesothelioma tumor organoids facilitate patient-centric therapeutic screening. *Sci Rep* **8**, 2886 (2018). doi: 10.1038/s41598-018-21200-8.

29. Votanopoulos, K. I. et al. Appendiceal cancer patient-specific tumor organoid model for predicting chemotherapy efficacy prior to initiation of treatment: A feasibility study. *Ann Surg Oncol* **26**, 139–147 (2019). doi: 10.1245/s10434-018-7008-2.

30. Skardal, A., Zhang, J., McCoard, L., Oottamasathien, S. & Prestwich, G. D. Dynamically cross-linked gold nanoparticle: Hyaluronan hydrogels. *Adv Mater* **22**, 4736–4740 (2010). doi: 10.1002/adma.201001436.

31. Skardal, A. et al. A hydrogel bioink toolkit for mimicking native tissue biochemical and mechanical properties in bioprinted tissue constructs. *Acta Biomater* **25**, 24–34 (2015). doi: 10.1016/j.actbio.2015.07.030.

32. Mazzocchi, A., Devarasetty, M., Huntwork, R., Soker, S. & Skardal, A. Optimization of collagen type I-hyaluronan hybrid bioink for 3D bioprinted liver microenvironments. *Biofabrication* **11**, 015003 (2018). doi: 10.1088/1758-5090/aae543.

33. Clark, C. C., Aleman, J., Mutkus, L. & Skardal, A. A mechanically robust thixotropic collagen and hyaluronic acid bioink supplemented with gelatin nanoparticles. *Bioprinting* **16** (2019).

34. Ahmed, T. A., Dare, E. V. & Hincke, M. Fibrin: A versatile scaffold for tissue engineering applications. *Tissue Eng Part B Rev* **14**, 199–215 (2008). doi: 10.1089/ten.teb.2007.0435.

35. Skardal, A. et al. Bioprinted amniotic fluid-derived stem cells accelerate healing of large skin wounds. *Stem Cells Transl Med* **1**, 792–802 (2012). doi: 10.5966/sctm.2012-0088.

36. Hoare, T. R. & Kohane, D. S. Hydrogels in drug delivery: Progress and challenges. *Polymer* **49**, 1993–2007 (2008). doi: 10.1016/j.polymer.2008.01.027.

37. Hoffman, A. S. Hydrogels for biomedical applications. *Adv Drug Delivery Revi* **54**, 3–12 (2002).

38. Huynh, C. T., Nguyen, M. K. & Lee, D. S. Injectable block copolymer hydrogels: Achievements and future challenges for biomedical applications. *Macromolecules* **44**, 6629–6636 (2011). doi: 10.1021/ma201261.

39. Skardal, A. et al. A tunable hydrogel system for long-term release of cell-secreted cytokines and bioprinted in situ wound cell delivery. *J Biomed Mater Res B Appl Biomater* **105**, 1986–2000 (2017). doi: 10.1002/jbm.b.33736.

40. Anseth, K. & Lin, C.-C. PEG hydrogels for the controlled release of biomolecules in regenerative medicine. *Pharm Res* **26** (2009). doi: 10.1007/s11095-008-9801-2.

41. Jensen, M., Hansen, P. B., Murdan, S., Frokjaer, S. & Florence, A. T. Loading into and electro-stimulated release of peptides and proteins from chondroitin 4-sulphate hydrogels. *Eur J Pharm Sci* **15**, 139–148 (2001) doi: 10.1016/S0928-0987(01)00193-2.

42. Nicodemus, G. D. & Bryant, S. Cell encapsulation in biodegradable hydrogels for tissue engineering. *Tissue Eng Part B* **14** (2008). doi: 10.1089/ten.teb.2007.0332.

43. Dash, S., Murthy, P. N., Nath, L. & Chowdhury, P. Kinetic modeling on drug release from controlled drug delivery systems. *Acta Poloniae Pharm Drug Res* **67**, 217–223 (2010).

44. Benoit, D. S. W., Collins, S. D. & Anseth, K. Multifunctional hydrogels that promote osteogenic human mesenchymal stem cell differentiation through stimulation and sequestering of bone morphogenic protein 2. *Adv Funct Mater* **17**, 2085–2093 (2007). doi: 10.1002/adfm.200700012.

45. Pike, D. B. et al. Heparin-regulated release of growth factors in vitro and angiogenic response in vivo to implanted hyaluronan hydrogels containing VEGF and bFGF. *Biomaterials* **27**, 5242–5251 (2006).

46. Riley, C. M. et al. Stimulation of in vivo angiogenesis using dual growth factor-loaded crosslinked glycosaminoglycan hydrogels. *Biomaterials* **27**, 5935–5943 (2006).

47. Bertz, A. et al. Encapsulation of proteins in hydrogel carrier systems for controlled drug delivery: Influence of network structure and drug size on release rate. *J Biotechnol* **163** (2013). doi: 10.1016/j.jbiotec.2012.06.036.

48. Yi, H. et al. Tissue-specific extracellular matrix promotes myogenic differentiation of human muscle progenitor cells on gelatin and heparin conjugated alginate hydrogels. *Acta Biomater* **62**, 222–233 (2017). doi: 10.1016/j.actbio.2017.08.022.

49. Serra, L., Domenech, J. & Peppas, N. A. Drug transport mechanisms and release kinetics from molecularly designed poly(acrylic acid-g-ethylene glycol) hydrogels. *Biomaterials* **27**, 5440–5451 (2006). doi: 10.1016/j.biomaterials.2006.06.011.

50. Li, Y. et al. A G-quadruplex hydrogel via multicomponent self-assembly: Formation and zero-order controlled release. *ACS Appl Mater Interfaces* **9**, 13056–13067 (2017). doi: 10.1021/acsami.7b00957.

51. Wang, Y., Cooke, M. J., Morshead, C. M. & Shoichet, M. S. Hydrogel delivery of erythropoietin to the brain for endogenous stem cell stimulation after stroke injury. *Biomaterials* **33**, 2681–2692 (2012). doi: 10.1016/j.biomaterials.2011.12.031.

52. Hurler, J. et al. Improved burns therapy: Liposomes-in-hydrogel delivery system for mupirocin. *J Pharm Sci* **101**, 3906–3915 (2012).

53. Echeverria, C., Fernandes, S. N., Godinho, M. H., Borges, J. P. & Soares, P. I. P. Functional stimuli-responsive gels: Hydrogels and microgels. *Gels* **4** (2018). doi: 10.3390/gels4020054.

54. Peppas, N. A., Bures, P., Leobandung, W. & Ichikawa, H. Hydrogels in pharmaceutical formulations. *Eur J Pharm Biopharm* **50**, 27–46 (2000). doi: 10.1016/S0939-6411(00)00090-4.

55. Hill, L. K. et al. Thermoresponsive protein-engineered coiled-coil hydrogel for sustained small molecule release. *Biomacromolecules* (2019). doi: 10.1021/acs.biomac.9b00107.

56. Bhattarai, N., Ramay, H. R., Gunn, J., Matsen, F. A. & Zhang, M. PEG-grafted chitosan as an injectable thermosensitive hydrogel for sustained protein release. *J Controlled Release* **103**, 609–624 (2005). doi: 10.1016/j.jconrel.2004.12.019.

57. Gupta, P., Vermani, K. & Garg, S. Hydrogels: From controlled release to pH-responsive drug delivery. *Drug Discovery Today* **7**, 569–579 (2002).

58. Boehnke, N., Cam, C., Bat, E., Segura, T. & Maynard, H. D. Imine hydrogels with tunable degradability for tissue engineering. *Biomacromolecules* **16**, 2101–2108 (2015). doi: 10.1021/acs.biomac.5b00519.

59. Seliktar, D. Designing cell-compatible hydrogels for biomedical applications. *Science* **336**, 1124–1128 (2012). doi: 10.1126/science.1214804.

60. Fonseca, K. B. et al. Enzymatic, physiochemical and biological properties of MMP-sensitive alginate hydrogels. *Soft Matter* **9**, 3283–3292 (2013). doi: 10.1039/C3SM27560D.

61. Fonseca, K. B., Bidarra, S. J., Oliveira, M. J., Granja, P. L. & Barrias, C. C. Molecularly designed alginate hydrogels susceptible to local proteolysis as three-dimensional cellular microenvironments. *Acta Biomater* **7**, 1674–1682 (2011). doi: 10.1016/j.actbio.2010.12.029.

62. Lee, K. Y., Peters, M. C., Anderson, K. W. & Mooney, D. J. Controlled growth factor release from synthetic extracellular matrices. *Nature* **408**, 998–1000 (2000).

63. Bin, Y., Boyer, J.-C., Habault, D., Branda, N. R. & Zhao, Y. Near infrared light triggered release of biomacromolecules from hydrogels loaded with upconversion nanoparticles. *J Am Chem Soc* 134, 16558–16561 (2012). doi: 10.1021/ja308876j.

64. Robson, M. C., Steed, D. L. & Franz, M. G. Wound healing: Biologic features and approaches to maximize healing trajectories. *Curr Prob Surg* **38**, A1–140 (2001). doi: 10.1067/msg.2001.111167.

65. Lazarus, G. S. et al. Definitions and guidelines for assessment of wounds and evaluation of healing. *JAMA Dermatol* **130**, 489–493 (1994). doi: 10.1001/archderm.1994.01690040093015.

66. Robbins, J. M. et al. Mortality rates and diabetic foot ulcers: Is it time to communicate mortality risk to patients with diabetic foot ulceration? *J Am Podiatric Med Assoc* **98**, 489–493 (2008).

67. Lu, H. et al. Recent advances of on-demand dissolution of hydrogel dressings. *Burns Trauma* **6**, 35 (2018). doi: 10.1186/s41038-018-0138-8.

68. Dhivya, S., Padma, V. V. & Santhini, E. Wound dressings: A review. *Biomedicine (Taipei)* **5**, 22 (2015). doi: 10.7603/s40681-015-0022-9.

69. Baranoski, S. & Ayello, E. A. Wound dressings: An evolving art and science. *Adv Skin Wound Care* **25**, 87–92; quiz 92–84 (2012). doi: 10.1097/01.ASW.0000411409.05554.c8.

70. Winter, G. D. Formation of the scab and the rate of epithelization of superficial wounds in the skin of the young domestic pig. *Nature* **193**, 293–294 (1962). doi: 10.1038/193293a0.

71. Dabiri, G., Damstetter, E. & Phillips, T. Choosing a wound dressing based on common wound characteristics. *Adv Wound Care (New Rochelle)* **5**, 32–41 (2016). doi: 10.1089/wound.2014.0586.

72. Deutsch, C. J., Edwards, D. M. & Myers, S. Wound dressings. *Br J Hosp Med* **78**, C103–C109 (2017). doi: 10.12968/hmed.2017.78.7.C103.

73. Kamoun, E. A., Kenawy, E.-R. S. & Chen, X. A review on polymeric hydrogel membranes for wound dressing applications: PVA-based hydrogel dressings. *J Adv Res* **8**, 217–233 (2017). doi: 10.1016/j.jare.2017.01.005.

74. Madaghiele, M., Demitri, C., Sannino, A. & Ambrosio, L. Polymeric hydrogels for burn wound care: Advanced skin wound dressings and regenerative templates. *Burns Trauma* **2**, 153–161 (2014). doi: 10.4103/2321-3868.143616.

75. Cuttle, L., Pearn, J., McMillan, J. R. & Kimble, R. M. A review of first aid treatments for burn injuries. *Burns J Int Soc Burn Inj* **35**, 768–775 (2009). doi: 10.1016/j.burns.2008.10.011.

76. Ribeiro, M. P. et al. Development of a new chitosan hydrogel for wound dressing. *Wound Repair Regen* **17**, 817–824 (2009). doi: 10.1111/j.1524-475X.2009.00538.x.

77. Drury, J. L. & Mooney, D. J. Hydrogels for tissue engineering: Scaffold design variables and applications. *Biomaterials* **24**, 4337–4351 (2003).

78. Boateng, J. S., Matthews, K. H., Stevens, H. N. E. & Eccleston, G. M. Wound healing dressings and drug delivery systems: A review. *J Pharm Sci* **97**, 2892–2923 (2008). doi: 10.1002/jps.21210.

79. Francesko, A., Petkova, P. & Tzanov, T. Hydrogel dressings for advanced wound management. *Curr Med Chem* **25**, 5782–5797 (2018). doi: 10.2174/0929867324666170920161246.

80. Mathangi Ramakrishnan, K., Mathivanan, B. M., Jayaraman, V. & Shankar, J. Advantages of collagen based biological dressings in the management of superficial and superficial partial thickness burns in children. *Ann Burns Fire Disasters* **26**, 98–104 (2013).

81. Knapp, T. R., Kaplan, E. N. & Daniels, J. R. Injectable collagen for soft tissue augmentation. *Plast Reconstr Surg* **60**, 398–405 (1977).

82. Chattopadhyay, S. & Raines, R. T. Review collagen-based biomaterials for wound healing. *Biopolymers* **101**, 821–833 (2014). doi: 10.1002/bip.22486.

83. Reynolds, M., Kelly, D. A., Walker, N. J., Crantford, C. & Defranzo, A. J. Use of integra in the management of complex hand wounds from cancer resection and nonburn trauma. *Hand (New York)* **13**, 74–79 (2018). doi: 10.1177/1558944717692090.

84. Chua, A. W. C. et al. Skin tissue engineering advances in severe burns: Review and therapeutic applications. *Burns Trauma* **4**, 3 (2016). doi: 10.1186/s41038-016-0027-y.

85. Lee, K. Y. & Mooney, D. J. Alginate: Properties and biomedical applications. *Prog Polym Sci* **37**, 106–126 (2012). doi: 10.1016/j.progpolymsci.2011.06.003.

86. Aderibigbe, B. A. & Buyana, B. Alginate in wound dressings. *Pharmaceutics* **10**, 42 (2018). doi: 10.3390/pharmaceutics10020042.

87. Rao, K. M., Suneetha, M., Zo, S., Duck, K. H. & Han, S. S. One-pot synthesis of ZnO nanobelt-like structures in hyaluronan hydrogels for wound dressing applications. *Carbohydr Polym* **223**, 115124 (2019). doi: 10.1016/j.carbpol.2019.115124.

88. Murphy, S. V. et al. Solubilized amnion membrane hyaluronic acid hydrogel accelerates full-thickness wound healing. *Stem Cells Transl Med* **6**, 2020–2032 (2017). doi: 10.1002/sctm.17-0053.

89. Longinotti, C. The use of hyaluronic acid based dressings to treat burns: A review. *Burns Trauma* **2**, 162–168 (2014). doi:10.4103/2321-3868.142398.

90. Barski, D. et al. Human amniotic membrane dressing for the treatment of an infected wound due to an entero-cutaneous fistula: Case report. *Int J Surg Case Rep* **51**, 11–13 (2018). doi: 10.1016/j.ijscr.2018.08.015.

91. Haugh, A. M. et al. Amnion membrane in diabetic foot wounds: A meta-analysis. *Plast Reconstr Surg Glob Open* **5**, e1302 (2017). doi: 10.1097/GOX.0000000000001302.

92. Lee, S. H. & Shin, H. Matrices and scaffolds for delivery of bioactive molecules in bone and cartilage tissue engineering. *Adv Drug Delivery Rev* **59**, 339–359(2007). doi: 10.1016/j.addr.2007.03.016.

93. Zhang, K. et al. Advanced smart biomaterials and constructs for hard tissue engineering and regeneration. *Bone Res* **6**, 31 (2018). doi: 10.1038/s41413-018-0032-9.

94. Bai, X. et al. Bioactive hydrogels for bone regeneration. *Bioact Mater* **3**, 401–417 (2018). doi: 10.1016/j. bioactmat.2018.05.006.

95. Short, A. R. et al. Hydrogels that allow and facilitate bone repair, remodeling, and regeneration. *J Mater Chem B* **3**, 7818–7830 (2015). doi: 10.1039/c5tb01043h.

96. Karageorgiou, V. & Kaplan, D. Porosity of 3D biomaterial scaffolds and osteogenesis. *Biomaterials* **26**, 5474–5491 (2005). doi: 10.1016/j.biomaterials.2005.02.002.

97. Hutmacher, D. W. Scaffolds in tissue engineering bone and cartilage. *Biomaterials* **21**, 2529–2543 (2000). doi: S0142961200001216.

98. Bertassoni, L. E. et al. Direct-write bioprinting of cell-laden methacrylated gelatin hydrogels. *Biofabrication* **6**, 024105 (2014). doi: 10.1088/1758-5082/6/2/024105.

99. Veronese, F. M. & Pasut, G. PEGylation, successful approach to drug delivery. *Drug Discovery Today* **10**, 1451–1458 (2005). doi: 10.1016/s1359-6446(05)03575-0.

100. Makadia, H. K. & Siegel, S. J. Poly lactic-co-glycolic acid (PLGA) as biodegradable controlled drug delivery carrier. *Polymers* (*Basel*) **3**, 1377–1397 (2011). doi: 10.3390/polym3031377.

101. Lee, K. Y. & Mooney, D. J. Hydrogels for tissue engineering. *Chem Rev* **101**, 1869–1879 (2001).

102. Cornell, C. N. et al. Multicenter trial of Collagraft as bone graft substitute. *J Orthop Trauma* **5**, 1–8 (1991).

103. Yunus Basha, R., Sampath Kumar, T. S. & Doble, M. Design of biocomposite materials for bone tissue regeneration. *Mater Sci Eng C Mater Biol Appl* **57**, 452–463 (2015). doi: 10.1016/j.msec.2015.07.016.

104. Chen, Z. et al. Newly designed human-like collagen to maximize sensitive release of BMP-2 for remarkable repairing of bone defects. *Biomolecules* **9** (2019). doi: 10.3390/biom9090450.

105. Wu, J. et al. Micro-porous polyetheretherketone implants decorated with BMP-2 via phosphorylated gelatin coating for enhancing cell adhesion and osteogenic differentiation. *Colloids Surf B* **169**, 233–241 (2018). doi: 10.1016/j.colsurfb.2018.05.027.

106. Priddy, L. B. et al. Oxidized alginate hydrogels for bone morphogenetic protein-2 delivery in long bone defects. *Acta Biomater* **10**, 4390–4399 (2014). doi: 10.1016/j.actbio.2014.06.015.

107. Boontheekul, T., Kong, H. J. & Mooney, D. J. Controlling alginate gel degradation utilizing partial oxidation and bimodal molecular weight distribution. *Biomaterials* **26**, 2455–2465 (2005). doi: 10.1016/j. biomaterials.2004.06.044.

108. Montalbano, G. et al. Synthesis of bioinspired collagen/alginate/fibrin based hydrogels for soft tissue engineering. *Mater Sci Eng C* **91**, 236–246 (2018). doi: 10.1016/j.msec.2018.04.101.

109. Campoccia, D. et al. Semisynthetic resorbable materials from hyaluronan esterification. *Biomaterials* **19**, 2101–2127 (1998). doi: 10.1016/S0142-9612(98)00042-8.

110. Kutty, J. K. & Webb, K. Mechanomimetic hydrogels for vocal fold lamina propria regeneration. *J Biomater Sci Polym Ed* **20**, 737–756 (2009). doi: 10.1163/156856209x426763.

111. Hsieh, F.-Y., Tao, L., Wei, Y. & Hsu, S.-H. A novel biodegradable self-healing hydrogel to induce blood capillary formation. *NPG Asia Mater* **9**, e363 (2017). doi: 10.1038/am.2017.23.

112. Elia, R. et al. Stimulation of in vivo angiogenesis by in situ crosslinked, dual growth factor-loaded, glycosaminoglycan hydrogels. *Biomaterials* **31**, 4630–4638 (2010). doi: 10.1016/j.biomaterials.2010.02.043.

113. Peattie, R. A. et al. Effect of gelatin on heparin regulation of cytokine release from hyaluronan-based hydrogels. *Drug Delivery* **15**, 389–397 (2008). doi: 10.1080/10717540802035442.

114. Yun, Y. H., Lee, B. K. & Park, K. Controlled drug delivery: Historical perspective for the next generation. *J Controlled Release* **219**, 2–7 (2015). doi: 10.1016/j.jconrel.2015.10.005.

115. Abu-Thabit, N. Y. & Makhlouf, A. S. H. (eds) *Stimuli Responsive Polymeric Nanocarriers for Drug Delivery Applications*, Vol. **1**, pp. 3–41. Elsevier: Cambridge (2018).

116. Fosgerau, K. & Hoffmann, T. Peptide therapeutics: Current status and future directions. *Drug Discovery Today* **20**, 122–128 (2015). doi: 10.1016/j.drudis.2014.10.003.

117. Tibbitt, M. W., Dahlman, J. E. & Langer, R. Emerging frontiers in drug delivery. *J Am Chem Soc* **138**, 704–717 (2016). doi: 10.1021/jacs.5b09974.

118. Norouzi, M., Nazari, B. & Miller, D. W. Injectable hydrogel-based drug delivery systems for local cancer therapy. *Drug Discovery Today* **21**, 1835–1849 (2016). doi: 10.1016/j.drudis.2016.07.006.

119. Bessa, P. C., Casal, M. & Reis, R. L. Bone morphogenetic proteins in tissue engineering: The road from laboratory to clinic, part II (BMP delivery). *J Tissue Eng Regen Med* **2**, 81–96, (2008). doi: 10.1002/term.74.

120. Oliveira, J. M. et al. Hydrogel-based scaffolds to support intrathecal stem cell transplantation as a gateway to the spinal cord: Clinical needs, biomaterials, and imaging technologies. *NPJ Regen Med* **3**, 8 (2018). doi: 10.1038/s41536-018-0046-3.

121. Tan, H. & Marra, K. G. Injectable, biodegradable hydrogels for tissue engineering applications. *Materials* **3**, 1746–1767 (2010). doi: 10.3390/ma3031746.

122. Banks, S. R., Enck, K., Wright, M. W., Opara, E. C. & Welker, M. E. Chemical modification of alginate for controlled oral drug delivery. *J Agric Food Chem* (2019). doi: 10.1021/acs.jafc.9b01911.

123. Quick, D. J., Macdonald, K. K. & Anseth, K. S. Delivering DNA from photocrosslinked, surface eroding polyanhydrides. *J Controlled Release* **97**, 333–343, doi:10.1016/j.jconrel.2004.03.001 (2004).

124. Sharma, A. et al. Nanogel--an advanced drug delivery tool: Current and future. *Artif Cells Nanomed Biotechnol* **44**, 165–177 (2016). doi: 10.3109/21691401.2014.930745.

125. Lee, J. I., Kim, H. S. & Yoo, H. S. DNA nanogels composed of chitosan and Pluronic with thermo-sensitive and photo-crosslinking properties. *Int J Pharm* **373**, 93–99 (2009). doi: 10.1016/j.ijpharm.2009.01.016.

126. Gao, C. et al. Stem cell membrane-coated nanogels for highly efficient in vivo tumor targeted drug delivery. *Small* **12**, 4056–4062 (2016). doi: 10.1002/smll.201600624.

127. Narayanaswamy, R. & Torchilin, V. P. Hydrogels and their applications in targeted drug delivery. *Molecules* **24** (2019). doi: 10.3390/molecules24030603.

128. Basso, J. et al. Hydrogel-based drug delivery nanosystems for the treatment of brain tumors. *Gels* **4** (2018). doi: 10.3390/gels4030062.

129. Kostenuik, P. & Mirza, F. M. Fracture healing physiology and the quest for therapies for delayed healing and nonunion. *J Orthop Res* **35**, 213–223 (2017). doi: 10.1002/jor.23460.

130. Boot, W. et al. Hyaluronic acid-based hydrogel coating does not affect bone apposition at the implant surface in a rabbit model. *Clin Orthop Relat Res* **475**, 1911–1919 (2017). doi: 10.1007/s11999-017-5310-0.

131. Indolfi, L. et al. Microsphere-integrated drug-eluting stents: PLGA microsphere integration in hydrogel coating for local and prolonged delivery of hydrophilic antirestenosis agents. *J Biomed Mater Res A* **97**, 201–211 (2011). doi: 10.1002/jbm.a.33039.

132. Semmling, B., Nagel, S., Sternberg, K., Weitschies, W. & Seidlitz, A. Impact of different tissue-simulating hydrogel compartments on in vitro release and distribution from drug-eluting stents. *Eur J Pharm Biopharm* **87**, 570–578 (2014). doi: 10.1016/j.ejpb.2014.04.010.

133. Kim, Y.-C., Park, J.-H. & Prausnitz, M. R. Microneedles for drug and vaccine delivery. *Adv Drug Delivery Rev* **64**, 1547–1568 (2012). doi: 10.1016/j.addr.2012.04.005.

134. Pearton, M. et al. Gene delivery to the epidermal cells of human skin explants using microfabricated microneedles and hydrogel formulations. *Pharm Res* **25**, 407–416 (2008). doi: 10.1007/s11095-007-9360-y.

135. Kim, M., Jung, B. & Park, J. H. Hydrogel swelling as a trigger to release biodegradable polymer microneedles in skin. *Biomaterials* **33**, 668–678 (2012). doi: 10.1016/j.biomaterials.2011.09.074.

136. Schlegel, P. N. Efficacy and safety of histrelin subdermal implant in patients with advanced prostate cancer. *J Urol* **175**, 1353–1358 (2006). doi: 10.1016/s0022-5347(05)00649-x.

137. Varghese, J. S., Chellappa, N. & Fathima, N. N. Gelatin-carrageenan hydrogels: Role of pore size distribution on drug delivery process. *Colloids Surf B* **113**, 346–351 (2014). doi: 10.1016/j.colsurfb.2013.08.049.

138. Censi, R. et al. Photopolymerized thermosensitive hydrogels for tailorable diffusion-controlled protein delivery. *J Controlled Release* **140**, 230–236 (2009). doi: 10.1016/j.jconrel.2009.06.003.

139. Tsuji, H. Poly(lactide) stereocomplexes: Formation, structure, properties, degradation, and applications. *Macromol Biosci* **5**, 569–597 (2005). doi: 10.1002/mabi.200500062.

140. Huang, H., Qi, X., Chen, Y. & Wu, Z. Thermo-sensitive hydrogels for delivering biotherapeutic molecules: A review. *Saudi Pharm J* (2019). doi: 10.1016/j.jsps.2019.08.001.

141. Shirakura, T., Kelson, T. J., Ray, A., Malyarenko, A. E. & Kopelman, R. Hydrogel nanoparticles with thermally controlled drug release. *ACS Macro Lett* **3**, 602–606 (2014). doi: 10.1021/mz500231e.

142. Ma, C., Shi, Y., Pena, D. A., Peng, L. & Yu, G. Thermally responsive hydrogel blends: A general drug carrier model for controlled drug release. *Angew Chem Int Ed Engl* **54**, 7376–7380 (2015). doi: 10.1002/anie.201501705.

143. Rezk, A. I., Obiweluozo, F. O., Choukrani, G., Park, C. H. & Kim, C. S. Drug release and kinetic models of anticancer drug (BTZ) from a pH-responsive alginate polydopamine hydrogel: Towards cancer chemotherapy. *Int J Biol Macromol* (2019). doi: 10.1016/j.ijbiomac.2019.09.013.

144. Shi, J. et al. Schiff based injectable hydrogel for in situ pH-triggered delivery of doxorubicin for breast tumor treatment. *Polym Chem* **5**, 6180–6189 (2014). doi: 10.1039/c4py00631c.

145. Nuttelman, C. R., Tripodi, M. C. & Anseth, K. S. Dexamethasone-functionalized gels induce osteogenic differentiation of encapsulated hMSCs. *J Biomed Mater Res A* **76**, 183–195 (2006).

146. Vepari, C. & Kaplan, D. L. Silk as a biomaterial. *Prog Polym Sci* **32**, 991–1007 (2007). doi: 10.1016/j.progpolymsci.2007.05.013.

147. Tauro, J. R. & Gemeinhart, R. A. Matrix metalloprotease triggered delivery of cancer chemotherapeutics from hydrogel matrixes. *Bioconjugate Chem* **16**, 1133–1139 (2005).

148. Guo, J. et al. MMP-8-responsive polyethylene glycol hydrogel for intraoral drug delivery. *J Dent Res* **98**, 564–571 (2019). doi: 10.1177/0022034519831931.

149. Aimetti, A. A., Machen, A. J. & Anseth, K. S. Poly(ethylene glycol) hydrogels formed by thiol-ene photopolymerization for enzyme-responsive protein delivery. *Biomaterials* **30**, 6048–6054 (2009). doi: 10.1016/j.biomaterials.20 09.07.043.

150. Wang, J., Kaplan, J. A., Colson, Y. L. & Grinstaff, M. W. Mechanoresponsive materials for drug delivery: Harnessing forces for controlled release. *Adv Drug Delivery Rev* **108**, 68–82 (2017). doi: 10.1016/j.addr.2016.11.001.

151. Tan, L. et al. Synthesis and characterization of β-cyclodextrin-conjugated alginate hydrogel for controlled release of hydrocortisone acetate in response to mechanical stimulation. *J Bioact Compat Polym* **30**, 584–599 (2015). doi: 10.1177/0883911515590494.

152. Xiao, L. et al. Hyaluronic acid-based hydrogels containing covalently integrated drug depots: Implication for controlling inflammation in mechanically stressed tissues. *Biomacromolecules* **14**, 3808–3819 (2013). doi: 10.1021/bm4011276.

153. Zhang, Y., Chen, Q., Ge, J. & Liu, Z. Controlled display of enzyme activity with a stretchable hydrogel. *Chem Commun (Cambridge)* **49**, 9815–9817 (2013). doi: 10.1039/c3cc45837g.

154. Huebsch, N. et al. Ultrasound-triggered disruption and self-healing of reversibly cross-linked hydrogels for drug delivery and enhanced chemotherapy. *Proc Natl Acad Sci U S A* **111**, 9762–9767 (2014). doi: 10.1073/pnas.1405469111.

155. Zhang, D. et al. A magnetic chitosan hydrogel for sustained and prolonged delivery of Bacillus Calmette-Guerin in the treatment of bladder cancer. *Biomaterials* **34**, 10258–10266 (2013). doi: 10.1016/j.biomaterials.2013.09.027.

156. Anugrah, D. S. B., Ramesh, K., Kim, M., Hyun, K. & Lim, K. T. Near-infrared light-responsive alginate hydrogels based on diselenide-containing cross-linkage for on demand degradation and drug release. *Carbohydr Polym* **223**, 115070 (2019). doi: 10.1016/j.carbpol.2019.115070.

157. Qiu, M. et al. Novel concept of the smart NIR-light-controlled drug release of black phosphorus nanostructure for cancer therapy. *Proc Natl Acad Sci U S A* **115**, 501–506 (2018). doi: 10.1073/pnas.1714421115.

158. Merino, S., Martin, C., Kostarelos, K., Prato, M. & Vazquez, E. Nanocomposite hydrogels: 3D polymer nanoparticle synergies for on-demand drug delivery. *ASC Nano* **9**, 4686–4697 (2015).

159. Liu, Y. et al. An electric-field responsive microsystem for controllable miniaturised drug delivery applications. *Procedia Eng* **25**, 984–987 (2011). doi: 10.1016/j.proeng.2011.12.242.

4 The Effect of Glutathione Incorporated as Chain Transfer Agent in Thermosensitive Hydrogels for Controlled Release of Therapeutic Proteins

Victor Hugo Pérez-Luna
Illinois Institute of Technology

CONTENTS

4.1 INTRODUCTION

Hydrogels are an important class of materials highly suitable for diverse biomedical applications.[1–6] They have been commonly used as highly absorbent materials in hygiene products,[6] wound dressings,[7–19] scaffolds for tissue engineering applications,[20–43] barriers to prevent the formation of surgical adhesions,[11,12] as immunoprotective barriers,[29,44–48] components of biosensors,[49–55] materials for contact lenses,[1,4–6,17] encapsulation of cells and other biological materials,[19,52,56–69] and for drug delivery applications.[8,55,63,69–104] Their versatility in such wide range of biomedical applications stems from their unique properties and biocompatibility.[1,5,39,74,90,105–109]

Hydrogels consist of crosslinked polymer chains that have very high affinity for water. These two characteristics confer them with good mechanical properties and biocompatibility. The large water content would result in very small interfacial tensions in the aqueous environment of biological systems, which has been hypothesized to be one of the main reasons why they are highly biocompatible.[1] The crosslinked nature of these materials confers them with adequate mechanical properties for a number of biomedical applications and also allows adjusting the mechanical properties through control of the crosslink density of these materials for specific applications.[26,27,29,32,34,57,58,110–113] These two characteristics, their crosslinked nature, and high water content make hydrogels highly suitable materials for the controlled release of proteins and other biomolecules that are sensitive to changes in the aqueous environment. The large water content permits maintaining the three-dimensional structure (and hence biological activity) of encapsulated proteins. The crosslinked nature of hydrogels also presents a protective barrier against immune recognition and clearance of the encapsulated proteins. An additional advantage of a crosslinked barrier is that it can offer protection against degradation by proteases and allows for the concentration of proteins in a small volume for applications requiring localized drug delivery. Because the crosslink density of hydrogels can be adjusted easily, this permits tailoring mechanical properties, water content, and size exclusion capabilities for any specific requirement in a medical application.

4.2 HYDROGEL SYNTHESIS

Hydrogels can be synthesized with a variety of methods and components. This makes possible to design hydrogel systems with properties that can be adjusted according to prior knowledge of the components. Thus, the hydrogel precursors (monomers or macromers) and crosslinking agents can be selected according to the intended application. Usually, hydrogel components are selected to meet biocompatibility requirements,[39,90,105,107] mechanical and barrier properties,[11,29,44,45,110,114,115] degradability or chemical stability,[10,11,13,75,84,85,92,116–122] the ability to respond to environmental stimuli such as pH or temperature,[89,123–130] and whether they are intended to be polymerized *in situ* for minimally invasive applications.[38,71,104,108,131–138] Crosslinking in hydrogels is a very important property that can be accomplished by means of different mechanisms, and the hydrogel properties can be affected by the specific crosslinking method. Crosslinks created by means of hydrogen bonds can allow the formation of hydrogels exhibiting large elongation and mechanical toughness due to the reversible nature of these types of bonds.[139] Hydrogen bonds can also be combined with ionic interactions to form self-healing hydrogels.[113,139,140] Hydrophobic interactions as well as van der Waals interactions can be exploited to form hydrogel crosslinks. These latter approaches can sometimes be implemented by means of forming ABA triblock copolymers. Some examples in the literature involve cholesterol-functionalized carbonates with a central hydrophilic group that self-assemble into gels encapsulating drug-loaded polymeric micelles[67]; peptide end-capped poly ethylene glycols (PEGs) that assemble into gels with transition temperatures close to physiological temperature of 37°C[141]; fluoroalkyl-ended PEGs can also be made that assemble into gels at body temperature.[71,142,143] Ionic interactions can also form the crosslinks and, in combination with other types of intermolecular interactions such as hydrophilic interactions, can produce hydrogels with high toughness.[144] Thus, selecting the specific type of crosslinking interaction can oftentimes help design hydrogel with specific properties. Often, the crosslinks involve the formation of covalent bonds because it is relatively easy to incorporate bifunctional or multifunctional monomers in their synthesis. In a good number of cases the polymerization methods involve free radical polymerization. Although free radical polymerization provides a facile method for hydrogel synthesis, the covalent bonds will not break unless they incorporate a degradable moiety.[14,72,85,116–119,134,145–147] The degradation of the crosslinks is thus normally irreversible but it may allow gradual and controlled release of encapsulated molecules. A variety of water-soluble monomers, macromers, crosslinkers, and photoinitiators are available, permitting *in situ* formation of hydrogels under mild conditions of temperature and pH, which permits performing minimally invasive procedures involving implantation *in vivo* of hydrogel systems by polymerizing them *in situ*.[39,80,104,108,135,148]

The fact that hydrogels can be synthesized under mild conditions of temperature and pH makes them highly compatible with delicate biological molecules such as proteins. In fact, hydrogels even permit the encapsulation of living cells.[69] This makes hydrogels highly desirable for applications involving controlled release of proteins such as recombinant antibodies, which are widely used as therapeutic agents.[149–155] In addition to helping preserve the structure and function of these molecules within the aqueous environment of hydrogels, they also protect the encapsulated proteins against immune surveillance by cellular and humoral components of the immune system as well as protecting them against degradation by proteases (Figure 4.1). This allows for an optimal combination of proteins and drug delivery system that permits a more efficient and longer lasting therapeutic use of protein-based pharmaceuticals.

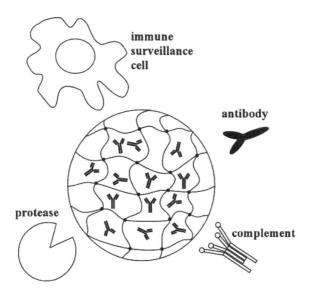

FIGURE 4.1 Biomolecules encapsulated within hydrogels maintain their structure and biological activity due to the high water content of the system. The crosslinked nature of the hydrogel prevents that encapsulated molecules diffuse away and become diluted; protects the encapsulated molecules from immune clearance by immune surveillance cells, antibodies, and complement factor molecules; and it also prevents degradation of the therapeutic biomolecule by proteases. All these factors help maximize the therapeutic effect of encapsulated biomolecules in these drug delivery systems.

4.3 THERMORESPONSIVE HYDROGELS

The properties of some polymeric and hydrogel materials can vary in response to changes in their environment. Many of these materials exhibit pronounced transition properties in response to pH, light, temperature, and other stimuli.[156,157] These are often referred to as "smart" or stimuli-responsive materials and can find use in many applications such as biosensing, as actuators, in bioseparations, chromatography, medical devices, minimally invasive surgery, and drug delivery. In the specific case of drug delivery, a particular type of smart materials consists of those exhibiting thermoresponsive behavior.[16,126,136,138,147,156–159] Materials that exhibit a transition in properties between room temperature and physiological temperature are of particular interest in medicine because they can be implemented in such a way that they are delivered into the body at room temperature and, when reaching the physiological temperature of 37°C, their properties can change significantly. This can offer advantages in medical applications that are not possible with other types of materials.

Among different stimuli-responsive polymers, poly(N-isopropylacrylamide) (PNIPAAm) is one of the most widely used thermoresponsive polymers. Because of its thermoresponsive properties, which allow switching its properties with temperature, it has been used in a wide variety of applications.[18,36,37,126,134,160–173] The chemical structure of this polymer is shown in Figure 4.2a and illustrates the origin of its thermoresponsive properties. The backbone of this polymer, as well as the pendant isopropyl group, are hydrophobic. In contrast, the amide group is hydrophilic and is capable of establishing hydrogen bonds with water molecules. Thus, in an aqueous environment, the state of this polymer is determined by competing hydrophilic and hydrophobic interactions of these groups. This hydrophilic/hydrophobic balance determines the state of the polymer. In an aqueous environment, such as that found in biological systems, when the hydrophilic interactions dominate, the polymer exists in a hydrated state. If the hydrophobic interactions dominate, the polymer chain collapses in order to minimize contact with water. These two factors determine the properties of

PNIPAAm in aqueous systems.[174] Since hydrogen bonds weaken with temperature, the state of the polymer can change from being hydrophilic to hydrophobic with increased temperature. As it turns out, for PNIPAAm, the change from the state where hydrophilic interaction dominates the state of the polymer to the state where hydrophobic interactions dominate occurs as a sharp transition at 32°C. At this temperature, PNIPAAm changes from being water soluble below this temperature, to being water insoluble above this temperature. This point is known as the lower critical solution temperature of the polymer or LCST.[172,175,176]

When PNIPAAm is crosslinked, it forms hydrogels that can take up large volumes of water below the transition temperature. In order to avoid confusion between solution properties, which are applicable to linear polymers, and swelling properties, which are applicable to crosslinked hydrogels, the term volume phase transition temperature (VPTT) is used when describing the thermal transition in crosslinked hydrogels.[172,177] As the temperature is increased, the polymer chains collapse and the hydrogel changes hydration state as it goes through the VPTT as shown in Figure 4.2b. This behavior of PNIPAAm hydrogels makes them very attractive for localized drug delivery applications.[130,178] As shown below, it is possible to make lightly crosslinked PNIPAAm hydrogels encapsulating proteins for localized drug delivery. Such light crosslinking is enough to entrap proteins but the hydrogel is highly deformable so that it can be extruded through a small gauge syringe needle. Upon reaching the body temperature, the lightly crosslinked hydrogel goes through the transition temperature, becomes dehydrated by expelling water, and acquires a more solid consistency. This results in a drug-loaded polymer system that "solidifies" at the site of injection, allowing for localized delivery of the encapsulated proteins. With the proper design of crosslinks, the polymer can slowly degrade over time and gradually release the encapsulated materials locally using these types of hydrogels.

Because PNIPAAm hydrogels require the addition of other components that can affect the properties of the system, it is important to discuss some of the effects that different process variables can have on the formed hydrogels. The amount of crosslink has an effect on the permeation characteristics and rigidity of the hydrogel. These are related to the crosslink density or molecular weight between crosslinks of the hydrogel. This is normally determined experimentally by measuring swelling ratio, which is defined as the fractional increase in the weight of the hydrogel due to water absorption.[180] The relationship between swelling ratios and crosslink density can be described, to a first approximation, by the Flory–Huggins equation:

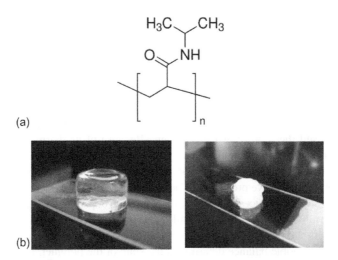

FIGURE 4.2   (a) Chemical structure of PNIPAAm. (b) PNIPAAm hydrogel below the LCST (left) and above the LCST (right). (Figure adapted with permission from Jiang et al.[179])

$$\ln\left(1-\phi_2\right)+\phi_2+\chi_{12}\phi_2^2+\frac{V_1}{\bar{v}M_c}\left(\phi_2^{1/3}-\frac{\phi_2}{2}\right)=0 \tag{4.1}$$

where ϕ_2 is the volume fraction of polymer in the hydrogel (estimated from swelling ratios), $\bar{v}$ is the specific volume of the polymer, χ_{12} is the polymer solvent interaction parameter, V_1 is the molar volume of the solvent, and M_c is the molecular weight between crosslinks.

Copolymerization of NIPAAm with other monomers or with the incorporation of crosslinkers can affect the LCST (or VPTT in the case of hydrogels) of the system.[174,181–183] In general, the addition of more polar or hydrophilic components tend to switch the transition temperatures to higher values, whereas more hydrophobic components lower the transition temperature.[181,183,184] The molecular weight of the linear polymer chains has an effect in the transition temperature only in the low molecular weight range,[185] and the effect could be due to the influence of the polarity of the end groups, which are dependent on the initiator used but such effects are only observed at low molecular weights.[184] The experimental observations being that the transition temperatures increase for very low molecular weights of PNIPAAm. This dependence of the transition temperatures on the polarity of copolymers and crosslinkers as well as molecular weights of the polymer chains can be useful to tailor the responsiveness of thermoresponsive drug delivery systems.

4.4 DRUG DELIVERY WITH THERMORESPONSIVE HYDROGELS

The capabilities to implement localized drug delivery using thermoresponsive hydrogels hold a great potential in many biomedical applications. Recently, this concept was explored towards developing drug delivery therapies for the treatment of macular degeneration.[130,178,179,186] In the wet form of macular degeneration, degeneration of the macula occurs when there is choroidal neovascularization. Thus, approaches at treating this condition consist in the injection of monoclonal antibodies (or Fab fragments) specific for vascular endothelial growth factor (VEGF), which would inhibit the interaction of VEGF with their receptors in endothelial cells, thus inhibiting neovascularization.[187] Current therapies consist in the intravitreal injection of the monoclonal antibody (or its Fab fragments) at high concentrations, which need to be repeated periodically.[187–189] For this particular application, the properties of thermoresponsive hydrogels are ideally suitable to improve the efficacy of monoclonal antibody-based treatments. The encapsulated antibodies are protected against immune recognition or degradation by proteases, and they remain concentrated within the hydrogel-based drug delivery system at the site where their effect is only needed. The latter can prevent the potentially undesirable systemic migration to other parts of the body. This improves the efficiency of the therapeutical agent, which would also be maintained for longer periods of time, and thus require less frequent administrations in the form of intravitreal injections. However, in order for thermoresponsive hydrogels to be a feasible solution for localized drug delivery in the treatment of macular degeneration, they also need to meet stringent conditions for biocompatibility. Some of the requirements are the following: (i) hydrogel formation needs to occur under mild conditions of temperature and pH that help preserve the structure and function of the encapsulated antibody; (ii) the hydrogel system needs to be biocompatible (nontoxic and not conducing to elicit and undesirable inflammatory response); (iii) the crosslink density must be such that it can entrap antibodies within the hydrogel while at the same time be deformable enough that it can be injected with a small gauge needle; (iv) the hydrogel needs to degrade in order to release the encapsulated molecules; (v) the released molecules need to show therapeutic activity; and (vi) the degradation products must be biocompatible and need to be cleared off once the function of the drug delivery system has been accomplished. Many of these requirements can be accomplished using fundamental knowledge of the physical chemistry of polymers. The last requirement, that the degraded hydrogel be cleared off the body is more difficult to accomplish, but it can be addressed with the use of chain transfer agents used during the polymerization process.

4.5 ENCAPSULATION AND DRUG RELEASE FROM PNIPAAM-BASED THERMORESPONSIVE HYDROGELS

Encapsulation of proteins within crosslinked PNIPAAm hydrogels can be accomplished under mild conditions of pH and temperature. Experimental details can be found elsewhere[130] and are summarized in Figure 4.3, which shows the synthesis procedure to make hydrogels encapsulating bovine serum albumin (BSA) as proof of concept demonstration. This polymerization involves water-soluble components, which are compatible with preserving the structure and biological activity of proteins. The monomer used was N-isopropylacrylamide, the crosslinker was based on poly(ethylene glycol) diacrylate (PEG-DA) (MW 575), ammonium persulfate as generator of free radicals, and N,N,N',N'-tetramethylethylenediamine (TEMED) as free radical stabilizer. The advantage of this system is that it permits polymerization to occur even at low temperatures (4°C in this case).

Although the transition temperature of PNIPAAm is 32°C, the copolymerization with other monomers or crosslinkers can shift the transition. Addition of the hydrophilic crosslinker PEG-DA increases the VPTT of hydrogels in a concentration-dependent manner. The VPPT of PNIPAAm hydrogels crosslinked with PEG-DA are ~32°C, 33.5°C, 34.5°C, 36°C, and 36.5°C for PEG-DA concentrations of 0, 4, 8, 12, and 16 mM respectively.[130] It is important to notice that the VPTT needs to be below physiological temperature for any relevant biomedical application, otherwise the injected hydrogel would not solidify after implantation in the body. Thus, the more suitable formulations were found to consist of concentrations of PEG-DA equal to 4, 8, and 12 mM.[130] As it turns out, these hydrogels were also easily deformable and could be extruded through a small gauge syringe needle. In fact, the hydrogel made with 8 mM PEG-DA could be injected through a 30-gauge needle.[186]

A potential problem with hydrogels based on PNIPAAm is the toxicity of the monomer, N-isopropylacrylamide. Since polymerization reactions do not occur to 100% completion, it is necessary to remove unreacted monomers through extraction procedures. Some of the encapsulated protein could also be lost during these extraction steps. Our work showed that these hydrogel systems retain between 84% and 90% of the encapsulated protein even after five extractions (in each extraction step, 5 mL of hydrogel was extracted with 40 mL of phosphate buffer at room

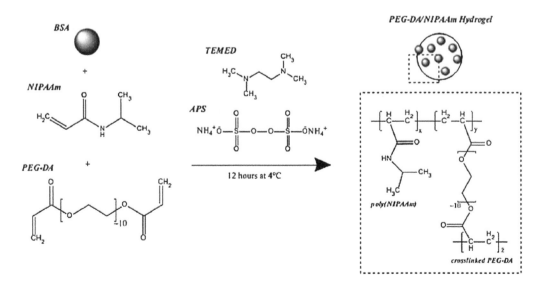

FIGURE 4.3 Formation of crosslinked PNIPAAm hydrogels encapsulating BSA. (Reproduced with permission from Drapala et al.[130])

temperature).[130] After this, it is important to test that the encapsulated protein can be released from the hydrogels. This could appear as a conundrum since the mesh structure of the hydrogel has to be small enough to retain the protein during the washing steps but large enough to allow diffusion out of the hydrogel during drug delivery. Release profiles of BSA above and below the VPTT from PEG-DA crosslinked PNIPAAm hydrogels showed similar behavior above and below the VPTT for all concentrations of crosslinker. Basically, there was a fast initial release of the encapsulated protein that proceeded at similar rates at 23°C (below VTT) and 37°C (above VPTT), indicating that the diffusion of encapsulated protein through the hydrogel was similar above and below the VPTT.[130] As time passed, the release of BSA was greater at 37°C than at 23°C. This could have been due to the higher concentration of encapsulated protein in the shrunk hydrogels (due to collapse of polymer chains above the VPTT) and possibly because, during hydrogel collapse, the proteins may have been redistributed within the hydrogel. At both temperatures, protein release reached a plateau after a couple of days. The plateau occurred at a larger fraction of released protein at 37°C than at 23°C.[130] These results indicated that there is always a fraction of protein that remains irreversibly entrapped within the hydrogel that cannot be released, and this fraction is larger below the VPTT and it appears to be independent of the degree of crosslinking of the hydrogels (within the range of PEG-DA concentrations tested[130]). The larger release from PNIPAAm hydrogels above the VPTT can also be explained in terms of the shrinkage that the hydrogel experiences above the VPTT. This translates in a larger concentration of proteins in the collapsed state, hence, a larger concentration gradient for diffusion. Additionally, during the shrinking process, convection effects are generated as the hydrogel expels water from its interior, which can promote transport of encapsulated proteins out of the hydrogel.[130]

The fact that the rates and amounts of protein released from the hydrogels are very much independent of the amount of crosslinker can be rationalized by examining the swelling ratios of hydrogels. By determining the equilibrium swelling ratios of BSA containing PNIPAAm hydrogels crosslinked with varying concentrations of PEG-DA it is possible to determine their degree of crosslinking using Flory–Huggins equation (equation 4.1). Using values for the specific volume of the polymer of $0.896\,\text{cm}^3/\text{g}$[190]; polymer–solvent interaction parameter is equal to 0.485 at 25°C,[191] and assuming the molar volume of the solvent to correspond to that of water, $18\,\text{cm}^3/\text{mol}$ the experimentally obtained values for swelling ratios[130] yielded molecular weight between crosslinks of 8.4×10^5, 5.0×10^5, and 2.6×10^5 g/mol, for PEG-DA concentrations of 8, 12, and 16 mM respectively. With the obtained values, the radii of gyration of PNIPAAm chains was estimated using published data for PNIPAAm,[190,192,193] assuming that the radii of gyration scaled linearly with the square root of the molecular weight of the polymer.[180] With these assumptions, the radii of gyration of PNIPAAm hydrogels made with 8, 12, and 16 mM PEG-DA were calculated as 31, 24, and 17 nm below the VPTT.[130] These dimensions are larger than the 8 nm size of BSA, which has a triangular prism shape with dimensions of $8 \times 8 \times 8 \times 3$ nm.[194,195] At these values, the sizes of the molecular mesh of hydrogels were found to have only a minor effect on the diffusion coefficients of BSA within the hydrogels as calculated[130] using models of diffusion based on the free-volume approach of Lusting and Peppas.[85,196] This explains why diffusion of BSA from these hydrogels did not differ significantly with the varying amounts of PEG-DA crosslinker employed. The fact that a significant portion of encapsulated BSA did not get released from the hydrogels could be because the size distribution of the molecular mesh of the hydrogels results in a fraction of the hydrogel with mesh sizes smaller than the BSA molecule.

What is significant about the results just described is that, at the crosslink densities used in these studies, the hydrogels can still be injected through a small diameter (gauge 30) syringe needle, and yet, the dimensions of the molecular mesh of the hydrogels compare well with the dimensions of encapsulated proteins. In fact, considering the collapse of hydrogel chains above the VPTT, the difference in swelling ratios above and below the VPTT permit to estimate the molecular mesh size in the collapsed states to be 15, 12, and 9 nm (assuming mesh size decreases in proportion to the cubic root of hydrogel volumes).[130] These dimensions are close to the size of antibody molecules.

As it turned out encapsulated BSA is readily released but the immunoglobulin (IgG) molecules remain for the most part trapped within these hydrogels.[130] Only a small burst release is initially observed for IgG without substantial amounts released subsequently. These results are consistent with the estimation of the molecular dimensions of the hydrogel mesh and the larger size of IgG (MW of 149 kDa) compared to BSA (66 kDa).

The results presented so far indicate the feasibility to make thermoresponsive and injectable hydrogels that can encapsulate therapeutic proteins (recombinant antibodies) for the localized treatment of macular degeneration. Other requirements that need to be met are the release of encapsulated molecules, the degradation and/or clearance of the hydrogel system from the body, and biocompatibility. Degradation of the hydrogel is necessary in order to release the encapsulated molecules. Since PNIPAAm is polymerized through free radical polymerization, it does not have groups in its backbone that can degrade under physiological conditions. However, it is possible to synthesize crosslinkers that degrade by hydrolysis. In this manner, as the crosslinks degrade, the hydrogel will release the encapsulated molecules. One approach at making degradable crosslinkers involves the synthesis of a central PEG moiety that is linked to poly(L-lactic acid) (PLLA) blocks on each side, which are further capped with diacrylate groups (Acry-PLLA-b-PEG-b-PLLA-Acry).[95,197] When Acry-PLLA-b-PEG-b-PLLA-Acry molecules are incorporated in the hydrogel, the PLLA blocks slowly degrade by hydrolysis and the crosslinks get broken, which allows release of encapsulated molecules. However, the PNIPAAm backbone left behind is not degraded, presenting a problem for its clearance from the body once the drug delivery system has accomplished its function. Without mechanisms to remove these PNIPAAm chains from the body, their bioaccumulation would present a potential deterrent to the use of PNIPAAm-based hydrogels in drug delivery. Clearance of PNIPAAm chains, even if they are linear polymers is problematic because, under physiological conditions, they would be insoluble in the aqueous environment of biological systems. However, it has been shown that PNIPAAm chains smaller than 32 kDa can be eliminated through renal clearance in rats.[182] Therefore, a feasible approach is to limit the size of the linear PNIPAAm segments in the hydrogel.

4.6 GLUTATHIONE AS A CHAIN TRANSFER AGENT TO LIMIT THE MOLECULAR SIZE OF PNIPAAM CHAINS

The size of the linear segments of PNIPAAm can be controlled through the addition of a chain transfer agent.[180] Being that thiols are very efficient chain transfer agents, these can be added to the polymerizing mixture in order to limit chain growth. The molecule selected to limit chain growth was glutathione because it is a naturally occurring antioxidant, and it is a tripeptide made up of three amino acids: cysteine, glycine, and glutamate.[198] This makes it highly biocompatible since it is naturally occurring in the body at millimolar concentrations.[199] Since it has a thiol group from the cysteine residue it is a very efficient chain transfer agent that can limit chain growth. Furthermore in the chain transfer process during polymerization, the newly formed chains will contain the tripeptide as end groups. Thus, limitation of chain growth during polymerization, as well as the transfer of the polar tripeptide group of glutathione to the growing chains during polymerization, would improve the solubility of linear PNIPAAm chains once the crosslinks in the polymer are degraded. The structure of glutathione and the potential mechanism of chain transfer during polymerization are shown in Figure 4.4.

Figure 4.5 shows the concept of forming hydrogels with encapsulated IgG molecules using hydrolytically degradable crosslinkers based on Acry-PLLA-b-PEG-b-PLLA-Acry and glutathione as a chain transfer agent that limits chain growth. The precursors for the formation of these hydrogels are all water soluble. Thus, they permit the incorporation of biomolecules in an aqueous environment that helps preserve protein structure and function. Furthermore, they can be polymerized at low temperatures (e.g. 4°C) using ammonium persulfate as generator of free radicals and TEMED as a free radical stabilizer.[178]

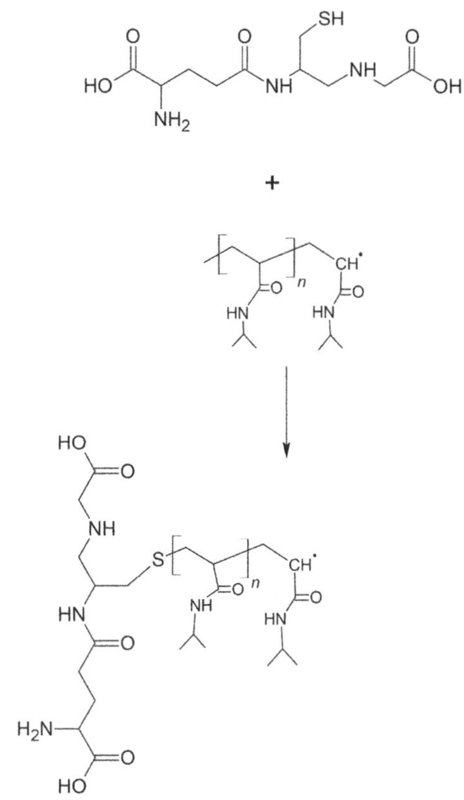

FIGURE 4.4 Chemical structure of glutathione and reaction mechanism occurring during chain transfer to monomer. Chain transfer results in newly initiated polymer chains that contain the glutathione tripeptide in one end.

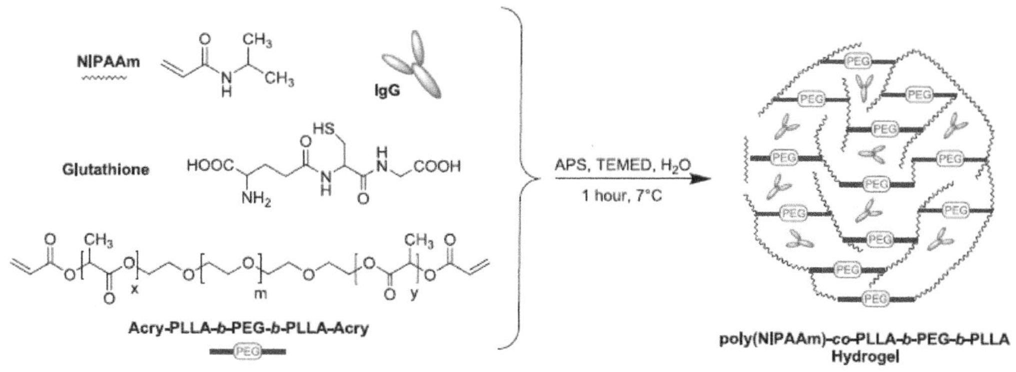

FIGURE 4.5 Process for the encapsulation of IgG molecules within thermoresponsive hydrogels containing a hydrolytically degradable crosslinker and glutathione as chain transfer agents. (Reproduced with permission from Drapala et al.[178])

The Acry-PLLA-b-PEG-b-PLLA-Acry used here was based on a PEG molecule with $\bar{M}_n = 3,350$ Da. This potentially can result in larger mesh size than with the hydrogels discussed previously, which were made with PEG of a molecular weight of 575 Da. This could result in a significant loss of encapsulated molecules during the extraction steps needed for the removal of unreacted monomers. As expected, the percentage loss of IgG from hydrogels prepared with

Acry-PLLA-b-PEG-b-PLLA-DA and varying amounts of glutathione were larger than when using the smaller PEG-DA (MW of 575 Da). However, the amount of IgG retained was still bigger than 70%, which still makes possible to use these hydrogels for drug delivery even if the encapsulation efficiency is slightly decreased.[178] The amount of protein lost during extraction was larger for the higher concentrations of glutathione, which can be explained by lower crosslink densities that result when chain transfer occurs with the Acry-PLLA-b-PEG-b-PLLA-Acry crosslinker.

Ensuring lack of toxicity is important in drug delivery applications involving biomaterials such as hydrogels. As mentioned above, even though the PNIPAAm polymer is biocompatible, there is always the concern about the cytotoxicity of unreacted monomers that may remain within the polymerized hydrogel. This is the reason why it was necessary to resort to extraction steps using buffer solutions. Although after five extraction steps there is still a large fraction (>70%) of remaining encapsulated protein, it is important to determine that these number of extraction steps is sufficient to decrease the cytotoxicity of the system to nondetectable levels. In order to determine cell viability, 3T3 fibroblast cells were exposed to solutions from each of the washing steps. After 2 days of exposure, cell viability was determined using a colorimetric method, which is based on the reduction of the compound (3-[4,5,dimethylthiazol-2-yl]-5-[3-carboxymethoxy-phenyl]-2-[4-sulfophenyl]-2H-tetrazolium, inner salt) (MTS) by nicotinamide adenine dinucleotide (phosphate) or NAD(P)H dependent dehydrogenase enzymes in metabolically active cells.[178] Such assay is more commonly referred to as the MTS assay. Although the first extraction solution showed significant cytotoxicity ($p < 0.05$, which was expected because of the presence of unreacted monomers and initiators), there were no significant differences after subsequent extraction steps. That is, two extraction steps decreased cytotoxicity significantly. To be safe, the number of extractions performed was always five in order to ensure complete absence of cytotoxicity.[178]

Release of encapsulated IgG molecules from these hydrogels are shown in Figure 4.6. In all cases there was a burst release of IgG molecules. This burst release amounted to more than 20% of the initially encapsulated protein, and it reached almost 50% for the largest glutathione concentration. The dependence of burst release amount with glutathione concentration can be interpreted in terms of the lower crosslink density for larger amounts of glutathione (chain transfer agent), which translates into a more open hydrogel mesh. During incubation of hydrogels above their VPPT, the chain collapse and dehydration expels water, which helps release entrapped molecules by convection. This convection enhanced release would be more significant for the more open mesh structures of hydrogels prepared with larger amounts of glutathione or chain transfer agent. After the burst effect there is a more gradual release of encapsulated molecules. This release shows differences in behavior for hydrogels prepared with or without glutathione. Without glutathione the release of encapsulated IgG reaches a plateau at about 70% with the remaining 30% remaining within the hydrogel even

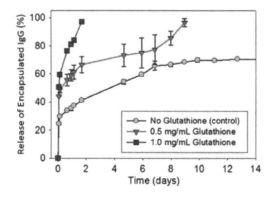

FIGURE 4.6   Release of encapsulated IgG molecules at 37°C from hydrogels prepared with different amounts of glutathione. (Reproduced with permission from Drapala et al.[178])

after 2 weeks. In contrast, release from hydrogels prepared with 0.5 and 1.0 mg/mL of glutathione released 100% of the encapsulated molecules after 9 and 2 days respectively. Furthermore, the release rate appeared to increase before 100% release rate was reached. This indicates that the addition of glutathione affects the degradation rate of hydrogels even when the crosslinker concentration used to make these systems was kept the same for all hydrogels.

There were also differences in the state of hydrogels after degradation. In the hydrogels prepared without glutathione, the hydrogels appeared to continue existing in the collapsed, dehydrated state and did not disintegrate after 3 weeks (release data is shown only up to 2 weeks). It is likely that the incomplete release observed in hydrogels prepared without glutathione was due to the hydrophobic nature of longer PNIPAAm chains in the hydrogel. Even though the Acry-PLLA-b-PEG-b-PLLA-Acry crosslinkers were degraded at that point, the encapsulated protein was still entrapped because, above the VPTT, the longer PNIPAAm chains created physical crosslinks due to hydrophobic interactions. In fact, when the hydrogels were left to degrade above the VPPT for several weeks, they appeared to remain intact. However, they disintegrated immediately when the temperature was lowered below the VPPT, which lends support to the hypothesis that longer PNIPAAm chains can establish physical crosslinks within the hydrogel by means of hydrophobic interactions.[178] Such crosslinks are not possible below the VPTT because the polymer chains solubilize, resulting in the loss of integrity of the hydrogels. The hydrogels that incorporated glutathione, in contrast, disintegrated slowly over time even though the temperature was above the VPPT. These observations indicate the following: (i) the incorporation of glutathione affects the amount of protein molecules that are released in the "burst" process; (ii) the release rate observed after the burst release is affected by the incorporation of glutathione; (iii) glutathione makes possible the complete release of encapsulated proteins; (iv) the time at which 100% release is obtained can be controlled by the incorporation of glutathione within the hydrogel; and (v) glutathione makes possible the complete disintegration of PNIPAAm hydrogels even above the VPTT.

The bottom part of Figure 4.7 shows schematic representations and photographs of a nondegraded hydrogel in the hydrated, swollen state (left); nondegraded hydrogel in the collapsed state (center); and partially degraded hydrogel above the VPTT (right). It is clear how the incorporation of glutathione permits disintegration of the hydrogel and solubilization of the degraded products above the VPTT as seen in the slow disintegration of the partially degraded hydrogel.

As shown, incorporation of glutathione in the synthesis of PNIPAAm-based thermoresponsive hydrogels has an effect in the degradability and drug release profiles from these materials. More importantly, glutathione permits the complete disintegration, above the VPTT, of the PNIPAAm based hydrogels studied here. This is important for drug delivery applications, where it is necessary that the degradation products get removed from the site of implantation, which is not possible in the absence of glutathione, where the resulting hydrogel remains in place due to nonphysical crosslinks formed by hydrophobic interactions above the VPTT. Since chain transfer agents also decrease the molecular weight of polymers, it should be possible to tailor their concentration in hydrogel formulations so that PNIPAAm chains remaining after degradation of crosslinks can be removed by the renal route. The latter is based on the observation that PNIPAAm chains smaller than 32 kDa can be removed by renal clearance in rats.[182]

The burst release observed in all hydrogels, which was increased by the addition of glutathione (Figure 4.6), can be eliminated by tethering the IgG molecules to the hydrogel by means of a PEG-based linker (Figure 4.7). Here a heterobifunctional PEG with an acrylate group on one end and a succinimidyl valeric acid (SVA) group on the other are used to tether the antibodies to the hydrogel. The SVA group of Acry-PEG-SVA reacts with the amine groups on the antibody while the acrylate group will tether the antibodies to the hydrogel during polymerization. In this manner, the antibody should not release immediately because the Acry-PEG-SVA tethers. Figure 4.8 shows the release profiles of tethered and nontethered IgG molecules from PNIPAAm-based thermoresponsive polymers that incorporate glutathione in their synthesis. Clearly, PEGylation of IgG with Acry-PEG-SVA can decrease significantly, or even eliminate almost completely, the burst release.

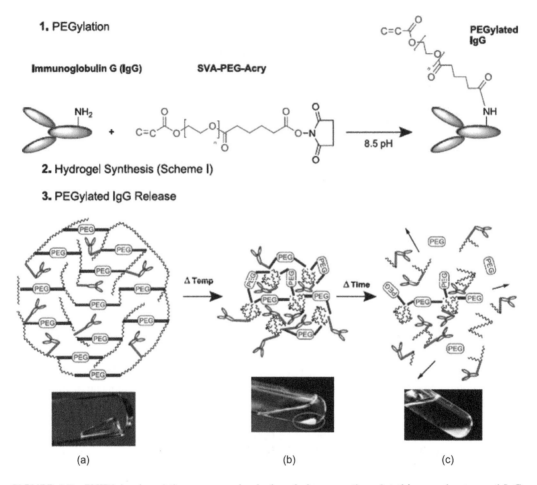

FIGURE 4.7 PNIPAAm-based thermoresponsive hydrogels incorporating glutathione and entrapped IgG molecules. (a) Postsynthesis hydrogel in the swollen state below the VPTT; (b) hydrogel in the hydrophobic, collapsed state at 37°C; and (c) hydrogel in the collapsed state at 37°C after partial degradation. (Reproduced with permission from Drapala et al.[178])

The release profiles observed when IgG molecules are tethered to the hydrogels are different in the sense that they appear to exhibit a delayed burst release, where there is very little release of molecules for a period of several days, after which there is a pronounced increase in the rate of release until 100% of the molecules are released. The point where the increased rate of release occurs corresponds to the point where disintegration of the hydrogel begins to become appreciable. The point where 100% of the IgG molecules have been released corresponds to the complete disintegration of the hydrogel. Such release behavior can be explained because the poly(lactic acid) moieties of the hydrogel crosslinks have a faster degradation than the ester groups of the Acry-PEG-SVA tether. Thus, release of the IgG molecules cannot occur until there is complete degradation of the hydrogel.

The lower part of Figure 4.7 shows the physical aspect of hydrogels at different stages. On the left side, the swollen, as prepared, nondegraded hydrogel is indicated. In the central part there is the nondegraded, collapsed hydrogel. Finally, the right side shows the hydrogel, above the VPTT in the stage where it is almost degraded. It can be seen that in the state of disintegration, the hydrogel products begin to dissolve. This is in contrast to hydrogels prepared without glutathione, which do not seem to disintegrate above the VPTT and appear identical to nondegraded hydrogels in the collapsed state (not shown).

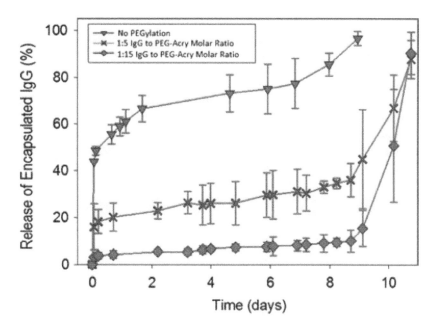

FIGURE 4.8 Release of IgG molecules tethered to hydrogels by means of an Acry-PEG-SVA linker. (Reproduced with permission from Drapala et al.[178])

The biomolecules released from hydrogels must show biological activity in order for the drug delivery system to be effective. Although glutathione could potentially reduce disulfide bridges, which could impact the bioactivity of proteins, it is expected that extraction procedures would also eliminate unreacted glutathione molecules. Thus, addition of glutathione does not require additional purification steps other than those already implemented in these systems. In order to test the bioactivity of encapsulated molecules, hydrogels consisting of PEGylated Avastin® and Lucentis® recombinant antibodies (1:5 molar ratio of protein to Acry-PEG-SVA) were encapsulated at concentrations of 0.1 mg/mL within thermoresponsive hydrogels prepared with the following composition: 350 mM N-isopropylacrylammide, 3 mM Acry-PLLA-b-PEG-b-PLLA-Acry crosslinker, 0.5 mg/mL gluthathione, 13 mM ammonium persulfate, and 168 mM TEMED. These compounds were dissolved in phosphate buffer at a pH of 7.4 and polymerized at 7°C for 1 h. As before, the hydrogels were subjected to five extraction steps in order to eliminate unreacted molecules.

In order to test for the potential cytotoxicity of the hydrogel degradation products, they were allowed to degrade completely. Hydrogel disintegration took place in 8–9 days at 37°C. Cytotoxicity was evaluated using 3T3 fibroblasts, to which hydrogel degradation products were added. The cytotoxicity of hydrogel degradation products was compared to that of phosphate buffer, Avastin® and Lucentis® solutions, as well as released non-PEGylated and PEGylated Avastin® and Lucentis® molecules from these hydrogels. There were no statistically significant differences ($p > 0.05$), which indicates that degradation products of these systems are also cytocompatible.[178]

Finally, the biological activity of Avastin® and Lucentis® molecules released from hydrogels prepared with glutathione must be tested for their biological activity. To this effect, human umbilical vein endothelial cells (HUVECs) were cultured on 96-well plates using endothelial growth medium (EGM) on fibronectin-coated multiwell plates. They were harvested and seeded below confluency (at 5,000 cells/well in 200 µL EGM with 0.5% v/v fetal bovine serum) for 24 h before adding test solutions. After 2 days of proliferation, they were tested for proliferation using a BrdU enzyme-linked immunosorbent assay (ELISA). The testing solutions consisted of phosphate buffer (negative control), and all the other solutions also contained VEGF at 10 ng/mL (positive control).

The released Avastin® and Lucentis® molecules (PEGylated and non-PEGylated were added together with VEGF in order to test their capability to inhibit the effect of VEGF. The results indicated the inhibition of VEGF activity by stock solutions of Avastin® and Lucentis® as well as PEGylated and non-PEGylated Avastin® and Lucentis® released from hydrogels.[178] Both stock solutions of Avastin® and Lucentis® showed statistically significant inhibition of VEGF-stimulated HUVECs growth ($p < 0.001$) as expected. Lucentis® was more effective at preventing HUVEC growth than Avastin® as reported before.[200] The hydrogel degradation products did not have an effect in inhibiting VEGF-stimulated cell growth and the differences were not statistically significant ($p > 0.05$).[178] Avastin® and Lucentis® released from hydrogels had an inhibitory effect in VEGF-stimulated cell growth whether they were PEGylated molecules or not. These results indicate that the biological activity of encapsulated molecules is maintained in the hydrogels studied and that the incorporation of glutathione did not have a deleterious effect in the bioactivity of encapsulated Avastin® and Lucentis®.

4.7 CONCLUSIONS

Thermoresponsive hydrogels based on N-isopropylacrylamide hold high potential for localized drug delivery applications. The transition temperature of PNIPAAm at 32°C makes it ideal for biomedical applications since this is between room temperature and body temperatures. As shown, it is possible to make lightly crosslinked hydrogels of PNIPAAm such that their mechanical properties at the crosslink densities explored permit them to be extruded through small gauge needles. This allows for the injection of thermoresponsive hydrogels that become more solid once they reach the physiological temperature of 37°C, which makes these systems ideal for localized drug delivery applications. Furthermore, at such low crosslink densities the hydrogel mesh size is still adequate to encapsulate most proteins, including recombinant antibodies. This makes them ideal for a large number of applications requiring the localized delivery of recombinant biomolecules. Potential deterrents for the application of these hydrogel systems are the toxicity of unreacted monomers, which can be addressed through the proper extraction procedures that allow removing potentially toxic components. Another potential problem, and probably the biggest problem for many applications involving thermoresponsive hydrogels made from PNIPAAm, is the bioaccumulation of this polymer once the hydrogel has degraded and released its therapeutic molecules. Here it was shown that the addition of chain transfer agents during polymerization can help address this problem. Since it has been shown elsewhere that PNIPAAm chains smaller than 32 kDa can be removed through glomerular filtration in rats,[182] it would be possible to limit the size of PNIPAAm chains by means of chain transfer agents. Glutathione is an effective chain transfer agent due to its thiol group. In contrast to some thiol compounds, glutathione does not present a toxicity problem since it is a natural antioxidant present in the body at millimolar concentrations. Not only glutathione permits to reduce the molecular weight of polymers but, as shown, it can help solubilize the degraded products of PNIPAAm-based hydrogels. This permits complete hydrogel disintegration and release of encapsulated molecules at body temperatures. In contrast, hydrogels that were prepared in the absence of glutathione appeared to remain intact and did not release the encapsulated molecules completely. This was probably due to the formation of physical crosslinks by longer PNIPAAm chains in the collapsed/hydrophobic state. Glutathione may contribute to the clearance of PNIPAAm chains not only by limiting the molecular size of the linear portions of polymer chains but also because it transfers the tripeptide molecule to polymer chains that get initiated during chain transfer. This, in addition to the smaller molecular dimensions, makes possible for the polymer chains to solubilize after the crosslinks in the hydrogel have degraded completely. Thus, the use of chain transfer agents such as glutathione may help increase the applications of PNIPAAm-based polymer systems in drug delivery. It is possible that other naturally occurring molecules that can act as chain transfer agents (e.g. cysteine) could be explored in order to improve the biocompatibility of PNIPAAm-based materials.

REFERENCES

1. Hoffman, A. S., Hydrogels for biomedical applications. *Advanced Drug Delivery Reviews* 2002, 54, 3–12.
2. Peppas, N. A.; Hilt, J. Z.; Khademhosseini, A.; Langer, R., Hydrogels in biology and medicine: From molecular principles to bionanotechnology. *Advanced Materials* 2006, 18(11), 1345–1360.
3. Maitra, J.; Shukla, V. K., Cross-linking in hydrogels: A review. *American Journal of Polymer Science* 2014, 4 (2), 25–31.
4. Ottenbrite, R. M.; Park, K.; Okano, T.; Peppas, N. A., *Biomedical Applications of Hydrogels Handbook*, 2010th ed. Springer: New York, 2010, p.432.
5. Ratner, B. D.; Hoffman, A. S., Synthetic hydrogels for biomedical applications. *ACS Symposium Series* 1976, 31, 1–36.
6. Ahmed, M.E., Hydrogel: Preparation, characterization, and applications: A review. *Journal of Advanced Research* 2015, 6 (2), 105–121.
7. Kim, G. H.; Kang, Y. M.; Kang, K. N.; Kim, D. Y.; Kim, H. J.; Min, B. H.; Kim, J. H.; Kim, M. S., Wound dressings for wound healing and drug delivery. *Tissue Engineering and Regenerative Medicine* 2011, 8 (1), 1–7.
8. Jain, E.; Sheth, S.; Dunn, A.; Zustiak, S. P.; Sell, S. A., Sustained release of multicomponent platelet-rich plasma proteins from hydrolytically degradable PEG hydrogels. *Journal of Biomedical Materials Research* 2017, 105 (12), 3304–3314.
9. Moura, L. I. F.; Dias, A. M. A.; Carvalho, E.; de Sousa, H. C., Recent advances on the development of wound dressings for diabetic foot ulcer treatment – A review. *Acta Biomaterialia* 2013, 9 (7), 7093–7114.
10. West, J. L.; Hubbell, J. A., Proteolytically degradable hydrogels. *23rd Proceedings of the International Symposium on Controlled Release of Bioactive Materials*, Kyoto, 1996, 224–225.
11. Sawhney, A. S.; Pathak, C. P.; van Rensburg, J. J.; Dunn, R. C.; Hubbell, J. A., Optimization of photo-polymerized bioerodible hydrogel properties for adhesion prevention. *Journal of Biomedical Materials Research* 1994, 28 (7), 831–838.
12. Halstenberg, S.; Panitch, A.; Rizzi, S.; Hall, H.; Hubbell Jeffrey, A., Biologically engineered protein-graft-poly(ethylene glycol) hydrogels: A cell adhesive and plasmin-degradable biosynthetic material for tissue repair. *Biomacromolecules* 2002, 3 (4), 710–723.
13. Hubbell, J. A.; Pathak, C. P.; Sawhney, A. S., In vivo photopolymerization of PEG-based biodegradable hydrogels for the control of wound healing. *Polymer Preprints* 1993, 34 (1), 846–847.
14. West, J. L.; Hubbell, J. A., Polymeric biomaterials with degradation sites for proteases involved in cell migration. *Macromolecules* 1999, 32 (1), 241–244.
15. Liu, Q.; Huang, Y.; Lan, Y.; Zuo, Q.; Li, C.; Zhang, Y.; Guo, R.; Xue, W., Acceleration of skin regeneration in full-thickness burns by incorporation of bFGF-loaded alginate microspheres into a CMCS-PVA hydrogel. *Journal of Tissue Engineering and Regenerative Medicine* 2017, 11 (5), 1562–1573.
16. Mostafalu, P.; Kiaee, G.; Giatsidis, G.; Khalilpour, A.; Nabavinia, M.; Dokmeci, M. R.; Sonkusale, S.; Orgill, D. P.; Tamayol, A.; Khademhosseini, A., A textile dressing for temporal and dosage controlled drug delivery. *Advanced Functional Materials* 2017, 27 (41), 1702399.
17. Holland, S.; Morck, D.; Schultz, C., Treatment of corneal defects with delayed re-epithelization with a medical device/drug delivery system for epidermal growth factor. *Clinical and Experimental Ophthalmology* 2012, 40 (7), 662–668.
18. Banerjee, I.; Mishra, D.; Das, T.; Maiti, T. K., Wound pH-responsive sustained release of therapeutics from a poly(NIPAAm-co-AAc) hydrogel. *Journal of Biomaterials Science, Polymer Edition* 2012, 23, 111–132.
19. Bean, J. E.; Alves, D. R.; Laabei, M.; Esteban, P. P.; Thet, N. T.; Enright, M. C.; Jenkins, A. T. A., Triggered release of bacteriophage K from agarose/hyaluronan hydrogel matrixes by Staphylococcus aureus virulence factors. *Chemistry of Materials* 2014, 26, 7201–7208.
20. Betre, H.; Setton, L. A.; Meyer, D. E.; Chilkoti, A., Characterization of a genetically engineered elastin-like polypeptide for cartilaginous tissue repair. *Biomacromolecules* 2002, 3, (5), 910–916.
21. Banerjee, A.; Arhaa, M.; Choudhary, S.; Ashton, R. S.; Bhatia, S. R.; Schaffer, D. V.; Kane, R. S., The influence of hydrogel modulus on the proliferation and differentiation of encapsulated neural stem cells. *Biomaterials* 2009, 30 (27), 4695–4699.
22. Mahoney, M. J.; Anseth, K. S., Three-dimensional growth and function of neural tissue in degradable polyethylene glycol hydrogels. *Biomaterials* 2006, 27 (10), 2265–2274.
23. Masters, K. S.; Shah, D. N.; Leinwand, L. A.; Anseth, K. S., Crosslinked hyaluronan scaffolds as a biologically active carrier for valvular interstitial cells. *Biomaterials* 2005, 26 (15), 2517–2525.

24. Masters, K. S.; Shah, D. N.; Walker, G.; Leinwand, L. A.; Anseth, K. S., Designing scaffolds for valvular interstitial cells: Cell adhesion and function on naturally derived materials. *Journal of Biomedical Materials Research, Part A* 2004, 71A (1), 172–180.

25. Rice, M. A.; Anseth, K. S., Encapsulating chondrocytes in copolymer gels: Bimodal degradation kinetics influence cell phenotype and extracellular matrix development. *Journal of Biomedical Materials Research, Part A* 2004, 70A (4), 560–568.

26. Bryant, S. J.; Anseth, K. S.; Lee, D. A.; Bader, D. L., Crosslinking density influences the morphology of chondrocytes photoencapsulated in PEG hydrogels during the application of compressive strain. *Journal of Orthopaedic Research* 2004, 22 (5), 1143–1149.

27. Bryant, S. J.; Bender, R. J.; Durand, K. L.; Anseth, K. S., Encapsulating chondrocytes in degrading PEG hydrogels with high modulus: Engineering gel structural changes to facilitate cartilaginous tissue production. *Biotechnology and Bioengineering* 2004, 86 (7), 747–755.

28. Bryant, S. J.; Anseth, K. S., Hydrogel properties influence ECM production by chondrocytes photoencapsulated in poly(ethylene glycol) hydrogels. *Journal of Biomedical Materials Research* 2002, 59 (1), 63–72.

29. Bryant, S. J.; Nuttelman, C. R.; Anseth, K. S., The effects of crosslinking density on cartilage formation in photocrosslinkable hydrogels. *Biomedical Sciences Instrumentation* 1999, 35, 309–314.

30. Mahoney Melissa, J.; Anseth Kristi, S., Three-dimensional growth and function of neural tissue in degradable polyethylene glycol hydrogels. *Biomaterials* 2006, 27 (10), 2265–2274.

31. Li, H.; Wijekoon, A.; Leipzig, N. D., 3D differentiation of neural stem cells in macroporous photopolymerizable hydrogel scaffolds. *PLoS One* 2012, 7 (11), e48824.

32. Zhu, J.; Marchant, R. E., Design properties of hydrogel tissue-engineering scaffolds. *Expert Review of Medical Devices* 2011, 8 (5), 607–626.

33. Rice Mark, A.; Anseth Kristi, S., Encapsulating chondrocytes in copolymer gels: Bimodal degradation kinetics influence cell phenotype and extracellular matrix development. *Journal of Biomedical Materials Research Part A* 2004, 70 (4), 560–568.

34. Bryant, S. J.; Chowdhury, T. T.; Lee, D. A.; Bader, D. L.; Anseth, K. S., Crosslinking density influences chondrocyte metabolism in dynamically loaded photocrosslinked poly(ethylene glycol) hydrogels. *Annals of Biomedical Engineering* 2004, 32 (3), 407–417.

35. Lanniel, M.; Huq, E.; Allen, S.; Buttery, L.; Williams, P. M.; Alexander, M. R., Substrate induced differentiation of human mesenchymal stem cells on hydrogels with modified surface chemistry and controlled modulus. *Soft Matter* 2011, 7 (14), 6501.

36. Stile, R. A.; Healy, K. E., Poly(N-isopropylacrylamide)-based semi-interpenetrating polymer networks for tissue engineering applications. 1. Effects of linear poly(acrylic acid) chains on phase behavior. *Biomacromolecules* 2002, 3 (3), 591–600.

37. Stile, R. A.; Healy, K. E., Thermo-responsive peptide-modified hydrogels for tissue regeneration. *Biomacromolecules* 2001, 2 (1), 185–194.

38. Stile, R. A.; Burghardt, W. R.; Healy, K. E., Synthesis and characterization of injectable poly(N-isopropylacrylamide)-based hydrogels that support tissue formation in vitro. *Macromolecules* 1999, 32 (22), 7370–7379.

39. Healy, K. E.; Rezania, A.; Stile, R. A., Designing biomaterials to direct biological responses. *Annals of the New York Academy of Sciences* 1999, 875 (Bioartificial Organs II), 24–35.

40. El-Sherbiny, I. M.; Yacoub, M. H., Hydrogel scaffolds for tissue engineering: Progress and challenges. *Global Cardiology Science and Practice* 2013, 2013 (38), 316–342.

41. Adeloew, C.; Segura, T.; Hubbell, J. A.; Frey, P., The effect of enzymatically degradable poly(ethylene glycol) hydrogels on smooth muscle cell phenotype. *Biomaterials* 2007, 29 (3), 314–326.

42. Fabiilli, M. L.; Wilson, C. G.; Padilla, F.; Martin-Saavedra, F. M.; Fowlkes, J. B.; Franceschi, R. T., Acoustic droplet-hydrogel composites for spatial and temporal control of growth factor delivery and scaffold stiffness. *Acta Biomaterialia* 2013, 9 (7), 7399–7409.

43. Bayer, E. A.; Jordan, J.; Roy, A.; Gottardi, R.; Fedorchak, M. V.; Kumta, P. N.; Little, S. R., Programmed platelet-derived growth factor-BB and bone morphogenetic protein-2 delivery from a hybrid calcium phosphate/alginate scaffold. *Tissue Engineering Part A* 2017, 23 (23–24), 1382–1393.

44. Pathak, C. P.; Sawhney, A. S.; Hubbell, J. A., Rapid photopolymerization of immunoprotective gels in contact with cells and tissue. *Journal of the American Chemical Society* 1992, 114 (21), 8311–8312.

45. Cruise, G. M.; Hegre, O. D.; Scharp, D. S.; Hubbell, J. A., A sensitivity study of the key parameters in the interfacial photopolymerization of poly(ethylene glycol) diacrylate upon porcine islets. *Biotechnology and Bioengineering* 1998, 57 (6), 655.

46. Cruise, G. M.; Hegre, O. D.; Lamberti, F. V.; Hager, S. R.; Hill, R.; Scharp, D. S.; Hubbell, J. A., In vitro and in vivo performance of porcine islets encapsulated in interfacially photopolymerized poly(ethylene glycol) diacrylate membranes. *Cell Transplantation* 1999, 8 (3), 293–306.

47. Kizilel, S.; Perez-Luna, V. H.; Teymour, F., Photopolymerization of poly(ethylene glycol) diacrylate on eosin-functionalized surfaces. *Langmuir* 2004, 20 (20), 8652–8658.

48. Koh, W.-G.; Revzin, A.; Pishko, M. V., Poly(ethylene glycol) hydrogel microstructures encapsulating living cells. *Langmuir* 2002, 18 (7), 2459–2462.

49. Itle, L. J.; Koh, W.-G.; Pishko, M. V., Multi-phenotypic cellular arrays for biosensing. *BioMEMS and Biomedical Nanotechnology* 2006, 3, 79–93.

50. Koh, W.-G.; Pishko, M. V., Fabrication of cell-containing hydrogel microstructures inside microfluidic devices that can be used as cell-based biosensors. *Analytical and Bioanalytical Chemistry* 2006, 385 (8), 1389–1397.

51. Itle, L. J.; Pishko, M. V., Multiphenotypic whole-cell sensor for viability screening. *Analytical Chemistry* 2005, 77 (24), 7887–7893.

52. Itle, L. J.; Zguris, J. C.; Pishko, M. V., Cell-based bioassays in microfluidic systems. *Proceedings of SPIE: The International Society for Optical Engineering* 2004, 5588 (Smart Medical and Biomedical Sensor Technology II), 9–18.

53. Yadavalli, V. K.; Koh, W.-G.; Lazur, G. J.; Pishko, M. V., Microfabricated protein-containing poly(ethylene glycol) hydrogel arrays for biosensing. *Sensors and Actuators, B: Chemical* 2004, B97 (2–3), 290–297.

54. Koh, W.-G.; Itle, L. J.; Pishko, M. V., Molding of hydrogel microstructures to create multiphenotype cell microarrays. *Analytical Chemistry* 2003, 75 (21), 5783–5789.

55. Russell, R. J.; Axel, A. C.; Shields, K. L.; Pishko, M. V., Mass transfer in rapidly photopolymerized poly(ethylene glycol) hydrogels used for chemical sensing. *Polymer* 2001, 42 (11), 4893–4901.

56. Harris, J. M., Introduction to biomedical and biotechnical applications of polyethylene glycol. *Polymer Preprints (American Chemical Society, Division of Polymer Chemistry)* 1997, 38 (1), 520–521.

57. Li, H.; Zheng, J.; Wang, H.; Becker, M. L.; Leipzig, N. D., Neural stem cell encapsulation and differentiation in strain promoted crosslinked polyethylene glycol-based hydrogels. *Journal of Biomaterials Applications* 2018, 32 (9), 1222–1230.

58. Cellesi, F.; Weber, W.; Fussenegger, M.; Hubbell, J. A.; Tirelli, N., Towards a fully synthetic substitute of alginate: Optimization of a thermal gelation/chemical cross-linking scheme ("tandem" gelation) for the production of beads and liquid-core capsules. *Biotechnology and Bioengineering* 2004, 88 (6), 740–749.

59. Cellesi, F.; Tirelli, N.; Hubbell, J. A., Towards a fully-synthetic substitute of alginate: Development of a new process using thermal gelation and chemical cross-linking. *Biomaterials* 2004, 25 (21), 5115–5124.

60. Zguris, J. C.; Itle, L. J.; Koh, W.-G.; Pishko, M. V., A novel single-step fabrication technique to create heterogeneous poly(ethylene glycol) hydrogel microstructures containing multiple phenotypes of mammalian cells. *Langmuir* 2005, 21 (9), 4168–4174.

61. Koh, W.-G.; Pishko, M., Cells in micropatterned hydrogels: Applications in biosensing. *Materials Research Society Symposium Proceedings* 2002, 723 (Molecularly Imprinted Materials--Sensors and Other Devices), 141–146.

62. Williams, C. G.; Malik, A. N.; Kim, T. K.; Manson, P. N.; Elisseeff, J. H., Variable cytocompatibility of six cell lines with photoinitiators used for polymerizing hydrogels and cell encapsulation. *Biomaterials* 2005, 26 (11), 1211–1218.

63. Murthy, N.; Xu, M. C.; Schuck, S.; Kunisawa, J.; Shastri, N.; Frechet, J. M. J., A macromolecular delivery vehicle for protein-based vaccines: Acid-degradable protein-loaded microgels. *Proceedings of the National Academy of Sciences of the United States of America* 2003, 100 (9), 4995–5000.

64. Skoumal, M.; Seidlits, S.; Shin, S.; Shea, L., Localized lentivirus delivery via peptide interactions. *Biotechnology and Bioengineering* 2016, 113 (9), 2033–2040.

65. Kim, S.-H.; Kim, B.; Yadavalli, V. K.; Pishko, M. V., Encapsulation of enzymes within polymer spheres to create optical nanosensors for oxidative stress. *Analytical Chemistry* 2005, 77 (21), 6828–6833.

66. Koh, W.-G.; Revzin, A.; Simonian, A.; Reeves, T.; Pishko, M., BioMEMs materials and fabrication technology: Control of mammalian cell and bacteria adhesion on substrates micropatterned with poly(ethylene glycol) hydrogels. *Biomedical Microdevices* 2003, 5 (1), 11–19.

67. Lee, A. L. Z.; Venkataraman, S.; Fox, C. H.; Coady, D. J.; Frank, C. W.; Hedrick, J. L.; Yang, Y. Y., Modular composite hydrogels from cholesterol-functionalized polycarbonates for antimicrobial applications. *Journal of Materials Chemistry B* 2015, 3 (34), 6953–6963.

68. Bowersock, T. L.; HogenEsch, H.; Torregrosa, S.; Borie, D.; Wang, B.; Park, H.; Park, K., Induction of pulmonary immunity in cattle by oral administration of ovalbumin in alginate microspheres. *Immunology Letters* 1998, 60 (1), 37–43.

69. Pérez-Luna, V. H.; González-Reynoso, O., Encapsulation of biological agents in hydrogels for therapeutic applications. *Gels* 2018, 4 (3), 61.

70. Zhao, X.; Harris, J. M., Novel degradable poly(ethylene glycol) esters for drug delivery. *ACS Symposium Series* 1997, 680 (Poly(ethylene glycol), 458–472.

71. Tae, G.; Kornfield, J. A.; Hubbell, J. A., Sustained release of human growth hormone from in situ forming hydrogels using self-assembly of fluoroalkyl-ended poly(ethylene glycol). *Biomaterials* 2005, 26 (25), 5259–5266.

72. Schoenmakers, R. G.; van de Wetering, P.; Elbert, D. L.; Hubbell, J. A., The effect of the linker on the hydrolysis rate of drug-linked ester bonds. *Journal of Controlled Release* 2004, 95 (2), 291–300.

73. Zisch, A. H.; Lutolf, M. P.; Ehrbar, M.; Raeber, G. P.; Rizzi, S. C.; Davies, N.; Schmoekel, H.; Bezuidenhout, D.; Djonov, V.; Zilla, P.; Hubbell, J. A., Cell-demanded release of VEGF from synthetic, biointeractive cell-ingrowth matrices for vascularized tissue growth. *FASEB Journal* 2003, 17 (15), 2260–2262. doi: 10 1096/fj 02-1041fje.

74. Zisch, A. H.; Lutolf, M. P.; Hubbell, J. A., Biopolymeric delivery matrices for angiogenic growth factors. *Cardiovascular Pathology* 2003, 12 (6), 295–310.

75. Zhao, X.; Harris, J. M., Novel degradable poly(ethylene glycol) hydrogels for controlled release of protein. *Journal of Pharmaceutical Sciences* 1998, 87 (11), 1450–1458.

76. Sosnik, A.; Seremeta, K. P., Polymeric hydrogels as technology platform for drug delivery applications. *Gels* 2017, 3 (3), 25.

77. Rwei, S. P.; Anh, T. H. N.; Chiang, W. Y.; Way, T. F.; Hsu, Y. J., Synthesis and drug delivery application of thermo- and pH-sensitive hydrogels: Poly(beta-CD-co-N-isopropylacrylamide-co-IAM). *Materials* 2016, 9 (12), E1003.

78. Graham, N. B., Poly(ethylene glycol) gels and drug delivery. *Poly(Ethylene Glycol) Chemistry* 1992, 263–281.

79. Elbert, D. L.; Pratt, A. B.; Lutolf, M. P.; Halstenberg, S.; Hubbell, J. A., Protein delivery from materials formed by self-selective conjugate addition reactions. *Journal of Controlled Release* 2001, 76 (1–2), 11–25.

80. Elisseeff, J.; McIntosh, W.; Fu, K.; Blunk, T.; Langer, R., Controlled-release of IGF-I and TGF-b1 in a photopolymerizing hydrogel for cartilage tissue engineering. *Journal of Orthopaedic Research* 2001, 19 (6), 1098–1104.

81. Elisseeff, J.; McIntosh, W.; Langer, R., Synthesis of succinic acid/poly(ethylene oxide) hydrogels and their use as controlled release vehicles. *Polymeric Materials Science and Engineering* 1997, 76, 228–229.

82. Quick, D. J.; Anseth, K. S., DNA delivery from photocrosslinked PEG hydrogels: Encapsulation efficiency, release profiles, and DNA quality. *Journal of Controlled Release* 2004, 96 (2), 341–351.

83. Burdick, J. A.; Mason, M. N.; Hinman, A. D.; Thorne, K.; Anseth, K. S., Delivery of osteoinductive growth factors from degradable PEG hydrogels influences osteoblast differentiation and mineralization. *Journal of Controlled Release* 2002, 83 (1), 53–63.

84. Anseth, K. S.; Metters, A. T.; Bryant, S. J.; Martens, P. J.; Elisseeff, J. H.; Bowman, C. N., In situ forming degradable networks and their application in tissue engineering and drug delivery. *Journal of Controlled Release* 2002, 78 (1–3), 199–209.

85. Mason, M. N.; Metters, A. T.; Bowman, C. N.; Anseth, K. S., Predicting controlled-release behavior of degradable PLA-b-PEG-b-PLA hydrogels. *Macromolecules* 2001, 34 (13), 4630–4635.

86. Lu, S.; Anseth, K. S., Release behavior of high molecular weight solutes from poly(ethylene glycol)-based degradable networks. *Macromolecules* 2000, 33 (7), 2509–2515.

87. Mellott, M. B.; Searcy, K.; Pishko, M. V., Release of protein from highly cross-linked hydrogels of poly(ethylene glycol) diacrylate fabricated by UV polymerization. *Biomaterials* 2001, 22 (9), 929–941.

88. Mellott, M.; Searcy, K.; Pishko, M. V., Transport properties of PEG gels. *25th Proceedings of the International Symposium on Controlled Release of Bioactive Materials,* Deerfield, IL, 1998, 900–901.

89. Kulkarni, R. V.; Biswanath, S., Electrically responsive smart hydrogels in drug delivery: A review. *Journal of Applied Biomaterials and Biomechanics.* 2007, 5 (3), 125–139.

90. Kopecek, J.; Yang, J., Hydrogels as smart biomaterials. *Polymer International* 2007, 56 (9), 1078–1098.

91. Elvira, C.; Abraham, G. A.; Gallardo, A.; San Roman, J., Chapter 26. Smart biodegradable hydrogels with applications in drug delivery and tissue engineering. In: *Biodegradable Systems in Tissue Engineering and Regenerative Medicine*, 1st ed., Reis, R. L.; Román, J. S. (Eds.) CRC Press: Boca Raton, FL, 2005, pp. 493–508.

92. Heller, J., Biodegradable polymers in controlled drug delivery. *Critical Reviews in Therapeutic Drug Carrier Systems* 1984, 1 (1), 39–90.

93. Rizzi, S. C.; Ehrbar, M.; Halstenberg, S.; Raeber, G. P.; Schmoekel, H. G.; Hagenmueller, H.; Mueller, R.; Weber, F. E.; Hubbell, J. A., Recombinant protein-co-PEG networks as cell-adhesive and proteolytically degradable hydrogel matrixes. Part II: Biofunctional characteristics. *Biomacromolecules* 2006, 7 (11), 3019–3029.

94. Sanchez-Diaz, J. C.; Martinez-Ruvalcaba, A.; Ortega-Gudino, P.; Gonzalez-Alvarez, A.; Mendizabal, E.; Puig, J. E., Determination of the diffusion coefficients in the ascorbic acid delivery from nanostructured-polyacrylamide hydrogels. *Polymer Bulletin (Heidelberg, Germany)* 2006, 56 (4–5), 437–446.

95. Sawhney, A. S.; Pathak, C. P.; Hubbell, J. A., Bioerodible hydrogels based on photopolymerized poly(ethylene glycol)-co-poly(alpha-hydroxyacid) diacrylate macromers. *Macromolecules* 1993, 26 (4), 581–587.

96. Lin, C. C.; Metters, A. T., Hydrogels in controlled release formulations: Network design and mathematical modeling. *Advanced Drug Delivery Reviews* 2006, 58 (12–13), 1379–1408.

97. Wu, X.; Wu, Y. D.; Ye, H. B.; Yu, S. J.; He, C. L.; Chen, X. S., Interleukin-15 and cisplatin co-encapsulated thermosensitive polypeptide hydrogels for combined immuno-chemotherapy. *Journal of Controlled Release* 2017, 255, 81–93.

98. Medina, S. H.; Li, S.; Howard, O. M. Z.; Dunlap, M.; Trivett, A.; Schneider, J. P.; Oppenheim, J. J., Enhanced immunostimulatory effects of DNA-encapsulated peptide hydrogels. *Biomaterials* 2015, 53, 545–553.

99. Hariyadi, D. M.; Ma, Y.; Wang, Y.; Bostrom, T.; Malouf, J.; Turner, M. S.; Bhandari, B.; Coombes, A. G. A., The potential for production of freeze-dried oral vaccines using alginate hydrogel microspheres as protein carriers. *Journal of Drug Delivery Science and Technology* 2014, 24 (2), 178–184.

100. Qi, X. L.; Wei, W.; Li, J. J.; Zuo, G. C.; Pan, X. H.; Su, T.; Zhang, J. F.; Dong, W., Salecan-based pH-sensitive hydrogels for insulin delivery. *Molecular Pharmaceutics* 2017, 14 (2), 431–440.

101. Gu, Z.; Dang, T. T.; Ma, M. L.; Tang, B. C.; Cheng, H.; Jiang, S.; Dong, Y. Z.; Zhang, Y. L.; Anderson, D. G., Glucose-responsive microgels integrated with enzyme nanocapsules for closed-loop insulin delivery. *ACS Nano* 2013, 7 (8), 6758–6766.

102. Mukerjee, A.; Pruthi, V., Oral insulin delivery by polymeric nanospheres. *Journal of Biomedical Nanotechnology* 2007, 3 (1), 68–74.

103. Raj, N. K. K.; Sharma, C. P., Oral insulin: A perspective. *Journal of Biomaterials Applications* 2003, 17 (3), 183–196.

104. Fletcher, N. A.; Babcock, L. R.; Murray, E. A.; Krebs, M. D., Controlled delivery of antibodies from injectable hydrogels. *Materials Science and Engineering C-Materials for Biological Applications* 2016, 59, 801–806.

105. Gibbs, D. M. R.; Black, C. R. M.; Dawson, J. I.; Oreffo, R. O. C., A review of hydrogel use in fracture healing and bone regeneration. *Journal of Tissue Engineering and Regenerative Medicine* 2016, 10 (3), 187–198.

106. Hoffman, A. S.; Stayton, P. S.; Bulmus, V.; Chen, G.; Chen, J.; Cheung, C.; Chilkoti, A.; Ding, Z.; Dong, L.; Fong, R.; Lackey, C. A.; Long, C. J.; Miura, M.; Morris, J. E.; Murthy, N.; Nabeshima, Y.; Park, T. G.; Press, O. W.; Shimoboji, T.; Shoemaker, S.; Yang, H. J.; Monji, N.; Nowinski, R. C.; Cole, C. A.; Priest, J. H.; Harris, J. M.; Nakamae, K.; Nishino, T.; Miyata, T., Founder's Award, Society for Biomaterials. Sixth world biomaterials congress 2000, Kamuela, HI, May 15–20, 2000. Really smart bioconjugates of smart polymers and receptor proteins. *Journal of Biomedical Materials Research* 2000, 52 (4), 577–586.

107. Hoffman, A. S.; Cohn, D.; Hanson, S. R.; Harker, L. A.; Horbett, T. A.; Ratner, B. D.; Reynolds, L. O., Application of radiation-grafted hydrogels as blood-contacting biomaterials. *Radiation Physics and Chemistry* 1983, 22 (1–2), 267–283.

108. Bidarra, S. J.; Barrias, C. C.; Granja, P. L., Injectable alginate hydrogels for cell delivery in tissue engineering. *Acta Biomaterialia* 2014, 10 (4), 1646–1662.

109. Nih, L. R.; Carmichael, S. T.; Segura, T., Hydrogels for brain repair after stroke: An emerging treatment option. *Current Opinion in Biotechnology* 2016, 40, 155–163.

110. Cruise, G. M.; Scharp, D. S.; Hubbell, J. A., Characterization of permeability and network structure of interfacially photopolymerized poly(ethylene glycol) diacrylate hydrogels. *Biomaterials* 1998, 19 (14), 1287–1294.

111. Pratt Alison, B.; Weber Franz, E.; Schmoekel Hugo, G.; Muller, R.; Hubbell Jeffrey, A., Synthetic extracellular matrices for in situ tissue engineering. *Biotechnology and Bioengineering* 2004, 86 (1), 27–36.

112. Burdick, J. A.; Khademhosseini, A.; Langer, R., Fabrication of gradient hydrogels using a microfluidics/photopolymerization process. *Langmuir* 2004, 20 (13), 5153–5156.

113. Hennink, W. E.; van Nostrum, C. F., Novel crosslinking methods to design hydrogels. *Advanced Drug Deliveries Review* 2002, 54 (1), 13–36.

114. Harris, J. M.; Bentley, M. D.; Zhoa, X.; Shen, X. Hydrolytically degradable polyoxyalkylene carbonate polymers and hydrogels made therefrom. Patent Application99-4593126348558, 19991210, 2002.

115. Sawhney, A. S.; Pathak, C. P.; Hubbell, J. A., Interfacial photopolymerization of poly(ethylene glycol)-based hydrogels upon alginate-poly(l-lysine) microcapsules for enhanced biocompatibility. *Biomaterials* 1993, 14 (13), 1008–1016.

116. Lee, S. H.; Miller, J. S.; Moon, J. J.; West, J. L., Proteolytically degradable hydrogels with a fluorogenic substrate for studies of cellular proteolytic activity and migration. *Biotechnology Progress* 2005, 21 (6), 1736–1741.

117. Dikovsky, D.; Bianco-Peled, H.; Seliktar, D., Proteolytically degradable photo-polymerized hydrogels made from PEG–fibrinogen adducts. *Advanced Engineering Materials* 2010, 12 (6), B200–B209.

118. Metters, A. T.; Bowman, C. N.; Anseth, K. S., Verification of scaling laws for degrading PLA-b-PEG-b-PLA hydrogels. *AIChE Journal* 2001, 47 (6), 1432–1437.

119. Metters, A. T.; Anseth, K. S.; Bowman, C. N., Predicting degradation behavior of PLA-b-PEG-b-PLA hydrogels. *Abstracts of Papers, 220th ACS National Meeting, Washington, DC, United States*, Washington, DC, August 20–24, 2000, POLY-233.

120. Metters, A. T.; Anseth, K. S.; Bowman, C. N., Fundamental studies of biodegradable hydrogels as cartilage replacement materials. *Biomedical Sciences Instrumentation* 1999, 35, 33–38.

121. Wade, R. J.; Bassin, E. J.; Rodell, C. B.; Burdick, J. A., Protease-degradable electrospun fibrous hydrogels. *Nature Communications* 2015, 6, 6639.

122. Gao, X. Y.; Cao, Y.; Song, X. F.; Zhang, Z.; Zhuang, X. L.; He, C. L.; Chen, X. S., Biodegradable, pH-responsive carboxymethyl cellulose/poly(acrylic acid) hydrogels for oral insulin delivery. *Macromolecular Bioscience* 2014, 14 (4), 565–575.

123. Dimitrova, I.; Trzebickab, B.; Müllerc, A. H. E.; Dworakb, A.; Tsvetanov, C. B., Thermosensitive water-soluble copolymers with doubly responsive reversibly interacting entities. *Progress in Polymer Science* 2007, 32, 1275–1343.

124. Yang, B. G.; Wang, C. Y.; Zhang, Y. B.; Ye, L.; Qian, Y. F.; Shu, Y.; Wang, J. M.; Li, J. J.; Yao, F. L., A thermoresponsive poly(N-vinylcaprolactam-co-sulfobetaine methacrylate) zwitterionic hydrogel exhibiting switchable anti-biofouling and cytocompatibility. *Polymer Chemistry* 2015, 6 (18), 3431–3442.

125. Lutolf, M. P.; Raeber, G. P.; Zisch, A. H.; Tirelli, N.; Hubbell, J. A., Cell-responsive synthetic hydrogels. *Advanced Materials* 2003, 15 (11), 888–892.

126. Pong, F. Y.; Lee, M.; Bell, J. R.; Flynn, N. T., Thermoresponsive behavior of poly(N-isopropylacrylamide) hydrogels containing gold nanostructures. *Langmuir* 2006, 22 (8), 3851–3857.

127. Velasco, D.; Elvira, C.; San Roman, J., New stimuli-responsive polymers derived from morpholine and pyrrolidine. *Journal of Materials Science: Materials in Medicine* 2008, 19 (4), 1453–1458.

128. Prabaharan, M.; Mano, J. F., Stimuli-responsive hydrogels based on polysaccharides incorporated with thermo-responsive polymers as novel biomaterials. *Macromolecular Bioscience* 2006, 6 (12), 991–1008.

129. Klouda, L.; Mikos, A. G., Thermo-responsive hydrogels in biomedical applications. *European Journal of Pharmaceutics and Biopharmaceutics* 2008, 68 (1), 34–45.

130. Drapala, P. W.; Brey, E. M.; Mieler, W. F.; Venerus, D. C.; Derwent, J. J. K.; Pérez-Luna, V. H., Role of thermo-responsiveness and poly(ethylene glycol) diacrylate cross-link density on protein release from poly(N-isopropylacrylamide) hydrogels. *Journal of Biomaterials Science, Polymer Edition* 2011, 22, 59–75.

131. Nuttelman, C. R.; Tripodi, M. C.; Anseth, K. S., In vitro osteogenic differentiation of human mesenchymal stem cells photoencapsulated in PEG hydrogels. *Journal of Biomedical Materials Research, Part A* 2004, 68A (4), 773–782.

132. Burdick, J. A.; Anseth, K. S., Photoencapsulation of osteoblasts in injectable RGD-modified PEG hydrogels for bone tissue engineering. *Biomaterials* 2002, 23 (22), 4315–4323.

133. Hasan, A.; Khattab, A.; Islam, M. A.; Hweij, K. A.; Zeitouny, J.; Waters, R.; Sayegh, M.; Hossain, M. M.; Paul, A., Injectable hydrogels for cardiac tissue repair after myocardial infarction. *Advanced Science* 2015, 2, 1500122.

134. Kim, S.; Healy, K. E., Synthesis and characterization of injectable poly(N-isopropylacrylamide-co-acrylic acid) hydrogels with proteolytically degradable cross-links. *Biomacromolecules* 2003, 4 (5), 1214–1223.

135. Coletta, D. J.; Ibanez-Fonseca, A.; Missana, L. R.; Jammal, M. V.; Vitelli, E. J.; Aimone, M.; Zabalza, F.; Issa, J. P. M.; Alonso, M.; Rodriguez-Cabello, J. C.; Feldman, S., Bone regeneration mediated by a bioactive and biodegradable extracellular matrix-like hydrogel based on elastin-like recombinamers. *Tissue Engineering Part A* 2017, 23 (23–24), 1361–1371.

136. Bobbala, S.; Tamboli, V.; McDowell, A.; Mitra, A. K.; Hook, S., Novel injectable pentablock copolymer based thermoresponsive hydrogels for sustained release vaccines. *AAPS Journal* 2016, 18 (1), 261–269.

137. Zhu, Y. J.; Wang, J. L.; Wu, J. J.; Zhang, J.; Wan, Y.; Wu, H., Injectable hydrogels embedded with alginate microspheres for controlled delivery of bone morphogenetic protein-2. *Biomedical Materials* 2016, 11 (2), 025010.

138. Seelbach, R. J.; Fransen, P.; Pulido, D.; D'Este, M.; Duttenhoefer, F.; Sauerbier, S.; Freiman, T.; Niemeyer, P.; Albericio, F.; Alini, M.; Royo, M.; Mata, A.; Eglin, D., Injectable hyaluronan hydrogels with peptide-binding dendrimers modulate the controlled release of BMP-2 and TGF-beta 1. *Macromolecular Bioscience* 2015, 15 (8), 1035–1044.

139. Song, G.; Zhang, L.; He, C.; Fang, D.-C.; Whitten, P. G.; Wang, H.; Jiang, L., Facile fabrication of tough hydrogels physically cross-linked by strong cooperative hydrogen bonding. *Macromolecules* 2013, 46 (18), 7423–7435.

140. Ren, Z.; Zhang, Y.; Li, Y.; Xua, B.; Liu, W., Hydrogen bonded and ionically crosslinked high strength hydrogels exhibiting Ca2+-triggered shape memory properties and volume shrinkage for cell detachment. *Journal of Materials Chemistry B* 2015, 3, 6347–6354.

141. Hamley, I. W.; Cheng, G.; Castelletto, V., A thermoresponsive hydrogel based on telechelic PEG end-capped with hydrophobic dipeptides. *Macromolecular Bioscience* 2011, 11 (8), 1068–1078.

142. Tae, G.; Kornfield, J. A.; Hubbell, J. A.; Johannsmann, D., Anomalous sorption in thin films of fluoroalkyl-ended poly(ethylene glycol)s. *Langmuir* 2002, 18 (21), 8241–8245.

143. Tae, G.; Kornfield, J. A.; Hubbell, J. A.; Johannsmann, D.; Hogen-Esch, T. E., Hydrogels with controlled, surface erosion characteristics from self-assembly of fluoroalkyl-ended poly(ethylene glycol). *Macromolecules* 2001, 34 (18), 6409–6419.

144. Chang, X.; Geng, Y.; Cao, H.; Zhou, J.; Tian, Y.; Shan, G.; Bao, Y.; Wu, Z. L.; Pan, P., Dual-crosslink physical hydrogels with high toughness based on synergistic hydrogen bonding and hydrophobic interactions. *Macromolecular Rapid Communications.* 2018, 1700806.

145. Metters, A. T.; Anseth, K. S.; Bowman, C. N., A statistical kinetic model for the bulk degradation of PLA-b-PEG-b-PLA hydrogel networks: Incorporating network non-idealities. *Journal of Physical Chemistry B* 2001, 105 (34), 8069–8076.

146. Metters, A. T.; Bowman, C. N.; Anseth, K. S., A statistical kinetic model for the bulk degradation of PLA-b-PEG-b-PLA hydrogel networks. *Journal of Physical Chemistry B* 2000, 104 (30), 7043–7049.

147. Kim, S.; Chung Eugene, H.; Gilbert, M.; Healy Kevin, E., Synthetic MMP-13 degradable ECMs based on poly(N-isopropylacrylamide-co-acrylic acid) semi-interpenetrating polymer networks. I. Degradation and cell migration. *Journal of Biomedical Materials Research Part A* 2005, 75 (1), 73–88.

148. Lutolf, M. P.; Lauer-Fields, J. L.; Schmoekel, H. G.; Metters, A. T.; Weber, F. E.; Fields, G. B.; Hubbell, J. A., Synthetic matrix metalloproteinase-sensitive hydrogels for the conduction of tissue regeneration: Engineering cell-invasion characteristics. *Proceedings of the National Academy of Sciences of the United States of America* 2003, 100 (9), 5413–5418.

149. Ferrandiz, C.; Carrascosa, J. M., Managing moderate-to-severe psoriasis with efalizumab: Experience at a single Spanish institute. *British Journal of Dermatology, Supplement* 2007, 156 (2), 24–29.

150. Hamilton, T. K., Clinical considerations of efalizumab therapy in patients with psoriasis. *Seminars in Cutaneous Medicine and Surgery* 2005, 24 (1), 19–27.

151. Scheinfeld, N., Efalizumab: A review of events reported during clinical trials and side effects. *Expert Opinion on Drug Safety* 2006, 5 (2), 197–209.

152. Joshi, A.; Bauer, R.; Kuebler, P.; White, M.; Leddy, C.; Compton, P.; Garovoy, M.; Kwon, P.; Walicke, P.; Dedrick, R., An overview of the pharmacokinetics and pharmacodynamics of efalizumab: A monoclonal antibody approved for use in psoriasis. *Journal of Clinical Pharmacology* 2006, 46 (1), 10–20.

153. Papp, K. A., EFALIZUMAB: Advancing psoriasis management with a novel, targeted T-cell modulator. *Drugs of Today* 2004, 40 (11), 889–899.

154. Saeed, A. F. U. H.; Wang, R.; Sumei L.; Wang, S., Antibody engineering for pursuing a healthier future. *Frontiers in Microbiology* 2017, 8, 495.

155. Bustamante-Córdova, L.; Melgoza-González, E. A.; Hernández, J., Recombinant antibodies in veterinary medicine: An update. *Frontiers in Veterinary Science* 2018, 5, 175.

156. Aguilar, M. R.; Román, J. S., *Smart Polymers and their Applications*, 2nd ed. Elsevier: Cambridge, MA, 2019, p.650.

157. Li, S.; Tiwari, A.; Prabaharan, M.; Aryal, S., *Smart Polymer Materials for Biomedical Applications*, 1st ed. Nova Science Publishers, Inc.: New York, 2010, p. 405.

158. Raula, J.; Shan, J.; Nuopponen, M.; Niskanen, A.; Jiang, H.; Kauppinen, E. I.; Tenhu, H., Synthesis of gold nanoparticles grafted with a thermoresponsive polymer by surface-induced reversible-addition-fragmentation chain-transfer polymerization. *Langmuir* 2003, 19, 3499–3504.

159. Wei, H.; Zhang, X.-Z.; Cheng, H.; Chen, W.-Q.; Cheng, S.-X.; Zhuo, R.-X., Self-assembled thermo- and pH responsive micelles of poly(10-undecenoic acid-b-N-isopropylacrylamide) for drug delivery. *Journal of Controlled Release* 2006, 116 (3), 266–274.

160. Ista, L. K.; Perez-Luna, V. H.; Lopez, G. P., Surface-grafted, environmentally sensitive polymers for biofilm release. *Applied and Environmental Microbiology* 1999, 65 (4), 1603–1609.

161. Pan, Y. V.; Wesley, R. A.; Luginbuhl, R.; Denton, D. D.; Ratner, B. D., Plasma polymerized N-isopropylacrylamide: Synthesis and characterization of a smart thermally responsive coating. *Biomacromolecules* 2001, 2 (1), 32–36.

162. Malmstadt, N.; Yager, P.; Hoffman Allan, S.; Stayton Patrick, S., A smart microfluidic affinity chromatography matrix composed of poly(N-isopropylacrylamide)-coated beads. *Analytical Chemistry* 2003, 75 (13), 2943–2949.

163. Mendez, S.; Ista, L. K.; Lopez, G. P., Use of stimuli responsive polymers grafted on mixed self-assembled monolayers to tune transitions in surface energy. *Langmuir* 2003, 19 (19), 8115–8116.

164. Rao, G. V. R.; Lopez, G. P., Encapsulation of poly(N-isopropylacrylamide) in silica: A stimuli-responsive porous hybrid material that incorporates molecular nano-valves. *Advanced Materials (Weinheim, Germany)* 2000, 12 (22), 1692–1695.

165. Chilkoti, A.; Dreher, M. R.; Meyer, D. E.; Raucher, D., Targeted drug delivery by thermally responsive polymers. *Advanced Drug Delivery Reviews* 2002, 54 (5), 613–630.

166. Liang, L.; Feng, X. D.; Martin, P. F. C.; Peurrung, L. M., Temperature-sensitive switch from composite poly(N-isopropylacrylamide) sponge gels. *Journal of Applied Polymer Science* 2000, 75 (14), 1735–1739.

167. Stile, R. A.; Chung, E.; Burghardt, W. R.; Healy, K. E., Poly(N-isopropylacrylamide)-based semi-interpenetrating polymer networks for tissue engineering applications. Effects of linear poly(acrylic acid) chains on rheology. *Journal of Biomaterials Science, Polymer Edition* 2004, 15 (7), 865–878.

168. Liu, S.-Q.; Yang, Y.-Y.; Liu, X.-M.; Tong, Y.-W., Preparation and characterization of temperature-sensitivity poly(N-isopropylacrylamide)-b-poly(D,L-lactide) microspheres for protein delivery. *Biomacromolecules* 2003, 4 (6), 1784–1793.

169. Meyer, D. E.; Shin, B. C.; Kong, G. A.; Dewhirst, M. W.; Chilkoti, A., Drug targeting using thermally responsive polymers and local hyperthermia. *Journal of Controlled Release* 2001, 74 (1–3), 213–224.

170. Serres, A.; Baudys, M.; Kim, S. W., Temperature and pH-sensitive polymers for human calcitonin delivery. *Pharmaceutical Research* 1996, 13 (2), 196–201.

171. Luchini, A.; Geho, D. H.; Bishop, B.; Tran, D.; Xia, C.; Dufour, R. L.; Jones, C. D.; Espina, V.; Patanarut, A.; Zhou, W.; Ross, M. M.; Tessitore, A.; Petricoin, E. F.; Liotta, L. A., Smart hydrogel particles: Biomarker harvesting: One-step affinity purification, size exclusion, and protection against degradation. *Nano Letters* 2008, 8 (1), 350–361.

172. Schild, H. G., Poly (N-isopropylacrylamide): Experiment, theory and application. *Progress in Polymer Science* 1992, 17 (2), 163–249.

173. Liu, G.; Ma, R. J.; Ren, J.; Li, Z.; Zhang, H. X.; Zhang, Z. K.; An, Y. L.; Shi, L. Q., A glucose-responsive complex polymeric micelle enabling repeated on-off release and insulin protection. *Soft Matter* 2013, 9 (5), 1636–1644.

174. Jain, K.; Vedarajan, R.; Watanabe, M.; Ishikiriyama, M.; Matsumi, N., Tunable LCST behavior of poly(N-isopropylacrylamide/ionic liquid) copolymers. *Polymer Chemistry* 2015, 6 (38), 6819–6825.

175. Heskins, M.; Guillet, J. E., Solution properties of poly(N-isopropylacrylamide). *Journal of Macromolecular Science Part A* 1968, A2 (8), 1441–1455.

176. Mendez, S.; Curro, J. G.; McCoy, J. D.; Lopez, G. P., Computational modeling of the temperature-induced structural changes of tethered poly(N-isopropylacrylamide) with self-consistent field theory. *Macromolecules* 2005, 38 (1), 174–181.

177. Wang, J.; Gan, D.; Lyon, L. A.; El-Sayed, M. A., Temperature-jump investigations of the kinetics of hydrogel nanoparticle volume phase transitions. *Journal of the American Chemical Society* 2001, 123 (45), 11284–11289.

178. Drapala, P. W.; Jiang, B.; Chiu, Y.-C.; Mieler, W. F.; Brey, E. M.; Kang-Mieler, J. J.; Pérez-Luna, V. H., The effect of glutathione as chain transfer agent in PNIPAAm-based thermo-responsive hydrogels for controlled release of proteins. *Pharmaceutical Research* 2014, 31, 742–753.

179. Jiang, B.; Larson, J.; Drapala, P.; Pérez-Luna, V. H.; Kang-Mieler, J. J.; Brey, E. M., Investigation of lysine acrylate containing poly (N-isopropylacrylamide) hydrogels as wound dressings in normal and infected wounds. *Journal of Biomedical Materials Research Part B: Applied Biomaterials* 2012, 100 (3), 668–676.

180. Flory, P. J., *Principles of Polymer Chemistry.* Cornell University Press: Ithaca, NY, 1953.

181. Kisselev, A. A.; Manias, E., Phase behavior of temperature-responsive polymers with tunable LCST: An equation-of-state approach. *Fluid Phase Equilibria* 2007, 261 (1–2), 69–78.

182. Bertrand, N.; Fleischer, J. G.; Wasan, K. M.; Leroux, J.-C., Pharmacokinetics and biodistribution of N-isopropylacrylamide copolymers for the design of pH-sensitive liposomes. *Biomaterials* 2009, 30 (12), 2598–2605.

183. Badiger, M. V.; Lele, A. K.; Bhalerao, V. S.; Varghese, S.; Mashelkar, R. A., Molecular tailoring of thermoreversible copolymer gels: Some new mechanistic insights. *Journal of Chemical Physics* 1998, 109 (3), 1175–1184.

184. Furyk, S.; Zhang, Y. J.; Ortiz-Acosta, D.; Cremer, P. S.; Bergbreiter, D. E., Effects of end group polarity and molecular weight on the lower critical solution temperature of poly(N-isopropylacrylamide). *Journal of Polymer Science, Part A: Polymer Chemistry* 2006, 44 (4), 1492–1501.

185. Pamies, R.; Zhu, K.; Kjøniksen, A.-L.; Nyström, B., Thermal response of low molecular weight poly-(N-isopropylacrylamide) polymers in aqueous solution. *Polymer Bulletin* 2009, 62 (4), 487–502.

186. Turturro, S. B.; Guthrie, M. J.; Appel, A. A.; Drapala, P. W.; Brey, E. M.; Pérez-Luna, V. H.; Mieler, W. F.; Kang-Mieler, J. J., The effects of cross-linked thermo-responsive PNIPAAm-based hydrogel injection on retinal function. *Biomaterials* 2011, 32 (14), 3620–3626.

187. Donati, G., Emerging therapies for neovascularage-related macular degeneration: State of the art. *Ophthalmologica* 2007, 221 (6), 366–377.

188. Rosenfeld, P. J., Intravitreal avastin: The low cost alternative to lucentis? *American Journal of Ophthalmology* 2006, 142 (1), 141–143.

189. Bhatnagar, P.; Spaide Richard, F.; Takahashi Beatriz, S.; Peragallo Jason, H.; Freund, K. B.; Klancnik James, M., Jr.; Cooney Michael, J.; Slakter Jason, S.; Sorenson John, A.; Yannuzzi Lawrence, A., Ranibizumab for treatment of choroidal neovascularization secondary to age-related macular degeneration. *Retina* 2007, 27 (7), 846–850.

190. Brandrup, J.; Immergut, E. H., Polymer Handbook, 3rd ed. Wiley: New York, 1989.

191. Gundogan, N.; Melekaslan, D.; Okay, O., Rubber elasticity of poly(N-isopropylacrylamide) gels at various charge densities. *Macromolecules* 2002, 35 (14), 5616–5622.

192. Wu, C.; Zhou, S., Thermodynamically stable globule state of a single poly(N-isopropylacrylamide) chain in water. *Macromolecules* 1995, 28 (15), 5388–5390.

193. Kubota, K.; Fujishige, S.; Ando, I., Single-chain transition of poly(N-isopropylacrylamide) in water. *The Journal of Physical Chemistry* 1990, 94 (12), 5154–5158.

194. Ferrer, M. L.; Duchowicz, R.; Carrasco, B.; de la Torre, J. G.; Acuña, A. U., The conformation of serum albumin in solution: A combined phosphorescence depolarization-hydrodynamic modeling study. *Biophysical Journal* 2001, 80 (5), 2422–2230.

195. He, X. M.; Carter, D. C., Atomic structure and chemistry of human serum albumin. *Nature* 1992, 358 (6383), 209–215.

196. Lustig, S. R.; Peppas, N. A., Solute diffusion in swollen membranes. IX. Scaling laws for solute diffusion in gels. *Journal of Applied Polymer Science* 1988, 36 (4), 735–747.

197. Chiu, Y.-C.; Larson, J. C.; Perez-Luna, V. H.; Brey, E. M., Formation of microchannels in poly(ethylene glycol) hydrogels by selective degradation of patterned microstructures. *Chemistry of Materials* 2009, 21 (8), 1677–1682.

198. Mari, M.; Morales, A.; Colell, A.; Garcia-Ruiz, C.; Fernandez-Checa, J. C., Mitochondrial glutathione, a key survival antioxidant. *Antioxidants and Redox Signaling* 2009, 11 (11), 2685–2700.

199. Wu, G.; Fang, Y.-Z.; Yang, S.; Lupton, J. R.; Turner, N. D., Glutathione metabolism and its implications for health. *Journal of Nutrition* 2004, 134 (3), 489–492.

200. Klettnerand, A.; Roider, J., Comparison of bevacizumab, ranibizumab, and pegaptanib in vitro: Efficiency and possible additional pathways. *Investigative Ophthalmology and Visual Science* 2008, 49, 4523–4527.

5 Controlled Vaccine Delivery

Kevin J. McHugh
Rice University

CONTENTS

5.1 INTRODUCTION

Vaccines are widely considered one of the greatest health innovations in human history, preventing an estimated 419 million illnesses over the past 25 years.[1,2] Using vaccines to elicit pathogen-specific immunity prior to exposure is associated with better patient outcomes and is typically far less expensive than postexposure treatment.[3] However, this prophylactic approach also requires that large populations receive doses multiple times, which has several key consequences. First, it increases the number of people that vaccines must be distributed to, second, it shifts the motivation profile, and most importantly, it requires the ability to access patients repeatedly over a long period of time to deliver the full series of doses. These factors have a particularly severe impact in low-resource environments, leading to localized pockets of underimmunization where the majority of 1.5 million vaccination-preventable deaths occur each year (Figure 5.1).

Despite the overwhelming success of the World Health Organization's Expanded Programme on Immunization, which has increased global vaccination coverage from just 5% in 1974 to 85% today,[4] distributing vaccines in rural and low-resource environments remains a challenge.[5] As a result, vaccination coverage has plateaued over the last 5 years, falling short of the 95% coverage needed for herd immunity against some of the most contagious infectious diseases, such as measles.[6] A number of logistical factors contribute to lowering the vaccination rates in the developing world including the difficulty of accessing patients, limited healthcare and transportation infrastructure (e.g., the cold chain), and inconsistent medical recordkeeping. As a result, one-in-seven infants worldwide (19.9 million) remain at risk for vaccine-preventable infectious diseases that are responsible for 29% of all deaths in children between 1 month and 5 years of age.[4,7] This chapter describes the controlled-release strategies being employed to overcome logistical barriers that limit vaccination coverage and hinder eradication efforts.

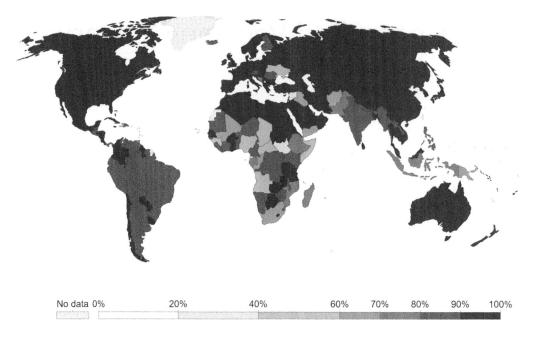

No data 0%   20%   40%   60% 70% 80% 90% 100%

FIGURE 5.1 Map depicting the percentage of children 12–23 months in age that have received a full three-dose regimen of the trivalent diphtheria, tetanus, and pertussis vaccine (DTP3) in each country based on 2017 reporting data. Figure is a derivative of an image by Samantha Vanderslott and Max Roser that originally appeared in OurWorldInData.org under a CC BY 4.0 license.

5.2 CONTROLLED-RELEASE VACCINES

The concept of controlled-release vaccines dates back to the 1970s when the release of macromolecules from polymers was first being explored.[8,9] Although the number of clinically approved vaccines has expanded over the past 50 years, there has been little modernization in their formulation and route of administration. Commercial vaccines are injected (usually intramuscularly) or administered orally and typically require multiple doses at least 4 weeks apart to be maximally effective at the population level.[10] With very few exceptions, current clinically approved vaccines exhibit very high seroconversion rates when administered on their recommended schedules, which are not considered difficult to follow in the developed world, since infants are seen regularly by their healthcare provider. As a result, most controlled vaccine delivery work to date has focused on the development of single-injection or "auto-boosting" vaccines for low-resource settings where regular access to patients cannot be taken for granted.[11,12] Although oral dosing is generally preferred by patients, it may not be appropriate for nonenteric pathogens and biodegradable particles given the harsh, variable gastrointestinal environment.[13] Therefore, a vast majority of controlled-release vaccines have been developed for parenteral injection.

The most common form of single-injection vaccines is biodegradable particles that exhibit degradation-mediated antigen release over the course of weeks or months. By delivering antigen over time, these vaccines seek to promote the formation of antigen-specific memory B cells, affinity maturation, long-lived plasma cells, and ultimately protective levels of neutralizing antibodies. More recently, the potential role of cellular immunity has also become better understood and appreciated, though current vaccines are largely considered to work by establishing humoral immunity. Lymph node-targeting nanoparticles have also been explored as an alternative delivery strategy to enhance the magnitude of the immune response via antigen persistence in an immune cell-rich environment, albeit delivering antigen over shorter time periods.[14,15] In order for single-injection vaccines to be clinically and ethically viable, they must confer immunity that is noninferior to current multidose regimens. Although there has been substantial preclinical work using controlled-release vaccines, this technology has yet to be commercialized due to challenges associated with biologics. The two key challenges facing single-injection vaccines today are release kinetics and antigen stability. These challenges are a consequence of multiple factors, including the type of vaccine, formulation method, encapsulating material, adjuvant load, and stabilizing excipients, which together determine the success of a controlled-release vaccine.

5.3 RELEASE KINETICS

Unfortunately, the ideal release kinetics for vaccine delivery remains unknown.[16–18] Current vaccination schedules have arisen because they were found to be safe and effective, but may not be truly optimized. However, evaluating alternative dosing regimens on populations with naïve immune systems raises ethical questions regarding the value of this knowledge compared with the risk of infectious disease for those enrolled in the study.[19] Within the field of controlled release, there are conflicting reports of the optimal kinetics for antigen release. For example, one group reported that the continuous release of gp120, an experimental vaccine for human immunodeficiency virus (HIV), led to a suppressed humoral response[20] while another observed an opposite effect.[21] Therefore, there is likely more complexity and nuance to these systems than currently appreciated.

As a result of this uncertainty, there has been an effort to create single-injection vaccines that release antigen in multiple discrete bursts, since those kinetics have demonstrated good efficacy and minimal side effects in the clinic (Figure 5.2).[11,16,22] It has also been suggested that continuous antigen exposure via controlled-release could induce immunological tolerance,[23–25] though more recent

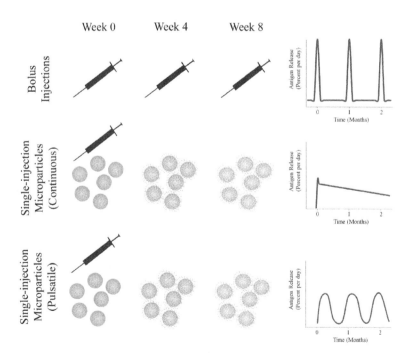

FIGURE 5.2 Current vaccination schedules consisting of multiple injections produce large, short-lived spikes in antigen concentration. Although some of the most common fabrication techniques used to produce controlled-release devices that result in continuous release that poorly mimics the current clinical standard, modified methods and specialized techniques have demonstrated the ability to create particles with pulsatile release kinetics. (Reprinted from McHugh, K. J, Guarecuco, R., Langer, R. & Jaklenec A. Single-injection vaccines: Progress, challenges, and opportunities. *J. Control. Release* **219**, 596–609 (2015), with permission from Elsevier.)

studies have not observed this outcome.[26,27] Regardless of the immunological necessity of pulsatile release, vaccine delivery systems that display this release profile may have an easier pathway to clinical approval because of their similarity to traditional vaccination regimens.

5.4   ENCAPSULATION STRATEGIES

Although many studies have tried to achieve pulsatile release, this profile is difficult to achieve using an emulsion/solvent evaporation or nanoprecipitation fabrication technique. Because vaccines are biological in nature, and therefore dispersible in water, this process is most often performed as a water-in-oil-in-water ($w_1/o_1/w_2$) double emulsion. Vaccine and stabilizing excipients (if applicable) are present in the first water phase (w_1), which is mixed in the oil phase (o_1) containing polymer dissolved in an organic solvent (e.g., poly(lactic-co-glycolic acid) (PLGA) in dichloromethane). This process is simple to perform and easily modified, but typically produces particles that exhibit biphasic release consisting of an initial burst followed by a period of slower continuous release and often damages the antigen.[11,28,29] However, with proper tuning, this method has been able to achieve triphasic release consisting of an initial burst followed by a period of little to no release and then a secondary period of accelerated release (Figure 5.3).[30] Further, triphasic particle populations with temporally shifted secondary bursts can be combined to approximate the three doses given currently (i.e., dose one from the initial burst from both populations, dose two from the secondary burst of one population, and dose three from the secondary burst of the other population). While these particles do not perfectly mimic the discrete pulses of antigen currently administered due to undesired leakage of antigen between bursts and broad secondary burst,[30–32] several formulations have demonstrated the ability to induce robust immune responses.[30]

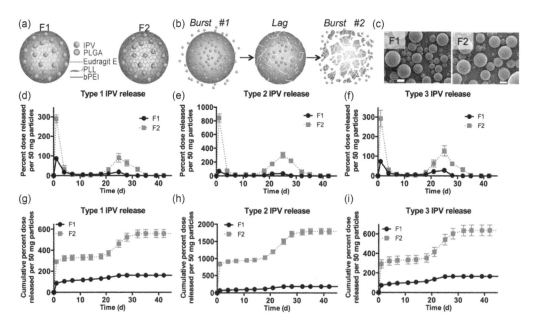

FIGURE 5.3   Encapsulation and release of trivalent inactivated polio vaccine (IPV) and stabilizing excipients using PLGA particles created using a double emulsion/solvent evaporation technique. (a) F1 and F2 microspheres were formulated with Eudragit E, poly(L-lysine) (PLL), and branched polyethylenimine (bPEI). (b) Diagram showing the hypothesized mechanism of triphasic antigen release. (c) Scanning electron microscopy image of each formulation. (d–f) Release and (g–i) cumulative release graphs for each strain of IPV released from particles as measured using an enzyme-linked immunosorbent assay (ELISA) for the immunity-conferring version of IPV. (Reprinted from Tzeng, S. Y. et al. Stabilized single-injection IPV elicits a strong neutralizing immune response. *Proc. Natl. Acad. Sci. USA* **115**(23), E5269–E5278 (2018) under CC BY 4.0 license.)

Nanoprecipitation, like emulsion/solvent evaporation, is a spontaneous formulation technique used to produce particles containing vaccine based on controlling solvent miscibility and material solubility. It also produces particles that exhibit continuous release and are usually smaller than emulsion-based techniques – typically on the order of hundreds of nanometers in diameter.[33] Due to the small size of particles produced, the encapsulating material must degrade very slowly to achieve release over durations that are relevant for vaccination. Extensive research evaluating vaccine release from surface eroding particles produced using this method have shown substantial promise for inducing robust immune responses, even though they exhibit continuous release.[34–40]

Recently, a new fabrication method, termed the StampEd Assembly of polymer Layers (SEAL), has been developed and used to create microparticles that exhibit pulsatile release both in vitro and in vivo.[12] This approach uses microfabrication, soft lithography, nanoliter dispensing, and thermal annealing under microscopic alignment to create particles with a polymeric shell surrounding a vaccine-filled core – a structure that is hypothesized to facilitate pulsatile release. When used with ovalbumin as a model antigen, microparticles produced using this method demonstrated not only noninferiority to multiple soluble injections, but a two-fold dose-sparing effect. Further development of this system is currently in progress.

PLGA has been the most common material used for controlled-release vaccines due to its biocompatibility, degradation over clinically meaningful periods of time, and precedence for use in Food and Drug Administration- (FDA) approved controlled-release formulations.[19,29,41–44] Additionally, PLGA has been reported to have an adjuvant effect, which could increase the immune response or generate a similar response using less antigen. Unfortunately, PLGA may not be ideal for delivering biologics, including vaccines, because it degrades into lactic acid and glycolic acid. These acidic species lower the pH of the local microenvironment, which can induce changes in protein conformation, aggregation, and degradation that may render the vaccine ineffective.[30] Other materials, such as collagen,[45] chitosan,[46] poly(lactic acid) (PLA),[47] polycaprolactone,[48] and polyanhydrides,[49] have also been used to create controlled-release devices with reasonable levels of success.

5.5 MAINTAINING ANTIGEN INTEGRITY

Antigen stability is a key parameter affecting the efficacy of both traditional soluble vaccines as well as controlled-release vaccines, especially for conferring humoral immunity. Due to their biological nature, most clinical vaccines degrade at elevated temperatures and must therefore remain refrigerated (4°C) or frozen (−20°C) prior to use.[50] When experiencing high temperatures or other environmental insults, antigens can change conformation, degrade, or aggregate, which can negatively impact their ability to evoke a protective immune response. For example, elevated temperatures cause the inactivated polio vaccine (IPV) to undergo a conformational change from the D-antigen conformation to the C-antigen conformation, which hides an epitope that is important for poliovirus neutralization.[51] Thus, although the immune system generates a response to the C-antigen, the immune memory and antibodies formed do not protect individuals from infection by the wild-type virus.[52]

Some antigens are inherently more resistant to environmental insults than others, with a trend that usually corresponds to their structural complexity. Whole-virus and whole-cell vaccines are generally the least stable because they may require higher order protein structure in order to generate a protective immune response.[33,53] Live vaccines have not been used frequently in controlled-release devices due to their high temperature sensitivity and generally low stability overall. In addition, since they are replication-competent, they do have the potential (albeit very small) to cause the disease itself, particularly in immunocompromised patients. Inactivated proteins do not have the potential to cause the disease, but are required in much larger amounts since they don't replicate in the host, which contributes to higher vaccine cost. The method of inactivation – formalin

TABLE 5.1
Potential Causes of Vaccine Instability

Fabrication	Storage	Post-administration
Solvent interactions	Drying	Prolonged exposure to 37°C
Heating	Freezing	Prolonged hydration
Physical perturbation	Formaldehyde-mediated aggregation	Acidic microenvironment
Polymer interactions	Removal from the cold chain	Polymer interactions

crosslinking – can also lead to stability issues as unreacted aldehyde groups on the formalin-inactivated antigen form bonds with the encapsulating material or other molecules of the antigen.[54] Nevertheless, whole-virus and whole-cell vaccines may be necessary when higher order structure is crucial for generating antibodies that neutralize the wild-type pathogen.[55]

Other vaccines, which tend to be more stable, are composed of only part of a pathogen, for example, a protein, peptide, polysaccharide, or an inactivated form of the toxin it produces (toxoids) because proper higher order is not required to confer immunity.[56] These vaccines are generally less immunogenic on a per-molecule basis, but often safer than their whole-pathogen counterparts.[57] Protein and peptide vaccines may also be produced recombinantly, which offers key manufacturing advantages.[58] Alternatively, conjugate vaccines that consist of a poorly immunogenic antigen conjugated to a highly immunogenic antigen may be more difficult to deliver in an immunity-conferring form since the bond must be maintained to have the vaccine remain effective.[50,59] Ultimately, to be clinically viable, a controlled-release vaccine must maintain antigen stability during all three stages of its life cycle: during device fabrication, "on-the-shelf" prior to use, and after administration into the body (Table 5.1), which may be easier to achieve for some antigens compared to others.

5.6   ANTIGEN STABILITY DURING FORMULATION

To minimize damage during formulation, storage, and after administration, excipients are often introduced to controlled-release vaccines. The most commonly used excipients include nonreducing sugars, salts, amino acids, polyols, and buffering agents.[31,60,61] Nonreducing sugars, such as trehalose, are thought to improve vaccine stability at several stages in the controlled-release vaccine product lifecycle by engaging in hydrogen bonding with the vaccine.[61–63] Depending on the fabrication process used to create controlled-release vaccines, the antigen may be subjected to a variety of physical, chemical, and thermal stressors that can cause vaccines to become ineffective. Degradation of vaccines at this stage can not only reduce efficacy but also cause toxicity due to the delivery of denatured or aggregated antigen.[64] Using an emulsion/solvent evaporation process results in antigen–solvent interactions at the interface of the oil and water phases, which can denature proteins.[65–68] Nanoprecipitation and microfluidic fabrication that use organic solvents may also suffer from this potential source of vaccine instability. Finer emulsions are also typically more at risk for damaging the vaccine since they present an increased surface area-to-volume ratio between the aqueous and organic phases.[65,69] Careful selection of solvents and surfactants, however, has been demonstrated to minimize these deleterious interactions. For example, hydrophobic solvents can produce a more well-defined oil–water interface, thereby reducing solvent–antigen interactions.[69–71] In addition, emulsions can also damage vaccines due to the physical perturbations associated with both high-speed mixing and local temperature elevation – particularly during sonication.[72]

New fabrication methods have been developed to avoid some of these potential environmental insults. The SEAL process avoids solvent interactions altogether in exchange for a short heating step, which can have a very minor effect on antigen stability provided that appropriate excipients are used.[12] A self-healing encapsulation method has also been developed to avoid solvent interaction.

In this process, antigen is loaded into porous particles after they have been created and then the particles are sealed using a gentle heating step to complete the devices. These approaches are also attractive because they allow the antigen to avoid harsh treatments, such as sterilization and residual solvent removal.[73–75]

5.7   ANTIGEN STABILITY DURING STORAGE

Vaccines must also be shelf-stable for a bare minimum of 1 year to be considered commercially viable.[76] This poses a problem for controlled-release vaccines stored in the liquid state because of both antigen and biomaterial degradation. In particular, degradation of the polymer on the shelf would advance the timeline to release after administration, potentially resulting in inadequate spacing between antigen release events.[19] As a result, particles are lyophilized or frozen to inhibit these processes. Both freezing and drying can be quite damaging to some vaccines, but once dry they are generally more stable, which could reduce reliance on cold chain transport.[77] Once again, non-reducing sugars are among the most common cryoprotectants used to maintain a favorable antigen conformation.[61,63,78–80] Formalinized antigens such as tetanus toxoid (TT) and IPV have also been reported to aggregate during lyophilization via formadehyde-mediated aggregation pathway—another possible source of reduced immunogenicity.[54]

5.8   ANTIGEN STABILITY IN THE BODY

Maintaining appropriate antigen structure for months in the hydrated, 37°C environment of the body remains a major challenge for single-injection vaccines. Further, PLGA and several other popular material choices can also cause local changes in pH during in vivo degradation due to the generation of acidic byproducts. A variety of carbohydrates, amino acids, and salts similar to those used to improve the thermostability of traditional vaccines have been used to successfully stabilize vaccines in particles.[31] Buffering excipients can also be incorporated into biodegradable materials that produce acidic products in order to neutralize the pH. This strategy is especially common for PLGA, given its degradation rate and the pKa of its degradation products.[30,46,81] Importantly, these buffering agents must be either minimally soluble or large in size to be effective, otherwise they will diffuse out of the particle long before vaccine release is complete. $Mg(OH)_2$ is perhaps the most widely used buffering excipient due to its low solubility at neutral pH, which allows it to act as a buffer reservoir that becomes more soluble in response to decreases in pH.[82,83] Fabricating smaller particles by changing processing parameters is another option to reduce acidification in these materials since it shortens the diffusion path length by which acidic species escape from the particle, though this will also likely affect release kinetics.[84] Surface-eroding polymers may also be attractive candidates for their ability to (1) confine acidic degradation products to the particle surface where the body's natural buffer can neutralize the environment and (2) their ability to maintain a dry interior promotes vaccine thermostability.

5.9   ADJUVANTS

Adjuvants, which can be added to vaccine formulations to enhance the immune response, have been used successfully in many controlled-release formulations.[85] The most common vaccine adjuvants include aluminum salts (e.g., $AlPO_4$, $Al(OH)_3$), CpG oligodeoxynucleotides, polycytidylic acid, and monophosphoryl lipid A (MPLA). These materials can be used to not only enhance the magnitude of the immune response but also guide it down specific response pathways via toll-like receptor (TLR) signaling.[86,87] The use of adjuvants is especially important to confer immunity while keeping the cost of goods low for recombinant and synthetic vaccines, which are typically less immunogenic.[87,88] Nonetheless, the inclusion of adjuvants in controlled-release devices adds another layer of complexity due to the high doses required (relative to the antigen dose) and dissimilar properties to the vaccine including hydrophobicity and molecular weight. In some cases, particle fabrication using solvents (i.e. emulsion/solvent evaporation, nanoprecipitation) may be advantageous as it allows for easy integration of water-insoluble adjuvants. In addition to dedicated adjuvants, the encapsulating material itself may act as an adjuvant. Many groups have reported PLGA adjuvancy even in the absence of controlled release, though the exact mechanism by which this occurs remains unknown.[12,27]

5.10   ELICITING NONINFERIOR IMMUNITY

Ultimately, the value of controlled-release vaccines will be determined by their ability to confer long-lived immunity against wild-type pathogens. Because infection challenge experiments are costly and difficult to perform, surrogate markers of success, such as neutralizing antibody titers, are often used to characterize the immune response.[89,90] Despite the challenges in achieving desirable release kinetics and maintaining vaccine stability in controlled-release devices, there have been successful demonstrations of preclinical noninferiority to three discrete injections for each diphtheria toxoid (DT) and the Hepatitis B surface antigen (HBsAg) using neutralizing antibody titers as a read out.[36–40] In these cases, PLGA or the closely related homopolymer, PLA, were used to encapsulate the vaccine using an emulsion process. Figure 5.4 displays the continuous release of DT from PLA microspheres and corresponding rise in antibody titers throughout the release window following injection into mice. Additional studies have also demonstrated that controlled release can be noninferior to two bolus doses for DT, HBsAg as well as TT and even IPV.[26,30,45,46,75] PLGA and PLA were again among the most common choices, but groups have also achieved this level of success using collagen,[45] chitosan,[46] and alginate[75] as part of the microparticle composition. The partial success of a controlled-release IPV vaccine is particularly notable since it is a whole-virus vaccine that is not as inherently stable as DT, TT, or HBsAg. Although these studies may not fully meet the three-fold reduction in administration requirements, they provide valuable insight into what strategies could accomplish this feat. Further improving the stability of more complex vaccines remains one of the main challenges facing the field of controlled-release vaccines today.

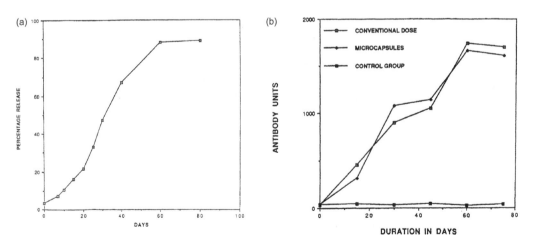

FIGURE 5.4 Controlled release of DT from PLA microparticles. (a) Cumulative in vitro release of DT from microspheres measured using an ELISA. (b) Immune response to three injections of soluble DT (open square), a single injection of microparticle-encapsulated DT (filled diamond), and unloaded microspheres (filled squares) in Balb/C mice. (Reprinted by permission from Springer Nature Customer Service Center GmbH: Springer, Pharmaceutical Research. Controlled delivery of DT using biodegradable poly(D,L-lactide) microcapsules. Singh, M., Singh, A. & Talwar, G. P. *Pharm. Res.* **8**(7), 958–961 (1991). Copyright 1991.)

5.11 POTENTIAL FOR CLINICAL TRANSLATION

In order to become clinically viable, controlled-release vaccines will need to meet a variety of criteria, including (i) noninferiority to current vaccines delivered on their recommended schedules, (ii) sufficient shelf-life, (iii) an acceptable cost versus value proposition, and (iv) a convenient administration route. Unlike most other drug delivery applications, controlled-release vaccines against infectious disease are prophylactics engineered primarily to improve vaccination feasibility in some of the poorest areas of the developing world. As a result, there is an extreme sensitivity to cost and an exceptionally low tolerance for negative side effects.[91]

Ideally, any solution would be a net neutral or beneficial from a cost perspective. However, an increase in the cost of the single-injection itself could theoretically be offset by reductions in the cost of cold chain transportation, healthcare worker time, materials (e.g., syringes, needles), and biohazardous waste disposal. Further, if these systems can exhibit dose-sparing effects through adjuvancy of the carrier, improved release kinetics, or anatomical targeting, they could reduce the amount of antigen required to confer immunity and thereby antigen cost. However, most vaccines in the developing world are already subsidized to at or near production cost-level that can be more than one-hundred times lower than the prices in the United States.[92]

These financial limitations extend to the vaccination process as well, since providing additional training or purchasing new supplies also requires financial support and may limit the adoption of controlled-release technology. Therefore, controlled-release vaccines should either use one of the current administration routes (intramuscular injection or oral) or require virtually no advanced training. This chapter has focused specifically on injectable particulate systems due to their compatibility with existing healthcare infrastructure in the developing world. Creating controlled-release vaccines for intramuscular injection imposes an upper bound on particle size since they must easily pass through 23- to 26-gauge needles (inner diameters of 337 and 260 µm, respectively) that are used for vaccination.[93] Fortunately, because these particles do not need to be transported in the blood to be effective, and can instead function at the site of injection, they do not need to be sufficiently small to pass through capillaries. Microneedle-based intradermal delivery has emerged as another possible route of administration for controlled release with promising potential for adoption due to its high patient acceptability during human ease-of-use trials.[74,94,95]

Lastly, the safety of controlled-release vaccines is paramount, perhaps even more so than controlled-release therapeutics because of the existence of safe alternatives and primary goal of increasing patient compliance rather than improving outcomes.[11,19] The use of a biomaterial to facilitate controlled release adds another component to the system with the potential to evoke a negative response, such as inflammation, that could potentially persist for months given the timeline of release and degradation. In order to limit the duration that this could occur, fully degradable systems are highly preferable over systems that release their vaccine payload, but never completely degrade. Some concern has also been expressed over the inability to easily retrieve devices prior to secondary antigen release if the primary dose of vaccine elicits an allergic response. Although true vaccine allergies are quite rare (about 1 in 450,000 vaccinations), this is nevertheless an issue that merits consideration.[96] Any negative outcomes resulting from controlled release must be outweighed by the benefits of improved vaccination coverage and reduced opportunity cost in order to justify the adoption of this new technology.

Nevertheless, the potential advantages of controlled vaccine delivery should not be understated. Truncating a two-, three-, or four-dose regimen into a single administration would revolutionize vaccine distribution, especially in the developing world. One could also imagine the corresponding reduction in healthcare reimbursement costs resulting from fewer doctor visits and reduced pain in the developed world. However, simply matching the efficacy of current vaccines may be shortsighted. Controlled vaccine delivery may be able to eliminate factors that prevent the implementation of new vaccines, such as poor immunogenicity. By extending the time window for antigen release and number of doses without increasing delivery complexity, controlled-release vaccines may be able to not only make existing vaccines easier to distribute but also improve seroconversion rates for existing and experimental vaccines alike.

REFERENCES

1. Sivakumar, S. M., Safhi, M. M., Kannadasan, M. & Sukumaran, N. Vaccine adjuvants - Current status and prospects on controlled release adjuvancity. *Saudi Pharm. J.* **19**, 197–206, doi:10.1016/j.jsps.2011.06.003 (2011).
2. Prevention, U. S. C. f. D. C. a. Protecting America's Children Every Day, <www.cdc.gov/vaccines/programs/vfc/protecting-children.html> (2019).
3. Rémy, V., Largeron, N., Quilici, S. & Carroll, S. The economic value of vaccination: Why prevention is wealth. *J. Mark. Access Health Policy* **3**, 29284, doi:10.3402/jmahp.v3.29414 (2015).
4. VanderEnde, K., Gacic-Dobo, M., Diallo, M. S., Conklin, L. M. & Wallace, A. S. Global routine vaccination coverage - 2017. *MMWR Morb. Mortal. Wkly. Rep.* **67**, 1261–1264, doi:10.15585/mmwr.mm6745a2 (2018).
5. Kaufmann, S. H. E. & Lambert, P. H. *The grand challenge for the future: Vaccines for poverty-related diseases from bench to field.* (Birkhäuser Verlag: Basel, Boston, 2005).
6. Orenstein, W. A. et al. Measles eradication: Is it in our future? *Am. J. Public Health* **90**, 1521–1525, doi:10.2105/ajph.90.10.1521 (2000).
7. World Health Organization, Global Immunization Data, <www.who.int/immunization/monitoring_surveillance/global_immunization_data.pdf> (2014).
8. Langer, R. & Folkman, J. Polymers for the sustained release of proteins and other macromolecules. *Nature* **263**, 797–800, doi:10.1038/263797a0 (1976).
9. Preis, I. & Langer, R. S. A single-step immunization by sustained antigen release. *J. Immunol. Methods* **28**, 193–197, doi:10.1016/0022-1759(79)90341-7 (1979).
10. National Center for Immunization & Respiratory Diseases. General recommendations on immunization --- recommendations of the Advisory Committee on Immunization Practices (ACIP). *MMWR Recomm. Rep.* **60**, 1–64 (2011).
11. Cleland, J. L. Single-administration vaccines: Controlled-release technology to mimic repeated immunizations. *Trends Biotechnol.* **17**, 25–29 (1999).
12. McHugh, K. J. et al. Fabrication of fillable microparticles and other complex 3D microstructures. *Science* **357**, 1138–1142, doi:10.1126/science.aaf7447 (2017).
13. Neutra, M. R. & Kozlowski, P. A. Mucosal vaccines: The promise and the challenge. *Nat. Rev. Immunol.* **6**, 148–158, doi:10.1038/nri1777 (2006).
14. Reddy, S. T. et al. Exploiting lymphatic transport and complement activation in nanoparticle vaccines. *Nat. Biotechnol.* **25**, 1159–1164, doi:10.1038/nbt1332 (2007).
15. Kelly, H. G., Kent, S. J. & Wheatley, A. K. Immunological basis for enhanced immunity of nanoparticle vaccines. *Expert Rev. Vaccines* **18**, 269–280, doi:10.1080/14760584.2019.1578216 (2019).
16. Plotkin, S. A., Orenstein, W. A. & Offit, P. A. *Vaccines.* Sixth edition. (Elsevier Saunders: Philadelphia, 2013).
17. Kissel, T., Koneberg, R., Hilbert, A. K. & Hungerer, K. D. Microencapsulation of antigens using biodegradable polyesters: Facts and phantasies. *Behring Inst. Mitt.* 172–183 (1997).
18. Shapiro-Shelef, M. & Calame, K. Regulation of plasma-cell development. *Nat. Rev. Immunol.* **5**, 230–242, doi:10.1038/nri1572 (2005).
19. McHugh, K. J., Guarecuco, R., Langer, R. & Jaklenec, A. Single-injection vaccines: Progress, challenges, and opportunities. *J. Control. Release* **219**, 596–609, doi:10.1016/j.jconrel.2015.07.029 (2015).
20. Cleland, J. L. et al. Development of a single-shot subunit vaccine for HIV-1. 3. Effect of adjuvant and immunization schedule on the duration of the humoral immune response to recombinant MN gp120. *J. Pharm. Sci.* **85**, 1350–1357, doi:10.1021/js960329b (1996).
21. Cirelli, K. M. et al. Slow delivery immunization enhances HIV neutralizing antibody and germinal center responses via modulation of immunodominance. *Cell* **177**, 1153–1171 e1128, doi:10.1016/j.cell.2019.04.012 (2019).
22. Sanchez, A., Gupta, R. K., Alonso, M. J., Siber, G. R. & Langer, R. Pulsed controlled-released system for potential use in vaccine delivery. *J. Pharm. Sci.* **85**, 547–552, doi:10.1021/js960069y (1996).
23. Dresser, D. W. & Gowland, G. Immunological paralysis induced in adult rabbits by small amounts of a protein antigen. *Nature* **203**, 733–736, doi:10.1038/203733a0 (1964).

24. Dixon, F. J. & Mauer, P. H. Immunologic unresponsiveness induced by protein antigens. *J. Exp. Med.* **101**, 245–257, doi:10.1084/jem.101.3.245 (1955).

25. Mitchison, N. A. Induction of immunological paralysis in two zones of dosage. *Proc. R. Soc. Lond. B Biol. Sci.* **161**, 275–292, doi:10.1098/rspb.1964.0093 (1964).

26. Gupta, R. K., Alroy, J., Alonso, M. J., Langer, R. & Siber, G. R. Chronic local tissue reactions, long-term immunogenicity and immunologic priming of mice and guinea pigs to tetanus toxoid encapsulated in biodegradable polymer microspheres composed of poly lactide-co-glycolide polymers. *Vaccine* **15**, 1716–1723, doi:10.1016/s0264-410x(97)00116-3 (1997).

27. Lofthouse, S. Immunological aspects of controlled antigen delivery. *Adv. Drug Deliv. Rev.* **54**, 863–870 (2002).

28. Tracy, M. A. Development and scale-up of a microsphere protein delivery system. *Biotechnol. Prog.* **14**, 108–115, doi:10.1021/bp9701271 (1998).

29. van de Weert, M., Hennink, W. E. & Jiskoot, W. Protein instability in poly(lactic-co-glycolic acid) microparticles. *Pharm. Res.* **17**, 1159–1167 (2000).

30. Tzeng, S. Y. et al. Stabilized single-injection inactivated polio vaccine elicits a strong neutralizing immune response. *Proc. Natl. Acad. Sci. U S A* **115**, E5269–E5278, doi:10.1073/pnas.1720970115 (2018).

31. Tzeng, S. Y. et al. Thermostabilization of inactivated polio vaccine in PLGA-based microspheres for pulsatile release. *J. Control. Release* **233**, 101–113, doi:10.1016/j.jconrel.2016.05.012 (2016).

32. Yang, J. & Cleland, J. L. Factors affecting the in vitro release of recombinant human interferon-gamma (rhIFN-gamma) from PLGA microspheres. *J. Pharm. Sci.* **86**, 908–914, doi:10.1021/js960480l (1997).

33. Bilati, U., Allemann, E. & Doelker, E. Nanoprecipitation versus emulsion-based techniques for the encapsulation of proteins into biodegradable nanoparticles and process-related stability issues. *AAPS PharmSciTech* **6**, E594–E604, doi:10.1208/pt060474 (2005).

34. Goodman, J. T., Mullis, A. S., Dunshee, L., Mitra, A. & Narasimhan, B. Automated high-throughput synthesis of protein-loaded polyanhydride nanoparticle libraries. *ACS Comb. Sci.* **20**, 298–307, doi:10.1021/acscombsci.8b00008 (2018).

35. Ulery, B. D. et al. Design of a protective single-dose intranasal nanoparticle-based vaccine platform for respiratory infectious diseases. *PLoS One* **6**, e17642, doi:10.1371/journal.pone.0017642 (2011).

36. Feng, L. et al. Pharmaceutical and immunological evaluation of a single-dose hepatitis B vaccine using PLGA microspheres. *J. Control. Release* **112**, 35–42, doi:10.1016/j.jconrel.2006.01.012 (2006).

37. Singh, M. et al. Controlled release microparticles as a single dose diphtheria toxoid vaccine: Immunogenicity in small animal models. *Vaccine* **16**, 346–352, doi:10.1016/s0264-410x(97)80912-7 (1998).

38. Singh, M. et al. Controlled release microparticles as a single dose hepatitis B vaccine: Evaluation of immunogenicity in mice. *Vaccine* **15**, 475–481, doi:10.1016/s0264-410x(97)00225-9 (1997).

39. Singh, M., Singh, A. & Talwar, G. P. Controlled delivery of diphtheria toxoid using biodegradable poly(D,L-lactide) microcapsules. *Pharm. Res.* **8**, 958–961 (1991).

40. Singh, M., Singh, O., Singh, A. & Talwar, G. P. Immunogenicity studies on diphtheria toxoid loaded biodegradable microspheres. *Int. J. Pharm.* **85**, R5–R8, doi:10.1016/0378-5173(92)90157-W (1992).

41. Gupta, R. K., Singh, M. & O'Hagan, D. T. Poly(lactide-co-glycolide) microparticles for the development of single-dose controlled-release vaccines. *Adv. Drug Delivery Rev.* **32**, 225–246 (1998).

42. Jiang, W., Gupta, R. K., Deshpande, M. C. & Schwendeman, S. P. Biodegradable poly(lactic-co-glycolic acid) microparticles for injectable delivery of vaccine antigens. *Adv. Drug. Delivery Rev.* **57**, 391–410, doi:10.1016/j.addr.2004.09.003 (2005).

43. Visscher, G. E. et al. Biodegradation of and tissue reaction to 50:50 poly(DL-lactide-co-glycolide) microcapsules. *J. Biomed. Mater. Res.* **19**, 349–365, doi:10.1002/jbm.820190315 (1985).

44. Cadee, J. A., Brouwer, L. A., den Otter, W., Hennink, W. E. & van Luyn, M. J. A comparative biocompatibility study of microspheres based on crosslinked dextran or poly(lactic-co-glycolic)acid after subcutaneous injection in rats. *J. Biomed. Mater. Res.* **56**, 600–609 (2001).

45. Higaki, M. et al. Collagen minipellet as a controlled release delivery system for tetanus and diphtheria toxoid. *Vaccine* **19**, 3091–3096, doi:10.1016/s0264-410x(01)00039-1 (2001).

46. Jaganathan, K. S. et al. Development of a single dose tetanus toxoid formulation based on polymeric microspheres: A comparative study of poly(D,L-lactic-co-glycolic acid) versus chitosan microspheres. *Int. J. Pharm.* **294**, 23–32, doi:10.1016/j.ijpharm.2004.12.026 (2005).

47. Pandit, S., Cevher, E., Zariwala, M. G., Somavarapu, S. & Alpar, H. O. Enhancement of immune response of HBsAg loaded poly (L-lactic acid) microspheres against hepatitis B through incorporation of alum and chitosan. *J. Microencapsul.* **24**, 539–552, doi:10.1080/02652040701443700 (2007).

48. Bansal, V., Kumar, M., Bhardwaj, A., Brahmne, H. G. & Singh, H. In vivo efficacy and toxicity evaluation of polycaprolactone nanoparticles and aluminum based admixture formulation as vaccine delivery system. *Vaccine* **33**, 5623–5632, doi:10.1016/j.vaccine.2015.08.076 (2015).

49. Petersen, L. K., Phanse, Y., Ramer-Tait, A. E., Wannemuehler, M. J. & Narasimhan, B. Amphiphilic polyanhydride nanoparticles stabilize Bacillus anthracis protective antigen. *Mol. Pharm.* **9**, 874–882, doi:10.1021/mp2004059 (2012).

50. Chen, D. & Kristensen, D. Opportunities and challenges of developing thermostable vaccines. *Expert Rev. Vaccines* **8**, 547–557, doi:10.1586/erv.09.20 (2009).

51. Ferguson, M., Wood, D. J. & Minor, P. D. Antigenic structure of poliovirus in inactivated vaccines. *J. Gen. Virol.* **74**(Pt 4), 685–690, doi:10.1099/0022-1317-74-4-685 (1993).

52. Sawyer, L. A., McInnis, J. & Albrecht, P. Quantitation of D antigen content in inactivated poliovirus vaccine derived from wild-type or sabin strains. *Biologicals* **21**, 169–177, doi:10.1006/biol.1993.1070 (1993).

53. Levine, T. P. & Chain, B. M. The cell biology of antigen processing. *Crit. Rev. Biochem. Mol.* **26**, 439–473, doi:10.3109/10409239109086790 (1991).

54. Jiang, W. & Schwendeman, S. P. Formaldehyde-mediated aggregation of protein antigens: Comparison of untreated and formalinized model antigens. *Biotechnol. Bioeng.* **70**, 507–517 (2000).

55. Scheiblhofer, S., Laimer, J., Machado, Y., Weiss, R. & Thalhamer, J. Influence of protein fold stability on immunogenicity and its implications for vaccine design. *Expert Rev. Vaccines* **16**, 479–489, doi:10.1080/14760584.2017.1306441 (2017).

56. Li, W., Joshi, M. D., Singhania, S., Ramsey, K. H. & Murthy, A. K. Peptide vaccine: Progress and challenges. *Vaccines (Basel)* **2**, 515–536, doi:10.3390/vaccines2030515 (2014).

57. Moyle, P. M. & Toth, I. Modern subunit vaccines: Development, components, and research opportunities. *ChemMedChem* **8**, 360–376, doi:10.1002/cmdc.201200487 (2013).

58. Nascimento, I. P. & Leite, L. C. Recombinant vaccines and the development of new vaccine strategies. *Braz. J. Med. Biol. Res.* **45**, 1102–1111, doi:10.1590/s0100-879x2012007500142 (2012).

59. Mahanty, S., Prigent, A. & Garraud, O. Immunogenicity of infectious pathogens and vaccine antigens. *BMC Immunol.* **16**, 31, doi:10.1186/s12865-015-0095-y (2015).

60. Singh, S. et al. Thermal inactivation of protective antigen of Bacillus anthracis and its prevention by polyol osmolytes. *Biochem. Biophys. Res. Commun.* **322**, 1029–1037, doi:10.1016/j.bbrc.2004.08.020 (2004).

61. Kraan, H., van Herpen, P., Kersten, G. & Amorij, J. P. Development of thermostable lyophilized inactivated polio vaccine. *Pharm. Res.* **31**, 2618–2629, doi:10.1007/s11095-014-1359-6 (2014).

62. Giri, J., Li, W. J., Tuan, R. S. & Cicerone, M. T. Stabilization of proteins by nanoencapsulation in sugar-glass for tissue engineering and drug delivery applications. *Adv. Mater.* **23**, 4861–4867, doi:10.1002/adma.201102267 (2011).

63. Alcock, R. et al. Long-term thermostabilization of live poxviral and adenoviral vaccine vectors at supraphysiological temperatures in carbohydrate glass. *Sci. Transl. Med.* **2**, 19ra12, doi:10.1126/scitranslmed.3000490 (2010).

64. Cleland, J. L., Powell, M. F. & Shire, S. J. The development of stable protein formulations: A close look at protein aggregation, deamidation, and oxidation. *Crit. Rev. Ther. Drug Carrier Syst.* **10**, 307–377 (1993).

65. Sah, H. Protein behavior at the water/methylene chloride interface. *J. Pharm. Sci.* **88**, 1320–1325, doi:10.1021/js9900654 (1999).

66. Lu, W. & Park, T. G. Protein release from poly(lactic-co-glycolic acid) microspheres: Protein stability problems. *PDA J. Pharm. Sci. Technol.* **49**, 13–19 (1995).

67. Morlock, M., Koll, H., Winter, G. & Kissel, T. Microencapsulation of rh-erythropoietin, using biodegradable poly(D,L-lactide-co-glycolide): Protein stability and the effects of stabilizing excipients. *Eur. J. Pharm. Biopharm.* **43**, 29–36, doi:10.1016/S0939-6411(96)00017-3 (1997).

68. Zambaux, M. F., Bonneaux, F., Gref, R., Dellacherie, E. & Vigneron, C. Preparation and characterization of protein C-loaded PLA nanoparticles. *J. Control. Release* **60**, 179–188 (1999).

69. Sah, H. Protein instability toward organic solvent/water emulsification: Implications for protein microencapsulation into microspheres. *PDA J. Pharm. Sci. Technol.* **53**, 3–10 (1999).

70. Alonso, M. J., Gupta, R. K., Min, C., Siber, G. R. & Langer, R. Biodegradable microspheres as controlled-release tetanus toxoid delivery systems. *Vaccine* **12**, 299–306, doi:10.1016/0264-410x(94)90092-2 (1994).

71. Rafati, H. et al. The immune response to a model antigen associated with PLG microparticles prepared using different surfactants. *Vaccine* **15**, 1888–1897, doi:10.1016/s0264-410x(97)00134-5 (1997).

72. Suslick, K. S., Hammerton, D. A. & Cline, R. E. The sonochemical hot-spot. *J. Am. Chem. Soc.* **108**, 5641–5642, doi:10.1021/ja00278a055 (1986).

73. Desai, K. G. & Schwendeman, S. P. Active self-healing encapsulation of vaccine antigens in PLGA microspheres. *J. Control. Release* **165**, 62–74, doi:10.1016/j.jconrel.2012.10.012 (2013).

74. Mazzara, J. M. et al. Self-healing encapsulation and controlled release of vaccine antigens from PLGA microparticles delivered by microneedle patches. *Bioeng. Transl. Med.* **4**, 116–128, doi:10.1002/btm2.10103 (2019).

75. Zheng, X., Huang, Y., Zheng, C., Dong, S. & Liang, W. Alginate-chitosan-PLGA composite microspheres enabling single-shot hepatitis B vaccination. *AAPS J.* **12**, 519–524, doi:10.1208/s12248-010-9213-1 (2010).

76. Izutsu, K. Stabilization of therapeutic proteins by chemical and physical methods. *Methods Mol. Biol.* **308**, 287–292, doi:10.1385/1-59259-922-2:287 (2005).

77. Anamur, C., Winter, G. & Engert, J. Stability of collapse lyophilized influenza vaccine formulations. *Int. J. Pharm.* **483**, 131–141, doi:10.1016/j.ijpharm.2015.01.053 (2015).

78. B'Hymer, C. Residual solvent testing: A review of gas-chromatographic and alternative techniques. *Pharm. Res.* **20**, 337–344 (2003).

79. Cleland, J. L. & Jones, A. J. Stable formulations of recombinant human growth hormone and interferon-gamma for microencapsulation in biodegradable microspheres. *Pharm. Res.* **13**, 1464–1475 (1996).

80. Shin, W. J. et al. Development of thermostable lyophilized sabin inactivated poliovirus vaccine. *mBio* **9**, e02287-18, doi:10.1128/mBio.02287-18 (2018).

81. Jaganathan, K. S., Singh, P., Prabakaran, D., Mishra, V. & Vyas, S. P. Development of a single-dose stabilized poly(D,L-lactic-co-glycolic acid) microspheres-based vaccine against hepatitis B. *J. Pharm. Pharmacol.* **56**, 1243–1250, doi:10.1211/0022357044418 (2004).

82. Shenderova, A., Burke, T. G. & Schwendeman, S. P. The acidic microclimate in poly(lactide-co-glycolide) microspheres stabilizes camptothecins. *Pharm. Res.* **16**, 241–248 (1999).

83. Varde, N. K. & Pack, D. W. Influence of particle size and antacid on release and stability of plasmid DNA from uniform PLGA microspheres. *J. Control. Release* **124**, 172–180, doi:10.1016/j.jconrel.2007.09.005 (2007).

84. Fu, K., Pack, D. W., Klibanov, A. M. & Langer, R. Visual evidence of acidic environment within degrading poly(lactic-co-glycolic acid) (PLGA) microspheres. *Pharm. Res.* **17**, 100–106 (2000).

85. O'Hagan, D. T. & Valiante, N. M. Recent advances in the discovery and delivery of vaccine adjuvants. *Nat. Rev. Drug Discov.* **2**, 727–735, doi:10.1038/nrd1176 (2003).

86. Cruz, L. J. et al. Controlled release of antigen and toll-like receptor ligands from PLGA nanoparticles enhances immunogenicity. *Nanomedicine (Lond)* **12**, 491–510, doi:10.2217/nnm-2016-0295 (2017).

87. Mohan, T., Verma, P. & Rao, D. N. Novel adjuvants & delivery vehicles for vaccines development: A road ahead. *Indian J. Med. Res.* **138**, 779–795 (2013).

88. Gupta, R. K. & Siber, G. R. Adjuvants for human vaccines--current status, problems and future prospects. *Vaccine* **13**, 1263–1276, doi:10.1016/0264-410x(95)00011-o (1995).

89. Weldon, W. C., Oberste, M. S. & Pallansch, M. A. Standardized methods for detection of poliovirus antibodies. *Methods Mol. Biol.* **1387**, 145–176, doi:10.1007/978-1-4939-3292-4_8 (2016).

90. Dunne, E. F., Markowitz, L. E., Taylor, L. D., Unger, E. R. & Wheeler, C. M. Human papilloma virions in the laboratory. *J. Clin. Virol.* **61**, 196–198, doi:10.1016/j.jcv.2014.06.014 (2014).

91. Dye, C. After 2015: Infectious diseases in a new era of health and development. *Philos. Trans. R. Soc. Lond. B Biol. Sci.* **369**, 20130426, doi:10.1098/rstb.2013.0426 (2014).

92. Vanderslott, S. & Roser, M. Vaccination, <https://ourworldindata.org/vaccination> (2018).

93. Beirne, P. V. et al. Needle size for vaccination procedures in children and adolescents. *Cochrane Database Syst. Rev.* **6**, CD010720, doi:10.1002/14651858.CD010720.pub2 (2015).

94. Norman, J. J. et al. Microneedle patches: Usability and acceptability for self-vaccination against influenza. *Vaccine* **32**, 1856–1862, doi:10.1016/j.vaccine.2014.01.076 (2014).

95. Rouphael, N. G. et al. The safety, immunogenicity, and acceptability of inactivated influenza vaccine delivered by microneedle patch (TIV-MNP 2015): A randomised, partly blinded, placebo-controlled, phase 1 trial. *Lancet* **390**, 649–658, doi:10.1016/S0140-6736(17)30575-5 (2017).

96. Wood, R. A. et al. An algorithm for treatment of patients with hypersensitivity reactions after vaccines. *Pediatrics* **122**, e771–e777, doi:10.1542/peds.2008-1002 (2008).

6 Controlled Release of Hormones by Pellet Implants

Sivanandane Sittadjody
Wake Forest Institute for Regenerative Medicine,
Wake Forest University School of Medicine

CONTENTS

6.1 INTRODUCTION: BACKGROUND ON HORMONE DELIVERY TO EXPERIMENTAL ANIMALS

Hormones are biological molecules secreted by the endocrine glands, circulate in the blood stream, and influence the target cell by using specific receptors. Almost every cell of our body is a target for one or more than one hormone. Hormones function as chemical messengers used by endocrine system to communicate and coordinate between various organ systems in the body. Hormones govern various physiological, morphological, and behavioral phenomena. The pleiotropic potential of hormones –that is their capacity to regulate multiple traits simultaneously – renders them particularly suited to control complex physiological and phenotype changes (Hau 2007). Studying the effect of a given hormone system in an experimental setup has been there for centuries. In one of the first endocrine experiments ever recorded, Professor Arnold A. Berthold (1803–1861) of Gottingen did a series of tests on roosters in 1849 while he was curator of the local zoo. Berthold found that a rooster's comb is an androgen-dependent structure. Following castration, the comb atrophies, aggressive male behavior disappears, and interest in the hens is lost. Importantly, Berthold also found that these castration-induced changes could be reversed by administration of a crude testicular extract (or prevented by transplantation of the testes). Similarly, in 1889 Brown-Séquard reported the effect of testicular extract from animals in humans (Brown 1889).

Ever since, the use of exogenous hormone for experimental purpose has been in practice to study the importance of a particular endocrine system or a specific hormone. Apart from classic endocrinology studies in laboratory animals, ecological and evolutionary studies also started using exogenous hormone administration in evaluating the effects of named hormones on change in behavior in addition to morphological changes. The pleiotropic potentials of hormones also qualify them as effective mediators of trade-offs in resource allocation, for example, the potential trade-off between reproduction and self-maintenance (Hau 2007, Ketterson and Nolan 1999, Zera, Harshman, and Williams 2007). This is the reason that the last two decades have seen a growing interest of evolutionary and ecological physiologists in hormones as a mechanistic link between changes in the environment and individual phenotypes. As a consequence, hormone manipulations in both laboratory and free-living field animals have become quite common in order to develop diagnostic and/or therapeutic tools for endocrine diseases and disorders using experimental animals, and to study the effect of hormones on fitness-relevant traits in free-living field animals.

6.2 HORMONE DELIVERY

The methods to administer hormones have been adopted from studies of classic endocrinology, which has been mainly concerned with the basic mechanisms of hormone action. In classic endocrinology, to study for example the effects of ovarian sex steroids such as 17 β-estradiol (E_2) and/or progesterone (P_4) in females one would remove the ovaries and investigate the pathophysiology. As a second step, one would administer E_2 and/or P_4 to restore the physiology (Gerard et al. 2017, Ingberg et al. 2012, Singh et al. 2008, Sittadjody et al. 2019, 2017, Strom et al. 2012). Often, the hormone dosages used in classic endocrinology studies have been in the pharmacological range, far beyond what an animal would experience under naturally relevant circumstances. The main problem in using a supraphysiological concentration of hormone is that it may not mimic the exact physiological scenario that naturally exists in either laboratory or field animals. Therefore, the focus recently has been to design an appropriate hormone delivery system to achieve the desired level of hormones in plasma as relevant to their respective studies.

The administration of exogenous hormones in general is referred to as hormone therapy (HT). When bioidentical hormones are used for therapeutic purpose to supplement the missing hormones in the body it is called hormone replacement therapy (HRT). However, the HRT regimens that are used in human cases are outside the scope of this chapter and hence the current chapter discusses the use and delivery of hormones in experimental animals that are used as preclinical animal models. The term drug delivery (in this context hormone delivery) can be defined as techniques that are used to get the therapeutic agents (hormones) into the body of the recipient (Lee and Robinson 2000). For most of the drugs, conventional method of administrations are effective, in contrast to hormones where many of the conventional methods are difficult as the hormones are unstable in solution and have narrow therapeutic indices. Some hormones have even solubility issues. For such cases, a continuous administration method of hormones is desirable to maintain plasma level of hormones (Barron-Peppas 1997).

6.2.1 Necessity for Controlled Hormone Delivery

Controlled hormone delivery system is one that delivers hormones at a rate determined by the need of body over a specific period of time (Lee and Robinson 2000). Ideally, the main objective of this system is to deliver hormone over an extended period of time during the treatment regimen. Sustained release, sustained action, prolonged action, controlled release, extended action, timed release, depot and repository dosage forms are terms used to identify drug delivery systems that are designed to achieve a prolonged therapeutic effect by continuously relapsing medication over an extended period of time after the administration of a single dose (Table 6.1 and Figure 6.1). As shown in Figure 6.1, in the case of injectable dosage forms, this period may vary from days to months. In the case of orally administered form, however, this period is measured in hours and critically depends on the transit time of the dosage form in the gastrointestinal (GI) tract. The term "Controlled Release" has become associated with those systems from which therapeutic agents may automatically be delivered at a predefined rate over a long period of time. Products of this type have been formulated for oral, injectable and topical use, and include inserts for the placement in subcutaneous (S.C.) regions as well (Lordi 1987).

6.3 HORMONE DELIVERY MODALITIES

Rodents, mainly rats and mice, are normally used to elucidate the effects of hormones in experimental studies. The commonly used hormone delivery system includes pellets, injections, creams, patches, and others. Like other drugs, the hormones also face the same challenges in delivering the desired dose to target organ in a timely fashion. Protein hormones cannot be administered orally since they get digested by the gastrointestinal enzymes before they bring about their biological effects, whereas steroid/thyroid/vitamin-D hormones could be delivered orally as they are small molecules and don't get digested by gut enzymes. In animal models, several routes of administration and delivery of hormones have been used, including oral formulations or food- or water-based delivery systems including addition of steroids to water supply (Gordon et al. 1986), oral gavage (Jung et al. 2004, Lee et al. 2004), intranasal administration (van den Berg et al. 2004), intravenous injection, S.C. injections (Strom, Theodorsson, and Theodorsson 2008, Theodorsson et al. 2005). Other modalities include S.C. slow-release pellets such as the ones provided by Innovative Research of America (IRA, Sarasota, FL) (Ingberg et al. 2012, Theodorsson et al. 2005) and Hormone pellet press (Li et al. 2004), S.C. Silastic® pellets (Bronson 1976, Elsaesser et al. 1989) or capsules (Dziuk and Cook 1966, Ingberg et al. 2012, Strom, Theodorsson, and Theodorsson 2008), and more recently per oral administration

---

TABLE 6.1

Advantages and Disadvantages of Sustained-Release System

Advantages of Sustained-Release System	Disadvantages of Sustained-Release System
i. Maintains the therapeutic effect for a longer period of time	i. Does not permit the prompt termination of therapy when it is desired or required.
ii. Reduction in dosing frequency	ii. Fixed dose by design, and the user has less flexibility to adjust the dosage regimens.
iii. Reduced fluctuation in circulating levels of hormones	iii. Dose dumping, where large quantity of hormones delivered as initial burst release.
iv. Avoidance of night time dosing	iv. Not all hormones are suitable for sustained-release system.
v. More uniform effect	v. Cost is high compared with other methods.
vi. Reduction in dose-related side effects	

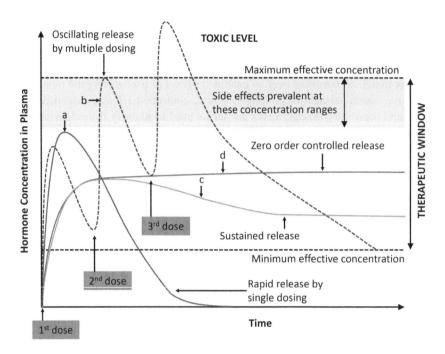

FIGURE 6.1 Release profile of various drug or hormone-release systems. A single dosing method such as one-time administration of hormones by injection reaches the therapeutic level and declines quickly as indicated by the line '**a**'. On the contrary, multiple dosing leads to peak and valley formation of plasma concentration of hormones and often reaches toxic level due to the cumulative effect as shown by the line '**b**'. However, the slow-release or sustained-release system reaches the therapeutic concentration and maintains the level for a prolonged time (shown by line '**c**'), which is closer to the ideal and desired zero-order controlled release as represented by the line '**d**'.

(Ingberg et al. 2012, Strom et al. 2010). S.C. implantation of Silastic® pellets and implantation of the "matrix-driven delivery (MDD)" pellet from IRA are the two methods that have been used with the intention of providing continuous delivery of hormones. The use of these pellets has been demonstrated to be effective in delivering a constant level of hormones over weeks (Dubal et al. 1998, Jung et al. 2002) to months (Singh, Meyer, and Simpkins 1995) in rats. However, there is a lack of consensus about the optimal means to reach the appropriate plasma concentration of hormones and maintenance of long-term steady-state plasma level of hormones. In this chapter each delivery system is briefly discussed along with their advantages and disadvantages.

6.3.1 ORAL ROUTE OF HORMONE DELIVERY

Steroid/thyroid hormones are usually administered orally to human. Several oral administration formulations have been developed for rodents and include gavage, food–mixture preparations (Ingberg et al. 2012, Isaksson et al. 2011), or supplemented in drinking water (Gordon et al. 1986, Levin-Allerhand, Sokol, and Smith 2003). The commonly used practice in delivering hydrophobic and/or small molecule hormones to animals by oral route is to train the experimental animal to consume the hormone-mixed food or drink *ad libitum*. The hormones are usually mixed in nutella powder paste or other food material to train the animals prior to the initiation of the experiment. However, the hydrophobic nature of these steroid/thyroid/vitamin-D hormones and their shorter half-life due to metabolic clearance poses another challenge in delivering these hormones. In addition, the delivery of desired dose is not possible in this method since the consumption of hormone-mixed food or drink cannot be controlled, and therefore the desired dose is not achieved most of the time. Additional difficulties in the administration of hormones orally to experimental animals include stressful animal handling, difficulty of mixing hydrophobic hormones in water, and difficulty to precisely control the individual intake.

6.3.2 INJECTABLE HORMONES

The second method of administering hormones to experimental animals is via S.C. injection. The low oral bioavailability and the short circulating half-life of many hormones create difficulties for its use in HT. To circumvent these limitations, various parenteral depot hormone preparations were developed. Among the earliest was injectable hormone. In order to deliver the desired dose of hormone irrespective of whether it is hydrophilic or hydrophobic hormone, the injectable form is preferred because the experimenter has control in this system (Strom, Theodorsson, and Theodorsson 2008, Theodorsson et al. 2005). The advantage of hormones delivered systemically is that hormones by nature are known to be released into the blood stream from their source and they reach their target on their own. Yet the practical disadvantage of injectable hormones include (i) discomfort to the experimental animal every time the animal is being poked with needle; (ii) labor intensiveness; (iii) hard to maintain the timely delivery; (iv) risk to users of accidental exposure to hormone while injecting the hormones.

6.3.3 HORMONE IMPLANTS

The third method is via S.C. slow-release hormone devices including pellets. The benefits of slow-release hormone pellets include the following: (i) they are easily inserted S.C. by a simple procedure, (ii) do not require daily stressful animal handling and manipulation, and (iii) they avoid pulsatile concentration observed by daily injections. The clearest advantage of the pellet-based delivery system is that they are easily administered and do not require daily attention, although the major drawback of most pellet systems is their high cost (Strom et al. 2010).

6.3.3.1 Materials Used for Implants

Various materials have been used to manufacture hormone delivery pellets. Polydimethylsiloxane (PDMS) is a silicone-based organic polymer present in silicone capsules and silicone adhesives (Silastic®, Dow corning). It has been proven to be useful in preparing steroid capsules or pellets, because Silastic® allows steroids to pass through its walls, providing a means of chronic administration of the drugs for long periods of time (Dziuk and Cook 1966, Elsaesser et al. 1989) and its chemical inertness avoids inflammatory reactions (Kivisaari and Niinikoski 1973). This component is also present in other low-cost, commercially available adhesives such as FASTIX® (Akapol SA, Argentina). Some manufacturers do not disclose the composition of the matrix in their hormone pellet and consider them as proprietary.

6.3.4 METHODS IN HORMONE IMPLANTS

Based on drug release mechanisms (Aulton and Taylor 2013), slow releasing hormone devices are classified into four categories: (i) osmotic systems, (ii) reservoir systems, (iii) matrix-based systems, and (iv) beeswax hormone pellets.

6.3.4.1 Osmotic Pump System

The AlZet® system is based on the osmotic pumping mechanism and consists of an osmotic compartment surrounded by a semipermeable membrane with a single delivery orifice. In an aqueous environment, water is imbibed through the semipermeable membrane, generates an osmotic flux, and builds up a hydrostatic pressure pushing the hormone solution out of the implant through the orifice. The drug release rate is generally constant. The maximum release time is 6 weeks for small animals (www.alzet.com). Although this system is mostly used for the delivery of steroids, this necessitates their prior solubilization in ethanol.

6.3.4.2   Reservoir-Based System

In the reservoir system, the hormone core is surrounded by a rate-controlling membrane. Hormone diffusion is driven by the concentration gradient of hormone across the membrane, according to the first-order law of Fick. As a large excess of hormone is present inside the reservoir to maintain saturation on the upstream side of the membrane, a constant rate of hormone release is preserved. Administration of steroids by reservoir system can be achieved either by the newly commercially available implants (www.belmatech.com/en/) or by home-made Silastic® capsules. However, the home-made Silastic® capsules imply the preparation of hormones dispersed in oil or mixed with cholesterol powder in various proportions and the filling of Silastic® tube (inner diameter ± 1.5 mm) (Ingberg et al. 2012, Isaksson et al. 2011, Strom et al. 2010). The use of a S.C. Silastic® tube filled with hormones has several advantages. It provides constant hormone release, and it can be prepared in the laboratory at a relatively low cost. The disadvantage is that it is time consuming and the consistency in the amount of hormone released will depend on the amount of hormone packed into the Silastic® tube, as well as the length, diameter, and permeability of the Silastic® tube. Other commonly employed methods for estradiol administration include S.C. insertion of commercial pellets (IRA, Sarasota, FL) or osmotic minipumps (for example Alzet™). Commercial pellets and Alzet minipumps are good alternatives to the Silastic® tubes, but are much more expensive.

6.3.4.3   MDD System

In a matrix device, the hormone is dissolved or dispersed in a polymeric carrier or lipid matrix. In this system, hormone molecules can elute out of the matrix by dissolution or erosion in the surrounding excipient and diffuse through the matrix structure, without any control of the release. As a consequence, the hormone release is not constant and decreases over time, proportional to the square root of time. Slow-release matrix pellet are commercially available for several hormones in a large range of concentrations, covering 21–90 days of release (www.innovrsrch.com). Another vendor who manufactures hormone pellets is Linshin located in Canada. They manufacture insulin pellets for experimental diabetic models mainly for rats and mice.

6.3.4.4   Beeswax-Based Hormone Pellets

Beeswax-based hormone pellets are usually made in the research laboratory by the user themselves. Briefly, beeswax is melted in a glass vial using a hotplate at 65°C, and the desired amount of steroid/thyroid hormone of interest is mixed until it turns clear. Using a glass Pasteur pipet, the hot mixture of beeswax hormone is dropped as small pellets on to an aluminum foil placed on dry ice (DeRose et al. 2013, Yang et al. 2015). Compared to Silastic® capsule implants, beeswax implants of hormones produced lower spike in plasma concentration of hormones 24 hours following implantation and more consistently elevated plasma concentration of hormones for 2 weeks following implantation (Beck et al. 2016, Quispe et al. 2015). Beeswax implants provide the additional advantage of dissolving inside the animal.

Some studies have compared the delivery of hormones by various release devices and reported that Silastic® tubing device had the fastest release, sustained-release matrix hormone pellets being an intermediate, and beeswax the slowest release of hormones. It is important to mention that steroid hormone manipulation carry some health hazards. Handling of hormones in crystalline powder form or in solution must occur in a functional fume hood with appropriate protection for the staff. Risks include fertility damage and carcinogenicity, in addition to clothes and environmental contamination (see safety data sheet such as www.caymaneurope.com/msdss/10006315m.pdf).

For all these reasons and because S.C. implantable devices must fulfill such criteria as sterility and apyrogenicity, ready-to-use commercial slow-releasing devices present significant advantages in terms of safety and represent the device of choice for experimental research on rodents.

Considering the pros and cons of various hormone delivery systems, subdermal or S.C. hormone pellet implants still offer the longest duration of hormone action with prolonged zero-order, steady-state delivery characteristics lasting 4–7 months.

6.4   HORMONE PELLETS

MDD hormone pellet system integrates the three main principles in drug delivery such as (i) diffusion, (ii) erosion, and (iii) concentration gradients. It generates a finished hormone pellet with a biodegradable matrix that effectively and continuously releases the active hormone in the experimental animal. Formulations of pellets are available for different durations of experiments ranging from 21 to 90 days, and the total concentration of hormone preparation in hormone pellet ranges from 0.001 to 200 mg/pellet. Based on the degradation rate, the dose of hormone released from pellet could be calculated based on the duration of the experimental study (21 or 60 or 90 days) and the total concentration of hormone preparation (0.001–200 mg) in the pellet. Some commercial vendors such as IRA provides an option of combining two or three hormones in one pellet, for example, combining a desired dose of 17 β-estradiol with a desired dose of progesterone.

6.4.1   IMPLANTATION OF HORMONE PELLETS

The hormone pellets are usually implanted S.C. using a sterile trochar. Different sizes of trochar are being used depending on the diameter or size of the hormone pellet. The implantation of hormone pellets is done cautiously to avoid any damage to muscular layer beneath the dermal layer and any unnecessary injury to the animal. The most ideal place to implant the hormone pellet is where there is maximal space between the skin and muscle, such as the lateral side of the neck between the ear and the shoulder. Some laboratories implant on the back of the animal. These regions are preferred because these implantation sites are out of reach for the experimental animals. Some manufacturers (e.g., IRA) advice not to expose the hormone pellets to any organic solvent or exogenous fluid, whereas others (e.g., LinShin, Canada) recommend to sterilize the pellet by briefly soaking the hormone pellet in iodine solution (www.linshincanada.com/linplant.html). The difference in the handling precaution is due to the fact that different proprietary matrix technologies are used by different manufacturers.

The standard implantation procedure is explained in Figure 6.2 as per the instructions from the commercial vendors (www.innovrsrch.com/trochar.asp; www.linshincanada.com/linplant.html; www.belmatech.com) as follows: This procedure is carried out while the experimental animal is under general anesthesia to avoid movement of the animal during the implantation process. After preparing the implantation site by removing hair followed by standard sterilizing procedures, a S.C. pocket of approximately 2 cm is created. The S.C. pocket could be created by either piercing the skin with sterile trochar itself or with a sterile appropriate-sized syringe needle or by making an incision. Then the hormone pellet is carefully placed well inside the S.C. pocket with the help of the trochar. Finally, the opening of the incision is closed if necessary.

This method provides solutions to

1. Consistency in timing for repeated hormone administration
2. Controlling the amount of hormone administered
3. Stability of hormone preparation (increased shelf-life up to 3 years)
4. Safety to the experimenter compared to other methods
5. Negligible neurophysiological trauma to the animal from excessive handling

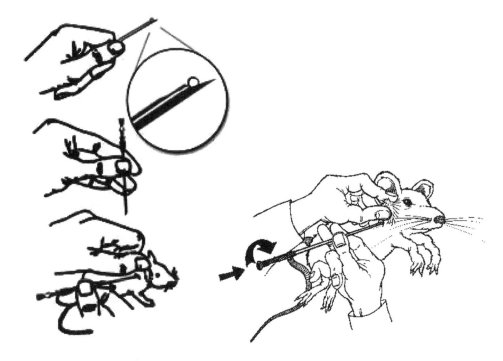

FIGURE 6.2 Implantation of S.C. hormone pellet or capsule. After preparing the implantation site, a S.C. pocket is made by either piercing or by making incision. The hormone is placed into the S.C. pocket with the help of a trochar of pair of forceps followed by the closure of incision if necessary. The preferred implantation sites include the side of the neck and the midline back of the experimental animal.

Advantages of the slow-release matrix-based hormone pellet delivery system:

a. They are often ready-to-use pellets, no necessity for hormone preparation
b. Long-term delivery of hormones in experimental animals
c. Better method to avoid peak and valley effect produced by conventional injectable delivery systems

6.5   COMMERCIALLY AVAILABLE HORMONE PELLETS

Provided here are the commercially available hormone pellets from vendors such as IRA, LinShin, BelmaTech, and others. Some hormone pellets are readily available as already formulated stocks while others are available as custom-made formulation hormone pellet based on request from the end user. Because of the limitation in space for each chapter it is impossible to provide the complete list of hormones available as pellets.

6.5.1   Androgen Pellets and Related Products

Any molecule that is capable of binding to androgen receptors (AR) and brings about the biological effect is termed as androgen. These compounds exhibit varying degrees of affinity towards AR, and the biological effects could be either positive or negative. Depending on the biological effect, the compound could be referred to as androgen or anti-androgen, or as androgen-receptor modulator (ARM). The use of androgen in laboratory animals or free-living field animals has been in practice in order to (i) test the preclinical therapeutic potentials or toxicity of androgens; (ii) study the influence of androgens on the behavioral changes or morphological change in the experimental animals

(Hau 2007, Fusani 2008, Handelsman, Conway, and Boylan 1990, Jockenhovel et al. 1996, Kelleher, Conway, and Handelsman 2001, Kelleher et al. 2004, Quispe et al. 2015). Some of the available ARMs as S.C. sustained-release pellets are listed in Table 6.2:

6.5.2 ADRENAL HORMONE PELLETS AND RELATED PRODUCTS

Adrenal gland is known to produce various steroid hormones that regulate a wide variety of physiological functions in the body ranging from glucose homeostasis to mineral homeostasis. The glucose regulation by steroids is mediated through glucocorticoid receptor (GR) and mineral regulation by mineralocorticoid receptor (MR) and the steroids from the adrenal cortex that bind to these receptors to bring about the physiological effects are called as glucocorticoids and mineralocorticoids, respectively. In addition, adrenal gland also secretes androgens and adrenalines. The adrenal androgens are listed along with other androgens in the above section. The medullary hormone pellet is listed along with other hormones in a separate section. The adrenal corticoids (cortex hormones) pellets are used in experimental animals to evaluate the physiological significance of these hormones and also study some of the behavioral changes (Beck et al. 2016, Bayorh et al. 2012, Chen, Blalock, et al. 2013, Frias-Dominguez et al. 2013, Muller-Fielitz et al. 2012, Diniz et al. 2013). Listed in Table 6.3 are some of the commercially available products related to adrenal cortex (adrenal medulla hormone pellet listed separately) hormone pellets.

6.5.3 PELLETS OF ESTROGEN RECEPTOR MODULATORS AND RELATED PRODUCTS

Similar to androgens, any molecule that binds to estrogen receptor alpha and/or beta (ERα, ERβ) and influences the physiology of the body is termed as estrogen. Estrogens exert widespread biological functions that reach far beyond their well-known role in reproduction. The effect caused by the molecules that bind to ER could be either positive or negative and hence they may be classified as estrogens or anti-estrogens. Whether the effect is positive or negative, those molecules that modulate the functions of either ERα or ERβ are generally termed as Selective Estrogen Receptor Modulators (SERMs). Exogenous administration of estradiol to ovariectomized experimental animals is of utmost importance in elucidating its mechanism of action. Estrogens are the subject

TABLE 6.2
Androgens and Related Products

19-Nortestosterone (nandrolone)	Gossypol acetate
19-Nortestosterone 17-decanoate	Mesterolone
19-Nortestosterone 17-propionate	Mesterone
5α-Androsterone	Methandriol
5α-Dihydrotestosterone	Methandriol dipropionate
5β-Androsterone	Methyl testosterone (see mesterlone)
5β-Dihydrotestosterone	Stanozolol
Androstenediol	Testosterone
Androstenedione	Testosterone 17β-hemisuccinate
Cyproterone acetate	Testosterone acetate
Dehydroepiandrosterone (DHEA)	Testosterone benzoate
Dehydroepiandrosterone acetate	Testosterone cypionate
Dehydroepiandrosterone sulfate	Testosterone enanthate
Fluoxymesterone	Testosterone propionate
Flutamide	

TABLE 6.3

Corticosteroids, Diuretics, and Related Products

Acetazolamide	Fludrocortisone
Adrenal cortex acetone powder	Fludrocortisone acetate
Adrenosterone	Flumethasone
Amcinonide	Flunisolide
Amiloride	Fluocinolone
Aminoglutethimide	Furosemide
Betamethasone	Hydrochlorothiazide
Cortexolone	Hydrocortisone
Cortexolone acetate	Hydrocortisone 21-acetate
Corticosterone	Hydrocortisone 21-hemisuccinate
Corticosterone	Hydrocortisone 21-phosphate
Cortisone	Methazolamide
Cortisone acetate	Methyl prednisolone
D-Aldosterone	Metyrapone
Demeclocycline	Prednisolone
Deoxycorticosterone (DOC)	Prednisone
Deoxycorticosterone acetate (DOCA)	Spironolactone
Desoximetasone	Triamcinolone
Dexamethasone	Triamcinolone acetonide
Dexamethasone 21-acetate	Triamcinolone diacetate
D-Mannitol	Triamterene
Ethacrynic acid	

of intensive researches aiming to elucidate their mechanism of action on the various tissues they target (Singh, Meyer, and Simpkins 1995, Jung et al. 2002, Jung et al. 2004, Lee et al. 2004, Dubal et al. 1998, Yang et al. 2001, Simpkins et al. 1997, Wen et al. 2004, Shi et al. 2001, Theodorsson and Theodorsson 2005, Levin-Allerhand, Sokol, and Smith 2003, Gordon et al. 1986, Isaksson et al. 2011, Strom et al. 2010, Bronson 1976, Li et al. 2004, Theodorsson et al. 2005, Strom et al. 2012, Ingberg et al. 2012, Sittadjody et al. 2019, 2017, Singh et al. 2008, Gottardis and Jordan 1988, Gerard et al. 2017, Yang et al. 2015). The use of ready-to-use slow releasing devices to administer steroids, especially estrogens, to small experimental animals remains the method of choice in terms of animal well-being and of safety for both the researcher and the animal. The development of SERMs, as an example tamoxifen, has provided important improvement for the treatment of ER-positive breast cancer (Fontaine et al. 2013, Bachelot et al. 2012). Listed in Table 6.4 are some (if not all) of the estrogens, anti-estrogens, and SERM pellets that are commercially available as ready-to-use sustained-release formulations for the animal research.

6.5.4 Progestin Pellets and Related Products

Progestins are molecules that bind to progesterone receptor (PR) and induce biological action. Progesterone is one of the precursor molecules from which many steroid hormones are derived biologically via the action of different steroidogenic enzymes. Progesterone is known for its protective role on uterine lining during the period of pregnancy and hence termed "Pro-gest-erone." In general, administration of progesterone and its related product is coupled with estrogen in studies elucidating the biological functions of ovarian sex steroids. This is because of its antagonistic properties against estrogens and protective effects over the adverse side effects of estrogens on estrogen-sensitive organs and tissues (Sittadjody et al. 2019, 2017, Singh et al. 2008). Some of the commercially available progestin pellets are listed in Table 6.5.

TABLE 6.4
Estrogens, Anti-Estrogens, and Related Products

17 β-Estradiol	Equilin
β-Estradiol 17-acetate	Equilin-methyl ether
β-Estradiol 17-cypionate	Estriol
β-Estradiol 17-valerate	Estriol 3-benzyl ether
β-Estradiol 3-benzoate	Estriol triacetate
β-Estradiol 3-methyl-ether	Estrone
β-Estradiol diacetate	Estrone 3-methyl ether
β-Estradiol dipropionate	Estrone 3-sulfate
β-Estradiol propionate	Estrone acetate
17α-Estradiol	Estrone hemisuccinate
17α-Ethynylestradiol	Hexestrol (Dihydro-DES)
Chlorotrianisene	Mestranol
D-equilenin	Nafoxidine
Dienestrol	Tamoxifen (Free base)
Dienestrol diacetate	Tamoxifen citrate
Diethylstilbestrol (DES)	

TABLE 6.5
Progestins and Related Products

11α-Hydroxyprogesterone	Ethisterone
16-Dehydropregnenolone	Medroxyprogesterone acetate
16-Dehydropregnenolone acetate	Megestrol acetate
16-Dehydroprogesterone	Norethindrone
17α-Hydroxypregnenolone	Norethindrone acetate
17α-Hydroxyprogesterone	Norethynodrel
Chlomadinone acetate	Norgestrel
Clomiphene citrate	Pregnenolone
Danazol	Progesterone

6.5.5 Thyroid Hormone Pellets and Related Products

Thyroid hormones are hydrophobic compounds like steroids. These hormones are derivatives of the amino acid, tyrosine, produced by the follicular cells of the thyroid. The iodination of tyrosine is possible at maximum four positions namely 3, 3', 5, 5'. However, it also produces iodinated product at three or two positions, which also can bind to the thyroid hormone receptor (TR) and carry out the biological action. Thyroid hormone has its receptor in almost every cell of the body making the whole body as target for this class of hormones. Apart from its pivotal role in controlling the basic metabolic rate (BMR) of body cells, these hormones regulate various other important functions. Thyroid hormone pellets are used to evaluate the physiological functions of this hormone ranging from embryonic development and growth to reproduction (Huffman et al. 2006, Nicolls et al. 2012, Al Husseini et al. 2013, Baliram et al. 2012, Chen, Weltman, et al. 2013). Listed in Table 6.6 are some of the commercially available pellets for thyroid hormones and their related products.

TABLE 6.6
Thyroid Hormones and Related Products

3,3',5-Triiodo-DL-thyronine	Methimazole
3,3',5-Triiodo-L-thyronine (T_3)	Methyl thiouracil
3,5-Diiodo-DL-thyronine	Potassium iodide
3,5-Diiodo-L-thyronine	Sodium iodide
6-N-Propyl-2-thiouracil	Thiobarbital
DL-thyronine	Thyroglobulin
D-thyroxine	Thyroid releasing hormone (TRH)
L-thyroxine (T_4)	Thyroid stimulating hormone (TSH)

6.5.6 PELLETS OF OTHER HORMONES AND RELATED PRODUCTS

Some other important hormone pellets used for research purpose are listed in Table 6.7. Among them, insulin is one of the widely used products in experimentally induced or genetically modified diabetes rodent models. It has been proven in several studies that these sustained-release insulin pellets are preferred over the injectable long-acting insulin to stabilize the glycemic level in the diabetic rodent models (Creque, Langer, and Folkman 1980, Schaschkow et al. 2016, Vaysburd, Lock, and McDevitt 1995, Brown and Sawchenko 1997, Friedman et al. 1993, Thompson et al. 2002, Bitar et al. 1987). Melatonin pellets are also used in place of other formulations to study its effect on behavior in experimental animals (Barcelo et al. 2016, van den Berg et al. 2004). S.C. implantable pellets are also available for various growth factors. Likewise, pellets for other hormones like Angiotensin-II (Weisberg et al. 2005), Epinephrine, Leptin (Barone et al. 2012), Luteinizing hormone (Wahjoepramono et al. 2011), all-trans Retinoic acid (Ablain et al. 2013), and Vitamin D_3 (Flanagan et al. 2003) are used in experimental animals for sustained release.

6.6 LIMITATIONS OF HORMONE PELLETS

The MDD has been used in rodents, especially rats and mice, and reported the delivery of hormones as the manufacturer claims, while a few researchers contradict the levels of hormones delivered by the MDD pellets. For example, IRA reports approximately 924 published papers using their 17 β-E_2 pellets and 142 reports using their P_4 pellets (www.innovrsch.com). Most of the published reports that utilized the 17 β-E_2 pellets from IRA cite either the IRA website (www.innovrsch.com) or other publications to support a continuous release of 17 β-E_2. However, Singh et al. 2008 have reported that these pellets have not been validated for the kinetic of release of the steroid in mice. Surprisingly, they further reported that these citations, in turn, lead to a single *ex vivo* dissolution study of one of the IRA pellets (Miller and Hunt 1998). Indeed, most studies assess levels of E_2 at the termination of their study and claim continuous release of the steroid at the reported concentration throughout the duration of treatment. The findings of Singh et al. 2008, however, in which they assessed the acute (up to 7 days) release characteristics of these steroid pellets suggest that this was

TABLE 6.7
Other Hormones and Related Products

Angiotensin-II	Luteinizing hormone (LH)
Epinephrine	Melatonin
Growth factors and peptides	Norepinephrine
Insulin	All trans-retinoic acid (atRA)
Leptin	Vitamin-D3 (Cholecalciferol)

not a valid assumption, and instead, show that both 17 β-E_2 and P_4 pellets produced a huge initial burst of hormone, followed by a gradual decline that even after 7 days is far less than the target mid-estrous cycle target levels of 50 pg/ml for 17 β-E_2 and 4 ng/ml for P_4.

Another study by Theodorsson and Theodorsson reported negative effects of estrogen, when delivered using the IRA pellet (1.5 mg), in a transient middle cerebral artery occlusion (MCAO) model of cerebral ischemia (Theodorsson and Theodorsson 2005). This is in sharp contrast to numerous reports that claim a benefit of estrogen treatment, where estrogen reduces the lesion size following experimental stroke (Shi et al. 2001, Simpkins et al. 1997, Wen et al. 2004, Yang et al. 2001).This discrepancy could be attributed to the differences in levels of estradiol to which the animal was exposed. The high concentrations may have desensitized the brain to the protective effects of estrogen (potentially through receptor down regulation). Thus, a more accurate conclusion that should have been made is that "high dose" estradiol is not beneficial in preventing damage associated with transient MCAO. Thus, these animal studies point to the importance of delivering the appropriate levels of hormones, and as such, question whether persistent delivery of a high dose of hormones (as is done in most HT regimens) is the appropriate means of delivering a therapeutic or protective dose of hormone. Based on these reports showing a large initial release of hormones after implantation of these pellets, it requires caution in the interpretation of results obtained from studies that use these hormone formulations.

6.7 CONCLUSIONS

Different hormone-release devices could induce variations in terms of drug pharmacokinetics and thus could influence the physiological endpoints being measured in an experimental setup. Previously, pharmacologic studies of hormone pellet implants have clearly established that circulating hormone levels rise rapidly into the physiological range where they are maintained at a stable level from day to day for months before gradual decrease to pretreatment levels between 4 and 7 months, depending upon dose, after implantations as pellets undergo full absorption *in vivo* (Handelsman, Conway, and Boylan 1990, Jockenhovel et al. 1996, Kelleher, Conway, and Handelsman 2001). Depending on the dose-dependent sensitivity of the physiological or pathological readout studied, careful attention should be paid to choosing a slow-releasing device that is most appropriate to a specific experiment. Several other novel approaches for delivering hormones to experimental animals have been developed and investigated recently, including bio-artificial organs such as pancreas (Opara, McQuilling, and Farney 2013, McQuilling, Sittadjody, Pareta, et al. 2017, McQuilling, Sittadjody, Pendergraft, et al. 2017) or cell/tissue-hormone delivery system (Sittadjody et al. 2013, 2019, 2017). Some of these delivery systems have been discussed separately in other chapters in this book. The advantages of choosing a bioartificial endocrine tissue or bioengineered endocrine tissue are that it not only integrates into the body but also regulates the endocrine loops via negative feedback mechanisms. In the context of ever-increasing legal requirement for the welfare and protection of animals used for scientific purposes, the judicious choice of a reliable and accurate drug release system will fulfill the three "R"s rule.

REFERENCES

Ablain, J., M. Leiva, L. Peres, J. Fonsart, E. Anthony, and H. de The. 2013. "Uncoupling RARA transcriptional activation and degradation clarifies the bases for APL response to therapies." *J. Exp. Med.* 210 (4):647–53. doi: 10.1084/jem.20122337.

Al Husseini, A., G. Bagnato, L. Farkas, J. Gomez-Arroyo, D. Farkas, S. Mizuno, D. Kraskauskas, A. Abbate, B. Van Tassel, N. F. Voelkel, and H. J. Bogaard. 2013. "Thyroid hormone is highly permissive in angioproliferative pulmonary hypertension in rats." *Eur. Respir. J.* 41 (1):104–14. doi: 10.1183/09031936.00196511.

Aulton, M.E., and K.M. Taylor. 2013. Aulton's Pharmaceutics: *The Design and Manufacture of Medicines.* 4th edition. Amsterdam, Netherlands: Churchill Livingstone Elsevier.

Bachelot, T., C. Bourgier, C. Cropet, I. Ray-Coquard, J. M. Ferrero, G. Freyer, S. Abadie-Lacourtoisie, J. C. Eymard, M. Debled, D. Spaeth, E. Legouffe, D. Allouache, C. El Kouri, and E. Pujade-Lauraine. 2012. "Randomized phase II trial of everolimus in combination with tamoxifen in patients with hormone receptor-positive, human epidermal growth factor receptor 2-negative metastatic breast cancer with prior exposure to aromatase inhibitors: A GINECO study." *J. Clin. Oncol.* 30 (22):2718–24. doi: 10.1200/JCO.2011.39.0708.

Baliram, R., L. Sun, J. Cao, J. Li, R. Latif, A. K. Huber, T. Yuen, H. C. Blair, M. Zaidi, and T. F. Davies. 2012. "Hyperthyroid-associated osteoporosis is exacerbated by the loss of TSH signaling." *J. Clin. Invest.* 122 (10):3737–41. doi: 10.1172/JCI63948.

Barcelo, P., C. Nicolau, A. Gamundi, M. A. Fiol, J. A. Tresguerres, M. Akaarir, and R. V. Rial. 2016. "Comparing the behavioural effects of exogenous growth hormone and melatonin in young and old wistar rats." *Oxid. Med. Cell. Longevity* 2016:5863402. doi: 10.1155/2016/5863402.

Barone, I., S. Catalano, L. Gelsomino, S. Marsico, C. Giordano, S. Panza, D. Bonofiglio, G. Bossi, K. R. Covington, S. A. Fuqua, and S. Ando. 2012. "Leptin mediates tumor-stromal interactions that promote the invasive growth of breast cancer cells." *Cancer Res.* 72 (6):1416–27. doi: 10.1158/0008-5472. CAN-11-2558.

Barron-Peppas, L. 1997. "Biomaterials: Polymers in controlled drug delivery." *Medical Plastics and Biomaterials Magazine.*

Bayorh, M., A. Rollins-Hairston, J. Adiyiah, D. Lyn, and D. Eatman. 2012. "Eplerenone inhibits aldosterone-induced renal expression of cyclooxygenase." J. Renin Angiotensin Aldosterone Syst. 13 (3):353–9. doi: 10.1177/1470320312443911.

Beck, M. L., S. Davies, I. T. Moore, L. A. Schoenle, K. Kerman, B. J. Vernasco, and K. B. Sewall. 2016. "Beeswax corticosterone implants produce long-term elevation of plasma corticosterone and influence condition." Gen. Comp. Endocrinol. 233:109–14. doi: 10.1016/j.ygcen.2016.05.021.

Bitar, M. S., M. Koulu, S. I. Rapoport, and M. Linnoila. 1987. "Adrenal catecholamine metabolism and myocardial adrenergic receptors in streptozotocin diabetic rats." *Biochem. Pharmacol.* 36 (7):1011–6. doi: 10.1016/0006-2952(87)90407-2.

Bronson, F. H. 1976. "Serum FSH, LH, and prolactin in adult ovariectomized mice bearing silastic implants of estradiol: Responses to social cues." *Biol. Reprod.* 15 (2):147–52. doi: 10.1095/biolreprod15.2.147.

Brown, S. C. 1889. "The effects produced on man by subcutaneous injections of a liquid obtained from the testicles of animals." *The Lancet* 134:105–7.

Brown, E. R., and P. E. Sawchenko. 1997. "Hypophysiotropic CRF neurons display a sustained immediate-early gene response to chronic stress but not to adrenalectomy." *J. Neuroendocrinol.* 9 (4):307–16. doi: 10.1046/j.1365-2826.1997.00586.x.

Chen, K. C., E. M. Blalock, M. A. Curran-Rauhut, I. Kadish, S. J. Blalock, L. Brewer, N. M. Porter, and P. W. Landfield. 2013. "Glucocorticoid-dependent hippocampal transcriptome in male rats: Pathway-specific alterations with aging." *Endocrinology* 154 (8):2807–20. doi: 10.1210/en.2013-1139.

Chen, Y. F., N. Y. Weltman, X. Li, S. Youmans, D. Krause, and A. M. Gerdes. 2013. "Improvement of left ventricular remodeling after myocardial infarction with eight weeks L-thyroxine treatment in rats." *J. Transl. Med.* 11:40. doi: 10.1186/1479-5876-11-40.

Creque, H. M., R. Langer, and J. Folkman. 1980. "One month of sustained release of insulin from a polymer implant." *Diabetes* 29 (1):37–40. doi: 10.2337/diab.29.1.37.

DeRose, Y. S., K. M. Gligorich, G. Wang, A. Georgelas, P. Bowman, S. J. Courdy, A. L. Welm, and B. E. Welm. 2013. "Patient-derived models of human breast cancer: Protocols for in vitro and in vivo applications in tumor biology and translational medicine." *Curr. Protoc. Pharmacol.* 60 (1):14–23. doi: 10.1002/0471141755.ph1423s60.

Diniz, L., T. B. dos Santos, L. R. Britto, I. C. Cespedes, M. C. Garcia, R. C. Spadari-Bratfisch, C. C. Medalha, G. M. de Castro, F. T. Montesano, and M. B. Viana. 2013. "Effects of chronic treatment with corticosterone and imipramine on fos immunoreactivity and adult hippocampal neurogenesis." *Behav. Brain Res.* 238:170–7. doi: 10.1016/j.bbr.2012.10.024.

Dubal, D. B., M. L. Kashon, L. C. Pettigrew, J. M. Ren, S. P. Finklestein, S. W. Rau, and P. M. Wise. 1998. "Estradiol protects against ischemic injury." *J. Cereb. Blood Flow Metab.* 18 (11):1253–8. doi: 10.1097/00004647-199811000-00012.

Dziuk, P. J., and B. Cook. 1966. "Passage of steroids through silicone rubber." *Endocrinology* 78 (1):208–11. doi: 10.1210/endo-78-1-208.

Elsaesser, F., S. Hayashi, N. Parvizi, and F. Ellendorff. 1989. "In vitro characterization of secretion rates from silastic micropellets containing estradiol." *Steroids* 54 (2):159–68. doi: 10.1016/0039-128x(89)90091-3.

Flanagan, L., K. Packman, B. Juba, S. O'Neill, M. Tenniswood, and J. Welsh. 2003. "Efficacy of vitamin D compounds to modulate estrogen receptor negative breast cancer growth and invasion." *J. Steroid Biochem. Mol. Biol.* 84 (2–3):181–92. doi: 10.1016/s0960-0760(03)00028-1.

Fontaine, C., A. Abot, A. Billon-Gales, G. Flouriot, H. Berges, E. Grunenwald, A. Vinel, M. C. Valera, P. Gourdy, and J. F. Arnal. 2013. "Tamoxifen elicits atheroprotection through estrogen receptor alpha AF-1 but does not accelerate reendothelialization." *Am. J. Pathol.* 183 (1):304–12. doi: 10.1016/j.ajpath.2013.03.010.

Frias-Dominguez, C., J. Garduno, S. Hernandez, R. Drucker-Colin, and S. Mihailescu. 2013. "Flattening plasma corticosterone levels increases the prevalence of serotonergic dorsal raphe neurons inhibitory responses to nicotine in adrenalectomised rats." *Brain Res. Bull.* 98:10–22. doi: 10.1016/j.brainresbull.2013.07.006.

Friedman, J. E., J. S. Yun, Y. M. Patel, M. M. McGrane, and R. W. Hanson. 1993. "Glucocorticoids regulate the induction of phosphoenolpyruvate carboxykinase (GTP) gene transcription during diabetes." *J. Biol. Chem.* 268 (17):12952–7.

Fusani, L. 2008. "Endocrinology in field studies: Problems and solutions for the experimental design." *Gen. Comp. Endocrinol.* 157 (3):249–53. doi: 10.1016/j.ygcen.2008.04.016.

Gerard, C., A. Gallez, C. Dubois, P. Drion, P. Delahaut, E. Quertemont, A. Noel, and C. Pequeux. 2017. "Accurate control of 17beta-estradiol long-term release increases reliability and reproducibility of preclinical animal studies." *J. Mammary Gland Biol. Neoplasia* 22 (1):1–11. doi: 10.1007/s10911-016-9368-1.

Gordon, M. N., H. H. Osterburg, P. C. May, and C. E. Finch. 1986. "Effective oral administration of 17 beta-estradiol to female C57BL/6J mice through the drinking water." *Biol. Reprod.* 35 (5):1088–95. doi: 10.1095/biolreprod35.5.1088.

Gottardis, M. M., and V. C. Jordan. 1988. "Development of tamoxifen-stimulated growth of MCF-7 tumors in athymic mice after long-term antiestrogen administration." *Cancer Res.* 48 (18):5183–7.

Handelsman, D. J., A. J. Conway, and L. M. Boylan. 1990. "Pharmacokinetics and pharmacodynamics of testosterone pellets in man." *J. Clin. Endocrinol. Metab.* 71 (1):216–22. doi: 10.1210/jcem-71-1-216.

Hau, M. 2007. "Regulation of male traits by testosterone: Implications for the evolution of vertebrate life histories." *Bioessays* 29 (2):133–44. doi: 10.1002/bies.20524.

Huffman, L. J., C. M. Beighley, D. G. Frazer, W. G. McKinney, and D. W. Porter. 2006. "Increased susceptibility of the lungs of hyperthyroid rats to oxidant injury: Specificity of effects." *Toxicology* 225 (2–3):119–27. doi: 10.1016/j.tox.2006.05.008.

Ingberg, E., A. Theodorsson, E. Theodorsson, and J. O. Strom. 2012. "Methods for long-term 17beta-estradiol administration to mice." Gen. Comp. Endocrinol. 175 (1):188–93. doi: 10.1016/j.ygcen.2011.11.014.

Isaksson, I. M., A. Theodorsson, E. Theodorsson, and J. O. Strom. 2011. "Methods for 17beta-oestradiol administration to rats." *Scand. J. Clin. Lab. Invest.* 71 (7):583–92. doi: 10.3109/00365513.2011.596944.

Jockenhovel, F., E. Vogel, M. Kreutzer, W. Reinhardt, S. Lederbogen, and D. Reinwein. 1996. "Pharmacokinetics and pharmacodynamics of subcutaneous testosterone implants in hypogonadal men." *Clin. Endocrinol. (Oxf)* 45 (1):61–71. doi: 10.1111/j.1365-2265.1996.tb02061.x.

Jung, E. Y., B. J. Lee, Y. W. Yun, J. K. Kang, I. J. Baek, M. Y. Jurg, Y. B. Lee, H. S. Sohn, J. Y. Lee, K. S. Kim, W. J. Yu, J. C. Do, Y. C. Kim, and S. Y. Nam. 2004. "Effects of exposure to genistein and estradiol on reproductive development in immature male mice weaned from dams adapted to a soy-based commercial diet." *J. Vet. Med. Sci.* 66 (11):1347–54. doi: 10.1292/jvms.66.1347.

Jung, M. E., S. H. Yang, A. M. Brun-Zinkernagel, and J. W. Simpkins. 2002. "Estradiol protects against cerebellar damage and motor deficit in ethanol-withdrawn rats." *Alcohol* 26 (2):83–93. doi: 10.1016/s0741-8329(01)00199-9.

Kelleher, S., A. J. Conway, and D. J. Handelsman. 2001. "Influence of implantation site and track geometry on the extrusion rate and pharmacology of testosterone implants." *Clin. Endocrinol. (Oxf)* 55 (4):531–6. doi: 10.1046/j.1365-2265.2001.01357.x.

Kelleher, S., C. Howe, A. J. Conway, and D. J. Handelsman. 2004. "Testosterone release rate and duration of action of testosterone pellet implants." *Clin. Endocrinol. (Oxf)* 60 (4):420–8. doi: 10.1111/j.1365-2265.2004.01994.x.

Ketterson, E. D., and V. Nolan, Jr. 1999. "Adaptation, exaptation, and constraint: A hormonal perspective." Am. Nat. 154 (S1):S4–25. doi: 10.1086/303280.

Kivisaari, J., and J. Niinikoski. 1973. "Use of silastic tube and capillary sampling technic in the measurement of tissue PO 2 and PCO 2." *Am. J. Surg.* 125 (5):623–7. doi: 10.1016/0002-9610(73)90149-9.

Lee, B. J., J. K. Kang, E. Y. Jung, Y. W. Yun, I. J. Baek, J. M. Yon, Y. B. Lee, H. S. Sohn, J. Y. Lee, K. S. Kim, and S. Y. Nam. 2004. "Exposure to genistein does not adversely affect the reproductive system in adult male mice adapted to a soy-based commercial diet." *J. Vet. Sci.* 5 (3):227–34.

Lee, T. W., and J. R. Robinson. 2000. *Remington: The Science and Practice of Pharmacy.* 2nd Edition. Baltimore: Lippincott Williams and Wilkins.

Levin-Allerhand, J. A., K. Sokol, and J. D. Smith. 2003. "Safe and effective method for chronic 17beta-estradiol administration to mice." *Contemp. Top. Lab. Anim. Sci.* 42 (6):33–5.

Li, J. J., S. J. Weroha, W. L. Lingle, D. Papa, J. L. Salisbury, and S. A. Li. 2004. "Estrogen mediates Aurora-A overexpression, centrosome amplification, chromosomal instability, and breast cancer in female ACI rats." *Proc. Natl. Acad. Sci. U S A* 101 (52):18123–8. doi: 10.1073/pnas.0408273101.

Lordi, N.G. 1987. "Sustained release dosage forms." In The Theory and Practice of Industrial Pharmacy, edited by Lachman, L., Lieberman, H. A., Kanig, J. L., 430–456. Bombay, India: Varghese Publishing House.

McQuilling, J. P., S. Sittadjody, R. Pareta, S. Pendergraft, C. J. Clark, A. C. Farney, and E. C. Opara. 2017. "Retrieval of microencapsulated islet grafts for post-transplant evaluation." *Methods Mol. Biol.* 1479:157–71. doi: 10.1007/978-1-4939-6364-5_12.

McQuilling, J. P., S. Sittadjody, S. Pendergraft, A. C. Farney, and E. C. Opara. 2017. "Applications of particulate oxygen-generating substances (POGS) in the bioartificial pancreas." *Biomater. Sci.* 5 (12):2437–47. doi: 10.1039/c7bm00790f.

Miller, L., and J. S. Hunt. 1998. "Regulation of TNF-alpha production in activated mouse macrophages by progesterone." *J. Immunol.* 160 (10):5098–104.

Muller-Fielitz, H., M. Lau, O. Johren, F. Stellmacher, M. Schwaninger, and W. Raasch. 2012. "Blood pressure response to angiotensin II is enhanced in obese Zucker rats and is attributed to an aldosterone-dependent mechanism." *Br. J. Pharmacol.* 166 (8):2417–29. doi: 10.1111/j.1476-5381.2012.01953.x.

Nicolls, M. R., S. Mizuno, L. Taraseviciene-Stewart, L. Farkas, J. I. Drake, A. Al Husseini, J. G. Gomez-Arroyo, N. F. Voelkel, and H. J. Bogaard. 2012. "New models of pulmonary hypertension based on VEGF receptor blockade-induced endothelial cell apoptosis." *Pulm. Circ.* 2 (4):434–42. doi: 10.4103/2045-8932.105031.

Opara, E. C., J. P. McQuilling, and A. C. Farney. 2013. "Microencapsulation of pancreatic islets for use in a bioartificial pancreas." *Methods Mol. Biol.* 1001:261–6. doi: 10.1007/978-1-62703-363-3_21.

Quispe, R., M. Trappschuh, M. Gahr, and W. Goymann. 2015. "Towards more physiological manipulations of hormones in field studies: Comparing the release dynamics of three kinds of testosterone implants, silastic tubing, time-release pellets and beeswax." Gen. Comp. Endocrinol. 212:100–5. doi: 10.1016/j.ygcen.2015.01.007.

Schaschkow, A., C. Mura, S. Dal, A. Langlois, E. Seyfritz, C. Sookhareea, W. Bietiger, C. Peronet, N. Jeandidier, M. Pinget, S. Sigrist, and E. Maillard. 2016. "Impact of the type of continuous insulin administration on metabolism in a diabetic rat model." *J. Diabetes Res.* 2016:8310516. doi: 10.1155/2016/8310516.

Shi, J., J. D. Bui, S. H. Yang, Z. He, T. H. Lucas, D. L. Buckley, S. J. Blackband, M. A. King, A. L. Day, and J. W. Simpkins. 2001. "Estrogens decrease reperfusion-associated cortical ischemic damage: An MRI analysis in a transient focal ischemia model." *Stroke* 32 (4):987–92. doi: 10.1161/01.str.32.4.987.

Simpkins, J. W., G. Rajakumar, Y. Q. Zhang, C. E. Simpkins, D. Greenwald, C. J. Yu, N. Bodor, and A. L. Day. 1997. "Estrogens may reduce mortality and ischemic damage caused by middle cerebral artery occlusion in the female rat." *J. Neurosurg.* 87 (5):724–30. doi: 10.3171/jns.1997.87.5.0724.

Singh, M., E. M. Meyer, and J. W. Simpkins. 1995. "The effect of ovariectomy and estradiol replacement on brain-derived neurotrophic factor messenger ribonucleic acid expression in cortical and hippocampal brain regions of female Sprague-Dawley rats." *Endocrinology* 136 (5):2320–4. doi: 10.1210/endo.136.5.7720680.

Singh, M., N. Sumien, C. Kyser, and J. W. Simpkins. 2008. "Estrogens and progesterone as neuroprotectants: What animal models teach us." *Front Biosci.* 13:1083–9. doi: 10.2741/2746.

Sittadjody, S., J. M. Saul, J. P. McQuilling, S. Joo, T. C. Register, J. J. Yoo, A. Atala, and E. C. Opara. 2017. "In vivo transplantation of 3D encapsulated ovarian constructs in rats corrects abnormalities of ovarian failure." *Nat. Commun.* 8 (1):1858. doi: 10.1038/s41467-017-01851-3.

Sittadjody, S., J. M. Saul, S. Joo, J. J. Yoo, A. Atala, and E. C. Opara. 2013. "Engineered multilayer ovarian tissue that secretes sex steroids and peptide hormones in response to gonadotropins." Biomaterials 34 (10):2412–20. doi: 10.1016/j.biomaterials.2012.11.059.

Sittadjody, S., K. M. Enck, A. Wells, J. J. Yoo, A. Atala, J. M. Saul, and E. C. Opara. 2019. "Encapsulation of mesenchymal stem cells in 3D ovarian cell constructs promotes stable and long-term hormone secretion with improved physiological outcomes in a syngeneic rat model." *Ann. Biomed. Eng.* doi: 10.1007/s10439-019-02334-w.

Strom, J. O., A. Theodorsson, E. Ingberg, I. M. Isaksson, and E. Theodorsson. 2012. "Ovariectomy and 17beta-estradiol replacement in rats and mice: A visual demonstration." J. Vis. Exp. (64):e4013. doi: 10.3791/4013.

Strom, J. O., E. Theodorsson, and A. Theodorsson. 2008. "Order of magnitude differences between methods for maintaining physiological 17beta-oestradiol concentrations in ovariectomized rats." Scand. J. Clin. Lab. Invest. 68 (8):814–22. doi: 10.1080/00365510802409703.

Strom, J. O., E. Theodorsson, L. Holm, and A. Theodorsson. 2010. "Different methods for administering 17beta-estradiol to ovariectomized rats result in opposite effects on ischemic brain damage." BMC Neurosci. 11:39. doi: 10.1186/1471-2202-11-39.

Theodorsson, A., and E. Theodorsson. 2005. "Estradiol increases brain lesions in the cortex and lateral striatum after transient occlusion of the middle cerebral artery in rats: No effect of ischemia on galanin in the stroke area but decreased levels in the hippocampus." Peptides 26 (11):2257–64. doi: 10.1016/j.peptides.2005.04.013.

Theodorsson, A., S. Hilke, O. Rugarn, D. Linghammar, and E. Theodorsson. 2005. "Serum concentrations of 17beta-estradiol in ovariectomized rats during two times six weeks crossover treatment by daily injections in comparison with slow-release pellets." Scand. J. Clin. Lab. Invest. 65 (8):699–705. doi: 10.1080/00365510500375206.

Thompson, C. I., J. W. Munford, E. H. Buell, R. J. Karry, C. T. Lee, B. L. Morgan, and A. J. Radnovich. 2002. "Plasma constituents and mortality in rat pups given chronic insulin via injection, pellet, or osmotic minipump." Can. J. Physiol. Pharmacol. 80 (3):180–92. doi: 10.1139/y02-020.

van den Berg, M. P., P. Merkus, S. G. Romeijn, J. C. Verhoef, and F. W. Merkus. 2004. "Uptake of melatonin into the cerebrospinal fluid after nasal and intravenous delivery: Studies in rats and comparison with a human study." Pharm. Res. 21 (5):799–802. doi: 10.1023/b:pham.0000026431.55383.69.

Vaysburd, M., C. Lock, and H. McDevitt. 1995. "Prevention of insulin-dependent diabetes mellitus in nonobese diabetic mice by immunogenic but not by tolerated peptides." J. Exp. Med. 182 (3):897–902. doi: 10.1084/jem.182.3.897.

Wahjoepramono, E. J., L. K. Wijaya, K. Taddei, K. A. Bates, M. Howard, G. Martins, K. deRuyck, P. M. Matthews, G. Verdile, and R. N. Martins. 2011. "Direct exposure of guinea pig CNS to human luteinizing hormone increases cerebrospinal fluid and cerebral beta amyloid levels." Neuroendocrinology 94 (4):313–22. doi: 10.1159/000330812.

Weisberg, A. D., F. Albornoz, J. P. Griffin, D. L. Crandall, H. Elokdah, A. B. Fogo, D. E. Vaughan, and N. J. Brown. 2005. "Pharmacological inhibition and genetic deficiency of plasminogen activator inhibitor-1 attenuates angiotensin II/salt-induced aortic remodeling." Arterioscler. Thromb. Vasc. Biol. 25 (2):365–71. doi: 10.1161/01.ATV.0000152356.85791.52.

Wen, Y., S. Yang, R. Liu, E. Perez, K. D. Yi, P. Koulen, and J. W. Simpkins. 2004. "Estrogen attenuates nuclear factor-kappa B activation induced by transient cerebral ischemia." Brain Res. 1008 (2):147–54. doi: 10.1016/j.brainres.2004.02.019.

Yang, C. H., A. Almomen, Y. S. Wee, E. A. Jarboe, C. M. Peterson, and M. M. Janat-Amsbury. 2015. "An estrogen-induced endometrial hyperplasia mouse model recapitulating human disease progression and genetic aberrations." Cancer Med. 4 (7):1039–50. doi: 10.1002/cam4.445.

Yang, S. H., Z. He, S. S. Wu, Y. J. He, J. Cutright, W. J. Millard, A. L. Day, and J. W. Simpkins. 2001. "17-beta estradiol can reduce secondary ischemic damage and mortality of subarachnoid hemorrhage." J. Cereb. Blood Flow Metab. 21 (2):174–81. doi: 10.1097/00004647-200102000-00009.

Zera, A. J., L. G. Harshman, and T. D. Williams. 2007. "Evolutionary endocrinology: The developing synthesis between endocrinology and evolutionary genetics." Annu. Rev. Ecol. Evol. Syst. 38:793–817.

7 Delivery of Ovarian Hormones for Bone Health

Justin M. Saul
Miami University

CONTENTS

7.1 INTRODUCTION

Bone health is a significant factor in overall health and quality of life.[1] Osteoporosis the most common bone disease and is a leading threat to bone and overall health. Clinical presentation with osteoporosis is associated with fractures of the wrist, hip, and spine as well as increased morbidity.[1] There are numerous factors that contribute to osteoporosis including genetics (via multiple genes),[118] diet (e.g., vitamin D and calcium intake),[81] and lifestyle (e.g., smoking and alcohol use).[81] However, given that women are at a four-fold greater risk of osteoporosis than men,[9] it is clear that there is a significant contribution from hormonal factors. The female ovaries are among the key components of the female endocrine system. The primary function of the ovaries can be associated with reproduction. However, both the direct systemic effects of the ovarian hormones as well as the effects of these hormones on other endocrine hormones from the hypothalamus and anterior pituitary have significant impacts on female physiology including bone. The loss of ovarian function due to genetic conditions, ablative therapies for diseases such as cancer, or menopause leads to alterations in the profiles of ovarian and associated hormones compared to normal, healthy individuals.

The use of hormone replacement therapy with estrogen alone or in combination with progesterone was a logical approach in the care and treatment of women in addressing not only bone health but also other systemic effects of the ovarian hormones such as cardiovascular health, libido, and neurological function. Hormone replacement therapy was widely used shortly after the discovery of the role of ovarian hormones on systemic female physiology until the early 2000s.[57] However, clinical studies in the late 1990s and early 2000s led to a large decline in the use of hormone therapy, primarily for reasons not related to bone health. Follow-up and follow-on studies in the past 20 years have shown that the use of ovarian hormone therapies is highly complex and depends on the individual, the timing of the therapy, the specific hormones used, the source of hormones, and the route of administration.[101]

In this chapter, we first consider the basic functions and hormones produced by the ovaries as well as the specific cell types involved. While the role of estrogen and progesterone will be clear, this discussion should also demonstrate that anterior pituitary hormones such as FSH play a significant role in bone health. Moreover, the role of ovarian hormones that is not included in hormone replacement therapy such as inhibin will also be discussed. A brief discussion on osteoporosis will help to highlight the key cellular and molecular mechanisms by which ovarian hormones impact bone health. Given the role of delivery route on safety and efficacy of the drugs, we then consider several mechanisms of controlled release of estrogen and progesterone. The net result of this discussion suggests that while estrogen and progesterone are critical ovarian hormones to consider, the impact of other ovarian hormones on bone or on hormones of the anterior pituitary is also important and yet is not considered in the formulation for pharmacological hormone therapy. We suggest that in order to achieve safer and more effective hormone therapies, cell-based approaches for the delivery of ovarian hormones should be considered. Cell-based approaches rely on strategies and knowledge developed from the fields of tissue engineering and regenerative medicine and offer a unique modality by which hormone therapy could be used in the future to safely enhance female bone health and overall quality of life.

7.2 THE FEMALE OVARY

The ovary is one of the key female sexual organs. The ovaries are connected to the uterus via the fallopian tubes. Within the ovary is found the individual ovarian follicles, which are the primary functional units of ovaries. The number of follicles varies over the course of the female's lifetime. During development, approximately 6×10^6 follicles are present, but this number declines to about 2×10^6 at birth and 300,000 at the onset of puberty. Although one ovum is expelled by an ovarian follicle each month, other follicles degenerate as well, such that by the onset of menopause, very few follicles remain. Indeed, even the few remaining follicles present at the onset of menopause ultimately degenerate. From birth until about the onset of puberty, follicles are in a primordial state where cells known as granulosa cells provide support for oocytes. At the onset of puberty, the granulosa cells undergo growth and proliferation. This, in turn, leads to an increase in follicular size to what is known as the primary follicle.[67]

Also at the onset of puberty, the anterior pituitary begins to produce large amounts of follicle stimulating hormone (FSH) and luteinizing hormone (LH). During the woman's monthly sexual cycle, some primary follicles (6–12 per month) exhibit additional growth via further granulosa cell proliferation. At this time, another class of cells called theca cells arise, some of which develop to a state in which they can secrete ovarian hormones. In a feedforward mechanism, granulosa cells respond to FSH from the anterior pituitary, and both granulosa and theca cells then undergo further growth and proliferation to form antral and then vesicular follicles. During this phase, both granulosa and theca cells become susceptible to LH. At this point, all but one of the follicles that had reached the antral or vesicular stage undergo atresia, which is the degeneration of the follicles. In turn, one of the follicles further matures into a mature follicle, which will be involved in ovulation via expulsion of the oocyte.[67]

Immediately before ovulation, a surge in LH as well as FSH leads to a further increase in the follicle size. The LH leads to increased levels of progesterone production from both the granulosa and theca cells. When the oocyte is expelled from the follicle during ovulation, the remaining cells of the mature follicle undergo luteinization and form what is known as the corpus luteum. During this period, both estrogen and progesterone are produced in increasing amounts by the granulosa cells while the theca cells produce androgens such as testosterone. Ultimately, ovulation followed by luteinization leads to degeneration of the remaining follicular cells.[67]

However, during the luteal phase and before degeneration, the production of estrogen and progesterone leads to feedback control over the anterior pituitary and the secretion of FSH and LH. In addition, other hormones are secreted by the ovaries. For example, during this period, inhibin is also secreted and is known to have inhibitory effects on both anterior pituitary (FSH and LH secretion) as well as hypothalamic secretion of gonadotropin-releasing hormone (GnRH) that is responsible, in part, for the stimulation of the anterior pituitary to secrete FSH and LH.

There are two main points to be noted here. First, when taken together, these processes of follicular growth and, ultimately, degeneration are responsible for the well-known cycles in estrogen and progesterone production during the monthly female sexual cycle. Second, in endocrine tissues, particular cell types are typically considered to have primary responsibility for the production of a particular hormone. Generally, granulosa cells are associated with estrogen production and theca cells with progesterone production. However, as can be seen from the discussion above, this is more complex in the ovaries as, for example, granulosa cells also produce progesterone. More specifically, the granulosa and theca cells cannot act independently of each other if proper function is to be achieved. Granulosa cells are responsive to FSH (and, to a lesser extent, LH) to produce progesterone. This progesterone from the granulosa cells as well as progesterone produced by the theca cells is used to produce androgens in the theca cell. These androgens are, in turn, secreted to the granulosa cells where they are converted to estrogen. Thus, in the absence of theca cells, granulosa cells have a greatly diminished ability to produce estrogen. As we will discuss at the end of this chapter, this interaction between these two cell types is part of the impetus for cell-based ovarian hormone replacement strategies.

As discussed earlier the number of follicles that a female has decreases from *in utero* to birth to puberty. This decrease continues not only during her reproductive years (approximately ages 13–51) due to the processes described above but also due resorption of other follicles. By the time a woman reaches *menopause*, very few follicles (~1,000) remain.[125] As a result, estrogen and progesterone levels decline to much lower levels following menopause. It should also be noted that there are numerous other causes for the loss of ovarian failure such as genetic conditions or ablation due to cancer therapy; conditions that are considered premature ovarian failure (POF). Whether via POF or menopause, this loss of ovarian hormones has profound systemic physiological effects. In the discussion throughout this chapter, we will focus on effects of ovarian-hormone loss on bone. However, we will also note several more systemic effects. It should also be noted that this chapter is strictly focused on the loss of ovarian hormones; as such the discussion is focused on women. However, men also produce these same hormones that are the focus of this chapter: estrogen, progesterone, activin, inhibin, and testosterone. Clearly, these hormones are not produced by the ovaries in men, but may be secreted from peripheral organs or from organs that make up the hypothalamus–pituitary–gonad (HPG) axis. Thus, although we are referring to these hormones as "ovarian hormones," they are not strictly produced by the ovaries and are also not strictly female hormones. Nonetheless, in women, the ovaries are the primary source of these hormones, and the loss of ovarian function ultimately impacts a woman's health, including susceptibility to loss of bone mineral density (BMD) and the onset of osteoporosis.

7.3 OSTEOPOROSIS

The ovarian hormones as well as other hormones from the hypothalamus–(anterior) pituitary–ovary (HPO) axis affect bone activity via osteoblasts, osteoclasts, and inflammatory cells. Osteoporosis literally means "porous bone." Osteoporosis affects ~10 million women in the U.S.[166] and over

200 million people worldwide.[35] Osteoporosis, in and of itself, is not problematic and is typically asymptomatic. However, it is when bone becomes so porous or fragile that collapse (e.g., of vertebra) or fracture (e.g., in wrist or femoral neck) occurs under conditions in which fracture would not ordinarily occur that it becomes problematic. Fractures of the vertebra, wrist, and femoral neck are most common.[158] The resulting pain is a quality of life issue, but the resulting effects (e.g., reduced mobility) can lead to the onset of secondary conditions, leading to an increased risk of death.[21]

Indeed, osteoporosis is the leading cause of bone fracture with direct costs alone expected to reach $25 billion by 2025.[5] BMD is widely used to determine whether a patient has osteoporosis and is prone to fracture risk. BMD is typically reported as a T-score, which normalizes BMD to the average BMD of a healthy, young adult. Per the World Health Organization, a T-score within ± standard deviation of 0 is considered normal. T-scores of −1 to −2.5 standard deviations below 0 indicate low bone mass, which is often considered osteopenia. T-scores of more than −2.5 standard deviations from 0 indicate osteoporosis and thus has an increased risk of fracture.[3] While BMD has been a traditional measure for osteoporosis, it is not particularly accurate in predicting risks of bone fracture.[31,91] The use of BMD in conjunction with analysis of other risk factors, such as age, smoking history, family history of hip fracture, glucocorticoid use, and arthritis, has led to a more accurate prediction of fracture risk known as the Fracture Risk Assessment Tool (FRAX) method.[154] Blood testing for bone turnover markers such as the C-telopeptide of collagen may allow further predictive capacity of osteoporosis and the likelihood of fracture.[137,161] Unfortunately, bone fracture remains the most likely clinical presentation of osteoporosis.[154]

Osteoporosis is four times more prevalent in women than in men, reflecting the underlying role of hormones in the condition. It is not surprising, then, that for women, hormone therapies were the first clinically used treatments for osteoporosis.

7.4 OVARIAN HORMONE MECHANISMS OF ACTION AND EFFECTS OF OVARIAN HORMONE LOSS ON BONE

7.4.1 Ovarian Hormone Systemic Effects

The ovaries are part of the complex HPO axis (Figure 7.1). This system operates through the secretion of GnRH from the hypothalamus to the anterior pituitary via the hypophyseal portal system of the infundibulum,[2] as triggered by upstream signals such as kisspeptin cells in the diencephalon.[90] GnRH, in turn, leads to secretion of FSH and LH from the anterior pituitaries, which enter the bloodstream to reach the ovaries, where they promote secretion of estrogen, progesterone, and other hormones. The secretion of estrogen and progesterone as well as hormones, including activin, inhibin, and testosterone, from the ovaries have feedforward and feedback control mechanisms on the secretion of the hypothalamic and pituitary hormones. As such, loss of the ovarian hormones due to loss of ovarian function has systemic effects not only on target tissues, to be discussed below, but also on the hormone levels of the hypothalamic and pituitary hormones. That is, the loss or change in ovarian hormone production (e.g., estrogen and inhibin) and blood concentrations also leads to changes in plasma concentrations of the anterior pituitary hormones before, during, and after menopause.[104,123] Although changes in the ovarian hormone levels affect hypothalamus and pituitary hormones, the converse is also true. Indeed, changes in plasma levels of FSH and changes in LH and GnRH are observed prior to decreases in estrogen and progesterone concentrations associated with the menopausal transition.[146]

It should be noted that the ovaries are not the only source of estrogens. Other cells with aromatase activity such as mesenchymal stem cells of adipose tissue, osteoblasts, vascular endothelial cells, and smooth muscle cells can also produce this hormone,[138] so estrogen is not completely eliminated during menopause. However, following menopause, the baseline levels in women is greatly reduced compared to the premenopausal period.

The ovarian hormones and, more broadly, hormones of the HPO axis have effects on numerous metabolic components and tissues throughout the body. As such, changes or disruption of these

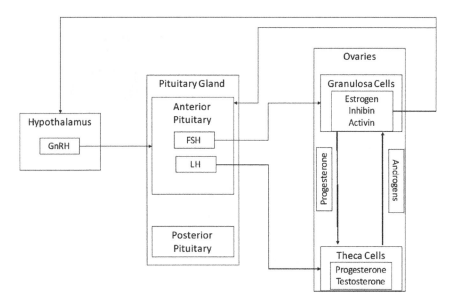

FIGURE 7.1 Schematic overview of the HPO axis. Shown are the key endocrine organs (hypothalamus, pituitary, and ovaries), the hormones secreted by each organ, and known feedback or interactions between the organs via secreted hormones. It should be noted that estrogen, inhibin, activin, progesterone, and testosterone can be secreted by both granulosa and theca cells, but they are shown with secretion from the cell that has primary responsibility for their secretion.

HPO axis hormones due to menopause cause observable changes in women. Well-known examples include increases in body weight and body fat composition, decreased libido, and decreases in bone mass and mineral density. Decreases in bone mass and mineral density commonly lead to osteoporosis or porous bone.

Prior to menopause or loss of ovarian function, the hormones of the HPO axis impact bone activity in several ways. The most prominent and well-understood effects are related to estrogen. Estrogen has effects on both osteoblasts responsible for mineralized bone deposition as well as osteoclasts responsible for bone deposition. Under homeostatic conditions, the rates of bone deposition and resorption are approximately equal. However, estrogen has impacts on other cell types that play a role in bone homeostasis including osteocytes and immune cells.[85]

7.4.2 Estrogen Mechanisms of Action in Bone

Estrogen has intracellular receptors in tissues throughout the body that can impact gene expression. As can be seen by its structure (Figure 7.2), estrogen is a lipophilic molecule readily capable of crossing the lipidic cellular membrane. Estrogen then binds to estrogen receptors, which achieve activity primarily through transcriptional control via direct binding to DNA after estrogen binding. However, the estrogen receptors also act indirectly through "tethering" effects to other transcription factors, nongenomically through estrogen-bound to extracellular receptors, or independent of ligands through the pathways of other growth factors.[72] Estrogen is known to have antiapoptotic effects on osteoblasts and osteocytes while also having proapoptotic effects on osteoclasts. Both of these promote an increase in bone mass. As such, the loss of estrogen due to menopause leads to decreased bone mass, as discussed above in regards to osteoporosis. Estrogen deficiency leads to increases in both osteoclast and osteoblast numbers and their related activities in bone resorption and deposition, respectively.[99] However, it is important to remember that it is the balance of resorption and deposition that ultimately dictates the total bone mass.

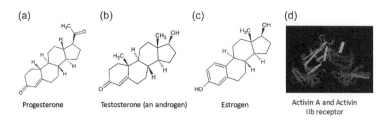

(a)	(b)	(c)	(d)
Progesterone	Testosterone (an androgen)	Estrogen	Activin A and Activin IIb receptor

FIGURE 7.2 Schematics of key ovarian hormones secreted by granulosa and/or theca cells. (a) Both granulosa and theca cells produce progesterone from cholesterol via CYP11A1 and 3β-hydroxysteroid dehydrogenase (HSD) enzymes. Granulosa cells secrete progesterone to theca cells. (b) Androgens such as testosterone are primarily formed in theca cells via conversion of progesterone via the CYP17A1 enzyme. Androgens are secreted from theca cells to granulosa cells. (c) Estrogens are primarily secreted by granulosa cells by conversion of androgens via the CYP19A1 (aromatase) enzyme. In addition to these cholesterol-derived hormones, ovarian cells (primarily granulosa cells) also secrete activin and inhibin. Structurally, activin and inhibin are similar and part of the TGF-β superfamily. (d) Activin A interacting with the activin IIb receptor is shown.[64] (Image from Cn3D software rendering of Protein Database ID 1SY4). Unlike the cholesterol-derived hormones, activin and inhibin are polypeptides that act on extracellular rather than intracellular receptors.

The two known receptors for estrogen are estrogen receptor α (ER-α) and estrogen receptor β (ER-β). Tissues with estrogen receptors include female-specific tissues, such as uterus and mammary glands, as well as other major organs/tissues including heart, liver, kidney, spleen, lung, components of the gastrointestinal tract, and skeletal muscle demonstrated estrogen receptors.[119] Given the role of estrogen in osteoporosis, it is not surprising that estrogen receptors are also found in bone tissue.

There are numerous mechanisms by which estrogen acts on bone tissue, and these are regulated by the relative actions and expression levels of ER-α and ER-β. It has been suggested that ER-α and ER-β have opposing effects to each other.[85] For example, knockout mice for the ER-β (i.e., mice without ER-β) have been shown to have longer femurs than wild type, whereas knockout mice for the ER-α have been shown to have shorter femurs than wild type. More globally, it has been shown that gene expression that is transcriptionally controlled by the ER-α in the presence of estrogen is higher when ER-β is inactivated, implying that ER-β inhibits ER-α transcription.[93] This so-called "ying-yang" effect[93] highlights the potentially opposing roles of ER-α and ER-β in bone.

Below, we discuss ER-α and ER-β expression in osteoblasts, osteocytes, osteoprogenitors, and osteoclasts. Because the two receptors have also been shown to be expressed in immune cells, which play a role in regulation of bone tissue, these are discussed as well. In each of these examples, the trend of opposing actions of the ER-α and ER-β will be highlighted. We will not discuss all possible mechanisms, but we do seek to show several of these as they relate to bone tissue deposition or resorption. In particular, we will discuss the role of FSH in osteoporosis (see Section 7.4.3).

7.4.2.1 Bone Deposition: Osteoblasts, Osteoprogenitors, and Osteocytes

The cells responsible for bone deposition are called osteoblasts. Osteoblasts are derived from osteoprogenitor cells, which in turn are derived from marrow-stromal cells or bone marrow-derived mesenchymal stem cells. Osteoblasts, in turn, ultimately differentiate into osteocytes, which are associated with sensing and responding to mechanical loading. Each of these cell types are thus, either directly or indirectly, involved in the deposition of the new bone matrix.

Estrogen itself has well-known effects on osteoblasts, which include inhibition of apoptosis. Loss of estrogen, therefore, leads to increases in osteoblastic apoptosis. As noted earlier, loss of estrogen actually leads to an increase in the formation of osteoblast cells in the bone marrow (known as osteoblastogenesis).[79] Intuitively, this would suggest the loss of estrogen would promote enhanced bone deposition, but it is again important to remember that it is the balance of bone deposition and resorption that dictates bone mass, and the activity of osteoblasts directly impacts osteoclasts through secretion of growth factors and cytokines.[99] In fact, osteoclastogenesis is also upregulated during estrogen loss, and the level of osteoclastogenesis outpaces osteoblastogenesis,[99] leading to greater overall bone turnover and loss of bone mass. Stated differently, there is a great deal of interplay between osteoblasts and osteoclasts, and their activities cannot (in a healthy individual) be decoupled.

Mature osteoblasts have been shown to express both ER-α and ER-β.[22,23] To investigate the effects of ER-α, the ER-α has been inactivated by using an osteocalcin-promoter regulated cyclic recombinase (known as the Cre system). Osteocalcin is produced only by mature osteoblasts, so this provides a system to selectively inactivate the ER-α in osteoblasts. Inactivation of the ER-α in osteoblasts led to reductions in bone volume for both trabecular and cortical bone, though effects in cortical bone were more pronounced.[98] The same osteocalcin-Cre system has also been shown to affect bone strength, which could have implications in osteoporotic fracture. Moreover, no effect on osteoclastic activity was observed in this model system, indicating that bone strength effects were associated with reduced osteoblast activity associated with ER-α inactivation.[105] It is important to reiterate that there are clearly sex-associated differences, and the effects noted above for bone mass were observed in female mice. In contrast, no effects of ER-α inactivation on bone mass were observed in young males, and only trabecular bone was affected in older male mice.

While estrogen receptors can act in conjunction with estrogen, they can also act independently of it. For example, both estrogen and mechanical strain have been shown to increase thymidine incorporation, indicating the ability to enhance cell proliferation. In addition, it was shown that epidermal growth factor (EGF), which interacts with estrogen receptors, enhanced mitosis. Conversely, truncated forms of insulin-like growth factor 1 and 2 (tIGF-1 and tIGF-2) and basic fibroblast growth factor (bFGF), which do not interact with estrogen receptors, did not have a mitogenic effect.[37,38] Again, sufficient numbers of osteoblasts must be present to balance bone resorption of osteoclasts, so the ability to promote osteoblast proliferation is important in hormone-based approaches to prevent osteoporosis.

Another way that sufficient numbers of osteoblasts can be achieved is through differentiation from osteoprogenitor cells, which have also been shown to express estrogen receptors.[113] The ER-α has been shown to enhance both proliferation (i.e., production of more osteoprogenitors) and differentiation (i.e., formation of osteoblasts) in osteoprogenitor cells, though this effect did not require estrogen. However, ER-α expression in osteoprogenitor cells also provides an estrogen-dependent protection in cortical bone resorption.[7] The net effect of both of these actions, then, is to increase cortical bone mass.

ER-α does not require the presence of estrogen, though estrogen does provide a beneficial effect and can operate on the receptor.[165] However, as with many other receptor–ligand systems, the presence or absence of estrogen does affect upregulation or downregulation of the receptor.[169] As noted earlier, osteoblasts do have aromatase activity and are capable of secreting small levels of estrogen, which adds a confounding effect to consider since autocrine activity becomes possible. Finally, although some studies suggest that one particular cell type (e.g., osteoprogenitors) has the primary role in the formation of particular types of bone (e.g., cortical bone), it is clear that interplay between osteoprogenitors, osteoblasts, and osteocytes as well as the interaction of each of these with osteoclasts is important in maintaining bone health and is responsible for the changes in bone health observed during osteoporosis.

7.4.2.2 Osteoclasts and Immune Cells

As noted above, it is the balance of osteoblast and osteoclast activity that ultimately determines loss of bone mass. Osteoclasts are derived from the same lineage as monocytes and macrophages. Given the known role of monocytes and macrophages in processes of phagocytosis, it is not surprising that osteoclasts are the cell types primarily responsible for bone resorption. The loss of estrogen leads to both decreased levels of osteoclastic apoptosis[75] and to increased osteoclastogenesis,[78] leading to increased numbers of osteoclasts following menopause. Osteoclastogenesis is partially controlled by interleukin 6 (IL-6), which has been shown to be suppressed by estrogen. Thus, loss of estrogen leads to increased levels of osteoclasts, though only in trabecular bone.[78] Both ER-α and ER-β have been reported in osteoclasts, implicating their role in bone resorption. Deletion of the gene encoding for

ER-α leads to increased production of osteoclasts as well as decreased levels of apoptosis in female osteoclasts, again with these effects being limited to trabecular rather than cortical bone.[102,109]

Osteoclast precursors circulate in peripheral blood[103] and differentiate in response to cytokines. Chief among these are macrophage colony-stimulating factor (M-CSF) and receptor activator of nuclear factor KB ligand (RANKL). RANKL is regulated, in part by cleavage of a soluble form of this ligand from osteoblasts via metalloproteinases,[24] highlighting communication between bone depositing and bone resorbing cells. Thus, the net result of reduced osteoclast apoptosis and increased osteoclast production shifts the balance of bone resorption and deposition toward resorption.

Inflammatory cells are not typically considered "bone cells." However, inflammatory cells can induce effects in each of the bone cell types through secretion of key cytokines.[55] For example, the secretion of IL-1, 3, 6, and 11 as well as leukocyte inhibitory factor (LIF) and tissue necrosis factor (TNF) are known to stimulate osteoclasts while IL-4, 10 and 18 as well as interferon (IFN) gamma are known to inhibit osteoclasts.[100] As noted above, IL-6 is a key mediator in these pathways, is inhibited by estrogen, and impacts osteoclastogenesis.[89] Thus IL-6 and these other cytokines may operate via indirect pathways on bone cells,[160] with their impacts being impacted by estrogen activity (or lack thereof) on the inflammatory cells that produce these cytokines. However, upstream stimulators of IL-6 such as TNF-α[120] also play a role in enhancing osteoclastogenesis. It has also been shown (in a rodent ovariectomy model) that estrogen loss, upregulated IFN-γ is upregulated, leading to enhanced activation and lifespan of T-cells responsible for TNF-α, ultimately leading to increased levels of bone loss.[32] Thus, although inflammatory cells are not directly responsible for bone deposition or resorption, they play an indirect role through cytokine release.

7.4.3 ROLE OF OTHER OVARIAN HORMONES ON BONE MASS

It is well established that estrogen has significant impacts on bone health and that the loss of estrogen through menopause or other ovarian failure leads to a decline in BMD and increased risk of fracture. The other ovarian hormones, however, more likely play both direct and indirect roles. The roles of ovary-secreted inhibin and anterior pituitary-secreted FSH are a good example of this. Menopause leads to clearly observed changes in the HPO axis. FSH levels increase significantly in the menopausal period, but it is known that these FSH increases begin about 5 years prior to the onset of estrogen decline due to depletion of ovarian follicles.[124] FSH levels are impacted further by the loss of estrogen, but inhibin[146] and specifically inhibin B[29] also play demonstrated roles, highlighting the role of nonestrogen ovarian hormones in the regulation of the HPO axis. The fact that FSH levels increase prior to estrogen decline, and the fact that BMD begins to decline during this time period, has led to the suggestion that FSH may directly impact bone mass[147] and a possible direct role for FSH. Through genetic knockout models, this was shown to occur primarily through increased osteoclastic resorption.[147] Later, antibodies to FSH not only verified the role of FSH acting on osteoclasts but also revealed that FSH may also act, by unknown mechanisms, on osteoblasts as well.[170] Nonetheless, there is little argument that estrogen plays a more significant role in bone loss than FSH.[129] The point is to recognize the complex interplay between the ovarian hormones (e.g., estrogen and inhibin) and the other hormones of the HPO axis (e.g., GnRH and FSH) and that perturbation of their functions near the time of menopause yields multiple mechanisms by which bone loss can occur.

7.5 HORMONE THERAPY AND CONTROLLED DELIVERY FOR PROMOTING IMPROVED BONE HEALTH

7.5.1 HORMONE REPLACEMENT THERAPY

Hormone therapy began in the 1930s in the U.S., shortly after the discovery of the role of hormones in menopause.[57] It grew in popularity through the 1990s,[34] with 85 million prescriptions written in 1999.[33] Use was typically short in duration and primarily focused on vasomotor symptoms, but longer-term use was not uncommon.[20] The two most common forms of therapy are estrogen alone or in combination with progesterone. Estrogen alone is typically given as conjugated equine estrogen (brand name Premarin), which consists of several estrogen salts. The progesterone component is typically given as medroxyprogesterone acetate, though other forms and sources of each are used.

The effects of estrogen were largely understood from the context of observational studies and meta-analyses indicated that hormone therapy promoted improved cardiovascular health,[145] improved neurological health,[168] reduced mortality from all causes,[65,71] and led to reduced bone loss[49] and risks of hip fracture.[12] A major shift in the use of hormone therapy occurred in the early 2000s with reports associated with the randomized, clinical trial studies of the Women's Health Initiative (WHI). Reports from the WHI showed that hormone therapy reduced osteoporosis and related fractures.[12,128] However, these studies also showed elevated risks of cardiovascular disease and certain cancers.[6,33,62] Thus, despite benefits to bone health, there was a precipitous decline in the use of hormone therapy following these studies.[27,153] Although other treatments for osteoporosis such as the bisphosphonates and selective estrogen receptor modulators (SERMS) existed, there was nonetheless a dramatic increase in fracture rates as well as overall mortality rates in women in the U.S.[77,82]

The topic of hormone therapy remains heavily debated, and the status of hormone therapy in the U.S. is controversial.[4] Currently, hormone therapy is not a first-line treatment for osteoporosis in the U.S.[59] However, it has been argued that an excess number of deaths have occurred by withholding hormone therapy from women without a uterus.[135] Further, consensus statements have concluded that hormone therapy is effective and appropriate for women who are at a particular risk for fracture.[42,43] In fact, more recent studies have suggested that the primary risks associated with hormone therapy (cardiovascular disease and cancer) are for women who are well into menopause,[59,60] and that hormone therapy may still be appropriate for treatment of peri- and postmenopausal treatment in healthy women.[97] Current recommendations for women taking hormone therapy are that they take the lowest effective dose.[111,142]

Following the reduction in hormone therapy use, it is also not surprising that the use of other therapeutic strategies has increased. The major players in treatment of osteoporosis besides hormone therapy include the bisphosphonates (e.g., alendronate or zoledronic acid), RANKL monoclonal antibodies (e.g., denosumab), teriparapeptide (PTH 1–34), and SERMS (e.g., raloxifene and bazedoxifine).[61] The pharmacodynamics of these drugs is beyond the scope of this chapter. However, there are several general principles that might be noted. First, hormone therapy is comparable to the beneficial effects of the bisphosphonates and SERMS in terms of bone health.[18] As such, from a benefit standpoint, it is likely that hormone therapies will continue to be part of the list of treatment options for menopause and osteoporosis. As noted above, there remains controversy over the use of hormone therapy, but even from a risk/drawback standpoint, the use of hormone therapy is likely a good treatment modality for some women. Second, both the bisphosphonates[50] and SERMS[36,39] have side effects or counterindications that can lead to noncompliance or inability to prescribe, respectively. Lack of compliance is not unique to bisphosphonates or SERMS; it is an issue for most user-delivered drug regimens.[80] Issues of noncompliance are part of the impetus for the use of controlled release delivery of estrogen therapy and other drugs, as will be discussed further below. Finally, these side effects vary from individual to individual. Thus, for some patients, side effects from hormone therapy may be more intolerable than those from the bisphosphonates or vice versa. For this reason, it is important to continue to develop new pharmacological approaches to treat menopause and/or osteoporosis (for a recent review, see Ref.[13]) and to improve on existing, known treatment modalities such that options are available to a physician who is working with the patient to identify the best method of disease treatment and prevention. In addition, treatments that make use of multiple therapies (e.g., bisphosphonates or SERMS in combination with hormone therapy) have also been shown to be beneficial for increasing BMD in patients with osteoporosis.[54,163,164]

One approach to improve upon existing hormone therapy strategies (estrogen alone or with progesterone) is through the use of novel delivery methods. The most prominent delivery method has traditionally been the oral route of administration. When given orally, hormone therapy can achieve systemic effects including those on genitourinary organs, libido, vasomotor, metabolic/weight gain/body fat composition, and bone. Hormone therapies can be tailored to the individual,[143] but use of the lowest effective dose is recommended.[111,142] One problem with oral delivery is first-pass hepatic clearance following absorption from the gastrointestinal tract. This first-pass effect necessitates higher doses than would typically be required if produced naturally (i.e., by the native ovaries).[44] It is thought that some of the systemic effects associated with hormone therapy, particularly effects on the cardiovascular system, can be associated with these high doses. Therefore, methods of delivery that can reduce the required dosage while achieving similar effects would be worthwhile. Further, if systemic effects are not required for a given patient, the oral route may not be desirable. For example, if the primary purpose of the hormone therapy is to prevent vulvovaginal atrophy or to prevent loss of BMD, the oral route may not be ideal. Stated differently, the use of oral delivery when only specific tissues are being targeted leads to systemic side effects with an unnecessary risk for potential adverse outcomes such as cardiovascular disease or cancer. The methods of delivery described below are geared towards reducing overall dose, minimizing systemic side effects, and/or improving outcomes.

Before we consider methods used to achieve controlled release of ovarian hormones for hormone therapy, there is a trend that should be noted. The use of polymeric delivery devices including nanoparticles, microparticles, or monolithic devices made from synthetic polymers, natural polymers, or combinations of these as methods to achieve controlled delivery of pharmacological agents has burgeoned since the 1990s. Examples include nanoparticle delivery for chemotherapy agents in the treatment of tumors,[115] polyanhydride wafers for local release of hydrophobic drugs to brain tumors,[26] drug-eluting stents for cardiovascular disease,[84] and microparticle's slow release of neurological drugs,[63] among others. Yet, a survey of the literature for controlled release of the ovarian hormones for therapeutic intervention shows relatively little progress in the past 15–20 years. Although it may be coincidental, it seems likely that the outcomes of the WHI and the sidelining of hormone therapies have impacted these research and development efforts. While understanding emerging trends is extremely important in the development of pharmaceutics, in the case of hormone therapy, this may represent an unnecessary setback given that the benefits of hormone therapy in early postmenopausal women (ages 50–59) are becoming clearer. For this reason, some of the examples described below have only been conducted *in vitro*, and their effects on bone have not been reported. Similarly, some of the studies have viewed hormone therapy as a potential use due to the hydrophobic nature of the drugs, but have used hydrophobic "model" drug molecules such as daidzein for their *in vitro* studies. This highlights that although there are limited examples of controlled release for ovarian hormones on bone, the developments in controlled release technology can be readily applied and/or modified for hormone therapies.

7.5.2 Transdermal Delivery

Estrogen and progesterone are lipophilic molecules and are therefore quite readily absorbed and transmitted through the skin, where they can be taken up via the subcutaneous vasculature. First-pass hepatic clearance issues can be avoided by this approach, potentially lowering the required dose and minimizing side effects.[30] However, the effects are still potentially systemic in nature. There are two general approaches to transdermal delivery: nonpatch and patch options.

For nonpatch delivery, the hormones are typically incorporated into gels, creams, or sprays. Gels and creams are composed largely of hydrophobic materials such as alcohols, glycerin, and/or mineral oil that allow the drugs to remain solubilized in the gel or cream until slowly absorbed through the skin. Patch delivery options are also widely used and are available as estrogen only (e.g., Alora, Climara Pro, Estroderm) or as estrogen and progesterone in combination (e.g., Combipatch). Clinical examples of these patches have been shown to increase BMDs in hip and lumbar spine.[48,52,112,159] These patch delivery systems are composed of three main parts: (i) a backing, (ii) an adhesive-containing hormone, and (iii) a protective liner. The backing is furthest from the skin and is composed of a translucent film such as polyolefin. The adhesive layer contains hormone as well as acrylic and silicone adhesives and components to aid in hormone suspension such as oleyl alcohol, polyvinyl-pyrrolidone (povidone) and dipropylene glycol. The protective liner is for packaging purposes and is removed prior to adhesion to the skin. These systems are typically replaced about twice per week,[56] potentially improving patient compliance compared to topical applications (gels/creams/sprays) or oral administration (pills).

These and similar transdermal system rely on diffusion of the hormones through the skin. Delivery of estrogen and progesterone via these techniques is largely successful due to their lipophilic nature. However, it is important to remember that estrogen and progesterone are not the only hormones secreted by the ovaries with high importance. In the Cell-Based Hormone Therapy section (see Section 7.6), we will consider how cells can play a role in improving outcomes by providing these other hormones. Should protein hormones such as activin and inhibin be given via such techniques, alternative patch systems are available that are suitable for hormone delivery. Alternatively, poly-meric systems for controlled release of estrogen and progesterone may also allow deduced dosages and minimization of side effects (see Sections 7.5.3–5.4, below). While polymeric nanoparticles may be delivered intravenously or implanted, transdermal delivery is also a possible route of administra-tion. For both protein (e.g., inhibin) or nanoparticle delivery, larger molecules that are less lipophilic must cross the skin. The primary limiting step is diffusion through the stratum corneum layer of the skin.[121] The electropotential energy (iontophoresis) has been used in an effort to enhance skin per-meability.[148,151] Others have used microneedles to overcome puncture through the stratum corneum with minimal pain/discomfort. This technology has been used for insulin delivery,[41,66] and could be useful for delivery of larger protein hormones such as activin and inhibin (Figure 7.3).

7.5.3 Polymeric Slow-Release Formulations

A general issue with all pharmacological agents, in general, and for osteoporosis treatments, specifi-cally, is patient compliance with the dosing regimen.[50,127] In the case of oral delivery, pills are typi-cally taken on a daily basis. However, other delivery methods may only be required several times

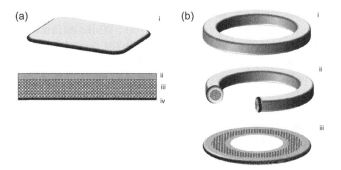

FIGURE 7.3 In addition to oral forms of pharmacological hormone therapy, there are several controlled delivery methods for delivery of ovarian hormones with a focus on estrogen and progesterone. (a) Transdermal systems and (b) silastic patches such as Vivelle and Estring, respectively, are shown schematically. Advantages of these systems include avoidance of first-pass hepatic clearance that occurs when drugs are taken orally. (a) Transdermal systems are a thin patch (i) that can be applied to the skin. These systems typically include a translucent film made of compounds such as polyolefins (ii). The middle layer (iii) is an adhesive formulation that may contain acrylic adhesives, silicone adhesives, and inactive ingredients to enhance solubility of the hormones, and the hormones themselves (cross-hatch pattern). These systems also contain a backing (iv) that is removed before application. (B) Silastic rings are implanted vaginally. Shown are the ring shape (i) and vertical (ii) or horizontal (iii) cross-sections showing the distribution of hormones within the rings (cross-hatch pattern).

per year. Consider the case of vaginal delivery of hormones, which can be done through the use of creams (e.g., Premarin),[126] tablets,[51] or silastic rings (e.g., Estring.).[155] Creams may be applied every day to every week while tablets may require biweekly application following a more frequent initial dosing. However, the silastic rings may achieve sustained release over the course of 3 months,[131] potentially providing the benefit of improved patient compliance. Here we consider several general approaches to controlled delivery of hormones. The goal with each of these approaches is to achieve sustained release of the hormones. Ideally, the release would be zero-order (time-independent), meaning that a constant level of hormone(s) could be supplied.

7.5.3.1   Diffusion-Based Release

Diffusion-based release relies on a reservoir system of drug incorporated into a polymeric network that relies on a concentration gradient. The surface area of the reservoir, molecular weight of the drug, thickness of the polymer, and the diffusivity of the drug also play a role in determining the rate of drug release. The polymeric network for these systems is typically nondegradable or degrades at a rate much slower than the rate of diffusion of the drug. The gel-based system for transdermal delivery is one example of this type of system. Alternatively, the polymer network can encapsulate another polymer or liquid core containing the drug. The drug must be released through the outer encapsulating polymer. These approaches are not exclusive to the examples noted above, as membrane-based systems have been applied to transdermal delivery.[122]

The vaginal silastic ring delivery system described above is one example of a system that uses a silicone polymer network to serve as the encapsulating material to control release.[134] Like other polymeric slow-release methods described in this section, the goal is to achieve a sustained, preferably zero-order release of the drug. The pharmacodynamics, though, may vary depending on the system. For example, the silastic rings are primarily designed to achieve their effects locally, whereas the transdermal systems seek to achieve blood distribution while avoiding first-pass hepatic clearance. At some point (depending on the size of the construct and the amount of drug loaded into the system) the drug will be depleted from the system such that sufficient quantities are no longer released. Because the system is nondegradable, it must then be removed and replaced if the therapy is to continue.

7.5.3.2   Polymer Degradation Release

In principle, polymer degradation draws on some of the same principles described above for diffusion-based release. A polymeric network can be used to encapsulate a drug reservoir or the drug can be distributed throughout the polymer network. While diffusion of the drug from the system may still occur, these approaches rely primarily on the degradation of the polymer network itself to allow drug release. For systems where the polymer acts as a membrane around the drug reservoir, degradation of the polymer may decrease the thickness of the membrane or increase the porosity of the polymer matrix, both of which lead to increased amounts of drug release. For systems in which the drug is distributed within the matrix, the degradation of the polymers leads to surface or bulk degradation or erosion, allowing release of the drug as the polymer matrix around the drug elutes from the system.

There are several FDA-approved polymers for such approaches, and these are primarily polyesters. These include poly(lactic acid), poly(glycol acid), poly(lactic-co-glycol acid), and polycaprolactone, which have been used for hormone release approaches.[92,107,149] Other classes of biodegradable polymers for slow release include the polyanhydrides (more rapid degradation than similarly structured polyesters) and polyamides (slower degradation than similarly structured polyesters), but there are no reports in the literature using these systems for ovarian hormone release. The polyesters, poly(anhydrides), and poly(amides) all rely on hydrolytic degradation of the polymer to achieve release.

A key advantage to such biodegradable systems is that, unlike the nondegradable polymers described in Section 7.5.3.1, there is no need to remove the system for subsequent dosings, though replacement would be needed for the therapy to continue. One of the drawbacks to these types of systems is a burst release that may occur due to initial swelling of the polymer upon placement in physiological fluids or an unequal distribution of the drug within the device such that more drug is present near the surface.

These systems may be used as monolithic devices, but there are numerous reports using microparticles[19,28] or nanoparticles[92] for hormone delivery. Again, although there is limited description of the effects of these controlled release systems on bone, two of these particulate-based delivery systems have been shown to enhance BMD when delivered via iontophoresis transdermally[149] or implanted subcutaneously.[114] It is also possible to incorporate microparticles into nondegradable matrices such as the silastic example above.[25] The principles of micro- or nanoparticle delivery are similar to those for monolithic devices, though the release profiles may differ.

In Section 7.5.4, we discuss targeted delivery that may employ systemic delivery (e.g., nanoparticles). It should be noted that carrier systems for systemic delivery are typically on the scale of tens to hundreds of nanometers to allow extravasation to the site of action. However, microparticulate controlled delivery systems for hormones are typically not suited to systemic delivery as they are too large to achieve extravasation to reach their site of action.

These hydrolytically driven systems may be considered "smart" release in that the polymer degrades in response to the local environment only under a set of desirable conditions. Other approaches to smart delivery that have been reported for hormone therapy include temperature[53] and pH[96] control, while enzymatically controlled delivery is also possible,[15,47] though not reported for ovarian hormone delivery.

7.5.4 TARGETED DELIVERY

When local (e.g., bone) rather than systemic effects are required, the ability to target the hormone therapy to its desired site of action may be beneficial. Clearly, in some situations such as libido, this is a complex system that involves both psychological and physical components that may require multiple targets. In other cases, such as bone, a more singular site of action may be suitable. It is important to recognize, however, that even in the case of enhancing bone formation and BMD, systemic effects from things such as diet and exercise will still impact outcomes. One example of targeting is the example of vaginal applications noted above. The rationale is that for women with genitourinary-specific conditions such as vulvovaginal atrophy, the hormone therapy can be applied locally, potentially reducing systemic concentrations of the hormones and mitigating side effects. With this approach, the hormones are targeted to their site of action simply by direct application at the site of action. However, given that the vagina is a mucous membrane, it is not surprising that hormones reach the blood stream in appreciable amounts, particularly at higher delivery concentrations.[131] As such, systemic effects can still be expected. This may not be problematic for some women, who may benefit from these systemic side effects, but it is likely that such effects will be reduced due to a lower systemic dosage. As such, the use of such vaginal creams may not be ideal for improving bone health. This concept of local or targeted delivery helps to reduce but does not eliminate the lack of selectivity for the target tissue, leading to off-target side effects. In addition, it is clearly more challenging for internal tissues such as bone, and other methods of targeting agents to the site of action are required.

As in the case of vaginal delivery, one goal for hormone therapy in bone could be selective delivery to bone tissue while decreasing impacts on brain, the cardiovascular system, and the genitourinary organs, all with the intention of reducing off-target effects that have led to questions regarding the utility of hormone therapy. One such approach is the use of liposomal encapsulation of the hormones. Liposomes consist of lipid bilayers and are typically composed primarily of phosphatidylcholine lipids, often with cholesterol. The internal region of the liposome is then an aqueous region, and liposomes can be sized to ~50–200 nm through processes such as extrusion or sonication. The loading of chemotherapy drugs into the internal aqueous region achieves a large "payload" of drug, and modification of the surfaces of liposomes with poly(ethylene glycol) (PEG) is known to achieve prolonged circulation that leads to greater accumulation in areas with loose vascular structures.[70] This so-called enhanced permeation and retention (EPR) effect then leads to slow release of drug from the liposomal carriers to improve therapeutic outcomes. Such an approach has been used for estrogen delivery, but the lipophilic nature of the estrogen leads to the drug partitioning primarily into the lipid bilayer of the liposomes rather than the internal core (it should be noted that some hydrophobic chemotherapy drugs such as bischloronitrosourea or BCNU partition in the same way[86]). This approach has been shown to lead to slow release of estrogen from the liposomes *in vitro* and improve body weight and BMD in ovariectomized rats, though only slightly better than free estrogen. It is not clear if this effect was due to enhanced delivery or deposition of the liposomes in the bone or via slow release, though PEG was not used in these studies. One approach to further enhance deposition in a particular tissue is to modify the PEG surface of the liposomes with targeting motifs that are selective for a tissue of interest.[46] Again, this work has been pioneered in the chemotherapy field, but could be readily adapted to targeting of bone tissue if the correct targeting motifs (or ligands) are conjugated to the surface of the carrier, though these approaches are more successful in areas of "leaky" vasculature such as tumors.[152]

This targeting approach does not require the use of liposome or other nanoparticles. The targeting motif can also be directly conjugated to drugs of interest such as estrogen. For example, tetracyclines are known to have high binding affinity to hydroxyapatite.[58,141] Tetracycline and tetracycline analogs have been used for conjugation to estrogen to improve bone targeting selectivity to bone compared to nontarget tissues that would be susceptible to estrogen effects, such as uterus.[110] Similarly, estrogens have also been conjugated to bisphosphonates. As described above, the bisphosphonates are a first-line treatment for osteoporosis. One reason that the bisphosphonates are successful in slowing the effects of osteoporosis through their antiresorptive effects is due to their high binding capacity for bone. Bisphosphonates can persist in bone tissue for months or years after deposition, likely due to their chemical similarity to hydroxyapatite.[162] Given their beneficial effects when given in conjunction with hormone therapy,[163,164] it is rational to use the bisphosphonates as targeting motifs to improve localization of hormone therapy, potentially providing the benefits of both with a greater degree of selectivity.[17,108]

As noted above, the bisphosphonates, SERMS, and RANKL inhibitors are the currently used clinical approaches to prevention and treatment of osteoporosis. In-depth discussion of these nonhormonal drugs is beyond the scope of this chapter, but excellent reviews on each are available.[45,106,117] At the preclinical level, tissue engineering and regenerative medicine techniques are being developed in which cells can be used for the production of ovarian hormones. Such approaches may offer some of the benefits of controlled release systems described above, but with the additional ability to participate in the HPO axis.

7.6   CELL-BASED HORMONE THERAPY

An unresolved issue associated with the use of hormone therapy is the time following menopause over which the therapy should be continued. It is known that cessation of hormone therapy will lead to a decrease in bone mass, and that approximately half of lifetime bone loss (as measured by BMD) occurs in the first 6 years of menopause.[144] However, the protective effects during the first 5–10 years of menopause may be sufficient to prevent formation of osteoporosis as this timeframe is the period when the most significant level of bone loss occurs. As noted earlier, while estrogen loss is the main reason for these effects, pituitary hormones such as FSH regulated by other ovarian hormones (e.g., inhibin) may also play a role in bone loss. Given the complexity of the female endocrine system, it is not surprising that non-ovarian aspects play a key role. In order to address these issues, more sophisticated delivery systems may be needed. However, it can be argued that the native ovaries themselves are the most sophisticated of systems due to their ability to respond to the pituitary hormones (FSH and LH) and secrete their own hormones that provide both feedforward and feedback control over the hypothalamus and anterior pituitary.

As discussed in the previous section, pharmacological hormone therapy is based on the restoration of ovarian hormones. While the introduction of estrogen alone or with progesterone does impact anterior pituitary hormone levels, particularly FSH, the levels of these hormones do not return to premenopausal (or ovarian failure) levels upon the introduction of hormone therapy. There are several possible reasons for this.

First, the process of aging has effects on the hypothalamus and anterior pituitary that seem to be largely independent of estrogen.[147] The reasons for this are not entirely understood, but because estrogen levels are still at normal, premenopausal levels, it is believed that this effect is related to other factors such as inhibin. Second, except for cases where hormone therapy is used to achieve conception (e.g., via *in vitro* fertilization or IVF),[133] hormone therapy regimens are generally designed to maintain hormone blood concentrations at constant (steady-state) values. Clearly, based on the discussion in Section 7.2, this does not follow the physiological pattern found in nature prior to menopause. During the reproductive years, the blood concentrations of estrogen and progesterone vary considerably over the course of the female sexual cycle. The fact that hormone levels remain constant during most forms of pharmacological hormone therapy, then, would lead to significant differences in the control mechanisms of estrogen and progesterone on the HPO axis. Finally, estrogen and progesterone are not the only hormones secreted by the ovaries. However, for the vast majority of pharmacological hormone replacement strategies, these are the only hormones that are given. Other hormones such as activin and inhibin are not included. Yet, it is well known that activin and inhibin have significant regulatory impacts on the hypothalamus and anterior pituitary. Because these are not included in pharmacological hormone therapies, then, there is no complete restoration of the HPO axis. During the reproductive years, there is clearly interaction and integration between the organs of the HPO axis that cannot be easily matched with pharmacological methods. Indeed, this is part of the impetus for the use of cell-based strategies for hormone delivery.

While this is not an exhaustive list for the possible reasons why the other hormones of the HPO axis do not return to premenopausal levels after introduction of pharmacological hormone therapy, these are likely to be the major players. Delivery of multiple hormones that vary in concentration over time and are required at different points in time is an extremely complex design challenge. Cell-based approaches in which the constructs and encapsulated cells integrate into the HPO axis offer, in concept, the ability to solve this complex problem.

There are a number of approaches that can be used to achieve encapsulation of cells. These include natural polymer methods, synthetic polymers, or combinations of the two. Of these, likely, the most well known and important is alginate (Figure 7.4a). The use of alginate for Type I diabetes treatment is described in a separate chapter by Dr Kendall in this book. Conceptually, its use for cell-based delivery of ovarian hormones for bone health is the same. Specifically, ovarian follicles

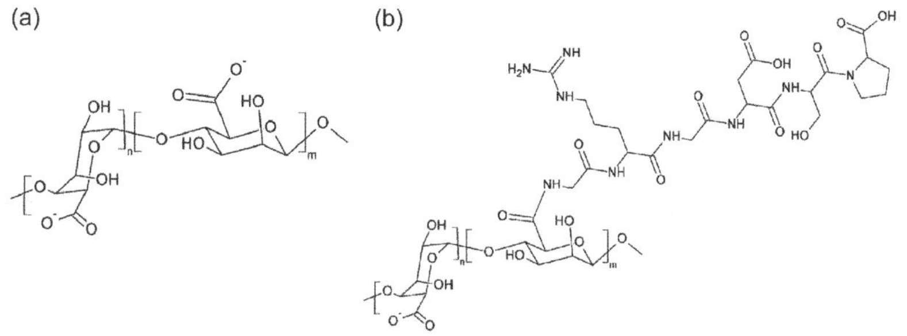

FIGURE 7.4 Schematic showing (a) the basic structure of alginate and (b) modification of the alginate with a GRGDSP amino sequence in which the RGD region supports integrin binding. (a) The two types of saccharide units that make up alginate is shown: guluronic (G; left) and mannuronic (M; right). The diagram depicts block copolymers of G and M for illustrative purposes only, but the G and M units are typically randomly arranged, though formulations can be enriched with either G or M units. (b) Modification of alginates can be achieved by the formation of amide bonds at the carboxyl group of either G or M units. The GRGDSP is shown, but the chemistry is compatible with other amino acid sequences or whole proteins such as collagen or laminin.

or cells can be placed in solution-phase alginate and then extruded or dropped into bivalent cation solutions (e.g., consisting of calcium, strontium, or barium ions) to gel the alginate, thus encapsulating the cells. The cells can be protected from immunological rejection if they come from allogeneic or xenogeneic sources by coating with poly-L-lysine, poly-ornithine, or other semipermeable polymers that prevent cell-based destruction of the encapsulated cells. Alginate can be readily modified with peptide sequences or proteins that promote cellular attachment or other cellular behaviors (Figure 7.4b shows modification with GRGDSP in which the arginine-glycine-aspartic acid (RGD) sequence is the functional, integrin-binding sequence).[8,87,130,132] Depending on the approach to cell or follicle encapsulation, the challenges associated with these strategies may vary.

There are two general approaches to ovarian hormone production through cell (or tissue) encapsulation strategies. These are the encapsulation of (i) whole (nondissociated) ovarian follicles from xenogeneic, allogeneic, or autologous sources (Figure 7.5a) and (ii) dissociated cells derived from ovarian follicles (Figure 7.5b). The focus of whole ovarian follicle encapsulation has largely been associated with a desire to preserve ovarian follicles for reproductive purposes in women interested in future pregnancies but who are undergoing, for example, ablative cancer therapies that could lead to later infertility due to destruction of ovarian tissue. A potential advantage of a dissociated cell approach would be the potential for long-term secretion of the hormones by avoiding luteinization that can occur via follicle maturation or ovulation. Clearly, however, a dissociated-cell approach is not appropriate for achieving reproduction. Both approaches could be used for hormone therapy, and allogeneic or even xenogeneic cell sources can theoretically be used if they are immunoisolated.

7.6.1 MATHEMATICAL MODEL OF DIFFUSION IN CELL ENCAPSULATION SYSTEMS

There are several challenges to cell encapsulation strategies. In the case of alginate, it is a polysaccharide derived from seaweed. Thus, it is clearly not a natural constituent of the extracellular matrix (ECM) to which islet cells or ovarian cells would attach. As such, cells are unlikely to take on a normal morphology which, in turn, could affect the behavior of the cells such that they secrete different levels of hormones in an encapsulated state compared to their native physiological state. As shown in Figure 7.4b, one approach to address this problem has been the incorporation of RGD sequences, collagen, fibronectin, or other native ECM constituents into alginate gels to facilitate cell adhesion and, thus, proper phenotype and product secretion.

Another key challenge associated with encapsulation strategies is fibrous encapsulation of the alginate due to the foreign body or inflammatory response of the host. One approach to limit these effects is to use "ultrapure" or "clinical-grade" alginate that has been purified of small molecules in order to reduce the inflammatory response.[16,150] As described in Dr Welker's chapter of this book and reported by others,[156] chemical modification of alginates is one approach to mitigate or minimize

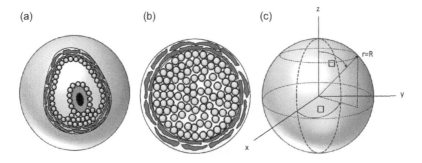

FIGURE 7.5 (a) Schematic showing whole follicle encapsulation where the oocyte, granulosa cells, and theca cells as well as other cells of the follicle are encapsulated in spherical alginate microparticles. (b) Schematic showing encapsulation of dissociated granulosa and theca cells from donor tissue. (c) Schematic showing the spherical coordinate system over an alginate bead for use in the mathematical model of diffusion.

the inflammatory response. Although material-related aspects might be mitigated, the encapsulated cells may also promote an inflammatory response to the constructs even if the encapsulated cells themselves are immunologically isolated. It is also noteworthy that much of the research associated with alginate encapsulation has focused on beta islet cell encapsulation for treatment of Type I diabetes. These cells have high metabolic demand and are typically clumps of cells. As such, they may also secrete danger-associated molecular patterns under oxygen-deprivation conditions.[116] It is not clear if such problems could also occur in the case of ovarian cell encapsulation but may be more likely in the encapsulation of whole follicles than of dissociated cells due to diffusional limitations associated with not only the alginate but also with the follicular tissue.

Thus, diffusional limitations in general are a potential challenge for all cell-encapsulation systems. The primary reasons for this are associated with the diffusion of oxygen and nutrients (e.g., glucose) into the cells within the encapsulation system and diffusion of metabolic waste products out of the encapsulation system. It is straightforward to mathematically model the system to determine a concentration profile for a given species (nutrient or waste product) based on the continuity equation in radial coordinates (see Figure 7.5c):

$$\frac{\partial G}{\partial t} + \left[\frac{1}{r^2} \frac{\partial}{\partial r} \left(r^2 N_{G,r} \right) + \frac{1}{r \sin \theta} \frac{\partial}{\partial \theta} \left(N_{G,\theta} \sin \theta \right) + \frac{1}{r \sin \theta} \frac{\partial N_{G,\varphi}}{\partial \varphi} \right] = \text{Rate of reaction}$$

where
   G is the concentration of some species (e.g., glucose)
   r represents the radial distance (from the center of the sphere)
   θ represents the polar angle
   φ the azimuthal angle
   t is the time
   r is the radial distance (from the center of the sphere)
   N_G is the flux of species G with the secondary subscript referring to flux of G in the radial (r),
      polar angular (θ), or azimuthal angular (φ) direction
   And the rate of reaction represents the consumption (in the case of a nutrient) or production
      (in the case of a waste product)

By making several common simplifying assumptions, the partial differential equation above can be reduced to an ordinary differential equation with an analytical solution. Specifically, if we assume that the system is operating at steady state (no time change) and that the change in the concentration of G occurs only in the radial direction (r), then

$$\frac{\partial G}{\partial t} = 0 \quad \text{by the steady-state assumption}$$

and

$$\frac{\partial}{\partial \theta} \left(N_{G,\theta} \sin \theta \right) = 0 \quad \text{by the radial direction assumption}$$

and

$$\frac{\partial N_{G,\varphi}}{\partial \varphi} = 0 \quad \text{by the radial direction assumption}$$

The resulting ordinary differential equation is

$$\frac{1}{r^2} \frac{d}{dr} \left(r^2 N_{G,r} \right) = \text{Rate of reaction}$$

The flux of G in the radial direction $N_{G,r}$ can be related to the diffusion coefficient (D_e) and the concentration gradient as

$$N_{G,r} = D_e \frac{dG}{dr}$$

to yield the equation as

$$\frac{1}{r^2}\frac{d}{dr}\left(r^2 D_e \frac{dG}{dr}\right) = \text{Rate of reaction}$$

If we then assume, in the case of a nutrient like glucose, that the cells are consuming G by first-order reaction kinetics, then

$$\text{Rate of reaction} = kG$$

where k is the rate constant for the reaction.

And we obtain

$$\frac{1}{r^2}\frac{d}{dr}\left(r^2 D_e \frac{dG}{dr}\right) = kG$$

This is a second-order, ordinary differential equation that can be solved analytically if two boundary conditions (BCs) are known. In this case, we can assume one BC is that the concentration of G (for a nutrient) is at a maximum at the edge of the sphere ($r = R$). We can also recognize that the concentration of G is at a minimum in the center of the sphere. As such, we can say

$$BC1: \text{at } r = R, G = G_{max}$$

where G_{max} is some known maximum concentration such as the concentration of glucose in the media.

$$BC2: \text{at } r = 0, \frac{dG}{dr} = 0$$

which indicates that the concentration of G is at a minimum at the center of the sphere.

Solving this differential equation and applying the BC yields the concentration profile of G in the radial direction:

$$G(r) = G_{max}\exp\left[\frac{k}{6D_e}\left(r^2 - R^2\right)\right]$$

So, from the above equation, it is possible to estimate the concentration at any distance from the center of the sphere. However, this equation can also be used to determine some critical radius of r at which point cell viability would be threatened due to low energy supply (glucose) or oxygen supply. It would only be necessary to know the rate constant, k, for consumption (or production in the case of waste products) and the diffusion coefficient, D_e.

A review of the literature provides some estimates for effective diffusion coefficients of various species in alginate (see Table 7.1). It is important to note that for these data, there are numerous variables from study to study, which include alginate composition (e.g., mannuronate:guluronate ratio), gel percentage, alginate purity, and temperature. In addition, the presence or absence of cells as well as the cell concentration within the gel will impact diffusion coefficients. Further, different cell or

TABLE 7.1

Effective Diffusion Coefficients of Various Chemical Species in Alginate

Chemical Species	Effective Diffusion Coefficient (D_e)	Alginate Composition (M:G Ratio and Weight Percentage)	Alginate Crosslinker	Temperature	References
Oxygen (32 g/mol)	0.175–$0.198 \times 10^{-8}\,m^2/s$	1%–3%; 4 mm	Calcium	Unknown	[76]
	$7.0 \times 10^{-6}\,cm^2/s$[a]	diameter	chloride	37°C	[73]
		2%	Barium chloride		
Urea	5×10^{-9} to $5 \times 10^{-11}\,m^2/s$	Alginate membrane; unknown concentration	Calcium chloride		[83]
Glucose	4.52–$7.38 \times 10^{-6}\,cm^2/s$	3%	Calcium	20°C–35°C	[68]
	$6.7 \times 10^{-6}\,cm^2/s$	3%	Calcium	30°C	[157]
	$6.23 \times 10^{-10}\,m^2/s$	3%	Calcium	30°C	[14]
	$6.8 \times 10^{-6}\,cm^2/s$	2%	Calcium	22°C–26°C	[69]
Estrogen (~272 g/mol)	N/A				
Progesterone (~314 g/mol)	N/A				
Testosterone (~288 g/mol)	N/A				
Ethanol (~46 g/mol)	$12.48 \times 10^{-10}\,m^2/s$	3%	Calcium	30°C	[14]
	$10.1 \times 10^{-6}\,cm^2/s$	2%	Calcium	30°C	[136]
	$1.0 \times 10^{-5}\,cm^2/s$	2%	Calcium (membrane)	22°C–26°C	[69]
Insulin (~5,800 g/mol)	$5.88 \times 10^{-12}\,m^2/s$ and $21.11 \times 10^{-12}\,m^2/s$		Calcium	pH = 5	[171]
Pepsin (~32,700 g/mol)	$5.63 \times 10^{-7}\,cm^2/s$	High G content, 1.3%	Calcium chloride	25°C	[10]
Ovalbumin (~44,000 g/mol)	$3.36 \times 10^{-7}\,cm^2/s$	High G content, 1.3%	Calcium chloride	25°C	[10]
Bovine serum albumin (~60,000 g/mol)	2.49×10^{-7} to $5.33 \times 10^{-7}\,cm^2/s$[a] $1.39 \times 10^{-7}\,cm^2/s$[a]	1%–6% High G content, 1.3%	Calcium chloride Calcium chloride	25°C 25°C	From Ref.[11] based on diffusion coefficient in water from Ref.[40] [10]
Beta-lactoglobulin (~146,940 g/mol)	$0.184 \times 10^{-7}\,cm^2/s$	High G content, 1.3%	Calcium chloride	25°C	[10]
Activin (~30,000 g/mol as dimer)	N/A				
Inhibin (~30,000 g/mol as dimer)	N/A				
FSH (~30,000 g/mol)	N/A				
LH	N/A				

[a] Indicates <75% of the diffusivity in water.

tissue types also have different susceptibilities to oxygen, nutrient, and waste product concentrations. Nonetheless, these values can be used as a guide for the diameter of the particles that would allow cell viability to ensure that cell diameters are not so large that diffusional limitations lead to cytotoxicity. It can be noted from the literature.

Species for which diffusion coefficients were available are clearly for common nutrients (e.g., glucose and oxygen) as well as cellular metabolic waste products (e.g., urea, ethanol). Some cell products such as insulin have documented diffusion coefficients due to the widespread use of cell encapsulation strategies for their delivery. However, literature values for the key ovarian hormones discussed in this chapter that would need to diffuse out of the alginate system (estrogen, progesterone, testosterone, activin, and inhibin) as well as the anterior pituitary hormones that would need to diffuse into the alginate system (FSH and LH) are unknown or unreported in the literature. For the protein peptides such as activin, inhibin, FSH, and LH, good estimates for their diffusion coefficients can likely be obtained based on the molecular weights of similar proteins (see insulin, pepsin, ovalbumin, bovine serum albumin, and beta-lactoglobulin in Table 7.1). Further, it is useful to note that the effective diffusion coefficients from most of the species in Table 7.1 were about 80%–90% of the values for the same species in water (with some noted exceptions in Table 7.1), suggesting that a first approximation could be made for the ovarian and pituitary hormones from their diffusion coefficients in water.

7.6.2 PRECLINICAL EXAMPLES OF CELL ENCAPSULATION STRATEGIES FOR OVARIAN HORMONE PRODUCTION AND EFFECTS ON BONE HEALTH

There are two general approaches to ovarian hormone delivery from encapsulated cells. The first is the use of encapsulated whole follicles and the second is the encapsulation of dissociated cells. In regards to the former, it was noted in Section 7.5 that the WHI reports also seem to have decreased the focus on controlled release of ovarian hormones. There are numerous reports reporting on the encapsulation of whole follicles, but much of this literature is focused on follicle encapsulation for reproductive purposes in which the follicles can be removed from a patient who, for example, will be undergoing an ablative chemotherapy regimen that could damage follicles and wishes to save her follicles for later use via IVF methods. These approaches have achieved functional success live births in rodents have been reported.[167] These approaches to whole follicle encapsulation have shown functionality of the encapsulated follicles by hormone production,[88] but the effects on bone have not been reported.

Approaches in which dissociated cells are used are unsuitable for reproductive purposes, but are more focused on hormone delivery. In considering dissociated cells, it is important to remember the interaction between granulosa and theca cells in the production/secretion of estrogen, progesterone, and other ovarian hormones. Interestingly, it has been shown that dissociated cells that are encapsulated in a two-layer system designed to mimic the native ovary (but without the oocyte) via an inner granulosa capsule and an outer theca capsule achieve more sustained levels of estrogen and progesterone secretion.[139] Importantly, these multilayer capsules have been shown to enhance bone architecture and repair in an ovariectomy model.[140] Further, this effect is superior to pharmacological delivery of estrogen or progesterone alone, and the effect is achieved at lower circulating levels of estrogen than the pharmacologically delivered hormones.[140] As such, this approach offers the potential to improve both safety and efficacy.

Currently, these strategies for cell-based delivery are at the preclinical level. Because these constructs consist of both cells (biologic) and materials (device), they would be classified as a combinatorial product, with related regulatory challenges. In addition, the source of cells to be used in the constructs is not trivial. For example, allogeneic or xenogeneic cells (as noted earlier) can be used if immunoisolated, but such strategies have not achieved the desired long-term success in other systems such as Type I diabetes. Autologous cells could also be used, but the use of primary ovarian cells is almost certainly not a possibility for women with menopause or other mechanisms of ovarian failure because there is no source for the primary cells. The use of autologous-induced pluripotent stem cells (iPSC) is a possibility, but fully functional granulosa cells have not been established from iPSC to date.[74,94,95] The use of pharmacological hormone therapy continues to be a complex issue, but it is becoming clearer that traditional, drug-based approaches that use estrogen alone or with progesterone may not be sufficient to safely replicate the native female ovary's function. The evaluation of cell-based constructs is at an early stage, but may provide an avenue to more safely deliver the fully array of ovarian hormones and allow more effective treatment of osteoporosis.

7.7 CONCLUSIONS

In this chapter, we have highlighted the effect of several hormones secreted by the female ovaries not only on bone but also on aspects of women's health. Ovarian failure due to menopause or other causes has profound implications on bone health. In particular, osteoporosis and related fracture is a major health problem for women stemming from roots associated with ovarian hormones. While hormone replacement therapy is not currently a first-line treatment for osteoporosis prevention, it is an important weapon in the arsenal for treatment of bone-related conditions in postmenopausal women. It may be the most appropriate treatment for some women such as those who do not respond well to the bisphosphonates or SERMs. Advances in controlled release and cell-based strategies to hormone therapy may help to overcome risks associated with traditional pharmacological hormone therapy. Indeed, hormone therapy is the only therapeutic method that finds its roots in the native physiology of the body, and improved methods for delivery that achieve favorable risk-benefit ratios could lead to a resurgence of hormone therapy in the future.

REFERENCES

1. Office of the Surgeon General (US). *Bone Health and Osteoporosis: A Report of the Surgeon General.* Rockville (MD): Office of the Surgeon General (US), 2004.
2. Section: 17.3 The pituitary gland and hypothalamus. In: *OpenStax. Anatomy and Physiology.* OpenStax CNX. Feb 26, 2016 http://cnx.org/contents/14fb4ad7-39a1-4eee-ab6e-3ef2482e3e22@8.24. Excerpt From: OpenStax. "Anatomy and Physiology." iBooks.
3. Assessment of fracture risk and its application to screening for postmenopausal osteoporosis. Report of a WHO Study Group. *World Health Organ Tech Rep Ser* 843: 1–129, 1994.
4. Editorial. HRT for menopause: A NICE treatment? *Lancet* 386: 2030, 2015.
5. Osteoporosis Fast Facts. https://cdn.nof.org/wp-content/uploads/2015/12/Osteoporosis-Fast-Facts.pdf, edited by N. O. Foundation, 2011.
6. Postmenopausal hormone replacement therapy: Ovarian cancer. *Prescrire Int* 25: 16, 2016.
7. Almeida M., S. Iyer, M. Martin-Millan, S. M. Bartell, L. Han, E. Ambrogini, M. Onal, J. Xiong, R. S. Weinstein, R. L. Jilka, C. A. O'Brien and S. C. Manolagas. Estrogen receptor-alpha signaling in osteoblast progenitors stimulates cortical bone accrual. *J Clin Invest* 123: 394–404, 2013.
8. Alsberg E., K. W. Anderson, A. Albeiruti, R. T. Franceschi and D. J. Mooney. Cell-interactive alginate hydrogels for bone tissue engineering. *J Dent Res* 80: 2025–2029, 2001.
9. Alswat K. A. Gender disparities in osteoporosis. *J Clin Med Res* 9: 382–387, 2017.
10. Amsden B. Solute diffusion in hydrogels. An examination of the retardation effect. *Polym Gels Networks* 6: 13–43, 1998.
11. Amsden B. and N. Turner. Diffusion characteristics of calcium alginate gels. *Biotechnol Bioeng* 65: 605–610, 1999.
12. Anderson G. L., M. Limacher, A. R. Assaf, T. Bassford, S. A. Beresford, H. Black, D. Bonds, R. Brunner, R. Brzyski, B. Caan, R. Chlebowski, D. Curb, M. Gass, J. Hays, G. Heiss, S. Hendrix, B. V. Howard, J. Hsia, A. Hubbell, R. Jackson, K. C. Johnson, H. Judd, J. M. Kotchen, L. Kuller, A. Z. LaCroix, D. Lane, R. D. Langer, N. Lasser, C. E. Lewis, J. Manson, K. Margolis, J. Ockene, M. J. O'Sullivan, L. Phillips, R. L. Prentice, C. Ritenbaugh, J. Robbins, J. E. Rossouw, G. Sarto, M. L. Stefanick, L. Van Horn, J. Wactawski-Wende, R. Wallace, S. Wassertheil-Smoller and Women's Health Initiative Steering Committee. Effects of conjugated equine estrogen in postmenopausal women with hysterectomy: The Women's Health Initiative randomized controlled trial. *JAMA* 291: 1701–1712, 2004.
13. Asafo-Adjei T. A., A. J. Chen, A. Najarzadeh and D. A. Puleo. Advances in controlled drug delivery for treatment of osteoporosis. *Curr Osteoporos Rep* 14: 226–238, 2016.

14. Axelsson A. and B. Persson. Determination of effective diffusion-coefficients in calcium alginate gel plates with varying yeast-cell content. *Appl Biochem Biotechnol* 18: 231–250, 1988.

15. Balmayor E. R., K. Tuzlakoglu, A. P. Marques, H. S. Azevedo and R. L. Reis. A novel enzymatically-mediated drug delivery carrier for bone tissue engineering applications: Combining biodegradable starch-based microparticles and differentiation agents. *J Mater Sci Mater Med* 19: 1617–1623, 2008.

16. Basta G. and R. Calafiore. Immunoisolation of pancreatic islet grafts with no recipient's immunosuppression: Actual and future perspectives. *Curr Diab Rep* 11: 384–391, 2011.

17. Bauss F., A. Esswein, K. Reiff, G. Sponer and B. Muller-Beckmann. Effect of 17beta-estradiol-bisphosphonate conjugates, potential bone-seeking estrogen pro-drugs, on 17beta-estradiol serum kinetics and bone mass in rats. *Calcif Tissue Int* 59: 168–173, 1996.

18. Bertonazzi A., B. Nelson, J. Salvador and E. Umland. The smallest available estradiol transdermal patch: A new treatment option for the prevention of postmenopausal osteoporosis. *Womens Health (London)* 11: 815–824, 2015.

19. Birnbaum D. T., J. D. Kosmala, D. B. Henthorn and L. Brannon-Peppas. Controlled release of beta-estradiol from PLAGA microparticles: The effect of organic phase solvent on encapsulation and release. *J Controlled Release* 65: 375–387, 2000.

20. Biscup P. Risks and benefits of long-term hormone replacement therapy. *Am J Health Syst Pharm* 60: 1419–1425, 2003.

21. Bliuc D., N. D. Nguyen, V. E. Milch, T. V. Nguyen, J. A. Eisman and J. R. Center. Mortality risk associated with low-trauma osteoporotic fracture and subsequent fracture in men and women. *JAMA* 301: 513–521, 2009.

22. Bonnelye E. and J. E. Aubin. Differential expression of estrogen receptor-related receptor alpha and estrogen receptors alpha and beta in osteoblasts in vivo and in vitro. *J Bone Miner Res* 17: 1392–1400, 2002.

23. Bord S., A. Horner, S. Beavan and J. Compston. Estrogen receptors alpha and beta are differentially expressed in developing human bone. *J Clin Endocrinol Metab* 86: 2309–2314, 2001.

24. Boyle W. J., W. S. Simonet and D. L. Lacey. Osteoclast differentiation and activation. *Nature* 423: 337–342, 2003.

25. Brannon-Peppas L. Controlled release of beta-estradiol from biodegradable microparticles within a silicone matrix. *J Biomater Sci Polym Ed* 5: 339–351, 1994.

26. Brem H., M. S. Mahaley, Jr., N. A. Vick, K. L. Black, S. C. Schold, Jr., P. C. Burger, A. H. Friedman, I. S. Ciric, T. W. Eller, J. W. Cozzens and J.N. Kenealy. Interstitial chemotherapy with drug polymer implants for the treatment of recurrent gliomas. *J Neurosurg* 74: 441–446, 1991.

27. Buist D. S., K. M. Newton, D. L. Miglioretti, K. Beverly, M. T. Connelly, S. Andrade, C. L. Hartsfield, F. Wei, K. A. Chan and L. Kessler. Hormone therapy prescribing patterns in the United States. *Obstet Gynecol* 104: 1042–1050, 2004.

28. Buntner B., M. Nowak, J. Kasperczyk, M. Ryba, P. Grieb, M. Walski, P. Dobrzynski and M. Bero. The application of microspheres from the copolymers of lactide and epsilon-caprolactone to the controlled release of steroids. *J Controlled Release* 56: 159–167, 1998.

29. Burger H. G., E. C. Dudley, J. L. Hopper, N. Groome, J. R. Guthrie, A. Green and L. Dennerstein. Prospectively measured levels of serum follicle-stimulating hormone, estradiol, and the dimeric inhibins during the menopausal transition in a population-based cohort of women. *J Clin Endocrinol Metab* 84: 4025–4030, 1999.

30. Carroll N. A review of transdermal nonpatch estrogen therapy for the management of menopausal symptoms. *J Womens Health (Larchmt)* 19: 47–55, 2010.

31. Cefalu C. A. Is bone mineral density predictive of fracture risk reduction? *Curr Med Res Opin* 20: 341–349, 2004.

32. Cenci S., G. Toraldo, M. N. Weitzmann, C. Roggia, Y. Gao, W. P. Qian, O. Sierra and R. Pacifici. Estrogen deficiency induces bone loss by increasing T cell proliferation and lifespan through IFN-gamma-induced class II transactivator. *Proc Natl Acad Sci U S A* 100: 10405–10410, 2003.

33. Chlebowski R. T., L. H. Kuller, R. L. Prentice, M. L. Stefanick, J. E. Manson, M. Gass, A. K. Aragaki, J. K. Ockene, D. S. Lane, G. E. Sarto, A. Rajkovic, R. Schenken, S. L. Hendrix, P. M. Ravdin, T. E. Rohan, S. Yasmeen, G. Anderson and W. H. I. Investigators. Breast cancer after use of estrogen plus progestin in postmenopausal women. *N Engl J Med* 360: 573–587, 2009.

34. Connelly M. T., M. Richardson and R. Platt. Prevalence and duration of postmenopausal hormone replacement therapy use in a managed care organization, 1990–1995. *J Gen Intern Med* 15: 542–550, 2000.

35. Cooper C., G. Campion and L. J. Melton, 3rd. Hip fractures in the elderly: A world-wide projection. *Osteoporos Int* 2: 285–289, 1992.

36. Cummings S. R., S. Eckert, K. A. Krueger, D. Grady, T. J. Powles, J. A. Cauley, L. Norton, T. Nickelsen, N. H. Bjarnason, M. Morrow, M. E. Lippman, D. Black, J. E. Glusman, A. Costa and V. C. Jordan. The effect of raloxifene on risk of breast cancer in postmenopausal women: Results from the MORE randomized trial. Multiple outcomes of raloxifene evaluation. *JAMA* 281: 2189–2197, 1999.

37. Damien E., J. S. Price and L. E. Lanyon. The estrogen receptor's involvement in osteoblasts' adaptive response to mechanical strain. *J Bone Miner Res* 13: 1275–1282, 1998.

38. Damien E., J. S. Price and L. E. Lanyon. Mechanical strain stimulates osteoblast proliferation through the estrogen receptor in males as well as females. *J Bone Miner Res* 15: 2169–2177, 2000.

39. Davies G. C., W. J. Huster, Y. Lu, L. Plouffe, Jr. and M. Lakshmanan. Adverse events reported by postmenopausal women in controlled trials with raloxifene. *Obstet Gynecol* 93: 558–565, 1999.

40. Davis H. E. and J. K. Leach. Designing bioactive delivery systems for tissue regeneration. *Ann Biomed Eng* 39: 1–13, 2011.

41. Davis S. P., W. Martanto, M. G. Allen and M. R. Prausnitz. Hollow metal microneedles for insulin delivery to diabetic rats. *IEEE Trans Bio-Med Eng* 52: 909–915, 2005.

42. de Villiers T. J., M. L. Gass, C. J. Haines, J. E. Hall, R. A. Lobo, D. D. Pierroz and M. Rees. Global consensus statement on menopausal hormone therapy. *Climacteric* 16: 203–204, 2013.

43. de Villiers T. J., A. Pines, N. Panay, M. Gambacciani, D. F. Archer, R. J. Baber, S. R. Davis, A. A. Gompel, V. W. Henderson, R. Langer, R. A. Lobo, G. Plu-Bureau, D. W. and Sturdee. Updated 2013 International Menopause Society recommendations on menopausal hormone therapy and preventive strategies for midlife health. *Climacteric* 16: 316–337, 2013.

44. Deady J. Clinical monograph: Hormone replacement therapy. *J Manag Care Pharm* 10: 33–47, 2004.

45. Deal C. Potential new drug targets for osteoporosis. *Nat Clin Pract Rheumatol* 5: 20–27, 2009.

46. Drummond D. C., K. Hong, J. W. Park, C. C. Benz and D. B. Kirpotin. Liposome targeting to tumors using vitamin and growth factor receptors. *Vitam Horm* 60: 285–332, 2000.

47. Ehrbar M., A. Metters, P. Zammaretti, J. A. Hubbell and A. H. Zisch. Endothelial cell proliferation and progenitor maturation by fibrin-bound VEGF variants with differential susceptibilities to local cellular activity. *J Controlled Release* 101: 93–109, 2005.

48. Ettinger B., K. E. Ensrud, R. Wallace, K. C. Johnson, S. R. Cummings, V. Yankov, E. Vittinghoff and D. Grady. Effects of ultralow-dose transdermal estradiol on bone mineral density: A randomized clinical trial. *Obstet Gynecol* 104: 443–451, 2004.

49. Ettinger B., H. K. Genant and C. E. Cann. Long-term estrogen replacement therapy prevents bone loss and fractures. *Ann Intern Med* 102: 319–324, 1985.

50. Ettinger M. P., R. Gallagher and P. E. MacCosbe. Medication persistence with weekly versus daily doses of orally administered bisphosphonates. *Endocr Pract* 12: 522–528, 2006.

51. Eugster-Hausmann M., J. Waitzinger and D. Lehnick. Minimized estradiol absorption with ultra-low-dose 10 microg 17beta-estradiol vaginal tablets. *Climacteric* 13: 219–227, 2010.

52. Evans S. F. and M. W. Davie. Low and conventional dose transdermal oestradiol are equally effective at preventing bone loss in spine and femur at all post-menopausal ages. *Clin Endocrinol (Oxford)* 44: 79–84, 1996.

53. Externbrink A., M. R. Clark, D. R. Friend and S. Klein. Investigating the feasibility of temperature-controlled accelerated drug release testing for an intravaginal ring. *Eur J Pharm Biopharm* 85: 966–973, 2013.

54. Fadanelli M. E. and H. G. Bone. Combining bisphosphonates with hormone therapy for postmenopausal osteoporosis. *Treat Endocrinol* 3: 361–369, 2004.

55. Faienza M. F., A. Ventura, F. Marzano and L. Cavallo. Postmenopausal osteoporosis: The role of immune system cells. *Clin Dev Immunol* 2013: 575936, 2013.

56. Files J. A., M. G. Ko and S. Pruthi. Bioidentical hormone therapy. *Mayo Clin Proc* 86: 673–680, quiz 680, 2011.

57. Fishman J. R., M. A. Flatt and R. A. Settersten, Jr. Bioidentical hormones, menopausal women, and the lure of the "natural" in U.S. anti-aging medicine. *Soc Sci Med* 132: 79–87, 2015.

58. Fujisaki J., Y. Tokunaga, T. Takahashi, T. Hirose, F. Shimojo, A. Kagayama and T. Hata. Osteotropic drug delivery system (ODDS) based on bisphosphonic prodrug. I: Synthesis and in vivo characterization of osteotropic carboxyfluorescein. *J Drug Target* 3: 273–282, 1995.

59. Gambacciani M. and M. Levancini. Hormone replacement therapy and the prevention of postmenopausal osteoporosis. *Prz Menopauzalny* 13: 213–220, 2014.

60. Gambacciani M. and M. Levancini. Hormone replacement therapy: Who should be treated? *Minerva Ginecol* 67: 249–255, 2015.

61. Gambacciani M. and M. Levancini. Management of postmenopausal osteoporosis and the prevention of fractures. *Panminerva Med* 56: 115–131, 2014.

62. Gambacciani M., P. Monteleone, A. Sacco and A. R. Genazzani. Hormone replacement therapy and endometrial, ovarian and colorectal cancer. *Best Pract Res Clin Endocrinol Metab* 17: 139–147, 2003.

63. Gefvert O., B. Eriksson, P. Persson, L. Helldin, A. Bjorner, E. Mannaert, B. Remmerie, M. Eerdekens and S. Nyberg. Pharmacokinetics and D2 receptor occupancy of long-acting injectable risperidone (Risperdal Consta) in patients with schizophrenia. *Int J Neuropsychopharmacol* 8: 27–36, 2005.

64. Greenwald J., M. E. Vega, G. P. Allendorph, W. H. Fischer, W. Vale and S. Choe. A flexible activin explains the membrane-dependent cooperative assembly of TGF-beta family receptors. *Mol Cell* 15: 485–489, 2004.

65. Grodstein F., M. J. Stampfer, G. A. Colditz, W. C. Willett, J. E. Manson, M. Joffe, B. Rosner, C. Fuchs, S. E. Hankinson, D. J. Hunter, C. H. Hennekens and F. E. Speizer. Postmenopausal hormone therapy and mortality. *N Engl J Med* 336: 1769–1775, 1997.

66. Gupta J., E. I. Felner and M. R. Prausnitz. Minimally invasive insulin delivery in subjects with type 1 diabetes using hollow microneedles. *Diabetes Technol Ther* 11: 329–337, 2009.

67. Guyton A. C. and J. E. Hall. *Textbook of Medical Physiology*. Philadelphia, PA: Elsevier Saunders, 2006, p. xxxv, 1116 p.

68. Hacimusalar M. and U. Mehmetoglu. Determination of the effective diffusion-coefficients of glucose and ethanol in calcium alginate gel by the moment analysis method. *Chem Eng Sci* 50: 3001–3004, 1995.

69. Hannoun B. J. and G. Stephanopoulos. Diffusion coefficients of glucose and ethanol in cell-free and cell-occupied calcium alginate membranes. *Biotechnol Bioeng* 28: 829–835, 1986.

70. Harris J. M. and R. B. Chess. Effect of pegylation on pharmaceuticals. *Nat Rev Drug Discov* 2: 214–221, 2003.

71. Henderson B. E., A. Paganini-Hill and R. K. Ross. Decreased mortality in users of estrogen replacement therapy. *Arch Intern Med* 151: 75–78, 1991.

72. Hewitt S. C. and K. S. Korach. Estrogen receptors: New directions in the new millennium. *Endocr Rev* 39: 664–675, 2018.

73. Hiemstra H., L. Dijkhuizen and W. Harder. Diffusion of oxygen in alginate gels related to the kinetics of methanol oxidation by immobilized hansenula-polymorpha cells. *Eur J Appl Microbiol Biotechnol* 18: 189–196, 1983.

74. Huang C. C., M. J. Chen, C. W. Lan, C. E. Wu, M. C. Huang, H. C. Kuo and H. N. Ho. Hyperactive CREB signaling pathway involved in the pathogenesis of polycystic ovarian syndrome revealed by patient-specific induced pluripotent stem cell modeling. *Fertil Steril*, 112 (3): 594–607, 2019.

75. Hughes D. E., A. Dai, J. C. Tiffee, H. H. Li, G. R. Mundy and B. F. Boyce. Estrogen promotes apoptosis of murine osteoclasts mediated by TGF-beta. *Nat Med* 2: 1132–1136, 1996.

76. Hulst A. C., H. J. H. Hens, R. M. Buitelaar and J. Tramper. Determination of the effective diffusion coefficient of oxygen in gel materials in relation to gel concentration. *Biotechnol Tech* 3: 199–204, 1989.

77. Islam S., Q. Liu, A. Chines and E. Helzner. Trend in incidence of osteoporosis-related fractures among 40- to 69-year-old women: Analysis of a large insurance claims database, 2000–2005. *Menopause* 16: 77–83, 2009.

78. Jilka R. L., G. Hangoc, G. Girasole, G. Passeri, D. C. Williams, J. S. Abrams, B. Boyce, H. Broxmeyer and S. C. Manolagas. Increased osteoclast development after estrogen loss: Mediation by interleukin-6. *Science* 257: 88–91, 1992.

79. Jilka R. L., K. Takahashi, M. Munshi, D. C. Williams, P. K. Roberson and S. C. Manolagas. Loss of estrogen upregulates osteoblastogenesis in the murine bone marrow. Evidence for autonomy from factors released during bone resorption. *J Clin Invest* 101: 1942–1950, 1998.

80. Jimmy B. and J. Jose. Patient medication adherence: Measures in daily practice. *Oman Med J* 26: 155–159, 2011.

81. Kanis J. A. Diagnosis of osteoporosis and assessment of fracture risk. *Lancet* 359: 1929–1936, 2002.

82. Karim R., R. M. Dell, D. F. Greene, W. J. Mack, J. C. Gallagher and H. N. Hodis. Hip fracture in postmenopausal women after cessation of hormone therapy: Results from a prospective study in a large health management organization. *Menopause* 18: 1172–1177, 2011.

83. Kashima K. and M. Imai. Impact factors to regulate mass transfer characteristics of stable alginate membrane performed superior sensitivity on various organic chemicals. *Chisa 2012* 42: 964–977, 2012.

84. Kastrati A., J. Mehilli, N. von Beckerath, A. Dibra, J. Hausleiter, J. Pache, H. Schuhlen, C. Schmitt, J. Dirschinger, A. Schomig and I.-D. S. Investigators. Sirolimus-eluting stent or paclitaxel-eluting stent vs balloon angioplasty for prevention of recurrences in patients with coronary in-stent restenosis: A randomized controlled trial. *JAMA* 293: 165–171, 2005.

85. Khalid A. B. and S. A. Krum. Estrogen receptors alpha and beta in bone. *Bone* 87: 130–135, 2016.

86. Kitamura I., M. Kochi, Y. Matsumoto, R. Ueoka, J. Kuratsu and Y. Ushio. Intrathecal chemotherapy with 1,3-bis(2-chloroethyl)-1-nitrosourea encapsulated into hybrid liposomes for meningeal gliomatosis: An experimental study. *Cancer Res* 56: 3986–3992, 1996.

87. Kreeger P. K., J. W. Deck, T. K. Woodruff and L. D. Shea. The in vitro regulation of ovarian follicle development using alginate-extracellular matrix gels. *Biomaterials* 27: 714–723, 2006.

88. Kreeger P. K., N. N. Fernandes, T. K. Woodruff and L. D. Shea. Regulation of mouse follicle development by follicle-stimulating hormone in a three-dimensional in vitro culture system is dependent on follicle stage and dose. *Biol Reprod* 73: 942–950, 2005.

89. Lam J., S. Takeshita, J. E. Barker, O. Kanagawa, F. P. Ross and S. L. Teitelbaum. TNF-alpha induces osteoclastogenesis by direct stimulation of macrophages exposed to permissive levels of RANK ligand. *J Clin Invest* 106: 1481–1488, 2000.

90. Lehman M. N., S. M. Hileman and R. L. Goodman. Neuroanatomy of the kisspeptin signaling system in mammals: Comparative and developmental aspects. *Adv Exp Med Biol* 784: 27–62, 2013.

91. Leslie W. D., S. R. Majumdar, S. N. Morin and L. M. Lix. Why does rate of bone density loss not predict fracture risk? *J Clin Endocrinol Metab* 100: 679–683, 2015.

92. Lim Soo P., J. Lovric, P. Davidson, D. Maysinger and A. Eisenberg. Polycaprolactone-block-poly(ethylene oxide) micelles: A nanodelivery system for 17beta-estradiol. *Mol Pharm* 2: 519–527, 2005.

93. Lindberg M. K., S. Moverare, S. Skrtic, H. Gao, K. Dahlman-Wright, J. A. Gustafsson and C. Ohlsson. Estrogen receptor (ER)-beta reduces ERalpha-regulated gene transcription, supporting a "ying yang" relationship between ERalpha and ERbeta in mice. *Mol Endocrinol* 17: 203–208, 2003.

94. Lipskind S., J. S. Lindsey, B. Gerami-Naini, J. L. Eaton, D. O'Connell, A. Kiezun, J. W. K. Ho, N. Ng, P. Parasar, M. Ng, M. Nickerson, U. Demirci, R. Maas and R. M. Anchan. An embryonic and induced pluripotent stem cell model for ovarian granulosa cell development and steroidogenesis. *Reprod Sci* 25: 712–726, 2018.

95. Liu T., Q. Li, S. Wang, C. Chen and J. Zheng. Transplantation of ovarian granulosalike cells derived from human induced pluripotent stem cells for the treatment of murine premature ovarian failure. *Mol Med Rep* 13: 5053–5058, 2016.

96. Liu Y. Y., Y. H. Shao and J. Lu. Preparation, properties and controlled release behaviors of pH-induced thermosensitive amphiphilic gels. *Biomaterials* 27: 4016–4024, 2006.

97. Lobo R. A., J. H. Pickar, J. C. Stevenson, W. J. Mack and H. N. Hodis. Back to the future: Hormone replacement therapy as part of a prevention strategy for women at the onset of menopause. *Atherosclerosis* 254: 282–290, 2016.

98. Maatta J. A., K. G. Buki, G. Gu, M. H. Alanne, J. Vaaraniemi, H. Liljenback, M. Poutanen, P. Harkonen and K. Vaananen. Inactivation of estrogen receptor alpha in bone-forming cells induces bone loss in female mice. *FASEB J* 27: 478–488, 2013.

99. Manolagas S. C. Birth and death of bone cells: Basic regulatory mechanisms and implications for the pathogenesis and treatment of osteoporosis. *Endocr Rev* 21: 115–137, 2000.

100. Manolagas S. C., C. A. O'Brien and M. Almeida. The role of estrogen and androgen receptors in bone health and disease. *Nat Rev Endocrinol* 9: 699–712, 2013.

101. Manson J. E. The role of personalized medicine in identifying appropriate candidates for menopausal estrogen therapy. *Metabolism* 62 (Suppl 1): S15–S19, 2013.

102. Martin-Millan M., M. Almeida, E. Ambrogini, L. Han, H. Zhao, R. S. Weinstein, R. L. Jilka, C. A. O'Brien and S. C. Manolagas. The estrogen receptor-alpha in osteoclasts mediates the protective effects of estrogens on cancellous but not cortical bone. *Mol Endocrinol* 24: 323–334, 2010.

103. Massey H. M. and A. M. Flanagan. Human osteoclasts derive from CD14-positive monocytes. *Br J Haematol* 106: 167–170, 1999.

104. Matt D. W., S. W. Kauma, S. M. Pincus, J. D. Veldhuis and W. S. Evans. Characteristics of luteinizing hormone secretion in younger versus older premenopausal women. *Am J Obstet Gynecol* 178: 504–510, 1998.

105. Melville K. M., N. H. Kelly, S. A. Khan, J. C. Schimenti, F. P. Ross, R. P. Main and M. C. van der Meulen. Female mice lacking estrogen receptor-alpha in osteoblasts have compromised bone mass and strength. *J Bone Miner Res* 29: 370–379, 2014.

106. Migliaccio S., M. Brama and G. Spera. The differential effects of bisphosphonates, SERMS (selective estrogen receptor modulators), and parathyroid hormone on bone remodeling in osteoporosis. *Clin Interv Aging* 2: 55–64, 2007.

107. Mofidfar M. and M. R. Prausnitz. Electrospun transdermal patch for contraceptive hormone delivery. *Curr Drug Delivery* 16(6): 577–583, 2019.

108. Morioka M., A. Kamizono, H. Takikawa, A. Mori, H. Ueno, S. Kadowaki, Y. Nakao, K. Kato and K. Umezawa. Design, synthesis, and biological evaluation of novel estradiol-bisphosphonate conjugates as bone-specific estrogens. *Bioorg Med Chem* 18: 1143–1148, 2010.

109. Nakamura T., Y. Imai, T. Matsumoto, S. Sato, K. Takeuchi, K. Igarashi, Y. Harada, Y. Azuma, A. Krust, Y. Yamamoto, H. Nishina, S. Takeda, H. Takayanagi, D. Metzger, J. Kanno, K. Takaoka, T. J. Martin, P. Chambon and S. Kato. Estrogen prevents bone loss via estrogen receptor alpha and induction of Fas ligand in osteoclasts. *Cell* 130: 811–823, 2007.

110. Neale J. R., N. B. Richter, K. E. Merten, K. G. Taylor, S. Singh, L. C. Waite, N. K. Emery, N. B. Smith, J. Cai and W. M. Pierce, Jr. Bone selective effect of an estradiol conjugate with a novel tetracycline-derived bone-targeting agent. *Bioorg Med Chem Lett* 19: 680–683, 2009.

111. North American Menopause Society. Estrogen and progestogen use in peri- and postmenopausal women: March 2007 position statement of The North American Menopause Society. *Menopause* 14: 168–182, 2007.

112. Notelovitz M., V. A. John and W. R. Good. Effectiveness of Alora estradiol matrix transdermal delivery system in improving lumbar bone mineral density in healthy, postmenopausal women. *Menopause* 9: 343–353, 2002.

113. Oreffo R. O., V. Kusec, S. Romberg and J. T. Triffitt. Human bone marrow osteoprogenitors express estrogen receptor-alpha and bone morphogenetic proteins 2 and 4 mRNA during osteoblastic differentiation. *J Cell Biochem* 75: 382–392, 1999.

114. Otsuka M., H. Uenodan, Y. Matsuda, T. Mogi, H. Ohshima and K. Makino. Therapeutic effect of in vivo sustained estradiol release from poly (lactide-co-glycolide) microspheres on bone mineral density of osteoporosis rats. *Biomed Mater Eng* 12: 157–167, 2002.

115. Papahadjopoulos D., T. M. Allen, A. Gabizon, E. Mayhew, K. Matthay, S. K. Huang, K. D. Lee, M. C. Woodle, D. D. Lasic, C. Redemann and F.J. Martin. Sterically stabilized liposomes: Improvements in pharmacokinetics and antitumor therapeutic efficacy. *Proc Natl Acad Sci U S A* 88: 11460–11464, 1991.

116. Paredes Juarez G. A., M. Spasojevic, M. M. Faas and P. de Vos. Immunological and technical considerations in application of alginate microencapsulation systems. *Front Bioeng Biotechnol* 2: 1–15, 2014.

117. Pavone V., G. Testa, S. M. C. Giardina, A. Vescio, D. A. Restivo and G. Sessa. Pharmacological therapy of osteoporosis: A systematic current review of literature. *Front Pharmacol* 8: 803, 2017.

118. Peacock M., C. H. Turner, M. J. Econs and T. Foroud. Genetics of osteoporosis. *Endocr Rev* 23: 303–326, 2002.

119. Pfaffl M. W., I. G. Lange, A. Daxenberger and H. H. Meyer. Tissue-specific expression pattern of estrogen receptors (ER): Quantification of ER alpha and ER beta mRNA with real-time RT-PCR. *APMIS* 109: 345–355, 2001.

120. Pfeilschifter J., R. Koditz, M. Pfohl and H. Schatz. Changes in proinflammatory cytokine activity after menopause. *Endocr Rev* 23: 90–119, 2002.

121. Prausnitz M. R. and R. Langer. Transdermal drug delivery. *Nat Biotechnol* 26: 1261–1268, 2008.

122. Rafiee-Tehrani M., N. Safaii-Nikui, H. Peteriet and T. Beckert. Acrylic resins as rate-controlling membranes in novel formulation of a nine-day 17beta-estradiol transdermal delivery system: In vitro and release modifier effect evaluation. *Drug Dev Ind Pharm* 27: 431–437, 2001.

123. Randolph J. F., Jr., M. Sowers, I. V. Bondarenko, S. D. Harlow, J. L. Luborsky and R. J. Little. Change in estradiol and follicle-stimulating hormone across the early menopausal transition: Effects of ethnicity and age. *J Clin Endocrinol Metab* 89: 1555–1561, 2004.

124. Rannevik G., S. Jeppsson, O. Johnell, B. Bjerre, Y. Laurell-Borulf and L. Svanberg. A longitudinal study of the perimenopausal transition: Altered profiles of steroid and pituitary hormones, SHBG and bone mineral density. *Maturitas* 61: 67–77, 2008.

125. Richardson S. J., V. Senikas and J. F. Nelson. Follicular depletion during the menopausal transition: Evidence for accelerated loss and ultimate exhaustion. *J Clin Endocrinol Metabol* 65: 1231–1237, 1987.

126. Rigg L. A., H. Hermann and S. S. Yen. Absorption of estrogens from vaginal creams. *N Engl J Med* 298: 195–197, 1978.

127. Ross S., E. Samuels, K. Gairy, S. Iqbal, E. Badamgarav and E. Siris. A meta-analysis of osteoporotic fracture risk with medication nonadherence. *Value Health* 14: 571–581, 2011.

128. Rossouw J. E., G. L. Anderson, R. L. Prentice, A. Z. LaCroix, C. Kooperberg, M. L. Stefanick, R. D. Jackson, S. A. Beresford, B. V. Howard, K. C. Johnson, J. M. Kotchen and J. Ockene. Risks and benefits of estrogen plus progestin in healthy postmenopausal women: Principal results From the Women's Health Initiative randomized controlled trial. *JAMA* 288: 321–333, 2002.

129. Rouach V., S. Katzburg, Y. Koch, N. Stern and D. Somjen. Bone loss in ovariectomized rats: Dominant role for estrogen but apparently not for FSH. *J Cell Biochem* 112: 128–137, 2011.

130. Rowley J. A. and D. J. Mooney. Alginate type and RGD density control myoblast phenotype. *J Biomed Mater Res* 60: 217–223, 2002.

131. Santen R. J. Vaginal administration of estradiol: Effects of dose, preparation and timing on plasma estradiol levels. *Climacteric* 18: 121–134, 2015.

132. Sapir Y., O. Kryukov and S. Cohen. Integration of multiple cell-matrix interactions into alginate scaffolds for promoting cardiac tissue regeneration. *Biomaterials* 32: 1838–1847, 2011.

133. Saple S., M. Agrawal and S. Kawar. Precycle estradiol in synchronization and scheduling of antagonist cycles. *J Obstet Gynaecol India* 66: 295–299, 2016.

134. Sarkar N. N. Low-dose intravaginal estradiol delivery using a Silastic vaginal ring for estrogen replacement therapy in postmenopausal women: A review. *Eur J Contracept Reprod Health Care* 8: 217–224, 2003.

135. Sarrel P. M., V. Y. Njike, V. Vinante and D. L. Katz. The mortality toll of estrogen avoidance: An analysis of excess deaths among hysterectomized women aged 50 to 59 years. *Am J Public Health* 103: 1583–1588, 2013.

136. Scott C. D., C. A. Woodward and J. E. Thompson. Solute diffusion in biocatalyst gel beads containing biocatalysis and other additives. *Enzyme Microb Technol* 11: 258–263, 1989.

137. Shetty S., N. Kapoor, J. D. Bondu, N. Thomas and T. V. Paul. Bone turnover markers: Emerging tool in the management of osteoporosis. *Indian J Endocrinol Metab* 20: 846–852, 2016.

138. Simpson E. R. Sources of estrogen and their importance. *J Steroid Biochem Mol Biol* 86: 225–230, 2003.

139. Sittadjody S., J. M. Saul, S. Joo, J. J. Yoo, A. Atala and E. C. Opara. Engineered multilayer ovarian tissue that secretes sex steroids and peptide hormones in response to gonadotropins. *Biomaterials* 34: 2412–2420, 2013.

140. Sittadjody S., J. M. Saul, J. P. McQuilling, S. Joo, T. C. Register, J. J. Yoo, A. Atala and E. C. Opara. In vivo transplantation of 3D encapsulated ovarian constructs in rats corrects abnormalities of ovarian failure. *Nat Commun* 8: 1858, 2017.

141. Skinner H. C. and J. Nalbandian. Tetracyclines and mineralized tissues: Review and perspectives. *Yale J Biol Med* 48: 377–397, 1975.

142. Skouby S. O., F. Al-Azzawi, D. Barlow, J. Calaf-Alsina Erdogan Ertungealp, A. Gompel, A. Graziottin, D. Hudita, A. Pines, S. Rozenberg, G. Samsioe, J. C. Stevenson, M. European and S. Andropause. Climacteric medicine: European Menopause and Andropause Society (EMAS) 2004/2005 position statements on peri- and postmenopausal hormone replacement therapy. *Maturitas* 51: 8–14, 2005.

143. Sood R., S. S. Faubion, C. L. Kuhle, J. M. Thielen and L. T. Shuster. Prescribing menopausal hormone therapy: An evidence-based approach. *Int J Womens Health* 6: 47–57, 2014.

144. Sowers M. R., H. Zheng, M. L. Jannausch, D. McConnell, B. Nan, S. Harlow and J. F. Randolph, Jr. Amount of bone loss in relation to time around the final menstrual period and follicle-stimulating hormone staging of the transmenopause. *J Clin Endocrinol Metab* 95: 2155–2162, 2010.

145. Stampfer M. J. and G. A. Colditz. Estrogen replacement therapy and coronary heart disease: A quantitative assessment of the epidemiologic evidence. *Prev Med* 20: 47–63, 1991.

146. Su H. I. and E. W. Freeman. Hormone changes associated with the menopausal transition. *Minerva Ginecol* 61: 483–489, 2009.

147. Sun L., Y. Peng, A. C. Sharrow, J. Iqbal, Z. Zhang, D. J. Papachristou, S. Zaidi, L. L. Zhu, B. B. Yaroslavskiy, H. Zhou, A. Zallone, M. R. Sairam, T. R. Kumar, W. Bo, J. Braun, L. Cardoso-Landa, M. B. Schaffler, B. S. Moonga, H. C. Blair and M. Zaidi. FSH directly regulates bone mass. *Cell* 125: 247–260, 2006.

148. Takeuchi I., K. Fukuda, S. Kobayashi and K. Makino. Transdermal delivery of estradiol-loaded PLGA nanoparticles using iontophoresis for treatment of osteoporosis. *Biomed Mater Eng* 27: 475–483, 2016.

149. Takeuchi I., S. Kobayashi, Y. Hida and K. Makino. Estradiol-loaded PLGA nanoparticles for improving low bone mineral density of cancellous bone caused by osteoporosis: Application of enhanced charged nanoparticles with iontophoresis. *Colloids Surf B* 155: 35–40, 2017.

150. Thanos C. G., R. Calafiore, G. Basta, B. E. Bintz, W. J. Bell, J. Hudak, A. Vasconcellos, P. Schneider, S. J. Skinner, M. Geaney, P. Tan, R. B. Elliot, M. Tatnell, L. Escobar, H. Qian, E. Mathiowitz and D. F. Emerich. Formulating the alginate-polyornithine biocapsule for prolonged stability: Evaluation of composition and manufacturing technique. *J Biomed Mater Res Part A* 83: 216–224, 2007.

151. Tomoda K., A. Watanabe, K. Suzuki, T. Inagi, H. Terada and K. Makino. Enhanced transdermal permeability of estradiol using combination of PLGA nanoparticles system and iontophoresis. *Colloids Surf B* 97: 84–89, 2012.

152. Torchilin V. Tumor delivery of macromolecular drugs based on the EPR effect. *Adv Drug Deliv Rev* 63: 131–135, 2011.

153. Tsai S. A., M. L. Stefanick and R. S. Stafford. Trends in menopausal hormone therapy use of US office-based physicians, 2000–2009. *Menopause* 18: 385–392, 2011.

154. Unnanuntana A., B. P. Gladnick, E. Donnelly and J. M. Lane. The assessment of fracture risk. *J Bone Joint Surg Am* 92: 743–753, 2010.

155. Vartiainen J., T. Wahlstrom and C. G. Nilsson. Effects and acceptability of a new 17 beta-oestradiol-releasing vaginal ring in the treatment of postmenopausal complaints. *Maturitas* 17: 129–137, 1993.

156. Vegas A. J., O. Veiseh, J. C. Doloff, M. Ma, H. H. Tam, K. Bratlie, J. Li, A. R. Bader, E. Langan, K. Olejnik, P. Fenton, J. W. Kang, J. Hollister-Locke, M. A. Bochenek, A. Chiu, S. Siebert, K. Tang, S. Jhunjhunwala, S. Aresta-Dasilva, N. Dholakia, R. Thakrar, T. Vietti, M. Chen, J. Cohen, K. Siniakowicz, M. Qi, J. McGarrigle, A. C. Graham, S. Lyle, D. M. Harlan, D. L. Greiner, J. Oberholzer, G. C. Weir, R. Langer and D. G. Anderson. Combinatorial hydrogel library enables identification of materials that mitigate the foreign body response in primates. *Nat Biotechnol* 34: 345–352, 2016.

157. Venancio A. and J. A. Teixeira. Characterization of sugar diffusion coefficients in alginate membranes. *Biotechnol Tech* 11: 183–185, 1997.

158. Warriner A. H., N. M. Patkar, J. R. Curtis, E. Delzell, L. Gary, M. Kilgore and K. Saag. Which fractures are most attributable to osteoporosis? *J Clin Epidemiol* 64: 46–53, 2011.

159. Weiss S. R., H. Ellman and M. Dolker. A randomized controlled trial of four doses of transdermal estradiol for preventing postmenopausal bone loss. Transdermal Estradiol Investigator Group. *Obstet Gynecol* 94: 330–336, 1999.

160. Weitzmann M. N. and R. Pacifici. Estrogen deficiency and bone loss: An inflammatory tale. *J Clin Invest* 116: 1186–1194, 2006.

161. Wheater G., M. Elshahaly, S. P. Tuck, H. K. Datta and J. M. van Laar. The clinical utility of bone marker measurements in osteoporosis. *J Transl Med* 11: 201, 2013.

162. Whitaker M., J. Guo, T. Kehoe and G. Benson. Bisphosphonates for osteoporosis--where do we go from here? *N Engl J Med* 366: 2048–2051, 2012.

163. Wimalawansa S. J. A four-year randomized controlled trial of hormone replacement and bisphosphonate, alone or in combination, in women with postmenopausal osteoporosis. *Am J Med* 104: 219–226, 1998.

164. Wimalawansa S. J. Prevention and treatment of osteoporosis: Efficacy of combination of hormone replacement therapy with other antiresorptive agents. *J Clin Densitom* 3: 187–201, 2000.

165. Windahl S. H., L. Saxon, A. E. Borjesson, M. K. Lagerquist, B. Frenkel, P. Henning, U. H. Lerner, G. L. Galea, L. B. Meakin, C. Engdahl, K. Sjogren, M. C. Antal, A. Krust, P. Chambon, L. E. Lanyon, J. S. Price and C. Ohlsson. Estrogen receptor-alpha is required for the osteogenic response to mechanical loading in a ligand-independent manner involving its activation function 1 but not 2. *J Bone Miner Res* 28: 291–301, 2013.

166. Wright N. C., A. C. Looker, K. G. Saag, J. R. Curtis, E. S. Delzell, S. Randall and B. Dawson-Hughes. The recent prevalence of osteoporosis and low bone mass in the United States based on bone mineral density at the femoral neck or lumbar spine. *J Bone Miner Res* 29: 2520–2526, 2014.

167. Xu M., P. K. Kreeger, L. D. Shea and T. K. Woodruff. Tissue-engineered follicles produce live, fertile offspring. *Tissue Eng* 12: 2739–2746, 2006.

168. Yaffe K., G. Sawaya, I. Lieberburg and D. Grady. Estrogen therapy in postmenopausal women: Effects on cognitive function and dementia. *JAMA* 279: 688–695, 1998.

169. Zaman G., H. L. Jessop, M. Muzylak, R. L. De Souza, A. A. Pitsillides, J. S. Price and L. L. Lanyon. Osteocytes use estrogen receptor alpha to respond to strain but their ERalpha content is regulated by estrogen. *J Bone Miner Res* 21: 1297–1306, 2006.

170. Zhu L. L., H. Blair, J. Cao, T. Yuen, R. Latif, L. Guo, I. L. Tourkova, J. Li, T. F. Davies, L. Sun, Z. Bian, C. Rosen, A. Zallone, M. I. New and M. Zaidi. Blocking antibody to the beta-subunit of FSH prevents bone loss by inhibiting bone resorption and stimulating bone synthesis. *Proc Natl Acad Sci U S A* 109: 14574–14579, 2012.

171. Villaverde Cendon F., R. M. Matos Jorge, R. Weinshutz, and A.L. Mathias, *J Microencapsul*, 35(1): 13–25, 2018.

8 Controlled Delivery Models of Bioactive Factors for the Maturation of Engineered Tissues

Ashkan Shafiee
Wake Forest Institute for Regenerative Medicine

Elham Ghadiri
Wake Forest Institute for Regenerative Medicine
Wake Forest University

Jareer Kassis and Anthony Atala
Wake Forest Institute for Regenerative Medicine

CONTENTS

8.1 INTRODUCTION

8.1.1 TISSUE ENGINEERING

The failure of tissues and organs is a significant present-day health challenge.[1,2] Such failure can be caused by diseases or injuries, and the unavailability of organ donors is a critical limitation.[3] Twenty-two people die every day while waiting for a new organ, while a new patient is added to the National Transplant Waiting List (https://optn.transplant.hrsa.gov) in the United States alone every "10 minutes". Tissue engineering is designed to remedy the problem of organ shortage, and involves combining life sciences, physical sciences, and engineering to restore, replace, and improve damaged tissues and organs.[4,5] Several successful clinical trials have been reported based on the engineered tissues and organs that are constructed in the laboratory and implanted into the patient.

Moreover, lab-grown human bladders,[6] vaginas,[7] and urethras[8] have been shown to maintain functionality for several years of follow-up. Currently, fabricated organs are limited to those that are flat (skin,[9] cartilage[10]), tubular (blood vessel[11]), or hollow nontubular (vagina,[7] bladder[6]), and solid organs such as the heart, liver, and kidney have not yet been successfully engineered. However, the rapid advancement of science and technology continuously produces new opportunities.

There are two main approaches to tissue engineering: scaffold-free[11,12] and scaffold-based.[13] The scaffold is an integral part of tissue regeneration and fabrication that replicates the extracellular matrix (ECM) of the cells to facilitate their proliferation, differentiation, reorganization, and maturation to tissues and organs.[2] Scaffolds can be made using natural or synthetic materials that must be compatible with tissue-specific cell types and with the anticipated native milieu in vivo.[14] A number of characteristics such as pore size, geometry, permeability, and spatial distribution must be optimized when developing an appropriate scaffold for a particular need.[15]

Nevertheless, scaffold-free tissue engineering involves the development of a near-physiological environment to permit cells to self-assemble and produce their own ECM, thereby constructing tissues and ultimately organs.[16] Regardless of the use of a scaffold, tissue engineers may stimulate cellular interactions and tissue regeneration using bioactive factors (a term used in this chapter to comprehensively denote any type of external stimulator and bioactive molecule, such as a small molecule, peptide, protein, growth factor, or cytokine).[17] Bioactive factors may enhance tissue regeneration and are sometimes essential for producing the final tissue-engineered products.[18] The types of bioactive factors used are dependent on the specific tissue, and should also be administered or released in an optimized and timely manner.[19] Consequently, controlled release and delivery of such bioactive factors are often needed during the engineering procedure to biofabricate a functional construct.[20] Herein, we review the delivery mechanisms of the most critical bioactive factors (i.e., growth factors, small molecules, and proteins) for different tissues, including cardiomyocytes and bone.

8.1.2 Bioactive Factors for Tissue Regeneration and Engineering

Tissue regeneration and organ engineering involve several different steps, starting from performing a cell biopsy on the patient (in the case of autologous tissue engineering), followed by cell culture to obtain a sufficient number of cells,[4] tissue fabrication using various biofabrication methods (including but not limited to bioprinting,[21,22] and electrospinning[23,24]), tissue/organ maturation in a designated bioreactor, and ultimately transplantation (Figure 8.1). While some processes that occur during this procedure are naturally innate, it is the responsibility of tissue engineers to investigate and understand the natural external stimuli in orders to both facilitate and accelerate the tissue engineering

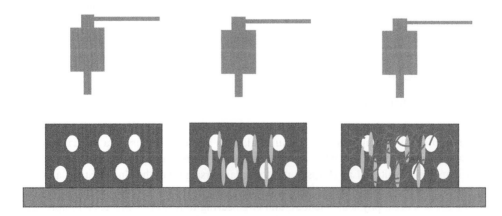

FIGURE 8.1 Biofabrication techniques such as bioprinting are able to make 3D scaffolds with different properties such as geometry and porous size. Scaffolds can be seeded by various cell types which communicate with each other through ECM.

procedure. For example, it has been shown that, during embryonic development, growth factors drive cells towards a particular behavior by providing essential signals that could also be used for tissue regeneration in an adult.[25] Such signaling molecules include mitogens that are responsible for cell division, growth factors that have multiple functions (the most important of which are proliferation), and morphogens that control tissue regeneration.[17]

Many different bioactive factors have been developed for tissue regeneration, such as growth factors, small molecule chemicals, peptides, proteins, cytokines, and other bioactive molecules. Nevertheless, numerous investigations have shown that the mere application of such bioactive factors is not sufficient; rather, delivery at the correct time points and to the correct locations is critical.[26,27] Therefore, an optimized spatiotemporally controlled release of bioactive agents may be needed for an optimal therapeutic effect, and this has been a topic of investigation for many years.[17,28]

8.2   GROWTH FACTORS

Growth factors are signaling molecules that regulate cellular behavior such as cell proliferation, differentiation, migration, and other activities that provide essential cell functionality.

8.2.1   Mechanisms of Growth Factor Function

The proper delivery of growth factors for purposes of tissue regeneration is important.[29] Cell adhesion, notch signaling, and traction-enabling adhesion, as well as proteoglycans, are all regulated by growth factors within the ECM. The diffusion of growth factors through the ECM is of limited range because of their slow diffusion and short half-lives; as such, they are only able to regulate proximal cells. Other than their ability to diffuse through the ECM, the performance of growth factors and their effects on a cell population also depend on the types of cell, the size of the target cell population, and the types of receptors targeted.[17,29] Figure 8.2 shows the general mechanism through which growth factors communicate with cells and regulate their interactions. Important growth factors during tissue regeneration are angiopoietin,[30] basic fibroblast growth factor,[31] epidermal

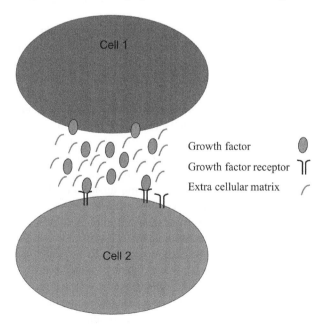

FIGURE 8.2   Growth factors are mediators for cross talk between cells. Cell 2 receptors can receive the growth factors made by cell 1 and translate to a particular cellular response. It is clear that the ECM plays an essential role to provide the environment for growth factors to transit from cell 1 to 2.

growth factor,[32] fibroblast growth factor,[33] hepatocyte growth factor,[34] insulin-like growth factor,[35] nerve growth factor,[36] platelet-derived growth factor,[37] transforming growth factor,[38] and vascular endothelial growth factor.[39] There are several delivery techniques that are being used to deliver growth factors for tissue regeneration. The techniques described in this section are also used for other bioactive factors, including proteins and small molecules.

8.2.2 PHYSICAL ENCAPSULATION

Tissue engineers can encapsulate growth factors in order to control their release; such encapsulation techniques include freeze-drying, phase emulsion, melt modeling, and gas foaming.[40] Researchers are attempting to either develop new techniques or enhance existing technologies to reduce the exposure time of growth factors to adverse agents such as solvents that are used in the encapsulation procedure.[17] Moreover, different investigative groups have reported combining two or more techniques for encapsulation and controlled delivery. In addition to the encapsulation technique, the selection of biomaterials is extremely important for optimal growth factor delivery. Various scaffold materials that are being manufactured from synthetic and natural polymers can be used by tissue engineers to encapsulate growth factors, and these are selected carefully by evaluating various criteria, including hydrophobicity. The hydrophilic interactions among biomaterials and growth factors play an essential role in successful delivery, and synthetic polymers such as poly(L-lactide), poly(glycoside), dextrin, poly(α-hydroxy acids), or a mixture of these materials are being used to encapsulate growth factors, as are natural polymers such as collagen, gelatin, fibrinogen, elastin, keratin, hyaluronic acid, cellulose, alginate, and chitosan. Importantly, the biocompatibility of these materials render them an excellent choice for drug delivery. Specific parameters, including gel degradation and growth factor diffusion dynamics, are important to optimize release requirements. For example, if a gel's degradation takes a long time, it can be used with a drug meant for slow release, whereas the opposite would be true for gels that possess fast degradation. Such degradation must be controllable and reproducible; therefore, chemical modification is often employed to obtain the desired delivery time when using natural polymers whose degradation times would otherwise be undesirable or unpredictable.

One of the most significant challenges for tissue engineering, particularly when fabricating solid organs, is tissue vascularization.[2] The diffusion lengths of oxygen and nutrients are $<200\,\mu m$ from any edge.[41] Therefore, in order to build tissues of more than a few hundred micrometers, vascularization is required.[42] To that end, proangiogenic growth factors are used to trigger vascularization of engineered tissues and organs implanted in vivo. Soluble molecules that regulate angiogenesis include vascular endothelial growth factor, insulin-like growth factor, basic fibroblast growth factor, and platelet-derived growth factor.[43] A drug delivery system for vascular endothelial growth factor was developed using heparin-functionalized hydrogels based on gelatin type A and albumin; these biomaterials are commonly used as matrices for tissue engineering, particularly for the storage and release of proangiogenic growth factors. The hydrogels were crosslinked using 1-ethyl-3-(3-dimethylaminopropyl) carbodiimide as the crosslinking agent, and their heparin functionalization was then evaluated using critical electrolyte concentration staining. The gelatin-based system showed a higher equilibrium degree of swelling than did the albumin-based system, and growth factor loading and release were found to be tunable via carbodiimide concentration. The delivery systems for both gels were stable for up to 21 days in terms of gel yield and degree of swelling, and osteogenic and chondrogenic regeneration could also be supported by a vascular network.[44] Moreover, 0.1 and 1 mg of vascular endothelial growth factor with a gene-activated matrix coated on a collagen sponge was shown to enhance both vascularization and bone regeneration.[45]

The encapsulation of stem cells and growth factors have shown promise for the field of tissue regeneration. Techniques such as extrusion, lithography, emulsion, microfluidics, and bioprinting as well as various materials including agarose, alginate, chitosan, and hyaluronic acid are used to encapsulate cells.[46] Bioprinting is one of the popular biofabrication methods that is used for drug delivery as well as in many medical fields.[47,48] Gasperini et al. provided a comprehensive overview of the different techniques and reported that an emulsion provides excellent scalability while extrusion, lithography, and microfluidics provide midrange benefits.[46]

Encapsulation of neural stem/progenitor cells is used to remedy the damaged or lost central neural system.[49] Hydrogels can play a critical role in the delivery of neural stem cells, which are naturally sensitive to their environment and substrate. Several previous experiments using agarose, collagen, or chitosan were reported for neural tissue engineering; however, the partially cytotoxic behavior of these systems towards neural stem/progenitor cells limited their capabilities. Therefore, novel delivery systems based on "click" hydrogels were developed using 4-dibenzocyclooctyno functionalized polyethylene glycol, tethered native protein attachment ligands, tethered potent neurogenic differentiation factor, and a polyethylene glycol tetraazide crosslinker. These systems maintained cell viability for almost twice the duration of other gels.[49] The effects of reactive oxygen species scavengers for neural resilience in neural damaged cells have also been investigated; these materials may have additional uses beyond the recovery of the cell functionality as they can also prevent damage.[50,51] Recently, manganese [III] 5, 10, 15, 20-tetra [4-pyridyl]-21H, 23H-porphine chloride tetrakis [methochloride], a semiconductor material that can be used for electronic device fabrication, was deposited using inkjet printing technology.[52] Interestingly, this material exhibits reactive oxygen species scavenger properties and can be used for repair, or else can prevent neural damaged caused by oxidative stress.

Cartilage regeneration is important for patients with damaged cartilage tissue because of trauma or disease, and the delivery of cells and growth factors to the damaged areas is critical for regeneration owing to the cartilage's inability to regenerate itself. Hydrogels based on κ-carrageenan were used to encapsulate chondrocyte cell lines, human nasal chondrocytes, and human-adipose-derived stem cells.[53] κ-carrageenan possesses high swelling characteristics as well as hydrophilic polysaccharide-based properties, making this hydrogel an excellent choice for encapsulation. While this delivery system showed cell viability and proliferation during long-term culture, the delivery of human adipose-derived stem cells had the highest efficacy of the delivery procedure. In another investigation, κ-carrageenan-based hydrogel was used to encapsulate transforming growth factor-β1.[54] Adipose-derived stem cells were also encapsulated, and were able to express specific cartilage matrix molecules within 2 weeks.

In addition to chemical and physical delivery approaches, other techniques exist that release growth factors at a particular location when combined with external stimuli. These delivery systems are preprogrammed to release the drug when a particular biological condition is met (i.e., at a specific pH or temperature, or upon exposure to an external magnetic field, voltage, or ultrasonographic beam). Free radical polymerization has also been used to fabricate thermoresponsive hydrogels.[55] In such cases, immunoglobulin G and recombinant proteins are encapsulated for local delivery, controlled degradation, and protein release using as-prepared thermoresponsive hydrogels. The most efficient temperature for immunoglobulin G encapsulation was shown to be 75%–87%, while the transition temperature was below the physiological temperature. The alginate matrices were combined with calcium phosphate scaffolds, and a programmed delivery system for platelet-derived growth factors and other "trigger molecules" for tissue regeneration (such as morphogenetic protein-2) were successfully developed.[56]

8.2.3 Chemical Immobilization

Two strategies are used when using growth factors for tissue regeneration: these are either physical encapsulation as part of a delivery system or chemical immobilization into/onto the ECM. The latter procedure can be accomplished via covalent and noncovalent techniques. The covalent method involves the direct covalent immobilization of growth factors in the matrix, whereas noncovalent approaches include the use of hydrophobicity or protein hydrogen bonding for the physical adsorption and immobilization of the growth factor onto the matrix. As an example of the latter method,

Xiong et al. applied quinone groups to facilitate the immobilization of vascular endothelial growth factor, given that substrates coated with these structures can covalently immobilize molecules with thiol or amine groups. Therefore, a functional coating with quinone groups was fabricated by first using amine-bearing plasma-polymerized allylamine, after which tannic acid was used to introduce phenolic hydroxylic hydroxyl/quinone groups. The immobilization was confirmed using surface energy measurements, X-ray photoelectron spectroscopy, and Fourier-transform infrared spectroscopy. This system produced a significant enhancement in the proliferation and functionality of human umbilical vein endothelial cells in the biological construct.

8.3 PROTEINS

Proteins are critical for tissue regeneration; therefore, tissue engineers have developed various techniques to deliver and release essential proteins to the appropriate locations within the tissues. These techniques are very similar to those described for growth factors above, including encapsulation, immobilization, and location-based delivery.

It has been shown that morphogenetic protein-2 incorporated into hydrogels may enhance bone regeneration.[57,58] Therefore, many delivery systems have been developed to release this protein. The delivery systems were fabricated using poly(phosphazene) hydrogels with different quantities and types of anionic side chains.[59] This provided the platform with several physical factors that enabled multitunable hydrogel systems to control the release of tissue regeneration biomolecules, including morphogenetic protein-2.

In addition to using various types of hydrogels individually, combinations of hydrogels that have different ratios and gelation levels have been used to control the delivery. To accomplish a sustained release of morphogenetic protein-2, a combination of alginate/hyaluronic acid hydrogels with controllable gelation rates were prepared using $CaSO_4$ and Na_2HPO_4 as crosslinking and retardation agents, respectively; this system's effect on human bone marrow stem cells and their osteogenic differentiation was investigated in vitro.[60] In addition, bone regeneration in pigs with mandibular defects was also investigated, with combinations of hydrogels releasing the protein over 5 weeks. Osteogenic differentiation of human bone marrow stem cells was significantly improved using a higher hyaluronic acid ratio, and the combination of stem cells and proteins in the hydrogels showed improved bone regeneration over either stem cells or proteins alone.

8.4 SMALL MOLECULES

While growth factors are ideal for triggering tissue regeneration and other cellular activities, they are subject to certain limitations, such as issues with contamination, unwanted immunogenic responses by the host, protein instability, and high cost. Therefore, small molecules are excellent substitutes for growth factors during tissue regeneration, and have already shown great promise for bone and cardiovascular tissue regeneration. In the case of the latter, small molecules have been used to treat ischemia and acute myocardial infarction[61]; they are also useful in cardiovascular tissue engineering, e.g., in terms of cardiac differentiation of pluripotent stem cells.[62] Moreover, sustained release of the prostaglandin I2 agonist ONO1301 over 10 days was accomplished in ischemic mice using microspheres constructed from polylactic-co-glycolic acid to encapsulate the drug.[63] The anti-inflammatory small molecule dexamethasone, which is also used as an osteoinductive agent, was covalently grafted to polyethylene glycol using a degradable lactic acid linker, and was released as the lactide bond degraded.[64] Moreover, the immunosuppressant small molecule FTY720 was found to trigger bone regeneration and microvascular formation in a rat model.[65] As such, FTY720 was used to address some postoperative complications (such as poor vascularization and mechanical instability) following massive bone allografts.

Sustained localized delivery of FTY720 was accomplished using a continuous polymer coating system. The FTY720 was encapsulated with polylactic-co-glycolic acid, which in turn was coated onto the devitalized bone allograft. This system showed a 64% delivery efficacy over a period of 14 days. Separately, prostaglandin E_2 has been found to be helpful for cardiovascular tissue regeneration[66] and bone regeneration. A drug delivery system using a cholesterol-bearing pullulan nanogel suspended in saline was fabricated to deliver prostaglandin E_2 locally.[67] The prostaglandin E_2 was also dissolved in saline, ethanol, and Tween-80, and was delivered as this composite.

8.5 FUTURE DIRECTIONS

Determining the essential bioactive molecules that trigger tissue regeneration is extremely important. Many researchers around the world are working to produce techniques that achieve optimized, reliable, and reproducible molecule delivery. However, the delivery techniques rely on precalculated and preprogrammed bioactive factor dosages that have been determined by tissue engineers for in vitro or in vivo settings. Therefore, a smart integrated system that can monitor tissue/organ functionality in real time and release the appropriate factors at the right dosage would be extremely helpful. This can be achieved using biosensors that are connected to the delivery systems. Biosensors are specific devices that can detect a particular bioanalyte in the environment.[68] This smart system would be capable of detecting any abnormal or dysfunctional behavior in the tissue and of controlling the delivery of the required bioactive factors in a fine-tuned manner. As such, the future of drug delivery is definitely heading towards smart monitoring and release based on tissue-related inputs.

8.6 CONCLUSION

Tissue engineering aims to address the current shortages in donated organs and tissues, which is a critical challenge in present-day healthcare. This encompasses multiple steps, including cell culture as well as tissue fabrication (using different methods such as bioprinting) and maturation in near-physiological conditions within bioreactors. Throughout this tedious and lengthy process, many bioactive molecules can be used to facilitate tissue regeneration. In this chapter, we reviewed the most common of these molecules, including growth factors and proteins used for the regeneration of various tissues such as bone and cartilage. Although marked advancements have been achieved in the local delivery of bioactive factors – at exact dosages – for tissue regeneration, a smart integrated system that incorporates biosensors and delivery systems is needed for more complex experiments. The future holds great promise for tissue engineering while these parallel technologies of drug delivery and biosensing advance toward fully automated control and delivery platforms.

REFERENCES

1. Langer, R. Editorial: Tissue engineering: Perspectives, challenges, and future directions. *Tissue Engineering* **13**, 1–2 (2007).
2. Shafiee, A. & Atala, A. Tissue engineering: Toward a new era of medicine. *Annual Review of Medicine* **68**, 29–40 (2017).
3. Atala, A. Engineering organs. *Current Opinion in Biotechnology* **20**, 575–592 (2009).
4. Langer, R. & Vacanti, J. Tissue engineering. *Science* **260**, 920–926 (1993).
5. Lanza, R., Langer, R. & Vacanti, J. P. *Principles of Tissue Engineering.* Academic Press: Cambridge, MA (2013).
6. Atala, A., Bauer, S. B., Soker, S., Yoo, J. J. & Retik, A. B. Tissue-engineered autologous bladders for patients needing cystoplasty. *The Lancet* **367**, 1241–1246 (2006).
7. Raya-Rivera, A. M. et al. Tissue-engineered autologous vaginal organs in patients: A pilot cohort study. *The Lancet* (2014). doi: 10.1016/S0140-6736(14)60542-0.
8. Raya-Rivera, A. et al. Tissue-engineered autologous urethras for patients who need reconstruction: An observational study. *The Lancet* **377**, 1175–1182 (2011).
9. Centanni, J. M. et al. StrataGraft skin substitute is well-tolerated and is not acutely immunogenic in patients with traumatic wounds. *Annals of Surgery* **253**, 672–683 (2011).
10. Jiang, Y. et al. Human cartilage-derived progenitor cells from committed chondrocytes for efficient cartilage repair and regeneration. *Stem Cells Translational Medicine* **5**, 1–12 (2016).

11. Norotte, C., Marga, F. S., Niklason, L. E. & Forgacs, G. Scaffold-free vascular tissue engineering using bioprinting. *Biomaterials* **30**, 5910–5917 (2009).

12. McCune, M., Shafiee, A., Forgacs, G. & Kosztin, I. Predictive modeling of post bioprinting structure formation. *Soft Matter* **10**, 1790–1800 (2014).

13. Moldovan, L., Babbey, C. M., Murphy, M. P. & Moldovan, N. I. Comparison of biomaterial-dependent and -independent bioprinting methods for cardiovascular medicine. *Current Opinion in Biomedical Engineering* **2**, 124–131 (2017).

14. Williams, D. F. Challenges with the development of biomaterials for sustainable tissue engineering. *Frontiers in Bioengineering and Biotechnology* **7**, 155 (2019).

15. Koh, Y.-G. et al. Optimal mechanical properties of a scaffold for cartilage regeneration using finite element analysis. *Journal of Tissue Engineering* **10** (2019). doi: 10.1177/2041731419832133.

16. Shafiee, A., Ghadiri, E., Williams, D. & Atala, A. Physics of cellular self-assembly: A microscopic model and mathematical framework for faster maturation of bioprinted tissues. *Bioprinting* **14**, e00047 (2019).

17. Lee, K., Silva, E. A. & Mooney, D. J. Growth factor delivery-based tissue engineering: General approaches and a review of recent developments. *Journal of the Royal Society Interface* **8**, 153–170 (2011).

18. Cheng, J., Amin, D., Latona, J., Heber-Katz, E. & Messersmith, P. B. Supramolecular polymer hydrogels for drug-induced tissue regeneration. *ACS Nano* **13**, 5493–5501 (2019).

19. Fathi-Achachelouei, M. et al. Use of nanoparticles in tissue engineering and regenerative medicine. *Frontiers in Bioengineering and Biotechnology* **7**, 173 (2019).

20. Cheng, G. et al. Controlled co-delivery of growth factors through layer-by-layer assembly of core: Shell nanofibers for improving bone regeneration. *ACS Nano* **13**, 6372–6382 (2019).

21. Shafiee, A., McCune, M., Forgacs, G. & Kosztin, I. Post-deposition bioink self-assembly: A quantitative study. *Biofabrication* **7**, 045005 (2015).

22. Shafiee, A. et al. Physics of bioprinting. *Applied Physics Reviews* **6**, 021315 (2019).

23. Liu, X. et al. An immunological electrospun scaffold for tumor cell killing and healthy tissue regeneration. *Materials Horizons* **5**, 1082–1091 (2018).

24. Kim, J. I., Kim, J. Y. & Park, C. H. Fabrication of transparent hemispherical 3D nanofibrous scaffolds with radially aligned patterns via a novel electrospinning method. *Scientific Reports* **8**, 6689 (2018).

25. Johnson, M. B., March, A. R. & Morsut, L. Engineering multicellular systems: Using synthetic biology to control tissue self-organization. *Current Opinion in Biomedical Engineering* **4**, 163–173 (2017).

26. Zhang, K. et al. Advanced smart biomaterials and constructs for hard tissue engineering and regeneration. *Bone Research* **6**, 1–15 (2018).

27. Strobel, H. A., Qendro, E. I., Alsberg, E. & Rolle, M. W. Targeted delivery of bioactive molecules for vascular intervention and tissue engineering. *Frontiers in Pharmacology* **9**, 1329 (2018).

28. Ekladious, I., Colson, Y. L. & Grinstaff, M. W. Polymer–drug conjugate therapeutics: Advances, insights and prospects. *Nature Reviews Drug Discovery*, 1–22 (2019). doi: 10.1038/s41573-018-0005-0.

29. Polo-Corrales, L., Latorre-Esteves, M. & Ramirez-Vick, J. E. Scaffold design for bone regeneration. *Journal of Nanoscience and Nanotechnology* **14**, 15–56 (2014).

30. Kang, J.-M., Yoon, J.-K., Oh, S.-J., Kim, B.-S. & Kim, S.-H. Synergistic therapeutic effect of three-dimensional stem cell clusters and angiopoietin-1 on promoting vascular regeneration in ischemic region. *Tissue Engineering Part A* **24**, 616–630 (2018).

31. Jia, Y.-Y. et al. Effect of optimized concentrations of basic fibroblast growth factor and epidermal growth factor on proliferation of fibroblasts and expression of collagen. *Chinese Medical Journal* **131**, 2089–2096 (2018).

32. Seonwoo, H. et al. Epidermal growth factor–releasing radially aligned electrospun nanofibrous patches for the regeneration of chronic tympanic membrane perforations. *Advanced Healthcare Materials* **5**, 1801160 (2018).

33. Endo, K., Fujita, N., Nakagawa, T. & Nishimura, R. Effect of fibroblast growth factor-2 and serum on canine mesenchymal stem cell chondrogenesis. *Tissue Engineering Part A* **25**, 901–910 (2019).

34. Zhang, Y. et al. Therapeutic effect of hepatocyte growth factor-overexpressing bone marrow-derived mesenchymal stem cells on CCl. *Cell Death and Disease*, 1–12 (2018). doi: 10.1038/s41419-018-1239-9.

35. Ziegler, A. N. et al. Insulin-like growth factor II: An essential adult stem cell niche constituent in brain and intestine. *Stem Cell Reports* **12**, 816–830 (2019).

36. Zhang, R., Zhang, Y. & Yi, S. Identification of critical growth factors for peripheral nerve regeneration. *RSC Advances* **9**, 10760–10765 (2019).

37. Joshi, A. A., Padhye, A. M. & Gupta, H. S. Platelet derived growth factor BB levels in gingival crevicular fluid of localized intrabony defect sites treated with platelet rich fibrin membrane or collagen membrane containing recombinant human platelet derived growth factor-BB-A randomized clinical. *Journal of Periodontology* **51**, 208 (2019).

38. Hsieh, H. H. S. et al. Coordinating tissue regeneration through transforming growth factor-β activated kinase 1 inactivation and reactivation. *Stem Cells* **37**, 766–778 (2019).

39. Karaman, S., Leppänen, V.-M. & Alitalo, K. Vascular endothelial growth factor signaling in development and disease. *Development* **145**, dev151019 (2018).

40. Wang, M. et al. Cold atmospheric plasma (CAP)-modified and bioactive protein-loaded core–shell nanofibers for bone tissue engineering applications. *Biomaterials Science* **7**, 2430–2439 (2019).

41. Jain, R. K., Au, P., Tam, J., Duda, D. G. & Fukumura, D. Engineering vascularized tissue. *Nature Biotechnology* **23**, 821–823 (2005).

42. Hu, M. et al. Facile engineering of long-term culturable ex vivo vascularized tissues using biologically derived matrices. *Advanced Healthcare Materials* **7**, 1800845 (2018).

43. Melincovici, C. S. et al. Vascular endothelial growth factor (VEGF): Key factor in normal and pathological angiogenesis. *Romanian Journal of Morphology and Embryology* **59**, 455–467 (2018).

44. Vo, T. N., Kasper, F. K. & Mikos, A. G. Strategies for controlled delivery of growth factors and cells for bone regeneration. *Advanced Drug Delivery Reviews* **64**, 1292–1309 (2012).

45. Geiger, F. et al. Vascular endothelial growth factor gene-activated matrix (VEGF165-GAM) enhances osteogenesis and angiogenesis in large segmental bone defects. *Journal of Bone and Mineral Research* **20**, 2028–2035 (2005).

46. Gasperini, L., Mano, J. F. & Reis, R. L. Natural polymers for the microencapsulation of cells. *Journal of the Royal Society Interface* **11**, 20140817 (2014).

47. Shafiee, A. & Atala, A. Printing technologies for medical applications. *Trends in Molecular Medicine* **22**, 254–265 (2016).

48. Shafiee, A., Norotte, C. & Ghadiri, E. Cellular bioink surface tension: A tunable biophysical parameter for faster maturation of bioprinted tissue. *Bioprinting* **8**, 13–21 (2017).

49. Li, H., Zheng, J., Wang, H., Becker, M. L. & Leipzig, N. D. Neural stem cell encapsulation and differentiation in strain promoted crosslinked polyethylene glycol-based hydrogels. *Journal of Biomaterials Applications* **32**, 1222–1230 (2018).

50. Yang, J.-L., Sykora, P., Wilson, D. M., III, Mattson, M. P. & Bohr, V. A. The excitatory neurotransmitter glutamate stimulates DNA repair to increase neuronal resiliency. *Mechanisms of Ageing and Development* **132**, 405–411 (2011).

51. Yang, J.-L., Tadokoro, T., Keijzers, G., Mattson, M. P. & Bohr, V. A. Neurons efficiently repair glutamate-induced oxidative DNA damage by a process involving CREB-mediated up-regulation of apurinic endonuclease 1. *Journal of Biological Chemistry* **285**, 28191–28199 (2010).

52. Shafiee, A., Ghadiri, E., Salleh, M. M., Yahaya, M. & Atala, A. Controlling the surface properties of an inkjet- printed reactive oxygen species scavenger for flexible bioelectronics applications in neural resilience. *IEEE Journal of the Electron Devices Society* **7**, 784–791 (2019).

53. Popa, E., Reis, R. & Gomes, M. Chondrogenic phenotype of different cells encapsulated in κ-carrageenan hydrogels for cartilage regeneration strategies. *Biotechnology and Applied Biochemistry* **59**, 132–141 (2012).

54. Rocha, P. M., Santo, V. E., Gomes, M. E., Reis, R. L. & Mano, J. F. Encapsulation of adipose-derived stem cells and transforming growth factor-β1 in carrageenan-based hydrogels for cartilage tissue engineering. *Journal of Bioactive and Compatible Polymers* **26**, 493–507 (2011).

55. Drapala, P. W. et al. The effect of glutathione as chain transfer agent in PNIPAAm-based thermoresponsive hydrogels for controlled release of proteins. *Pharmaceutical Research* **31**, 742–753 (2013).

56. Bayer, E. A. et al. Programmed platelet-derived growth factor-BB and bone morphogenetic protein-2 delivery from a hybrid calcium phosphate/alginate scaffold. *Tissue Engineering Part A* **23**, 1382–1393 (2017).

57. Pérez-Luna, V. & González-Reynoso, O. Encapsulation of biological agents in hydrogels for therapeutic applications. *Gels* **4**, 61 (2018).

58. Krishnan, L. et al. Hydrogel-based delivery of rhBMP-2 improves healing of large bone defects compared with autograft. *Clinical Orthopaedics and Related Research* **473**, 2885–2897 (2015).

59. Seo, B.-B., Koh, J.-T. & Song, S.-C. Tuning physical properties and BMP-2 release rates of injectable hydrogel systems for an optimal bone regeneration effect. *Biomaterials* **122**, 91–104 (2017).

60. Jung, S. W. et al. Multivalent ion-based in situ gelling polysaccharide hydrogel as an injectable bone graft. *Carbohydrate Polymers* **180**, 216–225 (2018).

61. Hastings, C. L. et al. Drug and cell delivery for cardiac regeneration. *Advanced Drug Delivery Reviews* **84**, 85–106 (2015).

62. Tsao, C. J. et al. Controlled release of small molecules for cardiac differentiation of pluripotent stem cells. *Tissue Engineering Part A* **24**, 1798–1807 (2018).

63. Nakamura, K. et al. A synthetic small molecule, ONO-1301, enhances endogenous growth factor expression and augments angiogenesis in the ischaemic heart. *Clinical Science* **112**, 607–616 (2007).

64. Nuttelman, C. R., Tripodi, M. C. & Anseth, K. S. Dexamethasone-functionalized gels induce osteogenic differentiation of encapsulated hMSCs. *Journal of Biomedical Materials Research* **76A**, 183–195 (2006).

65. Laurencin, C. T., Ashe, K. M., Henry, N., Kan, H. M. & Lo, K. W. H. Delivery of small molecules for bone regenerative engineering: Preclinical studies and potential clinical applications. *Drug Discovery Today* **19**, 794–800 (2014).

66. Hsueh, Y.-C., Wu, J. M. F., Yu, C.-K., Wu, K. K. & Hsieh, P. C. H. Prostaglandin E 2promotes post-infarction cardiomyocyte replenishment by endogenous stem cells. *EMBO Molecular Medicine* **6**, 496–503 (2014).

67. Kato, N. et al. Nanogel-based delivery system enhances PGE2 effects on bone formation. *Journal of Cellular Biochemistry* **101**, 1063–1070 (2007).

68. Shafiee, A., Ghadiri, E., Kassis, J., Pourhabibi Zarandi, N. & Atala, A. Biosensing technologies for medical applications, manufacturing, and regenerative medicine. *Current Stem Cell Reports* **4**, 105–115 (2018).

9 Controlled Delivery of Angiogenic Proteins

Binita Shrestha, Jacob Brown, and Eric M. Brey
The University of Texas at San Antonio

CONTENTS

9.1   INTRODUCTION

The ability to control the assembly of vascular networks is critical for the development of therapies in a number of areas of medicine. This includes the treatment of ischemic tissues (e.g., peripheral limbs, myocardium), enhancing healing of chronic wounds, improving survival of transplanted tissues and organs, and reconstruction or regeneration of tissues in the fields of tissue engineering and regenerative medicine (TERM). TERM is an interdisciplinary field that primarily focuses on the development of tissue substitutes to replace, repair, or regenerate tissues and organs. Over the past four decades, tissue engineering approaches have demonstrated a tremendous potential [1]. While TERM has found only limited clinical success, research in the field has resulted in significant advances in understanding biological processes such as identifying the ability of mesenchymal cells to induce tissue regeneration through the release of growth factors and cytokines [2,3].

Scalability, survival, and integration of engineered tissue are major challenges. A primary issue is limited or slow vascularization [4,5]. The tissue generated for TERM applications is greater than the approximate diffusion distance of oxygen in tissue (200 μm) [6,7]. This restrains the development of tissue constructs to a few hundred microns in the absence of a robust, extensive, and functional vascular network. Heterogeneity in vascular network formation results in spatial variations within the tissue (particularly in the core) in regards to oxygen and nutrient distribution [8]. Although a number of in vitro approaches have been designed to address this issue they are largely insufficient for engineering large tissues. In addition, after implantation tissue substitutes rely on vascularization from surrounding tissues. Inadequate blood supply results in poor host integration and subsequent cell death [9]. The importance of vascularization is clearly depicted in the literature and therefore is the heavily invested research topic in TERM [8,10–12]. Various strategies have been investigated for vascularization of engineered tissues which includes growth factor delivery, cell-based techniques, bioreactors, microfluidics, surgical techniques, and in vivo systems [8,13]. This chapter will focus on strategies that implement controlled delivery to stimulate vascularization.

9.2   VESSEL NETWORK FORMATION

The mechanisms of vessel network formation are generally placed in the following categories: vasculogenesis, angiogenesis, and arteriogenesis. Vasculogenesis is the process of de novo formation of blood vessels which is primarily responsible for primitive vascular network in the embryo. Angiogenesis is responsible for the expansion of this network by the formation of new capillaries from preexisting ones [14]. Vasculogenesis can also occur in adult organisms via an assembly of precursor cells but this typically occurs in coordination with angiogenesis. Arteriogenesis, or collateralization, is the maturation and enlargement of arteries through the recruitment and/or proliferation of vascular smooth muscle cells or pericytes [15]. Angiogenesis is a dynamic process that involves well-coordinated interactions of cells, soluble factors, and extracellular matrices (ECMs) [16]. The first step in angiogenesis is production of angiogenic growth factors triggered by pathology, damage, inflammation, etc. These growth factors activate endothelial cells (ECs) to produce metalloproteinases (MMPs) that degrade the underlying basement membrane [14]. ECs then migrate into the interstitial space led by tip cells forming sprout structures. These sprouts eventually connect with other vessels to form perfused networks [17]. Although angiogenesis occurs naturally following implantation of an engineered tissue or material, the process is often too slow to provide adequate vascularization for the survival of engineered tissues or regeneration of ischemic tissues [18]. The rapid development of vasculature is critical to achieve desirable therapeutic outcome for perfusion of large tissue beds.

Spatiotemporal control over the levels of angiogenic present in a tissue bed may enhance vascularization or increase the rate at which it forms. Growth factors are proteins that play a critical role in regulating the steps of cell proliferation, differentiation, and migration involved in angiogenesis. Growth factors function by binding with specific receptors present at the cell surface in a concentration-dependent manner [19]. The critical importance of growth factors in angiogenesis is well articulated in the literature, as they play a role in various stages of blood vessels development, from formation of new vessels to stabilization of the newly formed networks. Various strategies have been investigated to increase bioavailability of growth factors within a specific tissue or organ. For example, growth factors can be delivered systemically, locally, through encapsulation in polymer systems or by implanting cells that releasing growth factors. In order to exploit these methods, it is important to first understand the function of these naturally occurring proteins. Some of the more important growth factors regulating vascularization are discussed below.

9.2.1   VASCULAR ENDOTHELIAL GROWTH FACTORS (VEGF)

Vascular Endothelial Growth Factors (VEGFs) are a family of factors that are required for angiogenesis and/or lymphangiogenesis (formation of lymphatic vessels). The VEGF family consists of a number of members, including VEGF-A (which has many isoforms), VEGF-B, VEGF-C, VEGF-D, and placental growth factor (PIGF) [20]. Each of these members play important, but often different, roles in biological processes. For example, VEGF-A binds with VEGFR-1 to regulate normal and pathological angiogenesis. VEGF-A also binds with VEGFR-2 to modulate growth, migration, survival, and permeability of ECs [21] and stimulates ECs to release other growth factors essential to activate surrounding cells [22]. VEGF-C and VEGF-D and their receptor VEGFR-3 have been reported to regulate lymphangiogenesis. There is also a subgroup of VEGF isolated from snake venom, VEGF-F. VEGF-F regulates vascular permeability, angiogenesis, and blood pressure [23]. PIGF binds specifically to VEGFR-1 and regulates vascular events in both angiogenesis and vasculogenesis [24].

9.2.2 FIBROBLAST GROWTH FACTORS (FGF)

Fibroblast Growth Factors (FGFs) are generally heparin binding growth factors that are produced by a number of vascular cells, including vascular endothelial, smooth muscle cells, and fibroblasts. FGFs consists of over 20 members [25]. Among these, acidic FGF (FGF1) and basic FGF (FGF2) have received the most attention for therapeutic control of angiogenesis based on their fundamental role in this process [26]. FGF1 and FGF2 are potent angiogenic factors that stimulate EC proliferation, migration, and angiogenesis [27,28]. Using in vitro systems, both FGF1 and FGF2 have been shown to regulate EC proliferation and migration, ECM degradation, stimulate ECs invasion into collagen, and promote organization of ECs into vessel-like structures [27,29]. FGFs contribute to maturation of blood vessels through influence over the expression of various cell surface molecules, including cadherins and integrins. FGF2 is a promiscuous proteins, interacting with multiple cell types, ECM molecules, lipids, tyrosine kinase receptors, integrins, gangliosides, and proteoglycans [30–32]. These interactions influence protein integrity, stability, and bioavailability which relate directly to its ability to have a prolonged influence on angiogenesis.

9.2.3 PLATELET-DERIVED GROWTH FACTORS (PDGF)

Platelet-Derived Growth Factor (PDGF) includes PDGF-A, PDGF-B, PDGF-AB, PDGF-C, and PDGF-D [33]. PDGFs stimulate proliferation of mesenchymal and progenitor cells during early developmental stages of network formation and cellular differentiation and structural integrity required for later vessel maturation [34]. PDGF plays a crucial role in angiogenesis by recruiting bone marrow derived cells and mural cells. Pericytes, the mural cells of capillaries, are important regulators of morphological and functional aspects of vasculatures [35], including blood flow [36]. While the contribution of PDGFs to initial formation of blood vessels via angiogenesis appears limited [37], they are crucial for stabilization and maturation of newly formed vessels. PDGF-B promotes recruitment of mural cells which differentiate into vessel stabilizing cells, whereas PDGF C is involved in recruitment of both ECs and mural cells [38,39]. PDGF is also involved in regulation of platelet aggregation, a critical first step in healing, providing support for new vessel formation [40].

9.2.4 ANGIOPOIETINS

Angiopoietins is the family of growth factors that include Angiopoietin-1 (Ang-1), Angiopoietin-2 (Ang-2), Angiopoietin-3 (Ang-3), and Angiopoietin-4 (Ang-4). Tie-1 and Tie-2 are endothelial specific receptors for angiopoietins [41]. Angiopoietins and their receptors contribute to angiogenesis through maintenance of EC stability and vascular maturation [42]. Ang-1 and Ang-2 have both been investigated in therapies in angiogenesis. Ang-1 contributes to vessel maturation and stabilization through paracrine interactions with the endothelium that regulate migration, adhesion, and survival of ECs. In addition, Ang-1 is reported to exhibit anti-inflammatory effects [43,44]. While Ang-1 is essential for vascular formation [45], Ang-2 acts as a natural antagonist for Ang-1 and Tie-2 [45]. Ang-2 is indispensable for vascular modeling [46]. Hypoxia and pathological conditions upregulate Ang-2, and at high concentrations, the Ang-2/Tie-2 ligand receptor complex induces destabilization of blood vessels. Ang-2 promotes vascular regression by disrupting interactions between the endothelium and perivascular cells. In the presence of VEGF, the destabilization effects of Ang-2 are a critical step required for remodeling and growth of new vessels.

9.2.5 TRANSFORMING GROWTH FACTOR BETA PROTEINS (TGF-βs)

Transforming growth factors (TGFs) are cytokines that regulate cell growth, differentiation, motility, organization, inflammation, and morphogenesis. TGFα and TGFβ are known to contribute to angiogenesis, tissue development, and wound healing. The function of TGFβ is mediated by interactions with receptors TGFR-I, TGFR-II, and TGFR-III. TGFβ can stimulate or inhibit angiogenesis depending on temporal distribution and the presence/absence of other factors [47]. For example, TGFβ stimulates mesenchymal cells but exhibits antimitogenic properties for epithelial cells. TGFβ contributes to vascular morphogenesis based on regulation of ECM deposition and ECM remodeling. More importantly, TGF-β1 plays a fundamental role in stabilization of new vessels by inhibiting EC proliferation and inducing differentiation of recruited mural cells.

9.3 METHODS OF DELIVERY

Growth factors orchestrate a cascade of events critical in angiogenesis; from proliferation and migration of ECs, to the assembly of network structures and, finally, vessel maturation and stabilization. Controlled delivery of growth factors to promote or control angiogenesis is an attractive strategy for the treatment of ischemic tissues and for control of tissue development in TERM. Despite promising results in preclinical studies and clinical trials, large-scale clinical results have failed to find a significant and consistent therapeutic benefit. This calls for further research on parameters that influence angiogenesis including mode of administration, spatial and temporal profiles, concentration, and delivery of multiple growth factors simultaneously or sequentially. Growth factors typically exhibit short half-lives and act locally through diffusion-mediated transport. The ability of growth factor to instruct cells to perform specific tasks depends on concentration, time of delivery, bioavailability, and appropriate presentation and transport through the ECM. Therefore, the mode and timing of single or multiple growth factor delivery in addition to concentration and spatial distribution all play a role in the appropriate control over vascularization.

9.3.1 SYSTEMIC OR LOCALIZED DELIVERY

A wide range of growth factors have been investigated for therapeutic application as described in previous sections [48–51]. Initial clinical approaches exploited systemic delivery, via either intravenous or intra-arterial injection. This approach has been reported to improve myocardial function following ischemia [52–54].On comparing intravenous and intra-arterial delivery, several studies have reported intra-arterial delivery to have advantages in terms of increased bioavailability and reduced dose in the systemic circulation [55]. However, Intra-arterial infusion has a greater risk of embolization, arterial occlusion, and increased cost. Regardless of approach, systemic delivery has major limitations. Growth factors have a relatively short half-life and degrade rapidly in vivo due to denaturation and proteolysis [56,57]. Therefore, growth factors may not reach the target tissue or cells at sufficient levels or within the required timeframe to evoke an appropriate biological response when delivered systemically. [57]. Repeated administration and higher doses of growth factors are typically used in an attempt to overcome this issue [58,59], but high concentrations run the risk of side effects such as ectopic vessel formation or abnormal growth locally. Additionally, systemic delivery generally is unable to target specific cells or tissues. Taken together, the systemic delivery of growth factors may result in unsatisfactory therapeutic outcomes such as dose-associated side effects and transient or inadequate effects on neovascularization.

Localized administration or delivery via direct injection into a specific tissue, on the other hand, results in improved bioavailability of growth factors locally. This method may be invasive surgery or require specialized devices [53]. This delivery can be intramuscular, intramyocardial, pericardial, intracerebral, and so on depending on the targeted tissue. This method of delivery offers improved transfer and retention rates [60], and the growth factor levels necessary to achieve a sufficient biological response can be achieved with a lower dose relative to systemic delivery. While this is an improvement over systemic delivery, issues with nonspecific biological response, toxicity due to high local concentrations, and growth factor degradation are still significant challenges with direct injection into tissues [61].

9.3.2 CONTROLLED DELIVERY

Ongoing research in angiogenesis and drug delivery has determined that prolonged or sustained exposure of growth factors is likely necessary for the development and survival of newly formed tissues or vessels [60,62]. Systemic or bolus injection of growth factors results in an acute increase in local concentration that rapidly subsides, typically limiting the long-term impact of the therapy. Given this limitation, various strategies have been investigated to enhance bioavailability, stability and functionality of growth factors at the delivery site. One way to achieve this is to incorporate growth factors into synthetic or naturally occurring biomaterials, which serve to protect the proteins from the local environment and to slowly release the proteins into the tissue. This method allows sustained local delivery of growth factors and also preserves structure and function. Growth factors can be trapped in biomaterials by chemical attachment or physical encapsulation [63].

Physically encapsulating growth factors in polymeric systems is a simple yet prominent strategy. Once a growth factor is trapped in the material structure, it is released into the surrounding tissue through diffusion, degradation of the polymer, or a combination of both. Properties such as crosslink density, mesh size, porosity, and degradation kinetics can be fine-tuned to impart temporal control over release kinetics. Physical encapsulation methods include phase separation, phase emulsion, solvent casting, double emulsion, in situ polymerization, and gas foaming [64,65].

Growth factors can also be chemically attached to the biomaterial substrate through a variety of approaches. This includes direct covalent attachment, electrostatic interactions between the materials and proteins, or interactions with intermediate molecules such as heparin-derived proteins, gelatin, and fibronectin [66]. In the case of covalent incorporation, growth factors are conjugated to polymers through functional groups already present on the materials or introduced during polymer synthesis. Covalent bonding of growth factors generally provides improved long-term stability and release kinetics over physical entrapment [67,68]. Electrostatic interactions generally slow release relative to physical methods but do not offer the same level of control as covalent approaches. However, they do not require chemical modification of the growth factor which can influence folding and biological activity. The use of intermediates, such as heparin-derived molecules, can be used to present growth factors in a way that mimics in vivo when interacting with the ECM. This "natural" presentation can increase activity and prolong availability. Regardless of the types of conjugation, spatial and temporal control as well as stimuli-responsive delivery of growth factor release at the site of interest is critical to any tissue engineering application.

9.3.3 SPATIAL DELIVERY

Angiogenesis is influenced by both the concentration and spatial distribution of factors in the local microenvironment. Spatial gradients of substrate-immobilized molecules [69] and soluble molecules [70] influence the rate, direction, and structure of new vessel growth. Spatial gradients govern the directionality of vessel growth by directing EC and smooth muscle cell migration [71–73]. The diffusive properties and differential binding to ECM proteins of growth factors results in spatial gradient in vivo [74]. Various approaches have been studied to mimic the effect of spatial gradients. Both synthetic and natural polymeric biomaterials can be used as a depot for spatial delivery of growth factors [75]. One technique is to fabricate scaffolds containing a gradient of growth factors built in and designed to stimulate angiogenesis postimplantation [68, 76–79]. Polycaprolactone (PCL)/Pluronic F127 cylindrical scaffolds have also been developed with concentration gradients of BMP-7, TGFβ_2, and VEGF$_{165}$ along the longitudinal direction. Growth factors were immobilized on fibril-like PCL, and the surface area of the cylindrical scaffold was increased gradually by tailoring pore size along the longitudinal direction to produce a concentration gradient [80]. Although they did not explore the effect of growth factor gradients on angiogenesis, this study provides insight on how to develop scaffolds with spatial gradients in both longitudinal and radial directions. Another study developed scaffold with radial spatial gradient using point source method. In this method, Odedra et al. first activated VEGF and injected at the center of the scaffold to introduce gradient in a radial direction. This VEGF gradient resulted in enhanced EC migration to the center of the scaffold, as opposed to uniformly immobilized VEGF which showed relatively uniform cell distribution and free VEGF that showed sporadic distribution [81]. In another study, multilayer polymer hydrogels were generated with a persistent PDGF-B gradient. This method provided a persistent (21 day) gradient of PDGF in vivo and demonstrated dose- and gradient-dependent influences on the depth of tissue invasion and overall vessel density [82]. Guo et al stimulated angiogenesis by creating 3D of basic FGF (bFGF). They loaded gradient amount of bFGF in Poly(lactic-co-glycolic acid (PLGA) microspheres. Then they electrospin PCL fibers and electrospray bFGF-loaded PLGA microspheres simultaneously to form 3D constructs with bFGF gradient. They observed high density of vessel construct following 10 days of subcutaneous implantation. They reported vessel density as a function of gradient steepness (Figure 9.1) [83].

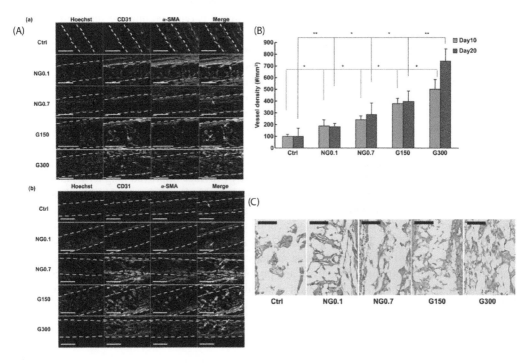

FIGURE 9.1 Angiogenesis in a 3D scaffold with bFGF growth factor gradient. Fibrous scaffolds were harvested on day 10 and 20 postimplantation. Control group (Ctrl) scaffolds fabricated without bFGF, nongradient scaffolds fabricated with injection rate of 0.1 ml/h (NG0.1) or 0.7 ml/h (NG0.7) of bFGF (150 μg/ml), gradient scaffolds fabricated with injection rate of 0.1–0.7 ml/h bFGF (150 μg/ml) (G150) or 0.7 ml/h bFGF (300 μg/ml) (G300) represent the different groups. (A) Immunohistological staining of scaffolds at (a) day 10 and (b) day 20. CD31 antibody staining was used for tubular structure and anti-αSMA antibody for vessel walls. Colocalized signals from CD31 and anti-αSMA are considered mature vessels. (B). Vessel density quantified for different groups at days 10 and 20. Significantly more vessel density was observed in nongradient and gradient scaffolds when compared with control group (*$p < 0.01$, **$p < 0.001$). (C) Histology of explanted scaffolds at day 10 showing functional vessels indicated by arrows. Values are the mean ± standard deviation for $n = 5$. Scale bar: A and $B = 200$ μm and; $D = 50$ μm. (Reprinted with permission from [83]. Copyright 2012, American Chemical Society.)

Recently, techniques such as microfluidics, photolithography, and electrospinning have been used as a tool to design materials with spatial gradients and to investigate their effects on cellular response [84–89]. For example, Barbick et al. explored localized presentation of VEGF and integrin ligand to accelerate angiogenic response of ECs. VEGF was covalently immobilized to the surface of hydrogel in patterned micron-scale regions [90]. In a similar study, VEGF was photopatterned in collagen–glycosaminoglycan scaffolds for spatial presentation resulting in increased cell infiltration and immature vessel formation [91].

9.3.4 TEMPORAL DELIVERY

Growth factors play crucial roles in angiogenesis and tissue repair; however, they are short-lived and fast-acting molecules. Since sustained delivery of growth factors have obvious advantage over its single or bolus administration in angiogenesis, various techniques have been developed to preserve the biological activity of growth factors for prolonged delivery [92,93]. For instance, sustained delivery of FGF-1 from alginate microbeads showed increased vascular density when compared to single bolus injection [94]. Growth factor concentration affects the morphology and stability of microvascular networks. Higher concentration of growth factors can negatively affect angiogenesis, whereas consistent long-term delivery of low concentration of growth factors has reported improved structural and functional aspects of vascular networks. Ozawa et al. reported aberrant vessel formation with higher dosages of VEGF, where lower dosages were reported to stimulate formation of mature capillary structures. This result supports the potential negative side effects of higher growth factor concentration, such as hyperpermeable vessels, hypotension, hypervascularity, and tumor growth [5,95]. In another study, high concentrations of FGF1 resulted in rapid and intense sprouts from ECs aggregates in vitro. However, these capillaries later began to regress. On the other hand, a lower concentration of FGF-1 promoted slower, but persistent and normal, capillary outgrowth [96]. Robinson et al. developed plasma lysate incorporated hydrogels for sustained release of PDGF-B over 20 days. This hydrogel system promoted EC sprouting when cultured alone and in combination with mesenchymal stem cells [97]. Similarly, gradual and consistent release of VEGF-A over the period of 30 days from a polyethylene glycol-fibrinogen hydrogel indicated significant improvement in arteriogenesis and cardiac performance [98]. Spatiotemporal release of growth factor also reported improved functionality of formed vessels indicated by restoration of normal tissue perfusion in addition to improved angiogenesis in hind limb ischemia by day 28. This was achieved by persistent and localized delivery of VEGF over the period of 15 days from an injectable hydrogel system [99].

9.3.5 TEMPORAL DELIVERY MULTIPLE GROWTH FACTORS

The formation of stable and functional blood vessels involves a complex interplay of multiple growth factors [100–102]. The research community has investigated controlled delivery of combinations of growth factors in an attempt to recapitulate the in vivo vascularization process. Recent studies show that some growth factors are critical in initiating blood vessel formation, while others are crucial for the stabilization and functionality of the formed vessels. For example, VEGF and FGF2 are involved in the initial phases of vessel development, while PDGF and Ang-2 are important in the stabilization of vessels at later stages [103]. Combinations of growth factors can work synergistically to induce angiogenesis [104–106]. Controlled dual- or multidelivery of growth factors has been reported to have significant positive effects on vessel density and stabilization over a single delivery [107]. Combined delivery of FGF2 and VEGF induced greater angiogenesis in vitro when compared to delivery of either factor alone [107]. This may be due to upregulation of VEGF in ECs by FGF [109,110]. A similar synergism has been reported with FGF1 and VEGF [111]. Increased vessel density has been shown with sequential delivery of FGF1 followed by PDGF-B, but not when PDGF-B delivery was followed by FGF-1 or either factor alone [112]. In another study, multiple proangiogenic and promaturation factors were delivered in a temporally controlled manner to enhance vessel formation and maturation [113]. In this study, rapid release of VEGF and Ang-2, proangiogenic factors, followed by delayed release of PDGF and Ang1, promoted vascular growth, maturation, and remodeling. In another recent study, VEGF was delivered in a sustained manner in conjunction with a localized injection of insulin growth factor-1 (IGF) for the treatment of hind limb ischemia. This combination of growth factors showed enhanced perfusion recovery at significantly lower doses in comparison to past studies [114]. Similarly, spatiotemporal release of VEGF and PDGF stimulated localized neovascularization [115]. Finally, sustained released of VEGF and Ang-1 from an injectable hydrogel over the period of 30 days resulted in improved cardiac function and arteriogenesis [116]. Although spatial and temporal control of growth factor delivery appears capable of stimulating angiogenesis, local or environmental conditions may result in the need to more precisely and specifically control the delivery process.

9.3.6 STIMULI-RESPONSIVE DELIVERY

Outside of controlling the rate and spatial distribution of drug delivery, there are many applications where it is necessary to limit drug release to only occur under specific conditions or at specific times. The class of biomaterials which release drugs only in the presence of a specific influence are considered "stimuli-responsive" biomaterials. There are many biological and chemical mechanisms that can be exploited to create materials which respond to a variety of stimuli, such as pH, temperature, magnetic fields, mechanical force, enzymatic activity, or electric fields, among others. These drug delivery systems can be broadly divided into those which respond to the native conditions that occur within a tissue, and those which respond to an external stimulus that is applied to the tissue.

Delivery systems which react to environmental cues that originate from the tissue of interest are either used to protect the drug until it is in the direct vicinity where repair is taking place, which is where the drug is most effective, or in response to a local change (e.g., an increase in inflammation). These systems exhibit little or no release until they encounter the stimuli, and then undergo a change to release their cargo. One application of this strategy is the targeted delivery of VEGF to wound sites using polymers that are degraded by specific enzymes. [117] VEGF is crucial to vascularization of healing tissue, and in the case of neural repair after a stroke, is normally applied repeatedly to wounds at very high concentration to induce revascularization. This is ineffective, however, as bolus injection of free VEGF contained within a bulk hydrogel has been shown to result in disordered and immature vessels, and not increase overall vascularization in the area of the wound. Restricting the activity of VEGF to areas where active remodeling is taking place allows the protein to function more effectively at much lower doses. Also, protecting the protein from the tissue environment until it is needed allows for a longer half-life in vivo. To accomplish this, one or two VEGF molecules are coated with a "nanogel" shell of acrylamide monomers crosslinked with Lys-Asn-Arg-Val-Lys peptides. These peptides exhibit chirality, and the ratio of L to D centers changes their reactivity with proteases present in remodeling tissue. The encapsulated VEGF is inactive once injected until it encounters activated plasmin, which is present where ECs are remodeling the surrounding matrix. Plasmin cleaves the peptide bonds crosslinking the gel, releasing VEGF into the system to signal nearby ECs. Delivery of VEGF to only specific areas where vessels are already developing results in significant increases in vascularization and pericyte coverage, which are important for vessel stability. This system can be further tuned with different peptides to change which protease causes release, as well as by changing the L to D ratio to affect the rate of release. The same study utilized this rate control to sequentially release VEGF followed by PDGF-BB, which was even more effective in stimulating vascularization, and showed that release in the other order was not as effective for pericyte coverage.

There are many other systems that react to the tissue environment to deliver proangiogenic proteins. VEGF-containing polymers have been functionalized with aptamer sequences that bind to molecules with a complimentary sequence and conformationally change, releasing the drug. [85,118]

Another study utilized a random terpolymer of N-isopropylacrylamide (NIPAAm), poly(acrylic acid) (PAA), and butyl acrylate (BA), which is both pH and temperature sensitive. The polymer is a liquid at room temperature and pH 7.4, but gels at 37°C and pH 6.8 in the acidic conditions of ischemic tissues. In its hydrogel form, it stabilizes and slowly releases contained VEGF and FGF to promote angiogenesis, and then is eliminated as the tissue stabilizes and returns to physiological pH. [119] A similar system of nanoparticles created from chitosan and poly(γ-glutamic acid) (γ-PGA) then coated with heparin were used as a pH-responsive reservoir that releases FGF2 into ischemic areas to stimulate angiogenesis. The relatively low pH of the ischemic area stabilizes the nanoparticles and allows slow release of FGF2, and when the area returns to normal pH, the nanoparticles degrade and release heparin, modulating any thrombosis or additional vascularization. [120]

In cases where there is no apparent endogenous condition to use as a release stimulus, exogenous stimulus can also be utilized to trigger the release of a drug from a biomaterial system. This generally gives control of the release to an operator who utilizes radiation, sound, or some other form of energy to initiate release of the drug at a specific time or location. There are a variety of stimuli which can be used to this effect including light, sound, heat, magnetic, and electric fields, and, in certain cases, other drugs. Materials that utilize external stimulus can be in the form of bulk materials that are implanted or injected, but frequently are deployed as nanomaterials that may be freely released into the system or localized to a specific area, either embedded in another bulk material or using a chemical receptor ligand to associate with a specific cell type.

External stimulus-responsive delivery systems can be effective in complex applications where a sensitive drug must be delivered to a specific area with precision. This is especially true in genetic transfection applications that target internal organs. Care must be taken when performing transfection to reduce the nonspecific alteration of genes outside of the area of interest and reduce systemic inflammation which can occur wherever plasmids are delivered. This can be accomplished several ways, but one study demonstrated the use of ultrasound-responsive microbubbles composed of perflutren as a carrier for plasmids containing the human VEGF165 gene that could be selectively ruptured in a chosen location. After coronary artery ligation to induce myocardial infarction in a mouse model, the microbubbles containing the plasmid were injected in the tail vein, allowed to perfuse, and then stimulated using an ultrasound probe directed at the heart for 20 minutes. Rupture of the microbubbles and delivery of the gene was confirmed using pulse sequencing imaging. After 14 days, delivery of the gene resulted in increased VEGF production, increased recruitment of progenitor cells to the area, increased vascular density, and improved cardiac function. Levels of VEGF production were also compared to remote regions of the left ventricle to confirm that the transfection occurred primarily in the area exposed to ultrasound. [121] Similar studies have also included magnetic targeting by coating the microbubbles with iron oxide magnetic nanoparticles. In one case, a magnet was placed over a targeted area of skin to accumulate nanoparticle-laden microbubbles which were injected systemically. This technique allows the ultrasound stimulus to affect a higher concentration of nanoparticles and release more plasmids. [122] Ultrasound is also a good candidate for controlled direct delivery of growth factors. Moncion et al. demonstrate the use of Pluronic F68 as a microbubble medium for delivery of bFGF to mice subcutaneously. bFGF is suspended within perfluorocarbon (PFC) using a PEG/Krytox fluorosurfactant, creating a double emulsion inside of the Pluronic microbubble. When stimulated by ultrasound, the PFC transitions to a gas, releasing the bFGF into the surroundings. This delivery method resulted in increased, stable perfusion in mice over a period of 2 weeks. (Figure 9.2) [123]

Each type of stimulus has its own advantages and limitations. Ultrasound is relatively safe, but there are limitations on the precision of stimulation, the range of materials which respond to it, and the applications that they can be used for. Other materials are limited by how the energy can be transmitted through the skin to the wound site. For example, light is an exogenous stimulus that can theoretically be used for controlled drug delivery. Photodegradable poly(ethylene glycol) di-photodegradable-acrylate microparticles were engineered by one group to contain TGF-β1. The polymer structure is cleaved when irradiated with 365 nm wavelength light, dissolving the particles

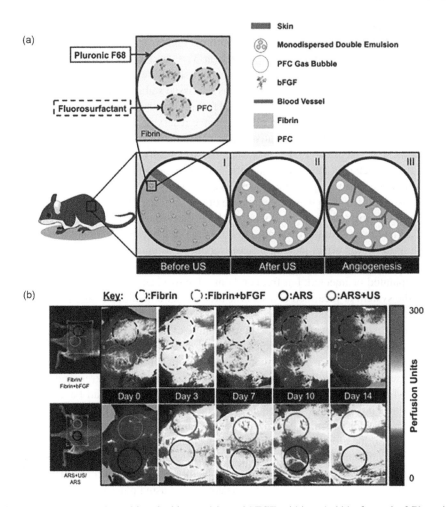

FIGURE 9.2 An ultrasound-sensitive double-emulsion of bFGF within a bubble formed of Pluronic filled with PFC. Under ultrasound stimulation, PFC transitions from liquid to gas and allows release of bFGF. (a) Acoustically responsive scaffolds (ARS) performed better at stimulating vascularization than control fibrin scaffolds with and without bFGF. Stimulation of the ARS resulted in higher vascularization than nonstimulated ARS. (b) Longitudinal LASCA images of two mice, each with two implants. The regions of interests (ROIs) were chosen based on the physical location of the implants, and are denoted by colored circles. The left most images are visible images of the mice. For all images, the caudal direction is left. ROI diameter: 0.9. cm. [124]

and releasing their payload. [125] Light-responsive systems, however, are limited by the penetration depth that can be achieved. Mechanical force has even been used as an external stimulus for drug release. One study utilized a calcium-crosslinked alginate hydrogel loaded with free VEGF which, when stimulated with compressive force, showed increased release of the contained drug based on increased convection of water out of the material. When implanted, the gel was physically manipulated by a custom external compression device, which regulated the rate of release of the contained drug. This allowed for control of the rate of release above normal diffusion. [126] In theory, similar systems could use a wide variety of materials and drugs, but applications would still be limited to areas where force can be safely applied through the skin at appropriate (i.e., safe) magnitudes. Restrictions encountered with some stimuli can be circumvented by using complex drug delivery systems that convert energy from one type to another. There are many thermally responsive polymers that could be used for drug delivery; however, the temperature threshold for pain in human skin is roughly 44°C, so only materials that show a significant change in properties above 37°C but below 44°C should be utilized for controlled drug delivery purposes. Also, because heating internal tissues still requires conductance of heat through the skin, this limits the depth at which responsive systems can operate. To get around this, a form of energy that can be directed throughout the body with little to no direct effect on the tissue is needed. One promising candidate is electromagnetism. Magnetic nanoparticles of specific composition can transduce alternating magnetic fields (AMF) into localized heat emission, and when coated with thermoresponsive polymers, can function as an externally controlled responsive drug delivery system. The field strength required to stimulate these nanoparticles is safe to use with living tissue and is not limited by the depth of implantation. No example of this kind of system was found which specifically delivered proangiogenic factors, but it has been utilized for other applications. One such study showed that allyl isothiocyanate (AITC) bonded to a poly(ethylenimine) (PEI) coating on iron oxide nanoparticles could be remotely triggered to release using an AMF of specific frequency and power. Once released, the AITC stimulated a response in nearby neurons in vitro.[127] This system can be adapted to release angiogenic growth factors such as VEGF and deployed in vivo within bulk polymers used for tissue regeneration. In combination with imaging techniques that can assess the density of blood vessels in vivo, this system could be used to directly intervene and support regenerating tissue with poor vascularization.

9.4 CONCLUSIONS AND FUTURE WORK

Angiogenesis is critical for nearly all applications of TERM. In addition, the ability to control angiogenesis can be used to treat pathological and surgical conditions. Growth factors are key regulators of the cascade of cellular events that initiate, develop, and stabilize new blood vessel formation. Appropriate control of growth factor availability can provide therapeutic efficacy over bolus administration of a single growth factor. These systems can be used in an attempt to recapitulate the actual biological processes available spatially and for prolong periods. While polymer delivery systems have demonstrated significant ability to control delivery of multiple growth factors in both space and time, these systems are still limited by the nature of biological processes. [128] In some cases, it is impractical to vascularize large tissue volumes in sufficient times. Combination of delivery strategies with cell or microvascular fragment-based prevascularization may move these approaches closer to success. In other cases, variability from one individual to the next may hinder strategies based on predetermined release kinetics. In this case, strategies that combine stimuli-responsive materials with noninvasive monitoring techniques could allow real-time monitoring and control over vascularization. Regardless of approach, the continued development of innovative controlled release systems has the potential for significant impact on medical practice.

REFERENCES

1. Berthiaume, F., T.J. Maguire, and M.L. Yarmush, Tissue engineering and regenerative medicine: History, progress, and challenges. *Annual Review of Chemical and Biomolecular Engineering*, 2011. **2**: pp. 403–430.
2. Yagi, H., et al., Mesenchymal stem cells: Mechanisms of immunomodulation and homing. *Cell Transplantation*, 2010. **19**(6–7): pp. 667–679.
3. Sordi, V., Mesenchymal stem cell homing capacity. *Transplantation*, 2009. **87**(9S): pp. S42–S45.
4. Phelps, E.A. and A.J. García, Engineering more than a cell: Vascularization strategies in tissue engineering. *Current Opinion in Biotechnology*, 2010. **21**(5): pp. 704–709.
5. Brey, E.M., et al., Therapeutic neovascularization: Contributions from bioengineering. *Tissue Engineering*, 2005. **11**(3–4): pp. 567–584.
6. Rouwkema, J., N.C. Rivron, and C.A. van Blitterswijk, Vascularization in tissue engineering. *Trends in Biotechnology*, 2008. **26**(8): pp. 434–441.
7. Kannan, R.Y., et al., The roles of tissue engineering and vascularisation in the development of microvascular networks: A review. *Biomaterials*, 2005. **26**(14): pp. 1857–1875.
8. Lovett, M., et al., Vascularization strategies for tissue engineering. *Tissue Engineering Part B: Reviews*, 2009. **15**(3): pp. 353–370.

9. Rouwkema, J. and A. Khademhosseini, Vascularization and angiogenesis in tissue engineering: Beyond creating static networks. *Trends in Biotechnology*, 2016. **34**(9): pp. 733–745.

10. Laschke, M.W., et al., Angiogenesis in tissue engineering: Breathing life into constructed tissue substitutes. *Tissue Engineering*, 2006. **12**(8): pp. 2093–2104.

11. Laschke, M. and M. Menger, Vascularization in tissue engineering: Angiogenesis versus inosculation. *European Surgical Research*, 2012. **48**(2): pp. 85–92.

12. Shrestha, B., DeLuna, F., Anastasio, M.A., Yong Ye, J., Brey, E.M. Photoacoustic imaging in tissue engineering and regenerative medicine. *Tissue Eng Part B Rev*, 2020. doi:10.1089/ten.TEB.2019.0296.

13. Santos, M. and R. Reis, Vascularization strategies in tissue engineering. In R.L. Reis, N.M. Neves, J.F. Mano, M.E. Gomes, A.P. Marques, and H.S. Azevedo (eds.) *Natural-Based Polymers for Biomedical Applications*. Elsevier: Amsterdam, Netherlands, 2008: pp. 761–780.

14. Patan, S., Vasculogenesis and angiogenesis as mechanisms of vascular network formation, growth and remodeling. *Journal of Neuro-Oncology*, 2000. **50**(1–2): pp. 1–15.

15. Heil, M., et al., Arteriogenesis versus angiogenesis: Similarities and differences. *Journal of Cellular and Molecular Medicine*, 2006. **10**(1): pp. 45–55.

16. D'amore, P. and R. Thompson, Mechanisms of angiogenesis. *Annual Review of Physiology*, 1987. **49**(1): pp. 453–464.

17. Yadav, L., et al., Tumour angiogenesis and angiogenic inhibitors: A review. *Journal of Clinical and Diagnostic Research: JCDR*, 2015. **9**(6): p. XE01.

18. Laschke, M.W., B. Vollmar, and M.D. Menger, Inosculation: Connecting the life-sustaining pipelines. *Tissue Engineering Part B: Reviews*, 2009. **15**(4): pp. 455–465.

19. Babensee, J.E., L.V. McIntire, and A.G. Mikos, Growth factor delivery for tissue engineering. *Pharmaceutical Research*, 2000. **17**(5): pp. 497–504.

20. Hoeben, A., et al., Vascular endothelial growth factor and angiogenesis. *Pharmacological Reviews*, 2004. **56**(4): pp. 549–580.

21. Holmes, K., et al., Vascular endothelial growth factor receptor-2: Structure, function, intracellular signalling and therapeutic inhibition. *Cellular Signalling*, 2007. **19**(10): pp. 2003–2012.

22. LeCouter, J., et al., Angiogenesis-independent endothelial protection of liver: Role of VEGFR-1. *Science*, 2003. **299**(5608): pp. 890–893.

23. Toivanen, P.I., et al., Snake venom VEGF Vammin induces a highly efficient angiogenic response in skeletal muscle via VEGFR-2/NRP specific signaling. *Scientific Reports*, 2017. **7**(1): p. 5525.

24. Torry, D.S., et al., Expression and function of placenta growth factor: implications for abnormal placentation. *Journal of the Society for Gynecologic Investigation*, 2003. **10**(4): pp. 178–188.

25. Itoh, N. and D.M. Ornitz, Evolution of the Fgf and Fgfr gene families. *TRENDS in Genetics*, 2004. **20**(11): pp. 563–569.

26. Chu, H. and Y. Wang, Therapeutic angiogenesis: Controlled delivery of angiogenic factors. *Therapeutic Delivery*, 2012. **3**(6): pp. 693–714.

27. Montesano, R., et al., Basic fibroblast growth factor induces angiogenesis in vitro. *Proceedings of the National Academy of Sciences*, 1986. **83**(19): pp. 7297–7301.

28. Folkman, J., et al., A heparin-binding angiogenic protein--basic fibroblast growth factor--is stored within basement membrane. *The American Journal of Pathology*, 1988. **130**(2): p. 393.

29. Presta, M., et al., Fibroblast growth factor/fibroblast growth factor receptor system in angiogenesis. *Cytokine & Growth Factor Reviews*, 2005. **16**(2): pp. 159–178.

30. Rusnati, M. and M. Presta, Interaction of angiogenic basic fibroblast growth factor with endothelial cell heparan sulfate proteoglycans. *International Journal of Clinical and Laboratory Research*, 1996. **26**(1): pp. 15–23.

31. Rusnati, M., et al., Interaction of fibroblast growth factor-2 (FGF-2) with free gangliosides: Biochemical characterization and biological consequences in endothelial cell cultures. *Molecular Biology of the Cell*, 1999. **10**(2): pp. 313–327.

32. Klein, S., et al., Basic fibroblast growth factor modulates integrin expression in microvascular endothelial cells. *Molecular Biology of the Cell*, 1993. **4**(10): pp. 973–982.

33. Fredriksson, L., H. Li, and U. Eriksson, The PDGF family: Four gene products form five dimeric isoforms. *Cytokine & Growth Factor Reviews*, 2004. **15**(4): pp. 197–204.

34. Hoch, R.V. and P. Soriano, Roles of PDGF in animal development. *Development*, 2003. **130**(20): pp. 4769–4784.

35. Armulik, A., G. Genové, and C. Betsholtz, Pericytes: Developmental, physiological, and pathological perspectives, problems, and promises. *Developmental Cell*, 2011. **21**(2): pp. 193–215.

36. Hirschi, K.K. and P.A. D'Amore, Pericytes in the microvasculature. *Cardiovascular Research*, 1996. **32**(4): pp. 687–698.

37. Heldin, C.-H. and B. Westermark, Mechanism of action and in vivo role of platelet-derived growth factor. *Physiological Reviews*, 1999. **79**(4): pp. 1283–1316.

38. Figg, W.D. and J. Folkman, *Angiogenesis: An Integrative Approach from Science to Medicine*. Springer Science & Business Media: New York. 2008.

39. Hellstrom, M., et al., Role of PDGF-B and PDGFR-beta in recruitment of vascular smooth muscle cells and pericytes during embryonic blood vessel formation in the mouse. *Development*, 1999. **126**(14): pp. 3047–3055.

40. Bryckaert, M., et al., Collagen-induced binding to human platelets of platelet-derived growth factor leading to inhibition of P43 and P20 phosphorylation. *Journal of Biological Chemistry*, 1989. **264**(8): pp. 4336–4341.

41. Fagiani, E. and G. Christofori, Angiopoietins in angiogenesis. *Cancer Letters*, 2013. **328**(1): pp. 18–26.

42. Thomas, M. and H.G. Augustin, The role of the angiopoietins in vascular morphogenesis. *Angiogenesis*, 2009. **12**(2): p. 125.

43. Tsigkos, S., M. Koutsilieris, and A. Papapetropoulos, Angiopoietins in angiogenesis and beyond. *Expert Opinion on Investigational Drugs*, 2003. **12**(6): pp. 933–941.

44. Fiedler, U. and H.G. Augustin, Angiopoietins: A link between angiogenesis and inflammation. *Trends in Immunology*, 2006. **27**(12): pp. 552–558.

45. Maisonpierre, P.C., et al., Angiopoietin-2, a natural antagonist for Tie2 that disrupts in vivo angiogenesis. *Science*, 1997. **277**(5322): pp. 55–60.

46. Gale, N.W., et al., Angiopoietin-2 is required for postnatal angiogenesis and lymphatic patterning, and only the latter role is rescued by Angiopoietin-1. *Developmental Cell*, 2002. **3**(3): pp. 411–423.

47. Chin, D., et al., What is transforming growth factor-beta (TGF-β)? *British Journal of Plastic Surgery*, 2004. **57**(3): pp. 215–221.

48. Li, X., et al., Revascularization of ischemic tissues by PDGF-CC via effects on endothelial cells and their progenitors. *The Journal of Clinical Investigation*, 2005. **115**(1): pp. 118–127.

49. Autiero, M., et al., Placental growth factor and its receptor, vascular endothelial growth factor receptor-1: Novel targets for stimulation of ischemic tissue revascularization and inhibition of angiogenic and inflammatory disorders. *Journal of Thrombosis and Haemostasis*, 2003. **1**(7): pp. 1356–1370.

50. Cai, L., et al., Suppression of hepatocyte growth factor production impairs the ability of adipose-derived stem cells to promote ischemic tissue revascularization. *Stem Cells*, 2007. **25**(12): pp. 3234–3243.

51. Sellke, F.W., et al., Angiogenesis induced by acidic fibroblast growth factor as an alternative method of revascularization for chronic myocardial ischemia. *Surgery*, 1996. **120**(2): pp. 182–188.

52. Lopez, J.J., et al., VEGF administration in chronic myocardial ischemia in pigs. *Cardiovascular Research*, 1998. **40**(2): pp. 272–281.

53. Laham, R.J., et al., Intracoronary and intravenous administration of basic fibroblast growth factor: Myocardial and tissue distribution. *Drug Metabolism and Disposition*, 1999. **27**(7): pp. 821–826.

54. Takeshita, S., et al., Therapeutic angiogenesis. A single intraarterial bolus of vascular endothelial growth factor augments revascularization in a rabbit ischemic hind limb model. *The Journal of Clinical Investigation*, 1994. **93**(2): pp. 662–670.

55. Eckman, W.W., C.S. Patlak, and J.D. Fenstermacher, A critical evaluation of the principles governing the advantages of intra-arterial infusions. *Journal of Pharmacokinetics and Biopharmaceutics*, 1974. **2**(3): pp. 257–285.

56. Bowen-Pope, D.F., et al., Platelet-derived growth factor in vivo: Levels, activity, and rate of clearance. *Blood*, 1984. **64**(2): pp. 458–469.

57. Eppler, S.M., et al., A target-mediated model to describe the pharmacokinetics and hemodynamic effects of recombinant human vascular endothelial growth factor in humans. *Clinical Pharmacology & Therapeutics*, 2002. **72**(1): pp. 20–32.

58. Henry, T.D., et al., The VIVA trial: Vascular endothelial growth factor in ischemia for vascular angiogenesis. *Circulation*, 2003. **107**(10): pp. 1359–1365.

59. Bethel, A., et al., Intravenous basic fibroblast growth factor decreases brain injury resulting from focal ischemia in cats. *Stroke*, 1997. **28**(3): pp. 609–616.

60. Simons, M. and J.A. Ware, Therapeutic angiogenesis in cardiovascular disease. *Nature Reviews Drug Discovery*, 2003. **2**(11): p. 863.

61. Sommer, A. and D.B. Rifkin, Interaction of heparin with human basic fibroblast growth factor: Protection of the angiogenic protein from proteolytic degradation by a glycosaminoglycan. *Journal of Cellular Physiology*, 1989. **138**(1): pp. 215–220.

62. Khurana, R. and M. Simons, Insights from angiogenesis trials using fibroblast growth factor for advanced arteriosclerotic disease. *Trends in Cardiovascular Medicine*, 2003. **13**(3): pp. 116–122.

63. Lee, K., E.A. Silva, and D.J. Mooney, Growth factor delivery-based tissue engineering: General approaches and a review of recent developments. *Journal of the Royal Society Interface*, 2010. **8**(55): pp. 153–170.

64. Lanza, R., R. Langer, and J.P. Vacanti, *Principles of Tissue Engineering*. Academic press: London. 2011.

65. Whitaker, M., et al., Growth factor release from tissue engineering scaffolds. *Journal of Pharmacy and Pharmacology*, 2001. **53**(11): pp. 1427–1437.

66. Reed, S. and B. Wu, Sustained growth factor delivery in tissue engineering applications. *Annals of Biomedical Engineering*, 2014. **42**(7): pp. 1528–1536.

67. DeLong, S.A., J.J. Moon, and J.L. West, Covalently immobilized gradients of bFGF on hydrogel scaffolds for directed cell migration. *Biomaterials*, 2005. **26**(16): pp. 3227–3234.

68. Roam, J.L., et al., The formation of protein concentration gradients mediated by density differences of poly (ethylene glycol) microspheres. *Biomaterials*, 2010. **31**(33): pp. 8642–8650.

69. Carter, S.B., Haptotaxis and the mechanism of cell motility. *Nature*, 1967. **213**(5073): p. 256.

70. Gerhardt, H., et al., VEGF guides angiogenic sprouting utilizing endothelial tip cell filopodia. *The Journal of Cell Biology*, 2003. **161**(6): pp. 1163–1177.

71. Tufró, A., VEGF spatially directs angiogenesis during metanephric development in vitro. *Developmental Biology*, 2000. **227**(2): pp. 558–566.

72. Cucina, A., et al., Vascular endothelial growth factor increases the migration and proliferation of smooth muscle cells through the mediation of growth factors released by endothelial cells. *Journal of Surgical Research*, 2003. **109**(1): pp. 16–23.

73. Gerhardt, H. and C. Betsholtz, How do endothelial cells orientate? In M. Clauss and G. Breier (eds.) *Mechanisms of Angiogenesis*. Springer: Berlin, Germany. 2005: pp. 3–15.

74. Ferrara, N., H.-P. Gerber, and J. LeCouter, The biology of VEGF and its receptors. *Nature Medicine*, 2003. **9**(6): p. 669.

75. Zisch, A.H., M.P. Lutolf, and J.A. Hubbell, Biopolymeric delivery matrices for angiogenic growth factors. *Cardiovascular Pathology*, 2003. **12**(6): pp. 295–310.

76. Cao, X. and M. Shoichet, Defining the concentration gradient of nerve growth factor for guided neurite outgrowth. *Neuroscience*, 2001. **103**(3): pp. 831–840.

77. Chung, B.G., et al., Human neural stem cell growth and differentiation in a gradient-generating microfluidic device. *Lab on a Chip*, 2005. **5**(4): pp. 401–406.

78. Kapur, T.A. and M.S. Shoichet, Immobilized concentration gradients of nerve growth factor guide neurite outgrowth. *Journal of Biomedical Materials Research Part A: An Official Journal of the Society for Biomaterials, the Japanese Society for Biomaterials, and the Australian Society for Biomaterials and the Korean Society for Biomaterials*, 2004. **68**(2): pp. 235–243.

79. Wang, X., et al., Growth factor gradients via microsphere delivery in biopolymer scaffolds for osteochondral tissue engineering. *Journal of Controlled Release*, 2009. **134**(2): pp. 81–90.

80. Oh, S.H., T.H. Kim, and J.H. Lee, Creating growth factor gradients in three dimensional porous matrix by centrifugation and surface immobilization. *Biomaterials*, 2011. **32**(32): pp. 8254–8260.

81. Odedra, D., et al., Endothelial cells guided by immobilized gradients of vascular endothelial growth factor on porous collagen scaffolds. *Acta Biomaterialia*, 2011. **7**(8): pp. 3027–3035.

82. Akar, B., et al., Biomaterials with persistent growth factor gradients in vivo accelerate vascularized tissue formation. *Biomaterials*, 2015. **72**: pp. 61–73.

83. Guo, X., et al., Creating 3D angiogenic growth factor gradients in fibrous constructs to guide fast angiogenesis. *Biomacromolecules*, 2012. **13**(10): pp. 3262–3271.

84. Lewallen, E.A., et al., Biological strategies for improved osseointegration and osteoinduction of porous metal orthopedic implants. *Tissue Engineering. Part B, Reviews*, 2015. **21**(2): pp. 218–230.

85. Kim, J.-S., et al., Tubing-electrospinning: A one-step process for fabricating fibrous matrices with spatial, chemical, and mechanical gradients. *ACS Applied Materials & Interfaces*, 2016. **8**(34): pp. 22721–22731.

86. Shirure, V.S., et al., Low levels of physiological interstitial flow eliminate morphogen gradients and guide angiogenesis. *Angiogenesis*, 2017. **20**(4): pp. 493–504.

87. Young, E.W., Advances in microfluidic cell culture systems for studying angiogenesis. *Journal of Laboratory Automation*, 2013. **18**(6): pp. 427–436.

88. Wade, R.J., et al., Nanofibrous hydrogels with spatially patterned biochemical signals to control cell behavior. *Advanced Materials*, 2015. **27**(8): pp. 1356–1362.

89. Baker, B.M., et al., Microfluidics embedded within extracellular matrix to define vascular architectures and pattern diffusive gradients. *Lab on a Chip*, 2013. **13**(16): pp. 3246–3252.

90. Leslie-Barbick, J.E., et al., Micron-scale spatially patterned, covalently immobilized vascular endothelial growth factor on hydrogels accelerates endothelial tubulogenesis and increases cellular angiogenic responses. *Tissue Engineering Part A*, 2010. **17**(1–2): pp. 221–229.

91. Alsop, A.T., et al., Photopatterning of vascular endothelial growth factor within collagen-glycosaminoglycan scaffolds can induce a spatially confined response in human umbilical vein endothelial cells. *Acta Biomaterialia*, 2014. **10**(11): pp. 4715–4722.

92. King, T.W. and C.W. Patrick Jr, Development and in vitro characterization of vascular endothelial growth factor (VEGF)-loaded poly (DL-lactic-co-glycolic acid)/poly (ethylene glycol) microspheres using a solid encapsulation/single emulsion/solvent extraction technique. *Journal of Biomedical Materials Research: An Official Journal of the Society for Biomaterials, the Japanese Society for Biomaterials, and the Australian Society for Biomaterials and the Korean Society for Biomaterials*, 2000. **51**(3): pp. 383–390.

93. Khanna, O., et al., Multilayered microcapsules for the sustained-release of angiogenic proteins from encapsulated cells. *The American Journal of Surgery*, 2010. **200**(5): pp. 655–658.

94. Moya, M.L., et al., Sustained delivery of FGF-1 increases vascular density in comparison to bolus administration. *Microvascular Research*, 2009. **78**(2): pp. 142–147.

95. Ozawa, C.R., et al., Microenvironmental VEGF concentration, not total dose, determines a threshold between normal and aberrant angiogenesis. *The Journal of Clinical Investigation*, 2004. **113**(4): pp. 516–527.

96. Uriel, S., E.M. Brey, and H.P. Greisler, Sustained low levels of fibroblast growth factor-1 promote persistent microvascular network formation. *The American Journal of Surgery*, 2006. **192**(5): pp. 604–609.

97. Robinson, S.T., et al., A novel platelet lysate hydrogel for endothelial cell and mesenchymal stem cell-directed neovascularization. *Acta Biomaterialia*, 2016. **36**: pp. 86–98.

98. Rufaihah, A.J., et al., Enhanced infarct stabilization and neovascularization mediated by VEGF-loaded PEGylated fibrinogen hydrogel in a rodent myocardial infarction model. *Biomaterials*, 2013. **34**(33): pp. 8195–8202.

99. Silva, E. and D.J. Mooney, Spatiotemporal control of vascular endothelial growth factor delivery from injectable hydrogels enhances angiogenesis. *Journal of Thrombosis and Haemostasis*, 2007. **5**(3): pp. 590–598.

100. Schiessl, B., et al., Localization of angiogenic growth factors and their receptors in the human placental bed throughout normal human pregnancy. *Placenta*, 2009. **30**(1): pp. 79–87.

101. Lalani, Z., et al., Spatial and temporal localization of transforming growth factor-β1, bone morphogenetic protein-2, and platelet-derived growth factor-A in healing tooth extraction sockets in a rabbit model. *Journal of Oral and Maxillofacial Surgery*, 2003. **61**(9): pp. 1061–1072.

102. Lash, G.E., et al., Localization of angiogenic growth factors and their receptors in the human endometrium throughout the menstrual cycle and in recurrent miscarriage. *Human Reproduction*, 2011. **27**(1): pp. 183–195.

103. Jiang, B. and E.M. Brey, Formation of stable vascular networks in engineered tissues. In *Regenerative Medicine and Tissue Engineering-Cells and Biomaterials*. Rijeka, Croatia: InTech, 2011: pp. 477–502.

104. Pepper, M.S., et al., Vascular endothelial growth factor (VEGF)-C synergizes with basic fibroblast growth factor and VEGF in the induction of angiogenesis in vitro and alters endothelial cell extracellular proteolytic activity. *Journal of Cellular Physiology*, 1998. **177**(3): pp. 439–452.

105. Cao, R., et al., Angiogenic synergism, vascular stability and improvement of hind-limb ischemia by a combination of PDGF-BB and FGF-2. *Nature Medicine*, 2003. **9**(5): p. 604.

106. Asahara, T., et al., Synergistic effect of vascular endothelial growth factor and basic fibroblast growth factor on angiogenesis in vivo. *Circulation*, 1995. **92**(9): pp. 365–371.

107. Chen, R.R., et al., Spatio–temporal VEGF and PDGF delivery patterns blood vessel formation and maturation. *Pharmaceutical Research*, 2007. **24**(2): pp. 258–264.

108. Sun, X.-T., et al., Angiogenic synergistic effect of basic fibroblast growth factor and vascular endothelial growth factor in an in vitro quantitative microcarrier-based three-dimensional fibrin angiogenesis system. *World Journal of Gastroenterology: WJG*, 2004. **10**(17): p. 2524.

109. Seghezzi, G., et al., Fibroblast growth factor-2 (FGF-2) induces vascular endothelial growth factor (VEGF) expression in the endothelial cells of forming capillaries: an autocrine mechanism contributing to angiogenesis. *The Journal of Cell Biology*, 1998. **141**(7): pp. 1659–1673.

110. Stavri, G.T., et al., Basic fibroblast growth factor upregulates the expression of vascular endothelial growth factor in vascular smooth muscle cells: Synergistic interaction with hypoxia. *Circulation*, 1995. **92**(1): pp. 11–14.

111. Xue, L. and H.P. Greisler, Angiogenic effect of fibroblast growth factor-1 and vascular endothelial growth factor and their synergism in a novel in vitro quantitative fibrin-based 3-dimensional angiogenesis system. *Surgery*, 2002. **132**(2): pp. 259–267.

112. Jiang, B., et al., Design of a composite biomaterial system for tissue engineering applications. *Acta Biomaterialia*, 2014. **10**(3): pp. 1177–1186.

113. Brudno, Y., et al., Enhancing microvascular formation and vessel maturation through temporal control over multiple pro-angiogenic and pro-maturation factors. *Biomaterials*, 2013. **34**(36): pp. 9201–9209.

114. Anderson, E.M., et al., VEGF and IGF delivered from alginate hydrogels promote stable perfusion recovery in ischemic hind limbs of aged mice and young rabbits. *Journal of Vascular Research*, 2017. **54**(5): pp. 288–298.

115. Tsao, C.J., et al., Electrospun patch functionalized with nanoparticles allows for spatiotemporal release of VEGF and PDGF-BB promoting in vivo neovascularization. *ACS Applied Materials & Interfaces*, 2018. **10**(51): pp. 44344–44353.

116. Rufaihah, A.J., et al., Dual delivery of VEGF and ANG-1 in ischemic hearts using an injectable hydrogel. *Acta Biomaterialia*, 2017. **48**: pp. 58–67.

117. Zhu, S., et al., Enzyme-responsive delivery of multiple proteins with spatiotemporal control. *Advanced Materials*, 2015. **27**(24): p. 3620–3625.

118. Battig, M.R., B. Soontornworajit, and Y. Wang, Programmable release of multiple protein drugs from aptamer-functionalized hydrogels via nucleic acid hybridization. *Journal of American Chemical Society*, 2012. **134**(30): pp. 12410–12413.

119. Garbern, J.C., et al., Delivery of basic fibroblast growth factor with a pH-responsive, injectable hydrogel to improve angiogenesis in infarcted myocardium. *Biomaterials*, 2011. **32**(9): pp. 2407–2416.

120. Tang, D.W., et al., Heparinized chitosan/poly(gamma-glutamic acid) nanoparticles for multi-functional delivery of fibroblast growth factor and heparin. *Biomaterials*, 2010. **31**(35): pp. 9320–9332.

121. Fujii, H., et al., Ultrasound-targeted gene delivery induces angiogenesis after a myocardial infarction in mice. *JACC Cardiovasc Imaging*, 2009. **2**(7): pp. 869–879.

122. Mannell, H., et al., Site directed vascular gene delivery in vivo by ultrasonic destruction of magnetic nanoparticle coated microbubbles. *Nanomedicine*, 2012. **8**(8): pp. 1309–1318.

123. Moncion, A., et al., Controlled release of basic fibroblast growth factor for angiogenesis using acoustically-responsive scaffolds. *Biomaterials*, 2017. **140**: pp. 26–36.

124. Moncion A. et al., Controlled release of basic fibroblast growth factor for angiogenesis using acoustically-responsive scaffolds. *Biomaterials*, 2017. 140: pp. 26–36, Copyright 2017, with permission from Elsevier.

125. Tibbitt, M.W., et al., Synthesis and application of photodegradable microspheres for spatiotemporal control of protein delivery. *Journal of Biomedical Materials Research. Part A*, 2012. **100**(7): p. 1647.

126. Lee, K.Y., et al., Controlled growth factor release from synthetic extracellular matrices. *Nature*, 2000. **408**(6815): p. 998.

127. Romero, G., et al., Localized excitation of neural activity via rapid magnetothermal drug release. *Advanced Functional Materials*, 2016. **26**(35): pp. 6471–6478.

128. Shrestha, B., L. Tang, and G. Romero, Nanoparticles-mediated combination therapies for cancer treatment. Advanced Therapeutics, 2019. 2(11).

10 Controlled Therapeutic Delivery in Wound Healing

Adam Jorgensen, Zishuai Chou, and Sean Murphy
Wake Forest Institute for Regenerative Medicine,
Wake Forest School of Medicine

CONTENTS

10.1 INTRODUCTION

Extensive burns and full-thickness skin wounds are devastating for patients, even when treated quickly in the clinic. There are an estimated 500,000 patients treated with full-thickness wounds in the United States every year, with an overall mortality rate of 4.9% between 1998 and 2007 [1,2]. The cost of burn injuries is very high. Specifically, studies have shown that the average cost per patient is over $15,250, and ranges as high as $46,069 [4,5], approaching $2 billion per year nationally [3]. Globally, there are over 11 million burn injuries per year, creating a significant demand for improved therapies [4].

Chronic wounds present an additional health burden and a significant resource drain. Venous ulcers, diabetic foot ulcers, and pressure ulcers are all chronic wounds with increasing prevalence, are difficult to heal, and can suffer many complications such as infection, amputation, or even death [5]. There are approximately 6.5 million patients with chronic wounds in the United States and the costs are approximately $37 billion. These costs are becoming unsustainable due to increasing healthcare costs, an aging population, and a sharp rise in the incidence of obesity and diabetes.

If a burn or chronic wound does finally close, the patient is often left with the burden of skin scarring, which alone accounts for a \$12 billion market each year. Moreover, the monetary costs of significant skin wounds do not include the additional costs associated with psychical trauma, pain, long-term rehabilitation, and, in some cases, prolonged time for society reintegration [6].

The gold standard for most wounds is the split-thickness autograft. Split-thickness autografts involve harvesting full-thickness fascia from a donor site and grafting over the compromised region. Unfortunately, this procedure has limitations, including scarring and contracture at the wound site, pain, donor-site infection, and limited donor sites for injuries that involve more than 20% of total body surface. The next available option is the allograft, but they have major disadvantages in that patients may need medication for immunosuppression in order to prevent immune rejection of the graft [7].

To overcome these limitations and to provide better treatment for burn and chronic wounds, new materials and techniques have been developed, including naturally derived hydrogels [8]. The addition of antibiotics and other antimicrobial materials to hydrogels provide a first step in hydrogel therapeutic delivery. Next, combinations of growth factors and cytokines incorporated in topical moisturizers and dressings administered in different combinations can be used to closely mimic the orchestration of the healing process. Rather than a passive gel dressing that will have a minimal role in the healing process, technologies have been developed that actively promote wound healing by acting as a substrate for endogenous cell migration and proliferation. Cell-based therapies, such as the application of stem cells, add an extra layer of complexity with clear therapeutic benefit. Finally, full-thickness skin can be generated through precise cell placement to be used as a replacement for autologous skin grafting.

Herein we will briefly discuss the current standard of care, wound dressings, and new wound healing materials. We will then explore key biomaterials and hydrogels which can be used as vehicles for therapeutic delivery, including antimicrobials, growth factors, and cells. This will be followed by the analysis of key cell-based therapies which promote wound healing. Finally we will discuss recent advances in the use of bioprinting and tissue engineering to recapitulate full-thickness skin.

10.2 CURRENT AND EVOLVING METHODS OF WOUND CARE

The gold standard therapy employed in the clinic is the autologous split-thickness skin graft. This requires removing a piece of skin from a secondary surgical site, stretching the skin under sterile conditions through meshing, and reapplying the graft at the primary site of injury. This approach has obvious limitations when dealing with large wounds, where a secondary surgical site may be limited, resulting in autografts being unusable in cases that require prompt, aggressive, and large-scale treatment measures to maintain the lives of wounded patients. Allografts, or skin grafts from other patients, are an additional option, but in many cases can suffer from the need of immunosuppressive drugs to prevent immune rejection of the allograft. As with any transplant surgery using allogeneic tissues, immunosuppressive drugs can have a variety of side effects on a patient, some of which can be negative [7].

These limitations have led to the development of noncellular dermal substitutes, which are generally a polymer scaffold-based membrane. These more advanced products are either dermal substitutes (INTEGRA ®Dermal Regeneration Template (Integra Life Sciences) and Biobrane® (UDL Laboratories) or tissue engineered products like complex biological skin equivalents that may yield more suitable wound treatment options for patients (Dermagraft® (Shire), Apligraf® (Organogenesis), and TransCyte® – Advanced BioHealing). However, these types of products are expensive to produce, and like allografts, can suffer from the same immunological drawbacks discussed above [9,10]. Development of more modern, functional approaches that permit immediate burn wound stabilization and support functional skin regeneration is needed. Unfortunately, because of the technical and regulatory requirements involved in culturing and maintaining these grafts prior to use, these grafts are expensive to produce, and as they are also allografts due to incorporation of nonautologous cells, they can suffer from the same immunological drawbacks of traditional skin allografts (Table 10.1).

TABLE 10.1

Current Treatments for Wound Healing

Type		Composition	Pros	Cons	Reference
Autologous split-thickness skin graft		Native skin	Gold standard for wound healing	Scarring and contracture at the wound site; limited donor sites	[7]
Allograft		Donor skin	More similar to patients' native skin	Immune rejection	[7]
Noncellular dermal substitutes	Integra® bilayer wound matrix	Bovine collagen and chondroitin-6-sulfate glycosaminoglycan; silicone polymer	Widely used for large burn wounds	Costly to produce, poor cosmetic outcomes	[11]
	Integra® dermal regeneration template	Polymer scaffold-based membrane	Improved healing	Costly to produce, poor cosmetic outcomes	[12,13]
	Biobrane®	Ultrathin silicone film; 3D nylon filament with type I collagen peptides	Controls water vapor loss from the wound; as effective as frozen human allografts	Costly to produce, poor cosmetic outcomes	[14]
Cellular dermal substitutes	Dermagraft®	Bioabsorbable polygalactin mesh matrix with human neonatal fibroblasts	Facilitates re-epithelialization	Expensive, immunological rejection	[15]
	Apligraf®	Bovine collagen gel seeded with neonatal foreskin fibroblasts and keratinocytes	Contains two cell types	Expensive, immunological rejection	[16]
	TransCyte®	Nylon mesh seeded with neonatal human foreskin fibroblasts that are destroyed before grafting	Contains ECM components and growth factors aid the healing process	Expensive, immunological rejection	[17]
Hydrogel-based dressings		Gels, sheets, and even impregnated in ordinary cotton gauze pads	Immunologically inert; aid fluid regulation and gas exchange; easy to use	Lack of biofunctionality	[18,19]

10.3 HYDROGELS FOR WOUND CARE

10.3.1 INERT HYDROGELS

Current commercially available hydrogel-based dressings have advantages in that they are often immunologically inert, can aid with regulation of fluid and gas exchange from the wound surface, and can be purchased as gels, sheets, and even impregnated in an ordinary cotton gauze pad/ordinary cotton gauze pads. [18,19] For relatively regular, shallow, and flat wounds, hydrogel sheets are quite easily employed as primary dressings and will remain in place for 4–7 days before fresh dressings are applied. For irregular and/or deep wounds, amorphous hydrogels can be used to fill the wound, but must be held in place with a secondary dressing or bandage that is usually changed once daily. Inert hydrogels are typically natural or artificial sources including collagen, fibrin, alginate, hyaluronic acid (HA), polyurethanes, and polyethylene glycol (PEG). They are either used alone or in combination with other materials.

Collagen is an abundant protein present in connective tissues, with collagen fibrils providing the primary component of extracellular matrix (ECM) responsible for maintaining its biological and structural integrity [20]. Collagen is a nontoxic, low antigenic, biodegradable material. It is a dynamic and flexible polymer that undertakes constant remodeling to regulate cellular behavior and tissue function [21]. Collagen plays a major role in hemostasis, which promotes fibroblasts and macrophage growth, attachment, and keratinocytes migration upon contact with wound tissue [22]. It was first used as an injectable material under the dermis, and was later used in many different forms such as sponges, foams, and wound dressings, but always in combination with other materials. Collagen-based hydrogels have been used for chronic wounds [23] and superficial partial thickness burns in children [24]. It is more practical and economical than growth-factor and cell-based treatments, and the combination of collagen and alginate has been shown to promote the inflammatory phase of wound healing and imparts mechanical strength, thanks to collagen fibrils [25]. However, permeability to bacteria and microorganisms is collagen's limitation.

Fibrin gel is another natural biopolymer made from fibrinogen, a natural blood clotting factor. It self-assembles into a similar polymer network by utilizing the coagulation process [26]. The crosslinked fibrin hydrogel adheres to native tissue to provide cells natural binding sites for attachment, migration, and proliferation [27]. Thus fibrin has been used widely for cellular and matrix interactions, inflammation, wound healing, angiogenesis, and neoplasia. Furthermore, fibrin hydrogel's mechanical properties, morphology, and degradation can be tuned by composition. Fibrin gel has been widely utilized as a bioadhesive for surgeries and wound closure [28]. It has also been utilized as a cell carrier to protect cells from the forces during cell delivery. However, fibrin hydrogel has a relatively slow crosslinking process and its mechanical strength is low (Table 10.2).

10.3.2 BIOACTIVE HYDROGELS

While hydrogel applications have advantages over traditional wound care regimes, the potential for hydrogels to promote wound healing is not limited to inert wound dressings. Wound healing is a complex process of interaction between epidermal and dermal cells, ECM, plasma-derived proteins in a controlled angiogenetic environment, and all of these components are being coordinated by multiple cytokines and growth factors [36]. The combination of these growth factors and cytokines incorporated in topical moisturizers or dressing may represent a future therapy in which growth factors can be administered in different combinations to more closely mimic the orchestration of the healing process [37]. Rather than passive and inert materials that have minimal contribution to the regenerative process, hydrogels can also be tuned to actively promote wound healing by either acting as a substrate for endogenous cell migration and proliferation or as a supportive delivery vehicle of potent cells and cytokines. The hydrogel must be not only nonimmunogenic but also able to facilitate desired cellular activities such as migration and secretion of trophic factors.

10.3.2.1 Antimicrobial Delivery

Topical antibiotics and antimicrobials can be used to prevent or combat infections in cutaneous wounds where the incidence of infections is elevated due to reduced antimicrobial resistance resulting from extreme trauma, diabetic foot ulcers, and surgery [38,39]. The use of dressings to deliver antibiotics to wound sites can provide tissue compatibility, low occurrence of bacterial resistance, and reduced interference with wound healing [40]. Furthermore, the lower antibiotic doses within the antimicrobial dressings reduce the risk of off-target toxicity which often results from the high antibiotic doses necessary to achieve systemic efficiency [41,42]. Local antibiotic delivery can also overcome the risk of ineffective systemic antibiotic therapy resulting from poor blood circulation at the extremities in wounds such as diabetic foot ulcers [43].

In some cases, the delivery of certain antibiotics from paraffin-based ointments such as bismuth subgallate has been shown to actively improve the wound healing process [44]. Common antibiotics incorporated into available dressings for delivery to wounds include dialkylcarbamoylchloride

TABLE 10.2
Inert Hydrogels in Wound Care

Type	Source	Pros	Cons	Use
Collagen	Connective tissues (Bovine; porcine; avian rodent marine)	Nontoxic; low antigenicity; biodegradable; stimulate macrophages and fibroblasts; promote cell attachment and migration	Permeable to bacteria and microorganisms; costly; fast degradation	Chronic wounds [23], superficial partial thickness burns in children [24], surgical adhesives [29]
Fibrin	Blood plasma	Easy to isolate; promote cell attachment; controllable degradation; tunable mechanical properties; and can be used as a cell carrier	Poor mechanical properties; slow crosslinking	Fibrin glue to stop bleeding and replace sutures [28]
Alginate	Marine brown algae and some soil bacteria	High strength; unique ion exchange crosslinking; limit wound exudates, minimize bacterial contamination; modulate macrophages to produce inflammation	May inhibit cell migration; lack cell attachment motifs, cannot apply to dry wounds	Moist, elastic, and biocompatible hydrogel wound dressing [30]
HA	Bacterial fermentation; extraction from animal tissues	Biodegradable; nonimmunogenic; nonthrombogenic; hydrophilic; antioxidant; facilitate cell motility and proliferation; stimulate inflammatory signals; accelerate wound closure	Costly; weak mechanical strength	Nasal wound dressing in sinusitis [31]; wound dressing with polyvinyl alcohol, hyaluronan and ampicillin [32]
Polyurethanes	Synthetic polymers produced by condensation	Nontoxic; high strength; tear resistant, nonallergenic; favor epithelialization; allow oxygen permeability	Nonbiodegradable; rarely used	An exterior film as an earlier epithelial cover to wound [33]
PEG	Synthetic	Nontoxic; biodegradable; transparent; cost-efficient; widely used; conjugated to many other polymers	Low mechanical strength	pH-modulating PEGDA/alginate hydrogel dressings [34]; PEG-based injectable, thermosensitive wound dressing [35]

which is incorporated into Cutisorb®, a highly absorbent cotton wool dressing, povidone-iodine used with fabric dressing, and silver used with most of the modern dressings [45]. Silver-impregnated modern dressings include Fibrous Hydrocolloid, Polyurethane Foam Film, and Silicone gels [45]. Other antibiotics delivered to wounds include gentamycin from collagen sponges, ofloxacin from silicone gel sheets and minocycline from chitosan film dressings [46–48]. Novel antimicrobial wound healing dressings include freeze-dried fibrin discs for the delivery of tetracycline and lactic acid based systems for the delivery of ofloxacin [49]. Treatment of dermal depth burn wounds using antimicrobial releasing silicone gel sheets which promote epithelization of superficial burns has been described [50]. A chitosan–polyurethane film dressing incorporating minocycline has also been developed for treating severe burn wounds [51].

10.3.2.2 Cytokine and Growth Factor Delivery

Antibacterials can prevent and treat infections, but they do not play an active role in the wound healing process. Cell division, migration, differentiation, protein expression, and enzyme production are all governed by complex cell–cell interactions governed by cytokines and growth factors. Growth factors necessary to wound healing stimulate angiogenesis and cellular proliferation, impact both the production and degradation of the ECM, and modulates cell inflammation and fibroblast activity [52]. Ultimately, growth factors impact the inflammatory, proliferation, and migratory phases of wound healing [53].

Many growth factors have been reported to participate in wound healing, including epidermal growth factor (EGF), fibroblast growth factor (FGF), granulocyte-macrophage colony-stimulating factor (GM-CSF), human growth hormone (HGH), insulin-like growth factor (IGF-1) platelet-derived growth factor (PDGF), and transforming growth factor (TGF-β1) [54,55]. In a study of the influence of GM-CSF in full-thickness wounds in transgenic mice, it was found that GM-CSF is of fundamental importance in the wound healing repair and a deficiency of this growth factor resulted in delayed wound healing and poor quality of newly formed scar tissue [56]. Further reports have demonstrated that silver sulphadiazine alone can impair wound healing and that EGF helps reverse this impairment when both are applied together [57].

A range of topical treatments have been used to administer some of the above growth factors to wound sites. These include hydrogel dressings for delivering TGF-β1, collagen film for delivering Platelet Derived Growth Factor- β (PDGF), and HGH alginate dressings in the form of beads used to deliver endothelial growth factor, polyurethane, and collagen film dressings for delivery of EGF [58–63]. A novel porous collagen–HA matrix, containing tobramycin, basic FGF, and PDGF was used to enhance wound healing compared with the matrix containing only the antibiotic [64]. Furthermore, it was reported that EGF when applied to partial thickness incisions as a cream stimulated epidermal regeneration [65].

10.3.3 Amniotic Membrane Hydrogels

One method that has been used to employ a large array of growth factors and cytokines is by utilizing highly bioactive antimicrobial and immunomodulatory biological products, including the amniotic membrane (AM). The AM develops from extraembryonic tissue and consists of a fetal component (the chorionic plate) and a maternal component (the decidua). The innermost layer of the AM nearest to the fetus is the amniotic epithelium, which is formed of a single layer of cells arranged on the basement membrane, one of the thickest membranes found among human tissues and which is known to have important roles in fetal development, immune regulation, and defense against infection [66]. The use of the amnion for wound healing purposes is well documented for the treatment of chronic and acute wounds [67–72]. It has been shown that amnion-treated burns demonstrated reduced scarring and faster healing times; moreover, there was less pain associated with changing the dressings in patients using amnion dressings, and wound exudation was also reduced [73]. One of the first studies using cultured amnion dressings was performed in 15 patients with chronic leg ulcers, which was conducted in 1980 by Fauk *et al.*, in which the amnion dressing improved the formation of profuse granulation tissue, increased capillary density compared to ulcers receiving standard treatments, and decreased connective tissue fibers [74]. Mohammadi *et al.* demonstrated a reduction in hypertrophic scar formation in the amnion dressing group compared to the conventional skin grafting group [69]. In a randomized trial in a pediatric population with second-degree burns, Branski *et al.* compared the standard topical treatment containing antibiotics to decellularized amnion dressings. They found that patients treated with AM experienced faster total healing times and fewer dressing changes. No differences were observed in scar formation and infection rates between the two groups [72].

The collective evidence of clinical trials using amnion has supported its use in burns and chronic wounds for the promotion of wound healing, as well as for increasing patient comfort and reducing the frequency of dressing changes [74]. Additionally, many of these studies demonstrated antimicrobial effects, pain relief, reduction of fluid, and reduced scar formation. Therefore, the use of amnion products is safe and effective, although the main challenges are the difficulty of handling and placing thin membrane sheets, as well as the moderate to high cost of fresh or cryopreserved AM products.

Murphy *et al.* manufactured a novel AM-based product that was processed to achieve a cell-free solution that still contains high concentrations of growth factors and cytokines [74]. They developed a variety of HA hydrogel supplemented with solubilized AM (SAM) that proved to be easy to produce, store, and apply to wounds. Briefly, they manually dissected the AM from the chorion membrane and washed it with sterile saline to remove blood clots, after which the membrane was cut into small pieces (5×5cm), washed in saline and sterile water, and lyophilized/freezer milled (-80°C). Next, the amnion underwent digestion in pepsin/HCl, and the resulting neutralized supernatant yielded the SAM solution. After incorporation with the hydrogel precursor components, hydrogel is then formed by thiol-ene photopolymerization chemistry, in which thiolated HA and gelatin are crosslinked with poly(ethylene oxide) (PEGDA) in the presence of a photoinitiator using UV light irradiation. To evaluate the potential of HA-SAM, they utilized a full-thickness murine model and compared the untreated group with HA-only and HA-SAM treatments. The evaluation included histological analysis, morphological, immunohistochemistry, and *in vivo* and *in vitro* observations. HA-SAM appeared to stimulate keratinocyte proliferation *in vivo*, which was demonstrated by the immunohistochemical analysis that identified higher numbers of proliferating keratinocytes for the HA-SAM group. Also, the histological analysis showed that HA-SAM treated wounds had thicker regenerated skin, increased number of blood vessels, especially newly formed vessels. An explanation of this phenomena could be the presence of growth factors known to promote neovascularization, including vascular endothelial growth factor (VEGF), human endocrine gland VEGF (EG-VEGF), EGF receptor (EGF-R), and members of the FGF family. Most importantly, HA-SAM proved to accelerate wound closure while reducing wound contraction. This study demonstrated the potential advantages of HA-SAM over frozen or fresh amnion products, facilitated by a novel processing methodology that preserves its efficacy as a wound treatment/dressing, but with long-term storage potential and ease of use [75].

10.4 CELL-BASED THERAPIES FOR WOUND HEALING

10.4.1 HYDROGEL CELL DELIVERY

We have explored promotion of endogenous cell migration and proliferation, as well as inclusion of autologous or allogeneic cell sources or cell or tissue-derived biologicals, employing the hydrogel bioink as a delivery vehicle as well. In the end, a hydrogel bioink needs to have suitable mechanical properties and swelling characteristics, short-term stability, be biodegradable over the long term, promote cell migration, proliferation and function, and facilitate robust engraftment in the endogenous wound site. An appropriate hydrogel bioink must also eventually meet appropriate regulatory, commercial, and financial considerations to provide affordable products that can be FDA approved, and be employed easily enough to be accepted by clinicians as an effective therapy in the clinic. In order to deliver cells, cell spraying and bioprinting technologies have recently been developed for wound treatment. In these approaches, cells are deposited over the wound, generally mixed in a hydrogel carrier vehicle, via a spray nozzle or printhead. Indeed, in our laboratory, we used a bioprinting device [76] to deposit amniotic fluid-derived stem cells in a full-thickness wound healing model with great success [77]. A wide range of cells have been used for this form of therapeutic delivery as described below.

10.4.1.1 Skin-Derived Stem Cells

Stem cells have an essential role in the maintenance of tissue homeostasis and regeneration following injury. More than 20 different cell types have been identified residing within the skin, each performing a number of critical functions necessary for tissue function [78]. These terminally differentiated, functional cell types are maintained by a pool of tissue-resident stem cells, which are capable of proliferating and differentiating to contribute new cells to the tissue. Skin stem cells are more quiescent than other skin cells, including keratinocytes, have a high proliferative potential, and can terminally differentiate into multiple differentiation lineages [79].

In the context of wound healing, stem cells capable of regenerating the epidermis have obvious therapeutic value. Epidermal stem cells have been identified and are characterized by a prolonged self-renewal and differentiation capacity into multiple skin cell lineages [80]. Isolation and functional assessment of epidermal stem cells have been evaluated in multiple studies [81,82]. These skin-derived stem cells have been shown to differentiate into all hair follicle lineages, including sebaceous gland, neuron, glial cells, Schwann cells, smooth muscle cells, dermal fibroblasts, melanocytes, and other cell types [83]. Epidermal stem cells have found some application in the development of skin equivalents [84].

An important repository of skin stem cells appears to be located at the bulge of the hair follicle, which does not degenerate during the hair cycle. The hair follicle contains multipotent stem cells that are activated at the start of the hair cycle and mobilized upon injury to stimulate regeneration of the damaged epidermis. Bulge stem cells respond rapidly to epidermal wounding during the acute wound repair phase and acquire an epidermal phenotype but interestingly, they are eliminated from the epidermis over several weeks after injury. This suggests that bulge stem cells contribute to the wound repair but not to the homoeostasis of the epidermis [85]. *In vitro,* bulge stem cells maintain their stem cell characteristics after propagation and can contribute to hair follicles, epidermis, and sebaceous gland formation when combined with neonatal dermal cells in culture [86].

Tissue-specific stem cells hold great promise to contribute to all phases of wound healing. However several limitations remain. Some limitations include difficulties in isolating, expanding, and differentiating these stem cells *in vitro*, as well as the potential that stem cells isolated from compromised patients, such as diabetics or the elderly may have limited effectiveness. Additionally, data on the application of skin stem cells for wound healing is not conclusive, and further investigation is warranted to ensure safety and effectiveness in wound healing therapies.

10.4.1.2 Adipose-Derived Stem Cells

Several nomenclatures have been used to describe plastic-adherent, multipotent, and self-renewal stem cells isolated from fat tissue including adipose-derived mesenchymal stem/stromal cells (MSCs), lipoblast, pericytes, preadipocyte, and many other names. While these names led to much confusion in the literature, the International Fat Applied Technology Society adopted the term "adipose-derived stem cells" (ADSCs) to identify stem cells isolated from fat tissue.

In addition to the fact that ADSCs can be easily isolated, possess immunomodulatory characteristics and a great potential of differentiation, they also have other attractive properties including protection, survival, and differentiation of a variety of endogenous cells and tissues [87]. These cells have broad secretory profiles of various angiogenic, hematopoietic, and proinflammatory growth factors and cytokines [88]. Fibroblast proliferation can be enhanced if cocultured with ADSCs due to the paracrine effect of ADSCs [89]. The secretory effect of ADSCs is still pronounced in the conditioned media used to culture fat tissue. It has been shown that the conditioned media of adipose tissue enhanced ADSC proliferation and induced cell sprouting of endothelial cells, which could be used as a safe topical treatment of skin wounds without the need to use cells [90]. The effect of conditioned media of ADSCs increases proliferation and migration of vascular endothelial cells, fibroblasts and keratinocytes, upregulates transcription of type I procollagen in fibroblasts, and increases the contraction of fibroblasts populated in a collagen lattice [91–93].

Despite the abundant source of stem cells from fat tissue, ease of isolation and high proliferation capacity, and secretion of proinflammatory and proangiogenic growth factors, the use of ADSCs as an autologous cell therapy option might not be attainable in some cases due to various reasons, such as patient age, current health, and comorbid diseases such as diabetes. The health status of ADSCs, whether they are harvested from a healthy or a diabetic subject, can affect their proliferation capacity, apoptosis rate, and secretory properties and could result in impaired vascular stabilization [94]. Diabetic ADSCs have lower expression of stem cell markers, lower amounts of secreted growth factors playing an important role in skin repair, and reduced capability to promote fibroblast and keratinocyte proliferation and migration [95]. The lack of local secretion of donor growth factors, not necessarily related to skin repair such as hepatocyte growth factors (HGF), can impair the function and potency of ADSCs [96].

10.4.1.3   Bone Marrow-Derived MSCs

MSCs have shown therapeutic potential for repair and regeneration of tissues damaged by injury or disease. A range of studies have demonstrated MSCs contribute to wound healing through multiple mechanisms, including (i) direct differentiation into keratinocytes [97–99], (ii) inducing angiogenesis through paracrine release VEGF, (iii) recruiting endothelial cells and endothelial progenitor cells (EPCs) to the wound, (iv) promoting regeneration of appendages by releasing cytokines such as EGF and keratinocyte growth factor (KGF), and (v) through anti-inflammatory mechanisms, such as releasing macrophage inflammatory protein-1 (MIP-1) and monocyte chemoattractant protein (MCP) [100,101].

In particular, MSC treatment of both acute and chronic wounds can result in accelerated wound closure, increases in re-epithelialization, formation of granulation tissue, and improved angiogenesis and neovascularization in the regenerated tissue [102]. MSCs play an important role in the host defense and inflammatory processes, matrix deposition principally collagen type I and III, angiogenesis, and recruitment of endogenous cells for dermal and epidermal reconstruction [103]. Others showed that the major source of deposited collagen is coming from the resident cells in the skin, and bone marrow-derived stem cells are contributing partially to collagen production during fibrogenesis [104,105]. MSCs have been found to accelerate wound healing in patients with chronic and acute wounds when delivered in a fibrin hydrogel [106]. Bone marrow-derived stem cells have been shown to improve dermal rebuilding and lead to closure of nonhealing chronic wounds, whether applied directly [107] or injected into the wound periphery [108].

In addition to their role in wound healing, bone marrow-derived MSCs may play an important role in enhancing the fibrotic behavior of deep dermal fibroblasts and have a possible involvement in the pathogenesis of hypertrophic scarring [109,110]. For example, MSCs from bone marrow secret high levels of VEGF, which is linked to excessive keloid scarring in patients who are susceptible to keloid scarring [111]. Several clinical trials have been conducted with different bone marrow-derived cells for chronic wounds and showed promising results [112,113]. MSCs have also recently been shown to be useful for improving *in vivo* skin expansion, an approach often used to establish space for surgical implants that induces tissue damage and requires treatment to heal the damaged tissue [114]. The specific mechanisms of how bone marrow-derived cells contribute to wound healing and regeneration are still under investigation. Additionally, further studies are needed to evaluate the optimal and selection, expansion and delivery mechanisms for these cells to acute and chronic wounds.

10.4.1.4   Placental MSCs

Placental MSCs share the characteristics of both embryonic and MSCs, including the ability to differentiate in all embryonic germ layers, while also exhibiting noncarcinogenic characteristics [94]. A large number of preclinical studies have demonstrated the use of placental MSCs in areas including neurological, cardiac, pulmonary, hepatic, pancreatic, muscular, and bone diseases, including tissue engineering applications [115–122]. The therapeutic potential of placental MSCs has also been investigated in wound and burn healing with the aim of mimicking the therapeutic properties of the amnion, as described in 1980 by Faulk *et al.* [68].

MSCs have been isolated from placental tissues as well as from the amnion and chorion [123,124]. The process of isolating stem cells from the placenta involves mechanically separating the fetal placental specimens from the maternal decidua by blunt dissection, followed by tissue homogenization and digestion with collagenase and dispase mixtures. Afterwards, the product is filtered and cells are placed into tissue culture [125]. The resulting placental MSCs resemble adult bone marrow-derived MSCs in terms of a spindle-shaped fibroblast appearance, the ability to adhere to plastic, and the ability to expand *ex vivo*. However, it has been reported that placental MSCs expand faster *in vitro* than adult MSCs, and appear to be less immunogenic and more immunosuppressive than their adult counterparts [126,127]. These properties make placental MSCs attractive as a potential clinical therapy for the treatment of burns and chronic nonhealing wounds. Kong *et al.* described a placental MSC treatment for wound healing in diabetic Goto-Kakizaki rats. They performed a full-thickness circular excisional wound, around which they delivered 1 million MSCs by intradermal injection. They found that MSC treatment increased the wound healing rate and reduced subsequent scarring. Additionally, a higher microvessel density was observed in the wound bed biopsy sites, and the transplanted MSCs were localized to the wound tissue and incorporated into the recipients' vasculature [127].

A recent study conducted by Mathew *et al.* demonstrated the use of hypoxia conditions for influencing the therapeutic potential of placental MSCs, taking into consideration that wound site is often under ischemic conditions. They employed perinatal MSCs that were isolated from full-term placenta and characterized them under normoxia and hypoxia conditions (2%–2.5% O_2). The study demonstrated that insulin secretion is not impeded under hypoxia, and in fact, the upregulation of glucose transporters under hypoxic conditions indicates enhanced glucose uptake needed to cater to the metabolic demands of proliferating cells. Also, the upregulation of adhesion molecules suggested hypoxic conditions induced an environment conducive for cell retention at the injury site. Furthermore, hypoxia also resulted in increased levels of angiogenesis-related markers in the placental MSCs. This confirmed that under hypoxia conditions, placental MSCs can modulate themselves by secreting insulin, exhibiting an increased angiogenic potential, and upregulating transporters and adhesion molecules, which could make them potentially more useful for wound healing therapies [128].

10.4.1.5 Amnion Epithelial Cells

Amniotic epithelial cells are a highly multipotent epithelial cell population isolated from the amnion. They develop from the epiblast 8 days after fertilization and prior to gastrulation. Due to this timing of development, amnion epithelial cells maintain the plasticity of pregastrulation embryonic cells [129].

Human amnion epithelial cells (hAECs) are currently used for many therapeutic applications, with reports that epithelial cells derived from human term amnion possess multipotent differentiation ability, low immunogenicity, and anti-inflammatory functions [130,131]. The procedure of separating and isolating hAECs starts with manually separating term human amnion from the chorion and washing it in a saline solution to remove the blood. Clinical grade amnion epithelial cells are isolated from the amnion by enzymatic digestion in TrypZean, which is an animal product-free recombinant trypsin. Approximately 120 million viable epithelial cells can be isolated from a single amnion, and these cells can be maintained in serum-free culture conditions. While hAECs lack the proliferative capacity of placental MSCs, they are highly multipotent and can differentiate into cells representing all 3 germ layers (specifically osteocytes, adipocytes, neurons, lung epithelial cells, cardiomyocytes, myocytes, hepatocytes, and pancreatic cells) [130]. Li and Hori characterized the immunosuppressive properties of hAECs both *in vitro* and *in vivo*, and it has been proposed that soluble factors produced by hAECs have anti-inflammatory effects and act to inhibit both the innate and adaptive immune systems [132,133].

A study conducted by Xing *et al.* evaluated the capability of hAECs to accelerate and improve laparotomy wound healing in rat abdominal walls [134]. They performed a standard laparotomy incision that they then repaired with a running suture. A proportion of the patients then received an injection of 1 million hAEC injected along the incision line in 200 μL of saline. Next, the wound's mechanical properties, as well as the incidence and severity of laparotomy wound failure, was measured over

28 days. Green fluorescent protein (GFP) labeled hAECs were identified in the wound area over the 28-day study, although the numbers of cells appeared to decrease over time. No GFP-expressing cells were found in the liver, lymph nodes, spleen, or testis, suggesting that no migration from the wound area occurred. Tensiometric analysis found that wounds treated with hAEC developed increased breaking strength in the early postoperative fascial incision. Additionally, amnion epithelial cell-treated wounds exhibited higher vascularization, more granulation tissue, and organized fibroproliferation.

10.4.1.6 Amniotic Fluid Stem Cells

Human amniotic fluid stem cells (AFSC) are obtained from the amniotic fluid that is extracted during amniocenteses performed to detect fetal congenital disorders. The role of amniotic fluid is to facilitate fetal growth. It contains nutrients and growth factors, provides mechanical cushioning, possesses antimicrobial properties that protect the fetus, and allows the assessment of fetal maturity and presence of disease [135]. Amniotic fluid also contains a mixture of different cell types of various origins, including those derived from the developing fetus, those sloughed from the fetal amnion and skin, and those derived from the alimentary, respiratory, and urogenital tracts [136].

AFSC shares some characteristics with MSCs; however, they can be considered more potent owing to their high proliferative capacity, lack of immunogenicity, immunomodulatory activity, and pluripotency since they are obtained at an early stage of the developmental timeline [137]. These cells also have a simpler isolation process (a high quantity of AFSC can be obtained from as little as 2 mL of amniotic fluid), a doubling time of 30–36 hours, and their lack of need for supportive feeder layers makes AFSC an effective "off-the-shelf" cell therapy product for wound healing. Additionally, they have been used in clinical studies to treat neurological, lung, heart, and kidney disease owing to their anti-inflammatory properties [138].

Skardal *et al.* have endeavored to isolate, characterize, and produce applications for AFSCs [139,140]. They utilized bioprinting technology to deliver 5 million AFSC to treat full-thickness mouse skin wounds [141]. In this process, multiple layers of a fibrin–collagen gel are deposited, the first consisting of thrombin plus fibrin/collagen, followed by a second layer of thrombin and fibrinogen/collagen, then a final layer of thrombin. This technique achieves a 100% uniform distribution of hydrogel over the wound bed. They followed the mice for 2 weeks using weekly imaging analysis. For each time point, wound closure and re-epithelialization were significantly better for the group treated with AFSC than the control group. Furthermore, histological examination showed increased microvessel density and capillary diameters, suggesting that AFSCs were promoting both wound healing and angiogenesis. Interestingly, tracking of fluorescently labeled AFSC revealed that they did not permanently integrate into the tissue, suggesting that the wound healing properties of the cells were more likely due to production of secreted paracrine factors rather than a direct cell contribution to new tissue formation. In subsequent work, they assessed a variety of hydrogels commonly used in various regenerative medicine and tissue engineering applications as alternatives to fibrin and collagen, evaluating gelation times, ease of use, biocompatibility, immunogenicity, and bioprinter compatibility. As expected, the different hydrogel materials exhibited differing pros and cons, again suggesting that a particular material should be chosen based on the particular target application. However, they did identify additional hydrogel formulations that were suitable for integration in the skin bioprinter and likely good choices for use as hydrogel bioinks in wound healing treatments. One such hydrogel, a UV-photopolymerizable HA and gelatin material, capable of elastic modulus modulation, cytokine loading, and cell delivery, is currently being employed in a variety of applications, including skin bioprinting [142] (Table 10.3).

10.4.2 Primary Skin Cells for Tissue Engineered Full-Thickness Skin

The cell source employed in cellularized wound healing therapies is an important component that has direct implications on cost, speed, and effectiveness of patient therapies. The widespread application of skin grafts have led researchers to explore delivering the cellular components of the grafts

TABLE 10.3
Cell Types for Wound Healing

Type	Source	Markers	Pros	Cons	Use
Skin-derived stem cells	Epidermis; dermis; hair follicle bulb	High α6-integrin, low CD71	Prolonged self-renewal; differentiation capacity into multiple skin cell lineages; can differentiate into all hair follicle lineages	Difficult to isolate, expand, and differentiate *in vitro;* limited effectiveness; need more conclusive investigations	Development of skin equivalents [84]
ADSC	Fat tissue	Many surface-positive and surface-negative antigens	Abundant source; easy to isolate; secrete proinflammatory and proangiogenic growth factors; high differentiation potential; minimize wound contraction	Prolonged expansion time, costly, and fragile; highly dependent on patient's health condition	Conditioned adipose tissue media can be used as a safe topical treatment of skin wounds [90]; enhance healing of diabetic ulcers, pressure ulcers, and full-thickness wounds [94–96]
Bone marrow-derived MSCs	Bone marrow		Differentiate into osteocytes, chondrocytes and adipocytes; accelerated wound closure; increases re-epithelialization; improve angiogenesis; host defense and inflammatory processes; matrix deposition	Pathogenesis of hypertrophic scarring; their specific mechanisms still unknown	Accelerate wound healing in chronic and acute wounds [129]; can be applied directly [108] or injected into the wound periphery [107]; improve in vivo skin expansion [114]
Amnion epithelial cells	Amnion		Multipotent differentiation ability; low immunogenicity and anti-inflammatory functions; easy to isolate	Lack the proliferative capacity of placental MSCs	
AFSCs	Amniotic fluid		Immunomodulatory activity; high pluripotency, high proliferation, and easy to isolate; promote angiogenesis	N/A	An effective "off-the-shelf" cell therapy product for wound healing; anti-inflammation for neurological, lung, heart, and kidney disease [138]

over a wider wound area, facilitating reduced donor site requirements through increased efficiency. Specifically, the harvesting of keratinocytes, fibroblasts, and other primary skin cell types and the distribution over the wound site through spraying or bioprinting has produced promising results in preclinical and clinical trials [143,144]. Human skin keratinocytes are one of the most obvious cell types used for wound healing, as one of the main goals of a given therapy is to regenerate the keratinocyte-based epithelial skin layer. Next, dermal fibroblasts are essential to a healing wound for producing a normal collagen ECM. As described above, the hair follicle bulb also contains a valuable stem cell niche which could be used for further enhancement of wound healing. One well-established method of using primary skin cells for grafting is the cultured epithelial autograft. Still other, more complex attempts to produce full-thickness skin through bioprinting and molding have also been performed.

10.4.2.1 Cultured Epithelial Autografts

Cultured epithelial autografts were first designed by O'Connor *et al.*, in 1981 for burn treatment, with the purpose of reducing pain and accelerating healing. The method involves a skin biopsy for cell harvesting, followed by *in vitro* cell expansion, harvesting sheets of epithelia by dissociation from the culture environment substrate with the enzyme dispase, and finally layering the cell sheets on the wound bed [145]. The benefit of such cultured autologous grafts is that they are appropriate for use to treat both acute and chronic wounds, provide a permanent skin replacement without the risk of graft rejection, are easy to apply – including spraying directly onto the wound using preconfluent cultured epidermal cells/grafts. However, the use of donor keratinocytes and cultured epithelial autografts also has limitations. For example, cell harvest success can be limited by the age of donor, as studies have shown that while newborn keratinocytes are highly proliferative, adult donor keratinocytes have a limited potential for proliferation *in vitro* [146]. These results demonstrated the inverse status of a donor cell line and aging, and therefore the time required for healing is increased in elderly populations [147]. Another drawback of this approach is the limited attachment of grafts to the basement membrane which is vital for the graft survival, the time required to culture and prepare the cell sheets for grafting, and the physiologically inaccurate polarity of cells grown on tissue culture plastic [148].

10.4.2.2 Bioprinted Full-Thickness Skin

Bioprinting has emerged as an exceedingly flexible tool in the broad field of regenerative medicine with potential in a wide variety of applications. Bioprinting has been described as robotic additive biofabrication approach that has the potential to build organs or viable tissues [149]. In general, bioprinting uses a computer-controlled 3D printing device to accurately deposit cells and biomaterials into precise and sometimes intricate geometries in order to fabricate anatomically correct tissue-like structures. These printing devices have the capability to print droplets of cells, cell aggregates, or cells encapsulated in hydrogels, – the "bioink", as well as cell-free polymers that provide structure [150,151]. Three-dimensional computer-assisted designs, or blueprints, can be used to guide the placement of specific types of cells and polymers into the appropriate geometries that mimic actual tissue construction, which can then be matured into a tissue or organ construct [152,153].To date, complete organs are still difficult to create, but creation of a whole functional human organ remains the primary long-term goal of bioprinting. A number of bioprinting approaches have been recently explored, many dealing the production of vascular structures, which are necessary if larger organs are to be fabricated. Cell aggregates and cell rods have been printed layer-by-layer into tubular formations, showing the feasibility of one method for printing cellularized vascular structures [154–157]. After printing, the property of tissue liquidity allows these aggregates and rods to fuse into singular seamless structures [158,159]. Other approaches have relied on the development of hydrogels with specific mechanical properties and crosslinking chemistries to facilitate extrusion from printing devices to build other cellularized tubular structures [160,161]. An area that has recently been explored is the application of bioprinting as a technique for treating open wounds and burns. Our team is currently utilizing novel bioprinting technology [162] to aid healing of dermal wounds and full-thickness burns by applying a layered gel and cells to the wound to promote appropriate cell regeneration and reduce inflammation and scarring.

However, autologous and allogeneic primary cells suffer from the same drawbacks and limitations as their autologous and allogeneic skin graft counterparts. Secondary surgical sites are required from which to harvest autologous cells and allogeneic cell-based treatment still have the potential for rejection by the immune system, respectively.

10.5   OUTLOOK AND CONCLUSIONS

Extensive burns and chronic wounds are a huge financial burden for the global health system and sometimes can become an unbearable invalidity for patients. Unfortunately, the numbers of chronic wounds that require treatment are increasing rapidly due to aging population, obesity, and increased number of diabetic patients. The gold standard treatment for wounds is currently autologous split-thickness skin graft despite its limitation. The studies discussed in this chapter serve as examples aiming to offer better solutions for both short- and long-term outcomes, seeking to address both health complications and cosmetic appeareance, and demonstrate that perinatal tissues and cells can be the basis of viable therapies when applied with the optimal carrier or biomaterial. Therefore, combinations of effective and versatile cell populations in tandem with reliable and easy-to-use biomaterial technologies may result in commercially available cell therapy products that will improve the quality of life for patients while decreasing costs associated with skin wounds.

Several types of stem cells have been isolated from various perinatal and adult human tissues and organs and show promising results as a cellular therapy for skin regeneration and repair. These cells differ in their proliferation capacity, immunomodulatory properties, secretory profile, tissue regeneration capacity, degree of reliability, ease of isolation, yield, expansion cost, clinical practicality, mode of delivery, etc. However, the underlying molecular and biological mechanisms of each stem cell type are still not fully defined. Despite the tremendous body of work available in the literature on the use of stem cells for skin tissue engineering and wound healing, there is no general consensus on the efficacy of each stem cell type in wound healing, and substantial discrepancies between studies can be seen. These discrepancies are attributed to many factors including the strain and species of the animal model used, the immunologic aspects of the donor and recipient cells, methods of cell isolation, propagation, storage/freezing, timing of cell delivery, route of delivery, and many other factors. Each of these factors has a tremendous potential to significantly impact the findings and conclusion of a given study. Lack of head-to-head studies comparing different sources of stem cells in a reliable preclinical model hinders the clinical translation of these therapies to patients. However, clinical trials using stem cells have already started for diseases that are particularly difficult to treat. Nonetheless, caution should be taken given that inadequate preclinical trials are all that is available for many applications of stem cells. Another important aspect to keep in mind during the development of a cell-based therapy is the regulatory pathway consisting of guidelines and manufacturing considerations. Early thoughts about the feasibility and cost of Good Manufacturing Practice will save substantial time and effort and expedite the transition into the clinic. Also, the engagement of end users at an early stage during the development of a product has proven to enhance proper and suitable utilization of the developed product on patients.

In the work in our laboratory, the primary limitation we have come across in our work towards building reliable skin substitutes is the inability to limit contraction during the wound healing process. In both of our studies described above, contraction contributed significantly to the overall wound closure. However, we believe that by incorporating the optimal delivery vehicle we can minimize healing by contraction, and rather induce re-epithelialization to be primarily responsible. Interestingly, when we employed HA above, the overall level of contraction did not decrease dramatically. However, the aspect ratio of the healing wound changed significantly. Specifically, wounds treated with HA healed uniformly resulting in roughly a square-shaped area of re-epithelialized skin. In contrast, control wounds and fibrin–collagen-treated wounds healed with a high aspect ratio, contracting more in the medial–lateral direction. This difference may be significant for limiting contraction and scar formation, but will require further investigation.

More general limitations, but limitations nonetheless, are those of regulatory hurdles associated with bringing any cell-based therapy or product to market and to patients in the clinic. The time and financial cost required to generate a simple drug molecule that is commercially available are staggering. Products that incorporate living cells are inherently more complex, resulting in a regulatory pathway that is therefore more complex, and not fully developed at this time. To that end, we have been exploring cell free, but bioactive biomaterials that can mimic the biological behavior of AFSC therapy in wounds. By using a cell-free, but AFS-like, approach we hope to address these issues.

REFERENCES

1. Cherry DK, Hing E, Woodwell DA, Rechtsteiner EA. National ambulatory medical care survey: 2006 summary. *Natl. Health Stat. Report* 2008:3;1–39.
2. Pitts SR, Niska RW, Xu J, Burt CW. National hospital ambulatory medical care survey: 2006 emergency department summary. *Natl. Health Stat. Report* 2008:3:1–38; volume 3.
3. Miller SF, Bessey P, Lentz CW, Jeng JC, Schurr M, Browning S. National burn repository 2007 report: A synopsis of the 2007 call for data. *J. Burn Care Res.* 2008;29:862–870; discussion 71.
4. Peck MD. Epidemiology of burns throughout the world. Part I: Distribution and risk factors. *Burns* 2011;37:1087–1100.
5. Section II. Placental and Placental Membrane-Derived Stem Cells Perinatal cells and biomaterials for wound healing.
6. Gurtner GC, Chapman MA. Regenerative medicine: Charting a new course in wound healing. *Adv. Wound Care* Jun 2016;5(7):314–328.
7. Holavanahalli RK, Helm PA, Kowalske KJ. Long-term outcomes in patients surviving large burns: The skin. *J. Burn Care Res.* 2010;31:631–639.
8. Skardal A, Murphy SV, Crowell K, Mack D, Atala A, Soker S. A tunable hydrogel system for long-term release of cell-secreted cytokines and bioprinted in situ wound cell delivery. *J. Biomed. Mater. Res. B Appl. Biomater.* Oct 2017;105(7):1986–2000.
9. Vyas KS, Vasconez HC. Wound healing: Biologics, skin substitutes, biomembranes, and scaffolds. In Healthcare (Vol. 2. No. 3). Multidisciplinary Digital Publishing Institute; 2014. pp. 356–400.
10. Davis JS. Skin transplantation. *Johns Hopkins Hosp. Rep.* 1910;15:307–396.
11. Branski LK, Herndon DN, Pereira C, Mlcak RP, Celis MM, Lee JO, Sanford AP, Norbury WB, Zhang XJ, Jeschke MG. Longitudinal assessment of Integra in primary burn management: A randomized pediatric clinical trial. *Crit. Care Med.* 2007;35:2615–2623. doi: 10.1097/01.CCM.0000285991.36698.E2.
12. Heimbach D, Luterman A, Burke J, Cram A, Herndon D, Hunt J, Jordan M, McManus W, Solem L, Warden G. Artificial dermis for major burns. A multi-center randomized clinical trial. *Ann. Surg.* 1988;208:313–320.
13. Heimbach DM, Warden GD, Luterman A, Jordan MH, Ozobia N, Ryan CM, Voigt DW, Hickerson WL, Saffle JR, DeClement FA, Sheridan RL, Dimick AR. Multicenter postapproval clinical trial of Integra dermal regeneration template for burn treatment. *J. Burn Care Rehabil.* Jan–Feb 2003;24(1):42–48.
14. Supp DM, Boyce ST. Engineered skin substitutes: Practices and potentials. *Clin. Dermatol.* Jul–Aug 2005;23(4):403–412.
15. Varkey M, Ding J, Tredget EE. Advances in skin substitutes-potential of tissue engineered skin for facilitating anti-fibrotic healing. *J. Funct. Biomater.* Jul 9 2015;6(3):547–563.
16. Curran MP, Plosker GL. Bilayered bioengineered skin substitute (Apligraf): A review of its use in the treatment of venous leg ulcers and diabetic foot ulcers. *BioDrugs* 2002;16(6):439–455.
17. Noordenbos J, Doré C, Hansbrough JF. Safety and efficacy of TransCyte for the treatment of partial-thickness burns. *J. Burn Care Rehabil.* Jul–Aug 1999;20(4):275–281.
18. Rahmanian-Schwarz A, Beiderwieden A, Willkomm LM, Amr A, Schaller HE, Lotter O. A clinical evaluation of biobrane((R)) and suprathel((R)) in acute burns and reconstructive surgery. *Burns* 2011;37:1343–1348.
19. Lloyd EC, Rodgers BC, Michener M, Williams MS. Outpatient burns: Prevention and care. *Am. Fam. Physician* 2012;85:25–32.

20. Chattopadhyay S, Raines RT. Review: Collagen-based biomaterials for wound healing. *Biopolymers* 2014;101(8):821–833.

21. Asz_odi A, Legate KR, Nakchbandi I, F€assler, R. What mouse mutants teach us about extracellular matrix function. *Annu. Rev. Cell Dev. Biol.* 2006;22:591–621.

22. Mian M, Beghe F, Mian E. Collagen as a pharmacological approach in wound healing. *Int. J. Tissue React.* 1992;14:1–9.

23. Thomas S, Loveless PA. A comparative study of twelve hydrocolloid dressings. *World Wide Wounds* 1997;1:1–12.

24. Thomas S. Hydrocolloids. *J. Wound Care* 1992;1:27–30.

25. Thomas A, Harding KG, Moore K. Alginates from wound dressings activate human macrophages to secrete tumour necrosis factor-a. *Biomaterials* 2000;21:1797–1802.

26. Noori A, Ashrafi SJ, Vaez-Ghaemi R, Hatamian-Zaremi A, Webster TJ. A review of fibrin and fibrin composites for bone tissue engineering. *Int. J. Nanomedicine* 2017;12:4937–4961. doi: 10.2147/IJN. S124671. Published 2017 Jul 12.

27. Litvinov RI, Weisel JW. Fibrin mechanical properties and their structural origins. *Matrix Biol.* 2017;60–61:110–123. doi: 10.1016/j.matbio.2016.08.003.

28. Miller R, Wormald JCR, Wade RG, Collins DP. Systematic review of fibrin glue in burn wound reconstruction. *Br. J. Surg.* Feb 2019;106(3):165–173. doi: 10.1002/bjs.11045.

29. Sekine T, Nakamura T, Shimizu Y, Ueda H, Matsumoto K, Takimoto Y, Kiyotani T. *J. Biomed. Mater. Res.* 2001;54:305–310.

30. Aderibigbe BA, Buyana B. Alginate in wound dressings. *Pharmaceutics* 2018;10(2):42. doi: 10.3390/pharmaceutics10020042. Published 2018 Apr 2.

31. Miller RS, Steward DL, Tami TA, Sillars MJ, Seiden AM, Shete M, Paskowski C, Welge J. The clinical effects of hyaluronic acid ester nasal dressing (Merogel) on intranasal wound healing after functional endoscopic sinus surgery. *Otolaryngol. Head Neck Surg.* Jun 2003;128(6):862–869.

32. Fahmy A., Kamoun EA, El-Eisawy R, El-Fakharany EM, Taha TH, El-Damhougy BK. Poly(vinyl alcohol)-hyaluronic acid membranes for wound dressing applications: Synthesis and in vitro bio-evaluations. *J. Braz. Chem. Soc.* 2015;26(7):1357–1366.

33. Wright KA, Nadire KB, Busto P, Tubo R, McPherson JM, Wentworth BM. Alternative delivery of keratinocytes using a polyurethane membrane and the implications for its use in the treatment of full-thickness burn injury. *Burns* 1998;24(1):7–17.

34. Koehler J, Wallmeyer L, Hedtrich S, Goepferich AM, Brandl FP. pH-modulating poly(ethylene glycol)/alginate hydrogel dressings for the treatment of chronic wounds. *Macromol. Biosci.* May 2017;17(5):1600369. doi: 10.1002/mabi.201600369. Epub 2016 Dec 20.

35. Lee JH. Injectable hydrogels delivering therapeutic agents for disease treatment and tissue engineering. *Biomater. Res.* 2018;22:27. doi: 10.1186/s40824-018-0138-6. Published 2018 Sep 26.

36. Yamada KM, Clark RAF. Provisional matrix. In Clark RAF, editor. *The Molecular and Cellular Biology of Wound Repair.* 2nd ed. London: Plenum Press; 1996. pp. 51–942.

37. Kamoun EA, Kenawy ES, Chen X. A review on polymeric hydrogel membranes for wound dressing applications: PVA-based hydrogel dressings. *J. Adv. Res.* 2017;8(3):217–233. doi: 10.1016/j.jare.2017.01.005.

38. O'Meara S, Callum N, Majid M, Sheldon T. Systematic reviews of wound care management (3) antimicrobial agents for chronic wounds (4) diabetic foot ulceration. *Health Technol. Assess.* 2000;4:1–237.

39. Nelson EA, O'Meara S, Craig D, Iglesias C, Golder S, Dalton J, Claxton K, Bell-Syer SE, Jude E, Dowson C, Gadsby R, O'Hare P, Powell J. A series of systematic reviews to inform a decision analysis for sampling treating infected diabetic foot ulcers. *Health Technol. Assess.* 2006;10:1–221.

40. Doillon CJ, Silver FH. Collagen-based wound dressing: Effect of hyaluronic acid and fibronectin on wound healing. *Biomaterials* 1986;7:3–8.

41. Chu HQ, Xiong H, Zhou XQ, Han F, Wu ZG, Zhang P, Huang XW, Cui YH. Aminoglycoside ototoxicity in three murine strains and effects on NKCC1 of stria vascularis. *Chin. Med. J.* 2006;119:980–985.

42. Patrick BN, Rivey MP, Allington DR. Acute renal failure associated with vancomycin- and tobramycin-laden cement in total hip arthroplasty. *Ann. Pharmacother.* 2006;40:2037–2042.

43. Boateng JS, Matthews KH, Eccleston HNESGM. Wound healing dressings and drug delivery systems: A review. *J. Pharm. Sci.* 2008;8(97):2892–2923.

44. Lee-Min Mai LM, Lin CY, Chen CY, Tsai YC. Synergistic effect of bismuth subgallate and borneol, the major components of Sulbogin1 on the healing of skin wound. *Biomaterials* 2003;24:3005–3012.

45. The Annual UK Drug Tariff. 1988 (Nov), 1998 (May), 2007 (Feb) *The Stationary Office*. London, UK: The UK Drug Tariff.

46. Rutten HJT, Nijhuis PHA. Prevention of wound infection in elective colorectal surgery by local application of gentamicin-containing collagen sponge. *Eur. J. Surg.* 1997;163:31–35.

47. Sawada Y, Tadashi O, Masazumi K, Kazunobu S, Koichi O, Sasaki J. An evaluation of a new lactic acid polymer drug delivery system: A preliminary report. *Br. J. Plast. Surg.* 1994;47:158–161.

48. Ganlanduik S, Wrigtson WR, Young S, Myers S, Polk HC, Jr. Absorbable, delayed-release antibiotic beads reduce surgical wound infection. *Am. J. Surg.* 1997;63:831–835.

49. Kumar TRS, Bai MV, Krishnan LK. A freeze-dried fibrin disc as a biodegradable drug release matrix. *Biologicals* 2004;32:49–55.

50. Sawada Y, Ara M, Yotsuyanagi T, Sone K. Treatment of dermal depth burn wounds with an antimicrobial agent-releasing silicone gel sheet. *Burns* 1990;16:347–352.

51. Aoyagi S, Onishi H, Machida Y. Novel chitosan wound dressing loaded with minocycline for the treatment of severe burn wounds. *Int. J. Pharm.* 2007;330:138–145.

52. Komarcevic A. The modern approach to wound treatment. *Med. Pregl.* 2000;53:363–368.

53. Dijke P, Iwata KK. Growth factors for wound healing. *Biotechnology* 1989;7:793–798.

54. Steenfos HH. Growth factors and wound healing Scand. *J. Plast. Reconstr. Surg.* 1994;28:95–105.

55. Greenhalgh DG. The role of growth factors in wound healing. *J. Trauma Inj. Infect. Crit. Care* 1996;41:159–167.

56. Mann A, Niekisch K, Schirmacher P, Blessing M. Granulocyte-macrophage colony-stimulating factor is essential for normal wound healing. *J. Investig. Dermatol. Symp. Proc.* 2006;11:87–92.

57. Lee ARC, Leem H, Jaegwan L, Park KC. Reversal of silver sulfadiadine-impaired wound healing by epidermal growth factor. *Biomaterials* 2005;26:4670–4676.

58. Puolakkainen P, Twardzik DR, Ranchalis JE, Pankey SC, Reed MJ, Gombotz WR. The enhancement in wound healing by transforming growth factor-b1 (TGF-b1) depends on the topical delivery system. *J. Surg. Res.* 1995;58:321–329.

59. Defail AJ, Edington HD, Matthews S, Lee WC, Marra KG. Controlled release of bioactive doxorubicin from microspheres embedded within gelatin scaffolds. *J. Biomed. Mater. Res.* 2006;79:954–962.

60. Koempel JA, Gibson SE, O'Grady K, Toriumi DM. The effect of platelet-derived growth factor on tracheal wound healing. *Int. J. Pediatr. Otorhinolaryngol.* 1998;46:1–8.

61. Maeda M, Kadota K, Kajihara M, Sano A, Fujioka K. Sustained release of human growth hormone (hGH) from collagen film and evaluation of effect on wound healing in mice. *J. Control. Release* 2001;77:261–272.

62. Gu F, Amsden B, Neufeld R. Sustained delivery of vascular endothelial growth factor with alginate beads. *J. Control. Release* 2004;96:463–472.

63. Grzybowski J, Oldak E, Antos-Bielska M, Janiak MK, Pojda Z. New cytokine dressings. I. Kinetics of the in vitro rhG-CSF, rhGM-CSF, and rhEGF release from the dressings. *Int. J. Pharm.* 1999;184:173–178.

64. Park S-N, Kim JK, Suh H. Evaluation of antibiotic loaded collagen-hyaluronic acid matrix as a skin substitute. *Biomaterials* 2004;25:3689–3698.

65. Brown G, Curtsinger L, White M, Mitchell RO, Pietsch J, Nordquis R, Fraunhofer A, Schultz GS. Acceleration of tensile strength of incisions treated with EGF and TGF-beta. *Ann. Surg.* 1988;208:788–794.

66. Tauzin H, Rolin G, Viennet C, Saas P, Humbert P, Muret P. A skin substitute based on human amniotic membrane. *Cell Tissue Bank.* 2014;15(2):257–265.

67. Bennett J, Matthews R, Faulk WP. Treatment of chronic ulceration of the legs with human amnion. *The Lancet* 1980;315:1153–1156.

68. Faulk WP, Stevens P, Burgos H, Matthews R, Bennett J, Hsi BL. Human amnion as an adjunct in wound healing. *The Lancet* 1980;315(8179):1156–1158.

69. Mohammadi AA, Mohammadi MK. How does human amniotic membrane help major burn patients who need skin grafting: New experiences. In Spear M., editor. *Skin Grafts—Indications, Applications and Current Research*. IntechOpen; 2011.

70. Singh R, Purohit S, Chacharkar M, Bhandari P, Bath A. Microbiological safety and clinical efficacy of radiation sterilized amniotic membranes for treatment of second-degree burns. *Burns* 2007;33(4):505–510.

71. Gajiwala K, Gajiwala AL. Use of banked tissue in plastic surgery. *Cell Tissue Bank.* 2003;4(2–4):141–146.

72. Branski LK, Herndon DN, Celis MM, Norbury WB, Masters OE, Jeschke MG. Amnion in the treatment of pediatric partial-thickness facial burns. *Burns* 2008;34(3):393–399.

73. Yang L, Shirakata Y, Tokumaru S, Xiuju D, Tohyama M, Hanakawa Y, Sayama K, Hashimoto K. Living skin equivalents constructed using human amnions as a matrix. *J. Dermatol. Sci.* 2009;56(3):188–195.

74. Murphy S, Skardal A, Atala A. Solubilized amnion membrane hyaluronic-acid hydrogel accelerates full thickness wound healing. *Stem Cell Transl. Med.* 2017;6(11):2020–2032.

75. Oliveira MS, Barreto-Filho JB. Placental-derived stem cells: Culture, differentiation and challenges. *World J. Stem Cells* 2015;7(4):769–775. doi: 10.4252/wjsc.v7.i4.769.

76. Yoo JJ, Atala A, Binder KW, et al. Delivery System. In: Office USPaT, ed. United States of America; 2011: 22.

77. Skardal A, Mack D, Kapetanovic E, Anthony A, Jackson JD, Yoo J, Soker S. Bioprinted amniotic fluid-derived stem cells accelerate healing of large skin wounds. *Stem Cells Transl. Med.* 2012;1:792–802.

78. Vagnozzi AN, Reiter JF, Wong SY. Hair follicle and interfollicular epidermal stem cells make varying contributions to wound regeneration. *Cell Cycle* 2015;23:0.

79. Tumbar T, Guasch G, Greco V, Blanpain C, Lowry WE, Rendl M, Fuchs E. Defining the epithelial stem cell niche in skin. *Science* 2004;303:359–363.

80. Blanpain C, Fuchs E. Epidermal stem cells of the skin. *Annu. Rev. cell Dev. Biol.* 2006;22:339–373.

81. Doucet YS, Owens DM. Isolation and functional assessment of cutaneous stem cells. *Methods Mol. Biol.* 2015;1235:147–164. doi: 10.1007/978-1-4939-1785-3_13.

82. Reiisi S, Esmaeili F, Shirazi A. Isolation, culture and identification of epidermal stem cells from newborn mouse skin. *In Vitro Cell. Dev. Biol. Anim.* 2010;46:54–59.

83. Lau K, Paus R, Tiede S, Day P, Bayat A. Exploring the role of stem cells in cutaneous wound healing. *Exp. Dermatol.* 2009;18:921–933.

84. Kim DS, Cho HJ, Choi HR, Kwon SB, Park KC. Isolation of human epidermal stem cells by adherence and the reconstruction of skin equivalents. *Cell. Mol. Life Sci.* 2004;61:2774–2781.

85. Ito M, Liu Y, Yang Z, Nguyen J, Liang F, Morris RJ, et al. Stem cells in the hair follicle bulge contribute to wound repair but not to homeostasis of the epidermis. *Nat. Med.* 2005;11:1351–1354.

86. Cotsarelis G. Epithelial stem cells: A folliculocentric view. *J. Invest. Dermatol.* 2006;126:1459–1468.

87. Salgado AJ, Reis RL, Sousa NJ, Gimble JM. Adipose tissue derived stem cells secretome: soluble factors and their roles in regenerative medicine. *Curr. Stem Cell Res. Ther.* 2010;5(2):103–110.

88. Kilroy GE, Foster SJ, Wu X, Ruiz J, Sherwood S, Heifetz A, Ludlow JW, Stricker DM, Potiny S, Green P, Halvorsen YDC. Cytokine profile of human adipose-derived stem cells: Expression of angiogenic, hematopoietic, and pro-inflammatory factors. *J. Cell. Physiol.* 2007;212(3):702–709.

89. Kim WS, Park BS, Sung JH, Yang JM, Park SB, Kwak SJ, Park JS. Wound healing effect of adipose-derived stem cells: A critical role of secretory factors on human dermal fibroblasts. *J. Dermatol. Sci.* 2007;48(1):15–24.

90. Kober J, Gugerell A, Schmid M, Zeyda M, Buchberger E, Nickl S, Hacker S, Ankersmit HJ, Keck, M. Wound healing effect of conditioned media obtained from adipose tissue on human skin cells: A comparative in vitro study. *Ann. Plast. Surg.* 2014;30:30.

91. Lee SH, Jin SY, Song JS, Seo KK, Cho KH. Paracrine effects of adipose-derived stem cells on keratinocytes and dermal fibroblasts. *Ann. Dermatol.* 2012;24(2):136–143.

92. Zhao J, Hu L, Liu J, Gong N, Chen L. The effects of cytokines in adipose stem cell-conditioned medium on the migration and proliferation of skin fibroblasts in vitro. *Biomed. Res. Int.* 2013;578479(10):15.

93. Hu L, Zhao J, Liu J, Gong N, Chen L. Effects of adipose stem cell-conditioned medium on the migration of vascular endothelial cells, fibroblasts and keratinocytes. *Exp. Ther. Med.* 2013;5(3):701–706.

94. Cronk SM, Kelly-Goss MR, Ray HC, Mendel TA, Hoehn KL, Bruce AC, Dey BK, Guendel AM, Tavakol DN, Herman, IM, Peirce, SM. Adipose-derived stem cells from diabetic mice show impaired vascular stabilization in a murine model of diabetic retinopathy. *Stem Cells Transl. Med.* 2015;4(5):459–467.

95. Cianfarani F, Toietta G, Di Rocco G, Cesareo E, Zambruno G, Odorisio, T. Diabetes impairs adipose tissue-derived stem cell function and efficiency in promoting wound healing. *Wound Repair Regen.* 2013;21(4):545–553.

96. Cai L, Johnstone BH, Cook TG, Liang Z, Traktuev D, Cornetta K, Ingram DA, Rosen ED, March KL. Suppression of hepatocyte growth factor production impairs the ability of adipose-derived stem cells to promote ischemic tissue revascularization. *Stem Cells* 2007;25(12):3234–3243.

97. Wu Y, Chen L, Scott PG, Tredget EE. Mesenchymal stem cells enhance wound healing through differentiation and angiogenesis. *Stem Cells* 2007;25:2648–2659.

98. Wu Y, Wang J, Scott PG, Tredget EE. Bone marrow-derived stem cells in wound healing: A review. *Wound Repair Regen.* 2007;15:S18–26.

99. Sasaki M, Abe R, Fujita Y, Ando S, Inokuma D, Shimizu H. Mesenchymal stem cells are recruited into wounded skin and contribute to wound repair by transdifferentiation into multiple skin cell type. *J. Immunol.* 2008;180:2581–2587.

100. Fathke C, Wilson L, Hutter J, Kapoor V, Smith A, Hocking A, Isik F. Contribution of bone marrow-derived cells to skin: Collagen deposition and wound repair. *Stem Cells* 2004;22:812–822.

101. Javazon EH, Keswani SG, Badillo AT, Crombleholme TM, Zoltick PW, Radu AP, Kozin ED, Beggs K, Malik AA, Flake, AW. Enhanced epithelial gap closure and increased angiogenesis in wounds of diabetic mice treated with adult murine bone marrow stromal progenitor cells. *Wound Repair Regen.* 2007;15:350–359.

102. Maxson S, Lopez EA, Yoo D, Danilkovitch-Miagkova A, LeRoux MA. Concise review: Role of mesenchymal stem cells in wound repair. *Stem Cells Transl. Med.* 2012;1:142–149.

103. Rea S, Giles NL, Webb S, Adcroft KF, Evill LM, Strickland DH, Wood, FM, Fear, MW. Bone marrow-derived cells in the healing burn wound--more than just inflammation. *Burns: J. Int. Soc. Burn Inj.* 2009;35:356–364.

104. Higashiyama R, Nakao S, Shibusawa Y, Ishikawa O, Moro T, Mikami K, Fukumitsu H, Ueda Y, Minakawa K, Tabata Y, Bou-Gharios G. Differential contribution of dermal resident and bone marrow-derived cells to collagen production during wound healing and fibrogenesis in mice. *J. Invest. Dermatol.* 2011;131:529–536.

105. Higashiyama R, Moro T, Nakao S, Mikami K, Fukumitsu H, Ueda Y, Ikeda K, Adachi E, Bou–Gharios G, Okazaki I, Inagaki Y. Negligible contribution of bone marrow-derived cells to collagen production during hepatic fibrogenesis in mice. *Gastroenterology* 2009;137:1459–1466.

106. Falanga V, Iwamoto S, Chartier M, Yufit T, Butmarc J, Kouttab N, Shrayer D, Carson P. Autologous bone marrow-derived cultured mesenchymal stem cells delivered in a fibrin spray accelerate healing in murine and human cutaneous wounds. *Tissue Eng.* 2007;13:1299–1312.

107. Badiavas EV, Falanga V. Treatment of chronic wounds with bone marrow-derived cells. *Arch. Dermatol.* 2003;139:510–516.

108. Rogers LC, Bevilacqua NJ, Armstrong DG. The use of marrow-derived stem cells to accelerate healing in chronic wounds. *Int. Wound J.* 2008;5:20–25.

109. Ding J, Ma Z, Shankowsky HA, Medina A, Tredget EE. Deep dermal fibroblast profibrotic characteristics are enhanced by bone marrow-derived mesenchymal stem cells. *Wound Repair Regen.* 2013;21:448–455.

110. Wang J, Dodd C, Shankowsky HA, Scott PG, Tredget EE. Deep dermal fibroblasts contribute to hypertrophic scarring. *Lab. Invest.* 2008;88:1278–1290.

111. Wilgus TA, Ferreira AM, Oberyszyn TM, Bergdall VK, Dipietro LA. Regulation of scar formation by vascular endothelial growth factor. *Lab. Invest.* 2008;88:579–590.

112. Yang M, Sheng L, Zhang TR, Li Q. Stem cell therapy for lower extremity diabetic ulcers: Where do we stand? *Biomed. Res. Int.* 2013;462179:18.

113. Kirby GT, Mills SJ, Cowin AJ, Smith LE. Stem cells for cutaneous wound healing. *Biomed. Res. Int.* 2015;285869:2.

114. Wang X, Li C, Zheng Y, Xia W, Yu Y, Ma X. Bone marrow mesenchymal stem cells increase skin regeneration efficiency in skin and soft tissue expansion. *Expert Opin. Biol. Ther.* 2012;12(9):1129–1139.

115. Cargnoni A, Di Marcello M, Campagnol M, Nassuato C, Albertini A, Parolini O. Amniotic membrane patching promotes ischemic rat heart repair. *Cell Transplant.* 2009;18:1147–1159.

116. Cargnoni A, Gibelli L, Tosini A, Signoroni PB, Nassuato C, Arienti D, Lombardi G, Albertini A, Wengler GS, Parolini O. Transplantation of allogeneic and xenogeneic placenta-derived cells reduces bleomycin-induced lung fibrosis. *Cell Transplant.* 2009;18:405–422.

117. Lee HJ, Jung J, Cho KJ, Lee CK, Hwang SG, Kim GJ. Comparison of in vitro hepatogenic differentiation potential between various placenta-derived stem cells and other adult stem cells as an alternative source of functional hepatocytes. *Differentiation* 2012;84:223–231.

118. Kadam S, Muthyala S, Nair P, Bhonde R. Human placenta-derived mesenchymal stem cells and islet-like cell clusters generated from these cells as a novel source for stem cell therapy in diabetes. *Rev. Diabet. Stud.* 2010;7:168–182.

119. Jin J, Wang J, Huang J, Huang F, Fu J, Yang X, Miao Z. Transplantation of human placenta-derived mesenchymal stem cells in a silk fibroin/hydroxyapatite scaffold improves bone repair in rabbits. *J. Biosci. Bioeng.* 2014;118:593–598.

120. Pozzobon M, Franzin C, Piccoli M, De Coppi P. Fetal stem cells and skeletal muscle regeneration: A therapeutic approach. *Front. Aging Neurosci.* 2014;6:222.

121. Wang Y, Guo G, Chen H, Gao X, Fan R, Zhang D, Zhou L. Preparation and characterization of polylactide/poly(ε-caprolactone)-poly(ethylene glycol)-poly(ε-caprolactone) hybrid fibers for potential application in bone tissue engineering. *Int. J. Nanomed.* 2014;9:1991–2003.

122. Alviano F, Fossati V, Marchionni C, Arpinati M, Bonsi L, Franchina M, Lanzoni G, Cantoni S, Cavallini C, Bianchi F, Tazzari PL. Term amniotic membrane is a high throughput source for multipotent mesenchymal stem cells with the ability to differentiate into endothelial cells in vitro. *BMC Dev. Biol.* 2007;7(1):11.

123. Bailo, M, Soncini, M, Vertua E, Signoroni PB, Sanzone S, Lombardi G, Arienti D, Calamani F, Zatti D, Paul P, Albertini, A Engraftment potential of human amnion and chorion cells derived from term placenta. *Transplantation* 2004;78(10):1439–1448.

124. Steigman SA, Fauza DO, Isolation of mesenchymal stem cells from amniotic fluid and placenta. *Curr. Protoc. Stem Cell Biol.* 2007;78(10):1E. 2.1–1E. 2.12.

125. Chang Dong L, Zhang WY, He Lian L, Jiang XX, Zhang Y, Tang PH, Ning MAO. Mesenchymal stem cells derived from human placenta suppress allogeneic umbilical cord blood lymphocyte proliferation. *Cell Res.* 2005;15(7):539–547.

126. Kern S, Eichler H, Stoeve J, Klüter H, Bieback K. Comparative analysis of mesenchymal stem cells from bone marrow, umbilical cord blood, or adipose tissue. *Stem Cells* 2006;24(5):1294–1301.

127. Kong P, Xie X, Li F, Liu Y, Lu Y. Placenta mesenchymal stem cell accelerates wound healing by enhancing angiogenesis in diabetic Goto Kakizaki (GK) rats. *Biochem. Biophys. Res. Commun.* 2013;438(2):410–419.

128. Mathew SA, Chandravanshi B, Bhonde R. Hypoxia primed placental mesenchymal stem cells for wound healing. *Life Sci.* 2017;182:85–92.

129. Miki T, Marongiu F, Dorko K, Ellis E, Strom SC. Isolation of amniotic epithelial stem cells. *Curr. Protoc. Stem Cell Biol.* 2010;12(1):1E. 3.1–1E. 3.10.

130. Murphy S, Wallace E, Jenkin G. Placental-derived stem cells: Potential clinical applications. In Appasani K, Appasani RK, editors. *Stem cells & regenerative medicine.* Humana Press; 2011. pp. 243–263.

131. Ilancheran S, Michalska A, Peh G, Wallace EM, Pera M, Manuelpillai, U. Stem cells derived from human fetal membranes display multilineage differentiation potential. *Biol. Reprod.* 2007;77(3):577–588.

132. Li H, Niederkorn JY, Neelam S, Mayhew E, Word RA, McCulley JP, Alizadeh H. Immunosuppressive factors secreted by human amniotic epithelial cells. *Invest. Ophthalmol. Visual Sci.* 2005;46(3):900–907.

133. Hori J, Wang M, Kamiya K, Takahashi H, Sakuragawa N. Immunological characteristics of amniotic epithelium. *Cornea* 2006;25:S53–S58.

134. Xing L, Franz MG, Marcelo CL, Smith CA, Marshall VS, Robson MC. Amnion-derived multipotent progenitor cells increase gain of incisional breaking strength and decrease incidence and severity of acute wound failure. *J. Burns Wounds* 2007;7:e5.

135. Underwood MA, Gilbert WM, Sherman MP. Amniotic fluid: Not just fetal urine anymore. *J. Perinatol.* 2005;25(5):341–348.

136. Medina-Gomez P. Del Valle M. The culture of amniotic fluid cells. An analysis of the colonies, metaphase and mitotic index for the purpose of ruling out maternal cell contamination. *Ginecol. Obstet. Mex.* 1988;56:122–126.

137. De Coppi P, Bartsch Jr G, Siddiqui MM, Xu T, Santos CC, Perin L, Mostoslavsky G, Serre AC, Snyder EY, Yoo JJ, Furth ME. Isolation of amniotic stem cell lines with potential for therapy. *Nat. Biotechnol.* 2007;25:100–106.

138. Moorefield EC, McKee EE, Solchaga L, Orlando G, Yoo JJ, Walker S, Furth ME, Bishop CE. Cloned, CD117 selected human amniotic fluid stem cells are capable of modulating the immune response. *PloS one* 2011;6(10):e26535.

139. Skardal A, Mack D, Atala A, Soker S. Substrate elasticity controls cell proliferation, surface marker expression and motile phenotype in amniotic fluid-derived stem cells. *J. Mech. Behav. Biomed. Mater.* 2013;17:307–316.

140. Guan X, Delo DM, Atala A, Soker S. In vitro cardiomyogenic potential of human amniotic fluid stem cells. *J. Tissue Eng. Regen. Med.* 2011;5(3):220–228.

141. Skardal A, Mack D, Kapetanovic E, Atala A, Jackson JD, Yoo J, Soker S. Bioprinted amniotic fluid-derived stem cells accelerate healing of large skin wounds. *Stem Cells Transl. Med.* 2012;1:792–802.

142. Xu T, Binder KW, Albanna MZ, Dice D, Zhao W, Yoo JJ, Atala A. Hybrid printing of mechanically and biologically improved constructs for cartilage tissue engineering applications. *Biofabrication* 2013;5:015001.

143. Murphy SV, Skardal A, Atala A. Evaluation of hydrogels for bio-printing applications. *J. Biomed. Mater. Res. A* 2013;101:272–284.

144. Gerlach JC, Johnen C, Ottomann C, Brautigam K, Plettig J, Belfekroun C, Münch S, Hartmann B. Method for autologous single skin cell isolation for regenerative cell spray transplantation with non-cultured cells. *Int. J. Artif. Organs* 2011;34:271–279.

145. Sood R, Roggy DE, Zieger MJ, Nazim M, Hartman BC, Gibbs JT. A comparative study of spray keratinocytes and autologous meshed split-thickness skin graft in the treatment of acute burn injuries. *Wounds: A Compend. Clin. Res. Prac.* 2015;27:31–40.

146. Pastar I, Stojadinovic O, Yin NC, Ramirez H, Nusbaum AG, Sawaya A, Patel SB, Khalid L, Isseroff RR, Tomic-Canic M. Epithelialization in wound healing: A comprehensive review. *Adv. Wound Care* 2014;3(7):445–464. PMC. Web. 10 Aug. 2017

147. Green H, Kehinde O, Thomas J. Growth of cultured human epidermal cells into multiple epithelia suitable for grafting *Proc. Natl. Acad. Sci. U. S. A.* 1979;76:5665–5668.

148. Lesher AP, Curry RH, Evans J, Smith VA, Fitzgerald MT, Cina RA, Streck CJ, Hebra AV. Effectiveness of Biobrane for treatment of partial-thickness burns in children. *J. Pediatr. Surg.* 2011;46:1759–1763.

149. Visconti RP, Kasyanov V, Gentile C, Zhang J, Markwald RR, Mironov V. Towards organ printing: Engineering an intra-organ branched vascular tree. *Expert Opin. Biol. Ther.* 2010;10:409–420.

150. Fedorovich NE, Alblas J, de Wijn JR, Hennink WE, Verbout AJ, Dhert WJ. Hydrogels as extracellular matrices for skeletal tissue engineering: State-of-the-art and novel application in organ printing. *Tissue Eng.* 2007;13:1905–1925.

151. Mironov V, Boland T, Trusk T, Forgacs G, Markwald RR. Organ printing: Computer-aided jet-based 3D tissue engineering. *Trends Biotechnol.* 2003;21:157–161.

152. Mironov V, Kasyanov V, Drake C, Markwald RR. Organ printing: Promises and challenges. *Regen. Med.* 2008;3:93–103.

153. Boland T, Mironov V, Gutowska A, Roth EA, Markwald RR. Cell and organ printing 2: Fusion of cell aggregates in three-dimensional gels. *Anat. Rec A Discov. Mol. Cell. Evol. Biol.* 2003;272:497–502.

154. Jakab K, Damon B, Neagu A, Kachurin A, Forgacs G. Three-dimensional tissue constructs built by bioprinting. *Biorheology* 2006;43:509–513.

155. Marga F, Neagu A, Kosztin I, Forgacs G. Developmental biology and tissue engineering. *Birth Defects Res., Part C* 2007;81:320–328.

156. Norotte C, Marga FS, Niklason LE, Forgacs G. Scaffold-free vascular tissue engineering using bioprinting. *Biomaterials* 2009;30:5910–5917.

157. Skardal A, Zhang J, Prestwich GD. Bioprinting vessel-like constructs using hyaluronan hydrogels crosslinked with tetrahedral polyethylene glycol tetracrylates. *Biomaterials* 2010;31:6173–6181.

158. Jakab K, Damon B, Marga F, Doaga O, Mironov V, Kosztin I, Markwald R, Forgacs G. Relating cell and tissue mechanics: Implications and applications. *Dev. Dyn.* 2008;237:2438–2349.

159. Jakab K, Neagu A, Mironov V, Markwald RR, Forgacs G. Engineering biological structures of prescribed shape using self-assembling multicellular systems. *Proc. Natl. Acad. Sci. U S A.* 2004;101:2864–2869.

160. Skardal A, Zhang J, McCoard L, Oottamasathien S, Prestwich GD. Dynamically crosslinked gold nanoparticle - hyaluronan hydrogels. *Adv. Mater.* 2010;22:4736–4740.

161. Skardal A, Zhang J, McCoard L, Xu X, Oottamasathien S, Prestwich GD. Photocrosslinkable hyaluronan-gelatin hydrogels for two-step bioprinting. *Tissue Eng. Part A* 2010;16:2675–2685.

162. Yoo JJ, Atala A, Binder KW, Zhao W, Dice D, Xu T. Delivery system. In *Office USPaT.* United States of America; 2011. p. 22.

11 Leveraging Plasma Insulin Estimates and Wearable Technologies to Develop an Automated Insulin Delivery System in Type 1 Diabetes

Iman Hajizadeh, Mudassir Rashid, Sediqeh Samadi, Mert Sevil, Nicole Hobbs, Rachel Brandt, Mohammad Reza Askari, and Ali Cinar
Illinois Institute of Technology

CONTENTS

11.1 INTRODUCTION

Throughout the world, one of the largest costs to the society is associated with the healthcare. Chronic diseases are on the rise in the world, increasing healthcare costs for covering care for patients with these expensive chronic conditions [1–3]. One of the most pressing medical problems in the world today is the growing epidemic of diabetes. This disease leads to complications such as cardiovascular problems, stroke, kidney failure, blindness, and lower limb amputation [4,5]. While many people acquire diabetes through an unhealthy lifestyle, some are born with genetic disorders leading to diabetes and require treatment from infancy in order to lead healthy, productive lives. People with Type 1 diabetes (T1D) have beta cells in the pancreas that do not produce any insulin while people with Type 2 diabetes (T2D) have insufficient insulin production and inefficient use of insulin. Consequently, people with T1D are unable to regulate their blood glucose concentration (BGC) without injecting appropriate amounts of insulin through either multiple daily injections or continuous subcutaneous insulin infusion (CSII) [6,7].

Improved glycemic control in individuals with T1D via the use of automated insulin delivery systems called artificial pancreas (AP) systems, which integrate a continuous glucose monitoring (CGM) sensor, CSII pump, and insulin dosing control algorithm, reduces the risks of immediate life-threatening conditions, such as severe hypoglycemia and ketoacidosis, and long-term health complications, such as cardiovascular disease, nephropathy, neuropathy, and retinopathy [8–11]. People with severe T2D are also taking additional insulin, and the AP technology may be beneficial for them as well.

Despite the proven advantages, design of a fully automated AP remains challenging because of the substantive requirements for (i) reliable models to accurately describe the patient-specific time-varying glucose–insulin dynamics; (ii) knowledge of insulin constraints to prevent an overdose and to improve patient safety; and (iii) efficient predictive control algorithms that regulate the BGC in the presence of unknown disturbances like meals and exercise [12–15].

AP systems require safety constraints to avoid aggressive control actions (insulin overdosing) to minimize the risk of hypoglycemia. This can significantly improve the performance of the AP system. The main limiting factor in quantifying the amount of active insulin present in the body is the lack of sensors to measure insulin concentrations in the bloodstream in real time. Determining the amount of available insulin in the body is difficult due to the inter- and intra-patient variabilities. Controlling the BGC in the target range requires AP systems to be aware of the quantity of insulin previously administrated, which if not appropriately incorporated into the control algorithm may cause overcorrection, especially for the postprandial rise in BGC. Such excessive insulin dosing can potentially lead to hypoglycemia. Hence, in addition to the current and target BGC, a constraint expressing an approximation of the insulin present in the body, such as the conventional insulin on board (IOB) estimates, is needed for insulin-dosing calculations. The IOB is an estimate of the amount of insulin present in the blood. It is typically determined through the approximation of the insulin decay curves, which represent the amount of insulin still remaining in the body due to prior insulin infusions. Static approximations of the insulin action curves are typically utilized in insulin pumps. The IOB calculations primarily rely on basic insulin decay profiles [16,17]. Furthermore, significant time-varying delays induced by the absorption and utilization of the subcutaneously administrated insulin as well as diurnal variations in the metabolic state of individuals have significant effects on the IOB. Therefore, the insulin action curves for IOB calculations, usually involving static models with basal and bolus insulin as inputs and active insulin as the output, are not accurate enough to be used in an AP control system. Regardless of the sophistication of the IOB calculation, the information obtained from insulin action curves is usually an approximation of the active insulin in the body. Other approaches to determine the bloodstream insulin concentration involve estimating plasma insulin concentrations (PICs) and calculating the amount of subcutaneously administered insulin present through insulin absorption models [18–22].

Accurate estimates of PIC can be obtained by using CGM measurements with adaptive estimators designed for simultaneous state and parameter estimation based on reliable glucose–insulin models [18–22]. In our previous studies, the design of adaptive and personalized PIC estimators that directly take into account the inter- and intrasubject variabilities in glucose–insulin dynamics is investigated using three different estimation techniques, including continuous-discrete extended Kalman filter (CDEKF), unscented Kalman filter (UKF), and moving horizon estimation (MHE) [21]. The results are based on clinical experiments conducted with adolescents at the Yale Children's Diabetes Clinic (New Haven, CT) involving 13 datasets from subjects with T1DM. We further analyzed the performance of the proposed individualized PIC estimation algorithm using 20 clinical datasets from closed-loop experiments conducted continuously over 60 h involving young adults with T1DM at the Kovler Diabetes Center, University of Chicago Medical Center, Chicago, IL [22]. The diversity of the subjects and the length of the clinical experiments allowed for a more comprehensive and critical evaluation of the performance of the PIC estimation method that will be incorporated into the AP system. The significant variability in data for various subjects is due to the different meals (amount and type of carbohydrate intake), varied daily basal rates, varied bolus insulin infusions, physical activity (PA) levels, and sleep characteristics. The discrete sampling nature of the CGM measurement output, the lack of knowledge on the exact time and amount of meals, the time-varying nature of human physiology, the unmeasured disturbances caused by exercise and sleep, the intersubject variability, the constraints on the state variables, and the rate of change of the model parameters are some of challenges addressed in this work. The PIC estimator is individualized using readily available demographic information, such as body weight, height, body mass index (BMI), and total daily insulin dose. The PIC estimation results are compared against those obtained through the conventional IOB curves to demonstrate the merits of the proposed individualized PIC estimator [21,22].

The core of the AP system is the control algorithm that computes the optimum amount of insulin. The control objective of regulating glucose concentrations is posed with constraints that avoid insulin overdosing. Model predictive control (MPC) formulations are a promising and effective approach for AP systems as they can handle multivariable systems and systematically deal with state and input constraints [12,13,23–32]. Since predictive controllers compute the optimal control actions by using a model and a cost function, the glucose control performance is affected by the accuracy of the glucose–insulin models. In fact, one of the main challenges to achieve a reliable AP is the lack of accurate glycemic models to describe the dynamic changes in the human body under various conditions. The future BGC values are difficult to predict accurately as glycemic dynamics vary substantially due to the effects of numerous factors such as meal consumptions, infused insulin, and exercise or PA levels. Moreover, metabolic processes vary substantially among subjects and temporally within people due to the diversified lifestyles and erratic routines of individuals. The diversity of physiology and behaviors in people causes the glucose–insulin dynamics and insulin sensitivities of individuals to vary over time, while large perturbations such as meals and PA cause significant excursions in glucose concentrations that may not be described accurately by generalized models. Hence, the necessity in AP systems of personalized glucose–insulin models rather than models with generalized parameters that do not reflect the dynamic characteristics of subjects in different situations [33–38]. In our previous work, an adaptive and personalized compartment model that translates the abrupt bolus and discrete basal changes into estimates of PIC is integrated with an adaptive system identification approach to characterize the transient dynamics of glycemic measurements. The adaptations by the recursive system identification assist in handling stochastic disturbances like the effects of meal consumption and physical activities. Furthermore, the system identification algorithm is extended to improve reliability for use in fully automated AP systems. The proposed approach involves the modification of the recursive predictor-based subspace identification (PBSID) algorithm to incorporate constraints on the fidelity and accuracy of the identified models, correctness of the sign of the input-to-output gains, and the integration of heuristics to ensure the stability of the recursively identified models. To achieve this, the proposed adaptive models also include estimated meal effects and the reported exercise-related biometric variables by wearable technology as additional inputs to automatically accommodate unannounced meals and exercise. The proposed adaptive and personalized modeling approach considering the effects of unannounced meals and exercise on the transient glycemic dynamics has been applied to 15 clinical datasets involving closed-loop experiments of the AP systems [39–42].

Motivated by the above considerations, an adaptive personalized multivariable AP system is proposed to effectively control the BGC and reject disturbances without manual user announcements for meals and exercise. The proposed AP uses physiological signals from wearable devices

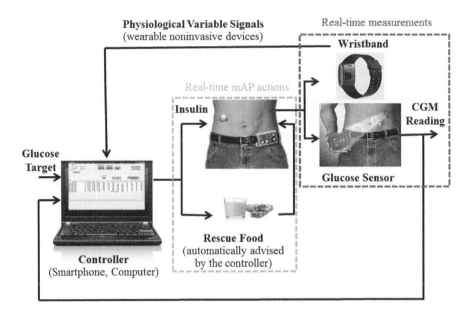

FIGURE 11.1   General flowchart of the proposed mAP system.

and estimates of unannounced meal effects and PIC in addition to glucose measurements with a CGM. A general flowchart of the proposed method is presented in Figure 11.1. A PIC estimator summarized in Section 11.3.1 generates estimates of the insulin concentration in the bloodstream. PIC estimates are used as an input, along with other physiological measurements such as energy expenditure (EE), in the identification of the controller model. The estimated PIC and EE are employed to identify adaptive models through recursive system identification techniques summarized in Section 11.3.2 to characterize the time-varying glucose–insulin dynamics. Then, the adaptive models are integrated with a physiological compartment model to build the models employed in Section 11.4 for the design of an adaptive MPC formulation. The multivariable adaptive MPC formulation is therefore aware of insulin available and the state of the subject. The adaptive controller parameters, dynamic plasma insulin constraint, addition of physiological measurements from wearable devices, and feature variables generated from the glucose measurements enable the multivariable AP (mAP) system to effectively compute the optimal insulin infusion over diverse diurnal variations without meal and exercise announcements. Simulation case studies using multivariable models illustrate the efficacy of the proposed mAP system in Section 11.5, followed by a discussion of the merits of the proposed multivariable adaptive MPC in Section 11.6. Finally, a few concluding remarks are given in Section 11.7.

11.2   METHODS

In this section, a brief overview of the adaptive and personalized PIC estimator is provided, followed by a review of the PBSID algorithm for the identification of linear, time-varying state-space models. Subsequently, the adaptive MPC formulation is presented. Figure 11.2 illustrates the proposed modeling and adaptive MPC algorithm. First, a UKF estimates the PIC value using the CGM data and infused insulin information. Then, the PIC estimates and CGM data are used to identify time-varying linear state-space model with the recursive PBSID technique. The estimated PIC and the identified state-space models form the basis of the adaptive MPC with dynamic constraint adjustment.

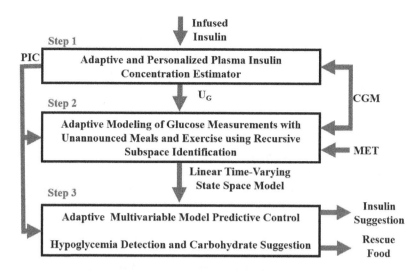

FIGURE 11.2   A summary of the developed techniques for the AP system.

11.2.1 PRELIMINARIES

We first provide brief descriptions of the nonlinear observer developed to estimate the physiological states. The estimates of the physiological states, including the estimates of the PIC, are used in dynamically constraining the insulin dosing control algorithm. Then we review the predictor-based subspace identification (PBSID) algorithm for the identification of linear, time-varying state-space models employed in the design of the predictive controller.

11.2.1.1 Adaptive and Personalized PIC Estimator

Hovorka's model, a glucose–insulin dynamics model, is used for designing the PIC estimator [21–23], which quantifies the available insulin in people with T1DM and is used to impose safety limits for the controller. A nonlinear observer based on the UKF algorithm for the simultaneous estimation of the state variables and the time-varying parameters is designed to provide accurate PIC estimates (I_k). The proposed PIC estimator can be individualized by appropriately initializing the time-varying parameters using partial least squares regression. To this end, the readily attainable demographic information of individuals, such as weight, BMI, and duration with diabetes, is used to estimate the initial values for the time-varying parameters in the model [21,22]. After initialization, the time-varying parameters and the state variables can be estimated online using an appropriate observer. The proposed PIC estimator is able to capture the inter- and intrasubject variabilities to provide accurate information on the amount of insulin present in the body. Furthermore, as information about the time and quantity of meals is difficult to ascertain and thus considered as unknown disturbances, the gut absorption rate is also included as an extended state to be estimated $(U_{G,k})$.

11.2.1.2 Recursive Subspace-Based System Identification

A stable, reliable, and computationally tractable dynamic model is essential for the design of model-based predictive control algorithms in AP systems. To this end, in this work, we use the recursive PBSID to identify a linear, time-varying model of the form

$$\tilde{x}_{k+1} = A_k\tilde{x}_k + B_ku_k + K_ke_k$$
$$y_k = C_k\tilde{x}_k + e_k \tag{11.1}$$

where $\tilde{x}_k$ denotes the states of the identified model, u_k is the input variable, and in this case the input is the estimates of the PIC, meal effects, and measured physiological signals, and y_k is the output CGM measurement. Further, A_k, B_k, and C_k are the system matrices of appropriate dimensions, K_k is the Kalman gain matrix, and e_k is the deviation between the measurement and estimate of the CGM output for feedback to correct the state variables [39–41,43].

11.2.2 ADAPTIVE PIC COGNIZANT MPC ALGORITHM

In this section, the insulin compartment model of Hovorka's model is incorporated with the recursive PBSID approach to build an appropriate form of the glycemic model for use in the AP control system. Then, we describe the glycemic and PIC risk indexes used in the MPC controller objective function. The safety constraints based on the PIC and a feature extraction method for manipulating these constraints during the meal consumption periods are presented. Subsequently, the adaptive mAP control formulation is presented.

11.2.2.1 Integrating Insulin Compartment Models with Subspace Identification

The manipulated variable of the AP control system is the injected insulin in the form of basal/bolus insulin. So, the identified state-space model using PBSID described by equation (11.1) cannot be used directly for the model-based control techniques since PIC is an input of the system [42]. In this subsection, we integrate the data-driven model determined from the PBSID technique with the insulin subsystem from Hovorka's model yielding

$$\bar{x}_{k+1} = D_k \bar{x}_k + E_k \bar{u}_k$$
$$\bar{y}_k = F_k \tag{11.2}$$

with the new state vector of $\bar{x}_k = \left[\tilde{x}_{k+3+d} S_{1,k} S_{2,k+1} I_{k+2} \right]$ and the output as $\bar{y}_k = y_{k+3+d}$. The state variables $S_{1,k}$ and $S_{2,k}$ denote the absorption rate of subcutaneously administered insulin and I_k is the PIC. Further, $\bar{u}_k$ includes delayed infused basal/bolus insulin information by a delay of order d, estimates of meal effects, and measured physiological signals.

11.2.2.2 Adaptive Glycemic and Plasma Insulin Risk Indexes

An adaptive glycemic risk index (GRI) is used to determine the weighting matrix for penalizing the deviations of the outputs (predicted CGMs) from their nominal set-point [12,13]. The GRI asymmetrically increases the set-point tracking weight when outputs diverge from the target range. Since hypoglycemic events have serious short-term implications, the set-point penalty increases rapidly in response to hypoglycemic excursions and more gradually in hyperglycemic excursions. Furthermore, a plasma insulin risk index (PIRI) is defined to manipulate the weighting matrix for penalizing the amount of input actuation (aggressiveness of insulin dosing) depending on the estimated PIC, thus suppressing the infusion rate if sufficient insulin is present in the bloodstream [12,13]. As it is impractical to directly consider the estimates of the PIC to define the parameters of the MPC due to the variability among subjects, the normalized value of the PIC is employed, which eliminates the dependency of the PIC estimates to a particular subject by standardizing with the known patient-specific basal PIC value.

11.2.2.3 PIC Bounds

In the proposed MPC, the estimated future PIC is dynamically bounded depending on the value of the CGM measurements. For instance, if the CGM values are elevated, the bounds on PIC are increased to ensure sufficient insulin is administered to regulate the glucose concentration. Furthermore, the PIC bounds also constrain the search space in the optimization problem, thus improving the computational tractability of the proposed MPC. The PIC bounds are determined based on the CGM measurements as $X_{\text{PIC}} = \left(P_{\text{fasting}} + P_{\text{meal}} \right) \times \bar{y}_k$, where X_{PIC} defines the lower and upper bounds and a desired target for the normalized PIC through the predicted CGM. P_{meal} is a parameter that modifies the PIC bounds when there is a rapid increase in the CGM measurements. P_{fasting} is a patient-specific parameter that defines the controller aggressiveness/conservativeness during the fasting period. These bounds and the reference target for the normalized PIC are defined as a function of the CGM measurement, and the MPC solution should satisfy the PIC constraints while maintaining the PIC close to the desired value. The nominal PIC bounds can be determined by multiplying the normalized PIC bounds with the basal PIC value. Therefore, appropriate PIC bounds can be determined based on each subject's basal PIC value and CGM measurement.

11.2.2.4 Feature Extraction for Manipulating Constraints

Meal consumption can be automatically detected using qualitative descriptions of glucose time series data, which is useful in modifying the aggressiveness of the adaptive MPC [44,45]. In this work, features are generated from the data to describe the recent trajectory of glycemic measurements. To this end, a p-order polynomial f is fitted to the most recent three glucose measurements $y_{k:k-2} = \left[y_k \, y_{k-1} \, y_{k-2} \right]$ at each sampling time using ordinary least squares. Then the derivatives of the polynomial are obtained and the first- and second-order derivatives, denoted f' and f'', are analyzed to derive parameter P_{meal} for detecting carbohydrate consumption as

$$
P_{\text{meal},k} = \left\{
\begin{array}{ll}
\dfrac{f_k'}{\delta_1} & \text{if } f_k' \geq \sigma \text{ and } f_k'' \geq 0 \\[2ex]
\dfrac{f_k'}{\delta_2} & \text{if } f_k' \geq \sigma \text{ and } f_k'' < 0 \\[2ex]
0 & \text{if } f_k' < \sigma
\end{array}
\right\}
\tag{11.3}
$$

where δ_1, δ_2, and σ are patient-specific threshold parameters. Detection of meals based on the P_{meal} parameter allows for the constraints of the adaptive MPC are modified when meals are to make the controller more aggressive to suggest a sufficient insulin dose.

11.2.2.5 Adaptive MPC Formulation

In this subsection, we propose a novel adaptive MPC algorithm cognizant of the PIC for computing the optimal insulin infusion rate. The proposed MPC formulation employs the glycemic and PIC risk indexes that manipulate the penalty weighting matrices in the cost function. To this end, the MPC computes the optimal insulin infusion over a finite horizon using the identified time-varying subspace-based models by solving at each sampling instant (k) the following quadratic programming problem

$$
\min_{\{\bar{u}_{k+j}\}_{j=0}^{N-1}} f,
$$

s.t.

$$
\bar{x}_{k+1+j} = D_k \bar{x}_{k+j} + E_k \bar{u}_{k+j}, \, j \hat{I} Z
$$

$$
\bar{y}_{k+j} = F_k \bar{x}_{k+j}, \, j \hat{I} Z
$$

(11.4)

with the objective function

$$\phi = \frac{1}{2}\sum_{j=0}^{N-1}\left(\overline{y}_{k+j+1} - r_{k+j+1}\right)^{T}\overline{Q}_{k}\left(\overline{y}_{k+j+1} - r_{k+j+1}\right) + \left(\overline{u}_{k+j} - u_{\text{ins,basal},k+j}\right)^{T}\overline{R}_{k}\left(\overline{u}_{k+j} - u_{\text{ins,basal},k+j}\right)$$

where $\overline{Q}_{k}$, $\overline{R}_{k}$, and $\overline{P}_{k}$ are the adaptive weights used in the MPC objective function, $Z = \{0...N\}$ and $u_{\text{ins,basal},k}$ is the patient-specific basal insulin rate.

11.3 RESULTS

The efficacy of the proposed mAP is demonstrated using a multivariable glucose–insulin-physiological variables simulator (mGIPsim) developed by our research group at Illinois Institute of Technology based on a modified Hovorka's glucose–insulin dynamic model that takes into account the effects of different physical activities [46]. In addition to the CGM values, mGIPsim generates physiological variable signals reported by noninvasive wearable devices. For this purpose, aerobic exercises with treadmill and bicycle are considered for testing the mAP system. Twenty virtual subjects are simulated for 3 days with varying times and quantities of meals consumed on each day and different types and times of physical activities as detailed in Tables 11.1 and 11.2. The meal and PA information are unannounced (no manual entries) to the AP system as the AP controller is designed to regulate the BGC in the presence of significant disturbances such as unannounced meals and exercises. The Metabolic Equivalent Task (MET) values computed by mGIPsim are used as physiological signals in the recursive system identification technique that predicts future glucose concentration values.

The quantitative and qualitative evaluations of the closed-loop results based on mAP are presented in Figure 11.3 and Table 11.3. Figure 11.3 presents detailed results using the first and third quartiles, median, minimum, maximum, and mean values of CGM for all 20 subjects. Table 11.3 also gives the percentage of samples in defined glycemic ranges and selected statistics for the glucose measurements of the mAP.

TABLE 11.1

Meal Scenario for 3 Days Closed-Loop Experiment Using the Multivariable Metabolic Simulator

Meal	Day 1 Time	Day 1 Amount (g)	Day 2 Time	Day 2 Amount (g)	Day 3 Time	Day 3 Amount (g)
Breakfast	07:00	50	08:00	60	07:30	55
Lunch	13:00	70	14:00	50	13:30	60
Dinner	19:00	60	20:00	70	19:30	50
Snack	21:30	30	23:00	25	22:00	20

TABLE 11.2

Exercise Scenario for 1 h Duration for 3 Days Closed-Loop Experiment Using the Multivariable Metabolic Simulator

Exercise	Day 1	Day 2	Day 3
Morning	Bicycling at 09:00	Treadmill at 10:00	Bicycling at 09:30
Afternoon	Treadmill at 15:00	Bicycling at 16:00	Treadmill at 15:30

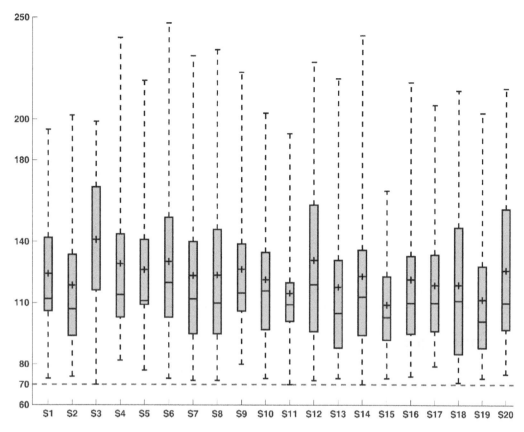

FIGURE 11.3 The mAP closed-loop results. The bottom and top of the boxes are the first and third quartiles and the line inside the box is the median. The ends of the whiskers represent minimum and maximum values and + indicates mean values.

TABLE 11.3
Closed-Loop Results for Percentage Time Spent in Different BGC Ranges and Various Statistics

| Subject | | Percent of Time in Range | | | | | Statistics | | | | Daily Insulin (U) | |
	<55	[55, 70)	[80, 140]	[70, 180]	[180, 250]	>250	Median	[Q1, Q3]	Min	Max	Total	Basal
1	0.0	0.0	73.5	94.3	5.7	0.0	112	[106, 142]	73	195	54.1	30.4
2	0.0	0.0	76.7	92.0	8.0	0.0	107	[94, 134]	74	202	47.5	23.8
3	0.0	0.0	45.0	88.3	11.7	0.0	141	[116, 167]	70	199	64.4	40.3
4	0.0	0.0	73.3	85.2	14.8	0.0	114	[103, 144]	82	240	71.5	26.4
5	0.0	0.0	73.6	89.3	10.7	0.0	111	[109, 141]	77	219	83.9	40.0
6	0.0	0.0	67.4	87.3	12.7	0.0	120	[103, 152]	73	247	63.0	25.6
7	0.0	0.0	71.7	87.7	12.3	0.0	112	[95, 140]	72	231	66.7	32.0
8	0.0	0.0	71.4	84.7	15.3	0.0	110	[95, 146]	72	234	66.4	31.3
9	0.0	0.0	76.1	89.1	10.9	0.0	115	[106, 139]	80	223	77.8	42.1
10	0.0	0.0	77.2	91.8	8.2	0.0	116	[97, 135]	73	203	65.5	37.2
11	0.0	0.0	77.8	97.7	2.3	0.0	109	[101, 120]	70	193	76.3	37.0
12	0.0	0.0	61.1	84.7	15.3	0.0	119	[96, 158]	72	228	62.5	30.1

(Continued)

TABLE 11.3 (*Continued*)

Closed-Loop Results for Percentage Time Spent in Different BGC Ranges and Various Statistics

Subject	Percent of Time in Range						Statistics				Daily Insulin (U)	
	<55	[55, 70)	[80, 140]	[70, 180)	[180, 250)	>250	Median	[Q1, Q3]	Min	Max	Total	Basal
13	0.0	0.0	76.01	87.5	12.5	0.0	105	[88, 131]	73	220	70.2	36.2
14	0.0	0.0	73.2	86.8	13.2	0.0	113	[94, 136]	70	241	70.0	40.8
15	0.0	0.0	80.5	100.0	0.0	0.0	103	[92, 123]	73	165	63.3	36.6
16	0.0	0.0	76.4	87.0	13.0	0.0	110	[95, 133]	74	218	91.8	44.0
17	0.0	0.0	79.8	93.0	7.1	0.0	110	[96, 134]	79	207	61.3	42.5
18	0.0	0.0	57.9	87.5	12.5	0.0	111	[85, 147]	71	214	82.7	47.4
19	0.0	0.0	74.8	95.0	5.0	0.0	101	[88, 128]	73	203	48.9	25.8
20	0.0	0.0	67.3	85.9	14.1	0.0	110	[97, 156]	75	215	53.9	36.1
Avg	0.0	0.0	71.5	89.7	10.3	0.0	112	[98, 140]	74	215	66.9	35.3

The Avg values refer to the mean value of each metrics over all subjects.

11.4 DISCUSSION

No hypoglycemia occurs for any subject, as the BGC is never below 70 mg/dL. The percentages of time spent in the target ranges are significantly high (71.5% and 89.7% for the [80–140] mg/dL and [70–180] mg/dL, respectively). Based on the average of maximum values of CGM (215 mg/dL) and median of CGM values (112 mg/dL), the feature extraction method for manipulating constraints when meal period is detected performs well in computing the required amount of insulin to avoid hyperglycemia. The CGM never goes below 55 or above 250 mg/dL. The percentage of time spent in the [180–250) mg/dL is significantly low (10.3%). The average of minimum values of CGM (74 mg/dL) shows that the mAP can perform safe against different unannounced disturbances such as meals and PA. The closed-loop CGM and infused insulin results of the mAP are presented in Figures 11.4 and 11.5.

The MET is a physiological measure expressing the energy cost of PA and is defined as the ratio of metabolic rate (and therefore the rate of energy consumption) during a specific PA to a reference metabolic rate. MET is used as a means of expressing the intensity and EE of activities in a way that is comparable among people. We have developed a real-time MET estimation algorithm by using noninvasive measurements of physiological variables [47].

A PIC estimator is used to estimate the PIC as well as the insulin compartmental model's time-varying parameters and the unannounced meal effects. The results for the proposed integrated compartment model with adaptive subspace identification techniques are promising. There are several benefits to the integration of insulin compartment model with recursively identified glycemic models.

First, the PIC estimates are adaptive and individualized to particular patients, thus providing accurate real-time estimates of the amount of active insulin present in the bloodstream. The PIC information can be readily used to impose constraints on the insulin dosing computation algorithm. Second, in contrast to the discrete basal and acute bolus insulin variations, the estimated PIC from the compartment model readily provides a more appropriate and filtered input variable for model identification. Third, the adaptive subspace identification technique renders the recursively identified glycemic models valid over a diverse range of daily activities without requiring onerous and obscure information such as the amount of carbohydrate consumption or quantification of PA levels. The proposed adaptive modeling approach with an integrated compartment

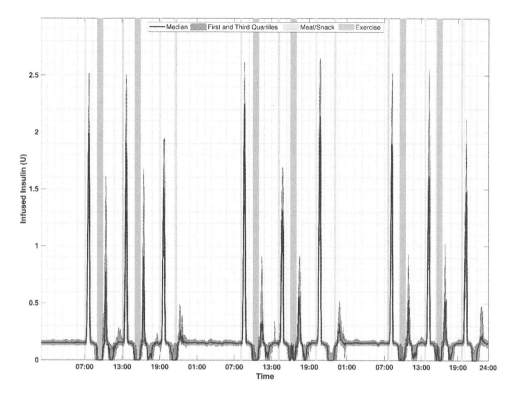

FIGURE 11.4   Closed-loop CGM results of the mAP.

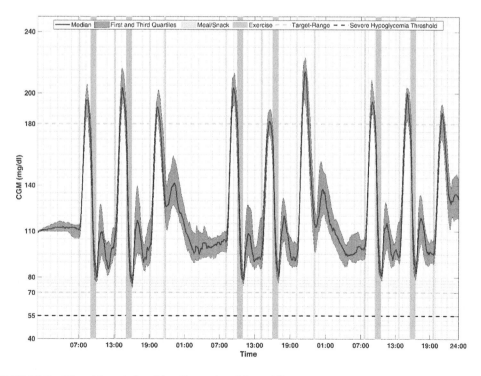

FIGURE 11.5   Closed-loop infused insulin results of the mAP.

model utilizes additional input variables such as the EE to consider the effects of PA on glycemic dynamics.

The PIRI is used to manipulate the penalty weights of the objective function and is specified using the PIC value normalized by the basal PIC. The PIC-bound constraints, along with the risk indexes, govern the aggressiveness of the controller. The insulin concentration in the bloodstream should be maintained within a safe range. If the PIC decreases to low values that characterize the PIC without disturbances and only steady basal insulin infusion), then the BGC may rise rapidly in response to meal consumption. The rapid increase in BGC due to carbohydrate consumption and low PIC may cause hyperglycemia, and consequently the controller may suggest a large bolus to derive the high BGC towards the set-point. However, the significant delays in the glucose–insulin dynamics may result in an overcorrection of the high glucose values, which may adversely lead to hypoglycemia. Such abrupt and counteracting behavior should be avoided for effective glucose regulation. One approach to ensure that such unfavorable dynamics are avoided is to effectively negotiate the trade-offs between the opposing criteria of the cost function. To this end, the glycemic and PIRIs are defined to maintain PIC close to the basal value under normal conditions and thus increase the effectiveness of the AP therapy.

11.5 CONCLUSIONS

An adaptive personalized mAP system is designed based on an MPC algorithm. PIC estimates and physiological variables are combined with a recursive subspace-based system identification approach to obtain the glycemic models. The MPC algorithm developed by using these adaptive models compute the optimal amount of insulin for AP systems without requiring any manual information on meal and PA specifications. The proposed mAP could be a reliable step towards improved glycemic control by individualizing the insulin computations and reducing the risk of hypoglycemia during and after exercise in the next-generation AP algorithms.

ACKNOWLEDGMENTS

This work is supported by the National Institutes of Health (NIH) under grants 1DP3DK10107701 and 1DP3DK101075-01, and JDRF award A18–0036-001 is made possible by funding provided through the collaboration between the JDRF and The Leona M. and Harry B. Helmsley Charitable Trust.

REFERENCES

1. R. DeVol, A. Bedroussian, A. Charuworn, A. Chatterjee, I. Kim, S. Kim, K. Klowden, *An Unhealthy America: The Economic Burden of Chronic Disease*, Santa Monica, CA: Milken Institute, 326 (2007) 2010–2060.
2. American Diabetes Association, Economic costs of diabetes in the us in 2007, *Diabetes Care* 31 (3) (2008) 596–615.
3. E. S. Huang, A. Basu, M. O'Grady, J. C. Capretta, Projecting the future diabetes population size and related costs for the us, *Diabetes Care* 32 (12) (2009) 2225–2229.
4. W. T. Cade, Diabetes-related microvascular and macrovascular diseases in the physical therapy setting, *Phys. Ther.* 88 (11) (2008) 1322–1335.
5. J. K. Snell-Bergeon, R. P. Wadwa, Hypoglycemia, diabetes, and cardiovascular disease, *Diabetes Technol. Ther.* 14 (S1) (2012) S51.
6. G. S. Eisenbarth, Type 1 diabetes mellitus, *Joslin's Diabetes Mellitus* 14 (2005) 399–424.
7. D. W. Cooke, L. Plotnick, Type 1 diabetes mellitus in pediatrics, *Pediatr. Rev.* 29 (11) (2008) 374–384.
8. K. Turksoy, N. Frantz, L. Quinn, M. Dumin, J. Kilkus, B. Hibner, A. Cinar, E. Littlejohn, Automated insulin delivery-the light at the end of the tunnel, *J. Pediat.* 186 (2017) 17–28.
9. T. Peyser, E. Dassau, M. Breton, J. S. Skyler, The artificial pancreas: Current status and future prospects in the management of diabetes, *Ann. N. Y. Acad. Sci.* 1311 (1) (2014) 102–123.

10. S. Esposito, E. Santi, G. Mancini, F. Rogari, G. Tascini, G. Toni, A. Argentiero, M. G. Berioli, Efficacy and safety of the artificial pancreas in the paediatric population with type 1 diabetes, *J. Transl. Med.* 16 (1) (2018) 176.

11. E. Bekiari, K. Kitsios, H. Thabit, M. Tauschmann, E. Athanasiadou, T. Karagiannis, A.-B. Haidich, R. Hovorka, A. Tsapas, Artificial pancreas treatment for outpatients with type 1 diabetes: Systematic review and meta-analysis, *BMJ* 361 (2018) k1310.

12. I. Hajizadeh, M. Rashid, S. Samadi, M. Sevil, N. Hobbs, R. Brandt, A. Cinar, Adaptive personalized multivariable artificial pancreas using plasma insulin estimates, *J. Process. Control* 80 (2019) 26–40.

13. I. Hajizadeh, M. Rashid, A. Cinar, Plasma-insulin-cognizant adaptive model predictive control for artificial pancreas systems, *J. Process. Control* 77 (2019) 97–113.

14. B. W. Bequette, Challenges and recent progress in the development of a closed-loop artificial pancreas, *Annu. Rev. Control* 36 (2) (2012) 255–266.

15. F. J. Doyle, L. M. Huyett, J. B. Lee, H. C. Zisser, E. Dassau, Closed-loop artificial pancreas systems: Engineering the algorithms, *Diabetes Care* 37 (5) (2014) 1191–1197.

16. C. Toffanin, H. Zisser, F. J. Doyle, E. Dassau, Dynamic insulin on board: Incorporation of circadian insulin sensitivity variation, *J. Diabetes Sci. Technol.* 7 (4) (2013) 928–940.

17. C. Ellingsen, E. Dassau, H. Zisser, B. Grosman, M. W. Percival, L. Jovanovic, F. J. Doyle, Safety constraints in an artificial pancreatic β cell: An implementation of model predictive control with insulin on board, *J. Diabetes Sci. Technol.* 3 (3) (2009) 536–544.

18. D. de Pereda, S. Romero-Vivo, B. Ricarte, P. Rossetti, F. J. Ampudia-Blasco, J. Bondia, Real-time estimation of plasma insulin concentration from continuous glucose monitor measurements, *Comput. Methods Biomech. Biomed. Eng.* 19 (9) (2016) 934–942.

19. C. Eberle, C. Ament, The unscented Kalman filter estimates the plasma insulin from glucose measurement, *Biosystems* 103 (1) (2011) 67–72.

20. C. Neatpisarnvanit, J. R. Boston, Estimation of plasma insulin from plasma glucose, *IEEE Trans. Biomed. Eng.* 49 (11) (2002) 1253–1259.

21. I. Hajizadeh, M. Rashid, K. Turksoy, S. Samadi, J. Feng, N. Frantz, M. Sevil, E. Cengiz, A. Cinar, Plasma insulin estimation in people with type 1 diabetes mellitus, *Ind. Eng. Chem. Res.* 56 (35) (2017) 9846–9857.

22. I. Hajizadeh, M. Rashid, S. Samadi, J. Feng, M. Sevil, N. Hobbs, C. Lazaro, Z. Maloney, R. Brandt, X. Yu, K. Turksoy, E. Littlejohn, E. Cengiz, A. Cinar, Adaptive and personalized plasma insulin concentration estimation for artificial pancreas systems, *J. Diabetes Sci. Technol.* 12 (3) (2018) 639–649.

23. R. Hovorka, V. Canonico, L. J. Chassin, U. Haueter, M. Massi-Benedetti, M. O. Federici, T. R. Pieber, H. C. Schaller, L. Schaupp, T. Vering, M. E. Wilinska, Nonlinear model predictive control of glucose concentration in subjects with type 1 diabetes, *Physiol. Meas.* 25 (4) (2004) 905.

24. W. L. Clarke, S. Anderson, M. Breton, S. Patek, L. Kashmer, B. Kovatchev, Closed-loop artificial pancreas using subcutaneous glucose sensing and insulin delivery and a model predictive control algorithm: The Virginia experience, *J. Diabetes Sci. Technol.* 3 (5) (2009) 1031–1038.

25. A. J. Laguna Sanz, F. J. Doyle III, E. Dassau, An enhanced model predictive control for the artificial pancreas using a confidence index based on residual analysis of past predictions, *J. Diabetes Sci. Technol.* 11 (3) (2017) 537–544.

26. R. Gondhalekar, E. Dassau, F. J. Doyle, Periodic zone-MPC with asymmetric costs for outpatient-ready safety of an artificial pancreas to treat type 1 diabetes, *Automatica* 71 (2016) 237–246.

27. A. Chakrabarty, S. Zavitsanou, F. J. Doyle, E. Dassau, Event-triggered model predictive control for embedded artificial pancreas systems, *IEEE Trans. Biomed. Eng.* 65 (3) (2018) 575–586.

28. F. Cameron, B. W. Bequette, D. M. Wilson, B. A. Buckingham, H. Lee, G. Niemeyer, A closed-loop artificial pancreas based on risk management, *J. Diabetes Sci. Technol.* 5 (2) (2011) 368–379.

29. C. Toffanin, M. Messori, F. D. Palma, G. D. Nicolao, C. Cobelli, L. Magni, Artificial pancreas: Model predictive control design from clinical experience, *J. Diabetes Sci. Technol.* 7 (6) (2013) 1470–1483.

30. D. Boiroux, A. K. Duun-Henriksen, S. Schmidt, K. Nørgaard, S. Madsbad, N. K. Poulsen, H. Madsen, J. B. Jørgensen, Overnight glucose control in people with type 1 diabetes, *Biomed. Signal Process. Control* 39 (2018) 503–512.

31. A. El Fathi, M. R. Smaoui, V. Gingras, B. Boulet, A. Haidar, The artificial pancreas and meal control: An overview of postprandial glucose regulation in type 1 diabetes, *IEEE Control Syst. Mag.* 38 (1) (2018) 67–85.

32. M. Messori, G. P. Incremona, C. Cobelli, L. Magni, Individualized model predictive control for the artificial pancreas: In silico evaluation of closed-loop glucose control, *IEEE Control Syst. Mag.* 38 (1) (2018) 86–104.

33. I. S. Dasanayake, D. E. Seborg, J. E. Pinsker, F. J. Doyle III, E. Dassau, Empirical dynamic model identification for blood-glucose dynamics in response to physical activity, *In IEEE Conference on Decision & Control*, Osaka, Japan, Vol. 2015, NIH Public Access (2015), pp. 3834–3839.

34. C. Toffanin, S. D. Favero, E. Aiello, M. Messori, C. Cobelli, L. Magni, Glucose-insulin model identified in free-living conditions for hypoglycaemia prevention, *J. Process Control* 64 (2018) 27–36.

35. A. Cinar, K. Turksoy, *Advances in Artificial Pancreas Systems: Adaptive and Multivariable Predictive Control*, Berlin, German: Springer (2018).

36. D. Boiroux, M. Hagdrup, Z. Mahmoudi, N. K. Poulsen, H. Madsen, J. B. Jørgensen, Model identification using continuous glucose monitoring data for type 1 diabetes, *IFAC-PapersOnLine* 49 (7) (2016) 759–764.

37. O. Silvia, V. Josep, C. Remei, A. Joaquim, A review of personalized blood glucose prediction strategies for T1DM patients, *Int. J. Numer. Methods Biomed. Eng.* 33 (6) (2017) e2833. doi: 10.1002/cnm.2833.

38. M. Messori, C. Toffanin, S. Del Favero, G. De Nicolao, C. Cobelli, L. Magni, Model individualization for artificial pancreas, *Comput. Methods Programs Biomed.* doi: 10.1016/j.cmpb.2016.06.006.

39. I. Hajizadeh, M. Rashid, K. Turksoy, S. Samadi, J. Feng, M. Sevil, N. Hobbs, C. Lazaro, Z. Maloney, E. Littlejohn, A. Cinar, Incorporating unannounced meals and exercise in adaptive learning of personalized models for multivariable artificial pancreas systems, *J. Diabetes Sci. Technol.* 12 (5) (2018) 953–966.

40. I. Hajizadeh, M. Rashid, A. Cinar, Ensuring stability and fidelity of recursively identified control-relevant models, *The 18th IFAC Symposium on System Identification (SYSID)*, Stockholm, Sweden (2018), pp. 927–932.

41. I. Hajizadeh, M. Rashid, K. Turksoy, S. Samadi, J. Feng, M. Sevili, N. Frantz, C. Lazaro, Z. Maloney, E. Littlejohn, A. Cinar, Multivariable recursive subspace identification with application to artificial pancreas systems, *IFAC-PapersOnLine* 41 (2017) 909–914.

42. I. Hajizadeh, M. Rashid, A. Cinar, Integrating compartment models with recursive system identification, *In American Control Conference (ACC)*, Milwaukee, WI, (2018), pp. 3583–3588.

43. I. Houtzager, J.-W. van Wingerden, M. Verhaegen, Recursive predictor-based subspace identification with application to the real-time closed-loop tracking of flutter, *IEEE Trans. Control Syst. Technol.* 20 (4) (2012) 934–949.

44. S. Samadi, K. Turksoy, I. Hajizadeh, J. Feng, M. Sevil, A. Cinar, Meal detection and carbohydrate estimation using continuous glucose sensor data, *IEEE J. Biomed. Health Inform.* 21 (3) (2017) 619–627.

45. S. Samadi, M. Rashid, K. Turksoy, J. Feng, I. Hajizadeh, N. Hobbs, C. Lazaro, M. Sevil, E. Littlejohn, A. Cinar, Automatic detection and estimation of unannounced meals for multivariable artificial pancreas system, *Diabetes Technol. Ther.* 20 (3) (2018) 235–246.

46. S. Samadi, M. Rashid, M. Sevil, I. Hajizadeh, N. Hobbs, P. Kolodziej, J. Feng, M. Park, L. Quinn, A. Cinar, Multivariable simulation platform for type 1 diabetes mellitus, *The 18th Annual Diabetes Technology Meeting*, Maryland (2018).

47. M. Sevil, M. Rashid, Z. Maloney, S. Samadi, C. Lazaro, N. Hobbs, I. Hajizadeh, J. Feng, R. Brandt, A. Cinar, Real-time estimation of energy expenditure using noninvasive wearable sensors for multivariable artificial pancreas system, *In 5th IEEE Conference on Biomedical and Health Informatics*, Las Vegas, NV, IEEE (2018).

12 New Developments in Oral Insulin Delivery

Alec Jost and Mmesoma Anike
Wake Forest School of Medicine
Wake Forest Institute for Regenerative Medicine

Emmanuel Opara
Wake Forest School of Medicine
Wake Forest Institute for Regenerative Medicine
Virginia Tech-Wake Forest School of Biomedical Engineering & Sciences

CONTENTS

12.1 INTRODUCTION

12.1.1 DISTINCTION BETWEEN THE TWO MAJOR TYPES OF DIABETES

Diabetes is one of the leading causes of chronic illness in America, and the costs associated with its treatment exceed $245 billion annually in the United States alone (Centers for Disease Control and Prevention 2017). Patients with diabetes are unable to produce adequate amounts of insulin, an important regulator of cellular metabolic pathways involved in glucose uptake and utilization

(Clark et al. 2017). The dysregulation of blood glucose that results from insufficient insulin can cause both micro- and macrovascular pathology, with complications including retinopathy, neuropathy (Vinik et al. 2000), nephropathy, and an increased risk of cardiovascular disease (Arieff 2000).

Speaking broadly, diabetes is divided into two types. While both result in insulin deficiency, their pathogeneses are markedly different. Type 1 diabetes results from autoimmune-mediated damage to pancreatic beta cells, evidenced by the presence of serum antibodies against beta cells, insulin, and/or various associated tyrosine phosphatases. It often affects children or adolescents but can occur at any age. As islets are damaged by autoimmune attack they lose their ability to produce insulin, resulting in hyperglycemia and other metabolic complications. While type 1 diabetes is often characterized by absolute insulin deficiency, this is not always the case, as patients in early stages of disease may still produce some level of endogenous insulin. Regardless, later stages of disease almost inevitably result in massive damage to islets and a complete lack of secreted insulin (Michels and Gottlieb 2000).

Type 2 diabetes, on the other hand, is characterized by insulin deficiency caused by peripheral insulin resistance without evidence of autoimmune-mediated destruction of pancreatic islets. It presents more often in adulthood and appears to have stronger genetic associations than type 1 diabetes. The pathogenesis of type 2 diabetes is less well understood than that of type 1, and multiple independent etiologies likely exist. This aside, type 2 diabetes is generally characterized by a relative (as opposed to absolute) insulin deficiency, in that while pancreatic islets still function and secrete insulin, blood glucose levels remain elevated. The discrepancy between seemingly adequate serum insulin levels and continually elevated blood glucose is explained by insulin resistance, wherein target tissues fail to uptake and process glucose appropriately in response to stimulation by insulin. As the disease and consequent resistance to insulin progresses, pancreatic islets secrete increasing amounts of insulin in response to persistently elevated blood glucose. This compensatory overactivity results in long-term damage to islets. As such, a significant number of patients with late-stage type 2 diabetes require exogenous insulin therapy similarly to those with type 1 diabetes, because the damaged islets lose their ability to function and secrete insulin. Thus, though the underlying etiologies differ, patients with both types 1 and 2 diabetes can become dependent on exogenous insulin to adequately regulate blood glucose levels (Cersosimo et al. 2000).

12.1.2 HISTORICAL PERSPECTIVES IN THE DEVELOPMENT OF ORAL INSULIN

Prior to 1920, and beginning with the seminal work of Mering and Minkowski in 1889 showing that total pancreatectomy induces severe diabetes, a hypothesis had been established that an internal secretion of the pancreas controlled glucose disposal. Subsequently, while doing routine autopsies, the American pathologist Moses Barron had observed in a rare case of the formation of a pancreatic stone (pancreatic lithiasis) that the stone had completely occluded the main pancreatic duct causing all the acinar cells to disappear through atrophy while most of the islet cells survived (Barron 1920). These findings were consistent with other observations made when pancreatic ducts were blocked by ligation, and all together laid the foundation for Frederick Banting's quest for the pancreatic internal secretion later named as "insulin." Also, it is known that, at the first meeting of Banting with J.J.R Macleod, the professor of physiology, in whose lab Banting and Best worked at the University of Toronto, part of their discussion was that many others had tried to prepare an extract of the pancreas which contained the internal secretion and failed. Both agreed that the problem with previous extracts was that they also contained potent digestive components of the external secretion, now known as enzymes, which may have destroyed the internal secretion (Bliss 1982).

One of the many frustrations of Banting and Best as they repeatedly tried to reduce the blood sugar of diabetic dogs, normal dogs, and normal rabbits, included the failed attempt to reduce the blood sugar levels in Joseph Gilchrist, a diabetic subject who was a classmate of Banting. To their chagrin the pancreatic extract that had worked in dogs was without any effect on Gilchrist's blood sugar (Bliss 1982). Of course, they were not aware of the fact at the time that the difference was the route of administration of the extract. While the administration of their extract in the dogs had been done parenterally, the extract was taken orally by Gilchrist. However, the extract was found to work subsequently when injected into the buttocks of another diabetic patient, Leonard Thompson, at the Toronto General Hospital. Thus, interest in oral insulin delivery dates back to the time of the discovery of insulin by the Toronto team.

Another, and perhaps the most difficult challenge that the Toronto team experienced early in the discovery of insulin was the extended period of failures in trying to make insulin after it had been announced to the whole world that they had discovered the magic treatment for insulin-dependent diabetes. It took many weeks and hours of endless tinkering with their extraction methods for the elusive pancreatic extract before the research team realized that the conditions that had proven successful in their small-scale procedure could not be used in large-scale production, as the substance was very sensitive to variations in temperature among other conditions (Bliss 1982). These experiences were compounded by the fact that the researchers had no idea of the biochemical nature of this elusive pancreatic extract. It took many more decades of additional research before the polypeptide nature of insulin was elucidated (Sanger 1959).

12.1.3 Need for Oral Insulin Delivery

Conventional insulin therapy has historically taken the form of a subcutaneous injectable product. While insulin formulations utilizing other therapeutic routes have been studied extensively and demonstrated some therapeutic benefit, none has yet been able to supersede injectable insulin as the standard of care.

Injectable insulin poses both advantages and disadvantages to the diabetic patient. A variety of formulations with vastly different release profiles are clinically available, allowing patients to make both gradual adjustments in blood insulin levels in anticipation of future metabolic changes, and more rapid changes to compensate for unforeseen or acutely concerning changes in blood glucose(Donner 2000). Additionally, injection allows for precise dosing and a consistent pharmacokinetic response, which reduce the chances of inadvertent pharmacologically induced hypoglycemia. On the other hand, injectable insulin therapy also comes with drawbacks. Compliance can be limited by needle fear or aversion, and patient quality of life is negatively impacted by the pain and inconvenience of daily needlesticks (Wagner et al. 2018). Injections come with an inherent risk of skin infection; while this risk is relatively low and can be minimized with good injection practices, the relatively high frequency of dosing associated with insulin therapy compounds this small risk significantly. In addition, long-term use of injected subcutaneous insulin in the management of diabetes has been associated with lipodystrophy, weight gain, edema, and hypoglycemia (Richardson and Kerr 2003).

Oral insulin has the potential to address many of the drawbacks of subcutaneous insulin. Without the need for injection, patient compliance issues related to needle aversion are no longer of concern. In the same vein, negative impacts on the quality of life associated with the pain/discomfort of injection would be eliminated. From a pharmacodynamic perspective, oral insulin is absorbed primarily through portal circulation and therefore creates a portosystemic gradient that closely resembles that generated by endogenous insulin secretion. The importance of this portosystemic gradient in insulin pharmacology is discussed in the next section.

12.1.4 Physiological Advantages of Oral over Parenteral Insulin Administration

Oral insulin may improve the quality of life and therapeutic adherence when compared to injectable preparations due to its more convenient and less traumatic route of administration. In conjunction, oral insulin is posited to offer physiologic advantages over parenteral preparations in two primary ways, namely, through the induction of a portosystemic insulin concentration gradient, and potentially the generation of immune tolerance to insulin.

When insulin is produced by the pancreas it primarily enters portal circulation and thereby passes through the liver before reaching the periphery. Hepatocytes rely on the uptake of insulin to induce appropriate metabolic changes associated with elevated blood glucose, and thus some amount (typically around 50%–60%) of insulin secreted from the pancreas is consumed by the liver before ever reaching peripheral circulation (Donner 2000). Thus, during endogenous secretion, the concentration of insulin in portal circulation is markedly higher than that in systemic circulation. This difference in concentrations is referred to as the portosystemic gradient. In contrast, subcutaneous injected insulin preparations enter peripheral circulation directly and consequently fail to create the portosystemic gradient characteristic of secreted insulin. Because the liver and peripheral tissues respond to insulin in unique ways, differences in regional insulin concentration represented by the portosystemic gradient impact the body's net response to a given dose of insulin. As such, the physiologic responses to injected and endogenously produced insulins are not the same (Madhav 2011). Indeed, it is suspected that many of the long-term complications of well-managed insulin-dependent diabetes may be at least in part due to the lack of an appropriate portosystemic gradient in insulin concentration associated with parenteral insulin administration (Kalra et al. 2010).

Figure 12.1 illustrates two potential routes for gastrointestinal tract (GI) uptake of oral insulin – the portal pathway and the immunolymphatic pathway. In the portal pathway, insulin passes through the liver before entering systemic circulation, generating a portosystemic gradient similar to that of pancreatic insulin. In the immunolymphatic pathway, insulin that enters M cells can then migrate through immune tissues called Peyer's Patches before reaching systemic circulation via the thoracic duct. Nanoparticle size, charge, and composition have all been shown to impact whether particles are absorbed via the portal or immunolymphatic pathway (Lopes et al. 2014). The immunolymphatic pathway is well-suited for many therapeutics (Jani et al. 1992), but may not be an ideal strategy for oral insulin formulations because it could compromise or reduce the creation of the portosystemic insulin gradient, creating a therapeutic profile akin to that of injectable insulins. On the other hand, oral insulin that enters enterocytes via the portal pathway passes through the liver before entering systemic circulation, creating portosystemic gradient similar to that of pancreatic insulin. Because the goal of insulin therapy in diabetes is to act as a surrogate for pathologically absent pancreatic

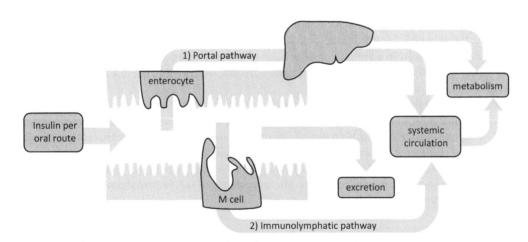

FIGURE 12.1 Illustrates two potential routes of insulin absorption in the GI tract. 1) The portal pathway describes insulin's absorption into enterocytes, portal circulation, and the liver (where some metabolism occurs) before reaching systemic circulation. 2) The immunolymphatic pathway describes insulin's absorption into M cells, Peyer's patches, and lymphatic vessels before directly entering systemic circulation via the thoracic duct. Once in systemic circulation insulin is metabolized by a variety of tissues. Some insulin may also be excreted from the GI tract without being absorbed.

insulin, uptake strategies that utilize the portal pathway and create a portosystemic gradient may prove advantageous.

Some published works support the theory that administration of oral insulin results in its presentation to the enteric immune system, ultimately generating some degree of immunomodulatory tolerance. Because autoantibodies to insulin are often associated with type 1 diabetes, it has been hypothesized that administration of oral insulin may attenuate the unwanted immune response and slow the progression of early type 1 diabetes (Bergerot et al. 1999). While various researches with animal models supported this theory in the early 2000s, the data from human trials presently suggests that such observations are yet to be replicated in human diabetic patients. Thus, while there may be some immunomodulatory benefit to oral insulin preparations, currently published studies do not yet provide any support for this notion (Chaillous et al. 2000).

While oral and injectable insulins may be chemically similar, their different routes of administration significantly impact local and regional drug concentrations within the body. Because various tissues respond to insulin in vastly different ways, differences in concentration between tissues have meaningful impacts on the overall pharmacologic action of the drug. By creating a portosystemic gradient mimicking that associated with pancreatic insulin secretion, oral insulin formulations may better approximate the endogenous physiologic response to insulin than their injectable counterparts.

12.1.5 BIODISTRIBUTION, PHARMACODYNAMICS, AND PHARMACOKINETICS OF INSULIN: ORAL VERSUS SUBCUTANEOUS ADMINISTRATION

Insulin is a double-chain polypeptide synthesized by beta cells in the pancreatic islets that serve primarily to regulate the storage and processing of surplus serum glucose. It is released from storage vesicles within the Golgi along with cleavage product C-peptide under stimulation by elevated serum glucose as well as a variety of other signaling compounds including glucagon-like peptide 1 and acetylcholine (Wilcox 2005). The level of insulin release in response to an intravenous glucose bolus typically occurs in two phases – an initial burst release followed by prolonged basal secretion. Insulin release following oral glucose stimulation is markedly less predictable, in part due to the influence of other signaling molecules which are implicated in gastrointestinal activity (Donner 2000).

Once released from beta cells, insulin potentiates changes in cellular activity via the insulin receptor, an intrinsic tyrosine kinase receptor. Binding and dimerization allow for the phosphorylation of multiple intracellular signaling molecules. In general, the changes associated with insulin receptor activation induce a cellular state favoring energy storage via protein, triglyceride, and glycogen synthesis. However, the specifics of insulin's action vary depending on target tissue. In muscle, insulin induces glycogen synthesis and suppresses protein catabolism, as well as upregulating cell surface glucose transporter-4 (GLUT4) receptors allowing for an increased uptake of extracellular glucose. Muscle plays a primary role in glucose clearance and storage; it is thought to be responsible for 60%–70% of insulin-mediated glucose uptake. In adipose tissue, insulin stimulates lipogenesis and GLUT4 translocation to the membrane, accounting for ~10% of glucose uptake mediated by insulin. In hepatic tissue, glycogen synthesis increases while gluconeogenesis and ketone body production are inhibited by insulin. The liver is responsible for up to 30% of postprandial glucose clearance, highlighting the importance of hepatic insulin delivery in the generation of appropriate glucose handling mechanisms and physiologic energy storage. Insulin also plays roles in the brain, kidneys, and vascular endothelium, and while these roles pertain less directly to serum glucose handling, they still may represent active contributors to the pathogenesis of diabetes (De Meyts 2000).

Insulin is metabolized by the liver and excreted by the kidneys. Peripheral tissues, which rely on insulin, like muscle and adipose tissue, also play some role in insulin degradation. Since pancreatic insulin reaches the liver first, more than half of it is typically degraded by the liver. In the case of subcutaneously administered insulin this ratio reverses owing to an elevated proportion of insulin in systemic instead of portal circulation (Duckworth et al. 1998).

12.2   APPROACHES TO ORAL INSULIN DEVELOPMENT

12.2.1   BARRIERS TO ORAL INSULIN DELIVERY

Oral insulin formulations face two major hurdles – degradation by gastrointestinal enzymes and transport barriers of the GI tract mucoepithelium. The mucous layer of the GI tract varies in composition and function across different regions of the gut, yet in general it serves as a barrier between the caustic and bacterial-laden lumen of the intestines and the surrounding epithelial brush border (Cornick et al. 2015). A variety of large and highly glycosylated proteins called mucins, broadly classified as either gel-forming or transmembrane, contribute to the mucous layer and are produced in region-dependent quantities by glands, goblet epithelial cells, and enterocytes. The constant secretion of mucus generates net movement into the lumen; this "current" drags small molecules such as insulin away from their potential site of uptake at the brush border and flushes them through the remainder of the GI tract. By employing strategies of adherence to and penetration through the gastrointestinal mucous layer, oral insulin formulations may increase their potential for bioavailability and efficacy.

Deep to the mucous layer is the gastrointestinal brush border and the underlying epithelium. Crossing either through (transcellular movement) or around (paracellular movement) these epithelial cells allows entrance into portal circulation, from where insulin can reach various sites of its activity. Transcellular uptake can be achieved via simple diffusion, facilitated diffusion, and carrier-mediated active transport. Simple diffusion relies on compounds passing directly through the nonpolar lipid cell membrane, and consequently the molecules that achieve this sort of uptake are generally small and lipophilic. Because peptides such as insulin are relatively large and typically carry surface charges, their ability to cross the cell membrane via simple diffusion is limited (Gedawy et al. 2018).

Carrier-mediated transport into enterocytes can occur via facilitated diffusion or active transport, but both require interactions between ligand and membrane receptor to achieve uptake. Insulin itself is not known to readily bind to any enterocyte membrane receptors associated with carrier-mediated transport and therefore is not usually absorbed via this mechanism with compelling efficiency through the GI epithelium (Renukuntla et al. 2013). While M cells absorb some amount of insulin through nonspecific phago- and endocytosis, this amount is insufficient for the regulation of blood glucose. As such, insulin exhibits very low levels of gastrointestinal absorption. If, and when transcellular uptake does occur, insulin must next cross the basolateral enterocyte cell membrane to enter into portal circulation. While no particular pathways of basolateral insulin transport have been elucidated it appears in preliminary studies that insulin, which is able to enter enterocytes, does cross this basolateral membrane and enter the bloodstream through one mechanism or another (Ziv and Bendayan 2000).

Paracellular diffusion relies on the movement of molecules through water-filled pores between cells. These pores are constrained primarily by tight junctions, which produce calcium-dependent adherence between neighboring cells. Because the interjunctional pores that facilitate paracellular transport are aqueous spaces, hydrophilic compounds including peptides are generally suited to this form of transport. However, pore size usually limits diffusivity to peptides smaller than approximately 700 Daltons, which is only a fragment of the size of insulin (Antosova et al. 2009).

One of the primary activities of the GI tract is to facilitate the degradation and metabolism of various macromolecules. Because proteins are absorbed as single amino acids and dipeptides, they are readily broken down by various enzymes secreted from the pancreas and glandular epithelium. Insulin acts as a substrate for many of these enzymes including trypsin, alpha chymotrypsin, and various carboxypeptidases (Gedawy et al. 2018). Recent studies have also demonstrated the presence of a specific insulin degrading enzyme (termed IDE) on the enterocyte brush border (Durham et al. 2015). In concert, these enzymes severely limit the amount of intact insulin present in the GI tract, thus reducing opportunities for oral delivery and consequent pharmacologic action.

The pH of the human GI tract ranges from strongly acidic (pH = 1–3 depending upon feeding state) to slightly alkaline (pH > 7) owing to the regional secretions of the stomach, gallbladder, pancreas, and intestinal glandular epithelium. These local environments themselves as well as the dramatic variations between them have the capacity to cause oxidation and deamination of peptides such as insulin (Cikrikci et al. 2018). Gastrointestinal pH also facilitates the enzymatic degradation of insulin because many of the previously discussed proteases are active only within a certain range of acidity or (more often) alkalinity. Thus, protecting insulin from local gastrointestinal pH has the potential to protect it from degradation both directly and indirectly.

12.2.2 STRATEGIES TO OVERCOME INSULIN TRANSPORT BARRIERS OF THE GI

For each of the previously described barriers to oral insulin delivery, researchers have developed preventative/circumventive strategies. Given that many barriers coexist in the GI tract, it is likely that multiple counterstrategies employed in combination may be advantageous in improving peroral insulin uptake and action (Zhu et al. 2016).

Without passing through the mucus barrier, insulin is unable to even reach the enterocyte brush border, much less pass through it. The addition of compounds which either enhance adhesion to the mucus layer or permeation through it has been employed in attempts to promote insulin transport across this barrier. Mucoadhesion can occur via a variety of mechanisms (many of which have not been well elucidated) but often relies on noncovalent bonding between a hydrophilic macromolecule and the secreted mucus layer. Current candidate macromolecules that are thought to function via this mechanism include alginate, chitosan, and polyacrylic acid, among others (Smart 2005). A second class of mucoadhesive molecules exploits covalent interactions and consequently exhibits higher levels of adhesion relative to the previously mentioned hydrophilic macromolecules. Among the molecules capable of forming covalent linkage with the mucus layer, the most researched are polylactic co-glycolic acid (PLGA) and thiomers (Gedawy et al. 2018). These biomolecules have been used in conjunction with first-generation mucoadhesive agents like alginate and chitosan to generate modified compounds that demonstrate increased residence time in the GI tract relative to unmodified controls due to increased mucoadhesion (Bernkop-Schnürch 2005). By increasing adherence to the GI mucosa and consequent transit time through the GI tract, mucoadhesive biomaterials are potentially advantageous additions to oral insulin formulations.

Along with enhanced adhesion, compounds that aim to increase penetration through the mucus barrier have also been developed. Some viruses are known to pass through mucus barriers at remarkably high velocities, a characteristic which they owe to their high concentrations of both positive and negative surface charges. Nanoparticles that mimic this characteristic have been created using positively charged chitosan and negatively charged chondroitin sulfate polymers (Pereira de Sousa et al. 2016). Another strategy for increasing mucus penetration involves generating microcapsules with a hydrophilic surface shell. The lipid content of mucus makes it relatively hydrophobic, and because microcapsules with a hydrophilic exterior do not interact as readily with surrounding mucus they are able to pass through it more readily. This is often accomplished using PEGylation (Ensign et al. 2012; Huckaby and Lai 2018). These strategies have been combined with some success to decrease the transit time of capsules intended for drug delivery through the mucus barrier. Table 12.1 includes biomaterials that have been studied with the intent of increasing mucoadhesion and/or mucopenetrance of oral insulin formulations.

If biomaterial constructs successfully pass through the mucus layer, the next transport barrier they face is the enterocyte membrane. This lipid bilayer can be either crossed by transcellular transport or circumvented by paracellular transport. Paracellular transport can be accomplished using the recently discovered zonula occludens toxin (Zot), isolated from various subspecies of the invasive enteric bacteria *Campylobacter*. The toxin disrupts tight junctions, allowing hydrophilic molecules such as insulin to pass between enterocytes into the interstitial space. In contrast, intercellular

TABLE 12.1

Compounds Used to Improve Drug Delivery via Mucoadhesion/Penetrance in Oral Insulin Formulations

Intended Role	Compound	Known Compatible Biomaterials	Specific Characteristics	References
Mucoadhesion	Alginate	Chitosan, PMAA	Hydrophilic, polyanionic, exhibits pH-dependent swelling	Sajeesh and Sharma (2004)
	Chitosan	Alginate, PMAA, PLGA, PLA	Hydrophilic, polycationic, exhibits pH-dependent swelling	Ma (2014) and Sajeesh and Sharma, (2011)
	Polyacrylic acid	Chitosan	Exhibits pH-dependent hydrogen bonding to mucosa	Ma (2014) and Ramdas et al. (1999)
	PLGA	Eudragrit, polyvinyl alcohol	pH-dependent hydrogen bonding to mucosa	Naha et al. (2008) and Sun et al. (2015)
	Thiomers	Alginate, chitosan, polyacrylic acid	Thiolation of biomaterial promotes thiol-cysteine bonding with mucus glycoproteins	Bernkop-Schnürch (2005)
Mucopenetrance	PEGylation	Chondroitin sulfate, Chitosan, PLGA	High surface charge variability	Casettari et al. (2010), Hinds and Kim (2002), and Pereira de Sousa et al. (2016)

transit can occur via receptor-mediated transport, endocytosis, or membrane disruption (Salama et al. 2006). Molecules that achieve transcellular transport are often peptides, including various immunoglobulins, cobalamin, penetratin, Tat, and oligopeptides of arginine and lysine among others (Rehmani and Dixon 2018). The specific mechanisms by which many of these cell penetrating agents function are still being elucidated. Cell penetrating agents can be conjugated directly to insulin, associated with it through noncovalent interactions, or added to a biomaterial carrier construct. It should be noted that cell penetrating agents which induce endocytosis must possess a mechanism to escape the endocytotic vesicle once they enter the cell, otherwise the insulin within will remain trapped and inactive. While most cell penetrating agents are peptides, some other molecules like ZnO are able to either interact with cell surface receptors or induce membrane disruption, and thus may be potentially useful in facilitating oral insulin delivery (Huang et al. 2017). Table 12.2 includes cell penetrating agents used in experimental studies on oral insulin formulations.

12.2.2.1 Paracellular Transport

The GI tract maintains a delicate biochemical balance to promote digestion without causing injury to the bowel. Under physiologic conditions, enzymes, specifically proteases, have potential activity against components of living tissue but the body uses counterenzymes and inhibitory factors to prevent unintentional damage. By isolating these counterregulatory compounds from plants and other animals and delivering them in conjunction with orally dosed peptide drugs, researches are able to reduce the rate of peptide degradation and improve oral administration of therapeutic peptides. Enzymes which are known to degrade insulin include trypsin, chymotrypsin, and insulin-degrading enzyme (Durham et al. 2015; Duckworth et al. 1998). Trypsin inhibitors are present in a number of biological mediums including human serum (alpha1-antitrypsin), bovine pancreas (aprotinin), and soybeans (Bowman-Birk trypsin inhibitor, Kunitz soybean trypsin inhibitor, etc.). In the pursuit of an oral administration of insulin, protease inhibitors specific to enzymes involved in insulin degradation are either conjugated directly to insulin or included in a biomaterial construct, potentially increasing the lifetime and consequent probability of absorption of insulin in the GI tract. Protease inhibitors commonly used for oral peptide delivery are included in Table 12.3.

TABLE 12.2

Compounds Used to Improve Drug Delivery via Cell Penetration in Oral Insulin Formulations

Intended Role	Compound	Known Compatible Biomaterials	Specific Characteristics	References
Transcytosis	Oligopeptides (lysine/arginine)	Conjugated directly to peptide, polyester amide, alginate, PLGA	Direct translocation (membrane disruption) and endocytosis	He et al. (2013), Mohy Eldin et al. (2015), Takeuchi and Futaki (2016), and Zhu et al. (2016)
	Penetratin	Chitosan, PLGA	Direct transport via membrane disruption	Almeida et al. (2016), Barbari et al. (2018), and Zhu et al. (2016)
	Cobalamin	Conjugated directly to peptide	Receptor-mediated endocytosis	Date et al. (2016)
	Tat	PLGA, chitosan	Arginine-rich, direct translocation, and/or endocytosis	Salatin and Yari Khosroushahi (2017) and Zhu et al. (2016)
	Immunoglobulin A	Chitosan	Receptor-mediated endocytosis	Sharma et al. (2013)
	Zinc oxide nanoparticles	Alginate, carboxymethyl cellulose	Direct transport via disruption of the cell membrane	Huang et al. (2017), Raguvaran et al. (2017), and Zare-Akbari et al. (2016)
Paracellular diffusion	Zot	Chitosan	Disrupts tight junctions	Lee et al. (2016)
	Chitosan	See above	Disrupts tight junctions	Škalko-Basnet (2014)

TABLE 12.3

Compounds Used to Improve Drug Delivery via Biochemical Protection in Oral Insulin Formulations

Intended Role	Compound	Known Compatible Biomaterials	Specific Characteristics	References
pH-sensitive behavior	Alginate	See above	pH-dependent shrinkage (positive correlation between particle diameter and pH)	Cikrikci et al. (2018)
	Chitosan	See above	Insoluble at neutral pH, soluble at acidic pH	Kondiah et al. (2017) and Zhu and Chen (2015)
	Zinc oxide nanoparticles	Alginate, carboxymethyl cellulose	Stable at physiologic pH, dissolve at pH < 5.5	Huang et al. (2017), Raguvaran et al. (2017), and Zare-Akbari et al. (2016)
Protease inhibition	Kunitz soybean trypsin inhibitor	Chitosan	Inhibits peptide degrading enzyme trypsin	Pechenkin et al. (2013)
	Bowman-Birk inhibitor	Chitosan	Inhibits trypsin and chymotrypsin	Marschütz and Bernkop-Schnürch (2000) and Pechenkin et al. (2013)
	Aprotinin	Chitosan, PLGA	Inhibits trypsin and other proteolytic enzymes	Morishita et al. (2006) and Pechenkin et al. (2013)

Both gastric and intestinal pH have the potential to damage the insulin peptide, as discussed previously. For oral drug delivery, this is typically prevented by use of a biomaterial construct that surrounds the target peptide and generates a protective local environment against gastrointestinal acidity or alkalinity. A wide variety of biomaterials are suited to this application, including alginate, chitosan, PLGA, and dextran. Alginate shrinks at low pH and expands with increased alkalinity, allowing it to exist as small, dense particles in the acidic stomach before expanding to promote cargo release in the alkaline small intestine (Zhu and Chen 2015). Biomaterials sensitive to pH used in experimental studies on oral insulin formulations are shown in Table 12.3.

Microfold (M) cells are specialized epithelial cells that overlie immune follicles in the gut, as mentioned earlier. They are responsible for the uptake of antigenic material from the lumen and presentation to follicular T cells (Williams and Owen 2015). Thus, M cells are constantly phagocytosing extracytosolic peptide fragments from the luminal side of the brush border. Researchers have exploited this characteristic for peptide drug delivery; since M cells phagocytose peptide fragments indiscriminately, pharmacologic proteins in the GI tract are taken up along with antigenic material. Interestingly, M cells are part of the lymphatic tissue and thus they drain into systemic circulation via the thoracic duct (Khan et al. 2013). As such, insulin taken up by M cells does not contribute to the portosystemic gradient but instead generates a uniform systemic concentration in the serum similar to that of injected subcutaneous insulin.

12.2.3 ROLE OF LIPOSOMES

Liposomes are manufactured vesicles bounded by a lipid bilayer. Like a cell membrane, this lipid bilayer sequesters the intervesicular space from the surrounding environment. Because of this protective effect liposomal systems have been developed for pharmacologic delivery of relatively fragile agents including peptides. Along with being inherently protective, liposomes can be modified with cell surface receptors and other compounds to generate tropic behavior and other unique characteristics (Niu et al. 2012). For instance, the addition of bile acids to liposomal phospholipids generates "bilosomes," which have been shown in preliminary research to offer greater resistance to degradation by bile in the gastrointestinal environment as well as an increased capacity to cross the enterocyte membrane (Wong et al. 2018). Bile salts integrated into the liposomal membrane appear to disrupt the enterocyte membrane at the brush border, allowing the liposome to become continuous with the cell membrane and deposit its contents intercellularly (Pavlović et al. 2018).

12.2.4 ROLE OF BIOMATERIALS AND NANOTECHNOLOGY-BASED DELIVERY

Before discussing the role of biomaterials and nanotechnologies in oral insulin delivery, both terms require definition. A biomaterial is any engineered substance that generates therapeutic or diagnostic effect on living tissues for medical purposes (Williams 2008). In the context of orally available insulin, biomaterials are often employed as carrier compounds in one form or another. Nanotechnologies are defined most fundamentally as engineered structures that exist on the scale of nanometers (Williams 2008). In the context of this chapter, nanotechnologies, like biomaterials, are mostly carriers for insulin delivery but may also comprise nanoparticles of insulin themselves. In general, biomaterials are defined by composition and application, whereas nanomaterials are defined by scale. Significant overlap exists between these two terms.

Our aim is to focus on biomaterials that have played interesting or important roles in the development of oral insulin formulations. Commonly employed biomaterials include alginate, chitosan, silica, resistant starches, hyaluronic acid, and PLGA, among others. Materials used in experimental studies involving oral insulin formulations are listed in Table 12.4. While specific agents differ, a general motif exists. Liquid polymers are formed into units of varying size and shape, and cured to become micro/nanoparticles constructs that carry peptide cargos, such as insulin. Methods of particle production vary between biomaterials, and many biomaterials can be processed in a variety

TABLE 12.4

Biomaterial Carriers Used in Oral Insulin Delivery

Biomaterial	Synthesis Method	Insulin Incorporation Method	Characteristics	References
Alginate	Ionotropic gelation	Added to biomaterial before construct formation	400–600 μm microspheres	Greimel et al. (2007)
	Emulsification/ internal gelation	Added to biomaterial before construct formation	4–135 μm microspheres	Reis et al. (2007) and Silva et al. (2006)
	Coacervation	Diffusion loading	260–680 μm microspheres	Builders et al. (2008)
	Piezoelectric ejection	Added to biomaterial before construct formation	1–20 μm particles	Kim et al. (2005)
	Extrusion/cold gelation	Diffusion loading	1.583 mm spherical particles	Déat-Lainé et al. (2013)
	Impinging aerosols, ionotropic gelation	Added to biomaterial before construct formation	32.9 μm particles	Martins et al. (2007)
	Membrane emulsification	Added to biomaterial before construct formation	7.5–16.7 μm particles	Zhang et al. (2015)
Chitosan	Free radical polymerization	Diffusion loading	1.2–4.7 μm particles	Kondiah et al. (2017)
	Ionotropic gelation	Diffusion loading	315 nm–1.09 μm particles	Rekha and Sharma (2009)
	Layer-by-layer electrostatic adhesion	Added to biomaterial before construct formation	3–12 μm particles	Balabushevich et al. (2011) and Pechenkin et al. (2013)
	Emulsion crosslinking	Added to biomaterial before construct formation	~30 μm particles	Jose et al. (2012 and 2013) and Ubaidulla et al. (2007b)
	Emulsion phase separation	Diffusion loading	~60 μm particles	Ubaidulla et al. (2007a)
Polymethacrylic acid	UV-initiated free radical solution polymerization	Diffusion loading	30–200 μm particles	Morishita et al. (2006)
	Free radical polymerization	Diffusion loading	1–100 μm particles	Mundargi et al. (2011)
	Ionic gelation	Diffusion loading		Sajeesh and Sharma (2011)
	Gamma radiation induced copolymerization	Diffusion loading	Porous 3D microstructure	Abou Taleb (2013)
Eudragit (PMMA-based proprietary enteric coating)	Oil in oil emulsion coacervation	Diffusion loading	10–50 μm particles	Kenechukwu and Momoh (2016) and Momoh et al. (2015)
	Water in oil emulsion solvent evaporation	Diffusion loading/added to biomaterial before construct formation	1–200 μm particles	Agrawal et al. (2017) and Marais et al. (2013)
Resistant starch	Extrusion spheronization	Added to biomaterial before construct formation	500 μm particles	Situ et al. (2014 and 2015)

(Continued)

TABLE 12.4 (*Continued*)
Biomaterial Carriers Used in Oral Insulin Delivery

Biomaterial	Synthesis Method	Insulin Incorporation Method	Characteristics	References
PLGA	Emulsion solvent diffusion	Diffusion loading	1–5 μm microspheres	Sun et al. (2015)
	Flow focusing	Diffusion loading	1.23 μm particles	Holgado et al. (2009)
	Direct membrane emulsion	Added to biomaterial before construct formation	Submicron-100 μm particles	Ma et al. (2000)
Silica	Sol–gel process	Added to biomaterial before construct formation	2.5–35 μm microspheres	Vanea et al. (2014)
Polyacrylic acid	Direct membrane emulsion	Added to biomaterial before construct formation	Submicron-100 μm particles	Ma et al. (2000)

of ways (Ma 2014). These methods are listed under their respective biomaterial in Table 12.4. Some constructs are loaded with insulin via diffusion loading, which involves storage of carrier particles in an insulin containing solution. In other instances, the insulin is mixed into the liquid polymer before processing. Biomaterials protect their cargo from premature degradation and can be modified with other effector compounds without necessitating conjugation directly to the drug itself. This is advantageous because conjugation directly to the drug entails chemical modification that can alter the drug's ability to bind to its receptors and produce consequent pharmacologic action (Zhang et al. 2009). Thus, biomaterial carriers are useful in oral insulin formulations because they not only surround and protect insulin but also provide a medium to which other advantageous compounds can be added without directly altering insulin's activity.

The fundamental advantage of nanomaterials is that they exist on a scale that facilitates direct interaction with living cells. Advances in manufacturing have allowed for the generation of remarkably small constructs with considerable consistency and specificity. Nanomaterials can be classified based on their structure; in oral drug delivery the most common iterations are nanocapsules, nanospheres, nanotubes and other nanofibers, and dendrimers (Ahlawat et al. 2018). Liposomes of adequately small size are also considered nanomaterials. Because of their size and structure, nanomaterials can often be pharmacologically loaded with high efficiency, modified for targeted delivery, and designed to facilitate uptake and consequent pharmacologic action. While many nanomaterials are biopolymer based, other compounds have also proven useful, e.g., zinc oxide. Some nanoparticles are even made entirely from pharmacologic agents (Zeng et al. 2018). Many of the bioparticles listed in Table 12.4 can be classified as nanomaterials based on their approximate size.

12.2.5 INNOVATIONS IN ORAL INSULIN FORMULATION

As discussed earlier, meaningful oral delivery of insulin has been hampered by the susceptibility of the peptide to enzymatic degradation and its poor permeability across the mucus and cellular membranes in the gastrointestinal tract. Cell-penetrating peptides have since emerged as permeability enhancers for hydrophilic macromolecules such as insulin and have included use with electrostatic or covalent conjugation with nanotechnology. One approach has been to exploit endogenous cellular uptake mechanisms by engineering peptide conjugates that transcytose – entering cells by endocytosis and leaving by exocytosis (Valainis et al. 1986). The caveat here is to get the hydrophilic therapeutic peptides to cross the digestive tract barrier with no adverse effect on gastrointestinal function. Thus, one group has developed low molecular weight protamine (LMWP) as a nontoxic but potent cell penetrating peptide, which with covalent linkage was capable of translocating protein cargos through the membranes of most cell types. The investigators subsequently developed an innovative strategy to formulate 1:1 monomeric insulin/LMWP conjugate by using succinimidyl-[(N-maleimidopropionamido)-polyethyleneglycol] ester (NHS-PEG-MAL) as an intermediate crosslinker during the coupling process. Cell culture studies demonstrated that transport of the insulin-PEG-LMWP conjugate across the intestinal mucosal layer was enhanced by about fivefold when compared with native insulin (Zhang et al. 2013). It remains to be determined if the biological activity of insulin would be affected by the conjugation to LMWP.

In a related development, a different research team has reported an oral insulin delivery system composed of mucoadhesive nanoparticles loaded with insulin conjugated to LMWP. The mucoadhesive N-trimethyl chitosan chloride-coated PLGA nanoparticles were loaded with the LMWP-insulin conjugates, which enhanced retention in the intestinal mucus layer. It was observed that insulin conjugates released from the mucoadhesive nanoparticles were protected from enzymatic degradation because of the proximity to the epithelial layer and their enhanced permeation through that layer. The investigators also found that this oral delivery system had significantly rapid and sustained blood glucose reduction effects in diabetic rats. However, the observed therapeutic effect of the oral delivery system for insulin was <20% of that achieved with subcutaneously delivered native insulin (Ru et al. 2016).

Another group has designed protamine nanocapsules as carriers for oral peptide delivery. The polymer shell of the nanocapsules was made of a single layer of protamine, a polycationic peptide, or a double protamine/polysialic (PSA) layer. Insulin glulisine-loaded protamine and protamine/PSA nanocapsules measuring 200–400 nm in size with a neutral surface charge were tested for colloidal stability in simulated intestinal media containing enzymes, and the results indicated that protamine nanocapsules were stable and capable of protecting insulin from degradation and that this protamine-mediated protection was further enhanced by the double protamine/PSA layer. When the insulin-loaded protamine nanocapsules were administered to diabetic rats via the intestinal route the treatment resulted in a sustained reduction of blood glucose level that was ~40% lower than was observed with subcutaneous insulin administration (Thwala et al. 2018).

It has been reported that poly(methacrylic acid-g-ethylene glycol) [P(MAA-g-EG)] hydrogels, which have a high insulin-loading efficiency, enzyme-inhibiting properties, and mucoadhesive properties rapidly release insulin in the intestine owing to their pH-dependent gelling. Thus, an oral insulin formulation based on a strategy of combined use of P(MAA-g-EG) hydrogels with hexa-arginine (R6) has been recently examined for improved intestinal absorption of insulin. The loading efficiency of insulin into crosslinked P(MAA-g-EG) hydrogels was ~96% while that of R6 was about 46%. In addition, an immediate release of the loaded insulin and R6 from these hydrogels was observed at pH 7.4 with 80% released in ~30 min. After coadministration of the insulin-loaded particles (ILP) and R6-loaded particles (ALP) into closed rat ileal segments ~18% reduction in blood glucose levels accompanied by improved insulin absorption was observed compared with ILP administration alone (Fukuoka et al. 2018).

An earlier review article by Carino et al. includes a previous study, which showed improved bioavailability of oral insulin by the synergistic effect of a combination of the permeation enhancer (sodium cholate) and protease inhibitor (aprotinin). A recent study has also described the development of an oral insulin formulation using choline and generate (CAGE) ionic liquid. The CAGE medium significantly enhanced paracellular transport of insulin, while protecting it from enzymatic degradation and by interacting with the mucus layer resulting in its thinning. When administered *in vivo*, an insulin-CAGE formula demonstrated exceptional pharmacokinetic and pharmacodynamic outcomes after jejunal administration in rats. Insulin doses in the range of 3–10 U/kg resulted in significant decreases in blood glucose levels, which were sustained for periods up to 12 h, in contrast to subcutaneous injection of insulin (Banerjee et al. 2018).

It is clear from the referenced studies that significant progress has recently been made in the development of oral insulin formulations that protect insulin from enzymatic degradation while promoting its transport across the intestinal barriers. These properties have been effectively demonstrated in *in vitro* studies and *in vivo* rodent models. What is desperately needed at the present time is assessment of the effectiveness of these different formulations in large animal and human studies. An approach that could enhance the potential development of an effective oral insulin formula may utilize the technology of engineered polymeric biomaterials that are sensitive to neutral-basic pH conditions under which insulin delivery vehicles would degrade to release their payload in the small intestine where absorption of orally delivered substances takes place. Such delivery vehicles would invariably improve the bioavailability of therapeutic agents including peptides such as insulin for improved efficacy. In particular, variations in the degrees of modifications of natural biopolymers such as alginate could provide new opportunities in the development of oral insulin formulations with potential for controlled release of payloads (Banks et al. 2019). In preliminary studies in our lab, we have found that 4-(2-aminoethyl)benzoic acid-modification of alginate enhances the loading efficiency of insulin in hydrogel microbeads made with the modified alginate by as much as 30% compared to the hydrogel made with unmodified alginate.

12.3 METHODS OF ASSESSMENT OF ORAL INSULIN FORMULA

Studies to assess oral insulin formulations generally fall into four major categories – pharmacokinetics, *in vitro* simulation, *in vivo*, and clinical trials. Pharmacokinetic studies examine the ability of carrier compounds to absorb and/or release insulin. *In vitro* studies examine the performance of carriers and modifying compounds in the context of cell cultures. *In vivo* studies apply oral insulin formulations to animal models, using blood insulin concentration or induced hypoglycemia as metrics of pharmacologic action. Lastly, clinical trials examine oral insulin formulations in the context of human subjects. Studies within each of these categories are summarized in Table 12.5.

TABLE 12.5
Studies on Oral Insulin Formulations

Class of Study	Model	Experimental variable	Effect measurement	Reference
In vitro	Caco2 epithelial cell coculture	Insulin-loaded PLGA nanoparticle	Nanoparticle labeling and flow cytometry	Czuba et al. (2018)
	Caco2 epithelial cell coculture	LMW protamine-insulin hybrid	Fluorescein isothiocyanate (FITC)-labeled insulin microscopy and fluorescence spectrophotometry	He et al. (2013)
In vivo	Diabetic rat	Insulin-loaded lipsomes	Blood glucose level	Niu et al. (2012)
		PLGA nanoparticle, chitosan chloride coating, LMW protamine conjugation	Blood glucose level	Sheng et al. (2016)
		Chitosan/poly(gamma glutamic acid) nanoparticles	Blood glucose level	Sonaje et al. (2010)
		Insulin-loaded CPP-g-chitosan microcapsules	Blood glucose level	Barbari et al. (2018)
		Insulin-loaded PLGA nanoparticle	Blood glucose level	Czuba et al. (2018)
	Nondiabetic rat	Choline and gerenate ionic liquid	Blood glucose level	Banerjee et al. (2018)
	Ileal Loop	PMAA nanoparticle with R8 cell penetrating peptide	Blood glucose level	Fukuoka et al. (2018)
		LMW protamine-insulin hybrid	Blood glucose level	He et al. (2013)

12.3.1 Phamacokinetics

Pharmacokinetic studies typically demonstrate drug loading by incubating empty biomaterial carriers designed for oral drug delivery in solutions containing insulin. By measuring the decrease in solution of insulin concentration over time, researchers are able to estimate the quantity of insulin absorbed into the construct. Likewise, by incubating insulin containing formulations in physiologic solutions that resemble environments within the GI tract and measuring the solution for insulin concentration over time, researches can examine the simulated release profile of the carrier. These studies offer rapidly accessible data regarding the capacity of carrier compounds to absorb and release insulin. However, they are limited by inherent differences between the simulated and physiologic gastrointestinal environment. In addition, these studies do not examine insulin uptake into circulation, only its release into the interstitial fluid.

12.3.2 In Vitro Studies

In vitro studies have been used to expose cultured enterocytes to oral insulin formulations to examine insulin's ability to cross the intestinal enterocyte membrane. Use of fluorescently labeled insulin allows for detection within enterocytes with fluorescence microscopy. Typically, cultured cells are exposed to labeled insulin for some intervals of time, after which insulin concentration in the media and within cells is measured. These studies offer insight into the performance of compounds, which aid in transcellular transport, but are limited by differences between enterocyte cell cultures and the physiologic gastrointestinal epithelium. In response to this disparity, some studies use cocultures to better simulate the intestinal environment. This paradigm of *in vitro* study also fails to account for the degradation of not only insulin itself but also the accompanying cell penetrating agents that may occur in regional environments that precede the intestine, such as the stomach.

12.3.3 In Vivo Studies

In vivo studies use animal models to examine the effects of oral insulin preparations on serum insulin concentrations and blood glucose levels. Many studies involve oral administration of the insulin formulation, while others use an ileal loop model wherein insulin is administered directly into the ileum while the animal subject is under anesthesia. Subsequent blood sampling allows for quantification of serum insulin and blood glucose levels. Studies using the ileal loop model have limitations similar to *in vitro* studies in that the influence of the preintestinal regions of the oral route on the processing of the formulation has been basically ignored. In addition to circumvention of the gastric environment, ileal infusion bypasses the duodenal loop and other regions of proximal small intestine by delivering therapeutics directly into the ileum. Studies that involve buccal administration of insulin formulations are not subject to these limitations. Interestingly, the human GI tract is significantly different from various animal GI tracts, and thus animal studies of oral therapeutic delivery are often limited in their generalizability (Hunter et al. 2012). With that said, animal models still represent a necessary step in characterizing the safety and effectiveness of experimental oral insulin formulations. It should be noted that serum concentrations of insulin may not be an ideal measure for comparing peroral to injectable subcutaneous insulin activity; because serum concentrations are measured in the systemic circulation, they fail to account for the portosystemic gradient generated by oral insulin formulations. Thus, serum insulin measurements may underestimate the pharmacologic action of oral preparations relative to their injectable counterparts. Portal venous serum insulin concentration or simply blood glucose reduction may be more suitable measures of therapeutic action.

12.3.4 CLINICAL TRIALS

Clinical trials represent the final stage of research for oral insulin formulations. Once formulations are shown to be safe and effective in animal models, they may be studied using human subjects. There is a scarcity of published clinical trials of oral insulin formulations to date. These trials offer superior evidence relative to other study designs because they take into consideration the preintestinal environment, and involve a truly physiologic human GI tract. They do however pose inherent risks of harm to human patients, and thus experimental therapies should be well characterized in preclinical large animal studies prior to human testing. Relevant studies can involve healthy human subjects or those with underlying pathology. However, because type 2 diabetes involves insulin resistance as well as beta cell dysfunction, results gathered in the context of healthy subjects may not be generalizable to patients with type 2 diabetes.

12.4 SUMMARY AND CONCLUSION

There is significant interest in the development of an effective oral insulin formulation. This interest is largely driven by the necessity for ease of administration and the physiological advantages of the oral route of insulin delivery over parenteral administration. In this chapter, we have discussed the current stage of oral insulin formula development. This discussion has highlighted the barriers to effective oral insulin formulation and the different strategies designed to overcome the barriers. The two major physiological barriers to oral insulin formulation are enzymatic degradation of the polypeptide insulin and its transport limitations across the gastrointestinal membrane and mucus layers. An effective oral insulin formulation would have to include components that address these two barriers. New areas of intense research have included the use of novel and engineered biomaterials as delivery vehicles for insulin and other substance, which are components of a viable oral insulin formula. Adequate characterization of delivery vehicle materials is critical prior to use in oral insulin formulation. Some of the key parameters necessary in the assessment of these materials are their loading efficiency for insulin and the other components in the formula, their release kinetics, and their physical properties including transport characteristics.

Important advances have been made in designing promising strategies to overcome the two major physiological barriers in the gastrointestinal tract. Effective approaches include use of protective polymeric hydrogels and nanoparticles to package insulin, the coupling of insulin to polymeric materials and copackaging of insulin with protease-resistant materials among others. However, considerable challenges remain in the development of a clinically viable formula. Among the critical barriers in the path of development of an effective oral insulin formulation is the absence of a validated and easily available animal model for preclinical testing of insulin formulations prior to clinical trials. The testing of insulin formulations in human subjects has the inherent risk of severe and debilitating hypoglycemia, which demands extreme care in the design of clinical testing protocols. This in itself constitutes another barrier to oral insulin formulation.

Still oral insulin formulation is not beyond reach. As we learn more of the inherent limitations involved, new strategies will be developed to address them, and one can certainly hope that successful oral delivery of insulin will someday become a clinical reality that will have a huge impact in the management of patients afflicted by diabetes.

ACKNOWLEDGEMENT

The authors would like to thank Dr Marks Welker and Dr Surya Bank for their collaboration that has generated novel materials for our laboratory to engage in research on this exciting subject. In addition we would like to thank Dr Kevin Enck for technical guidance of our research in this area.

REFERENCES

Abou Taleb, M. F. Radiation synthesis of multifunctional polymeric hydrogels for oral delivery of insulin. *International Journal of Biological Macromolecules*, vol. 62, 2013, pp. 341–47. doi: 10.1016/j.ijbiomac.2013.09.004.

Agrawal, G. R., et al. Formulation, physicochemical characterization and in vitro evaluation of human insulin-loaded microspheres as potential oral carrier. *Progress in Biomaterials*, vol. 6, no. 3, 2017, pp. 125–36. doi: 10.1007/s40204-017-0072-z.

Ahlawat, J., et al. Enhancing the delivery of chemotherapeutics: Role of biodegradable polymeric nanoparticles. *Molecules : A Journal of Synthetic Chemistry and Natural Product Chemistry*, vol. 23, no. 9, 2018. doi: 10.3390/molecules23092157.

Almeida, C., et al. Membrane re-arrangements and rippled phase stabilisation by the cell penetrating peptide penetratin. *Biochimica et Biophysica Acta (BBA): Biomembranes*, vol. 1858, no. 11, 2016, pp. 2584–91. doi: 10.1016/j.bbamem.2016.07.012.

Antosova, Z., et al. Therapeutic application of peptides and proteins: Parenteral forever? *Trends in Biotechnology*, vol. 27, no. 11, 2009, pp. 628–35. doi: 10.1016/j.tibtech.2009.07.009.

Arieff, A. I. Diabetic nephropathy and treatment of hypertension. In: *Endotext*, edited by Kenneth R. F. et al., MDText.com, Inc., 2000. www.ncbi.nlm.nih.gov/books/NBK279103/.

Balabushevich, N. G., et al. Mucoadhesive polyelectrolyte microparticles containing recombinant human insulin and its analogs aspart and lispro. *Biochemistry (Moscow)*, vol. 76, no. 3, 2011, pp. 327–31. doi: 10.1134/S0006297911030059.

Banerjee, A., et al. Ionic liquids for oral insulin delivery. *Proceedings of the National Academy of Sciences of the United States of America*, vol. 115, no. 28, 2018, pp. 7296–301. doi: 10.1073/pnas.1722338115.

Banks, S. R, et al. Chemical modification of alginate for controlled oral drug delivery. Journal of Agricultural and Food Chemistry, 2019. doi: 10.1021/acs.jafc.9b01911.

Barbari, G. R., et al. Synthesis and characterization of a novel peptide-grafted Cs and evaluation of its nanoparticles for the oral delivery of insulin, in vitro, and in vivo study. *International Journal of Nanomedicine*, vol. 13, 2018, pp. 5127–38. doi: 10.2147/IJN.S161240.

Barron, M. The relation of the islets of langerhanns to diabetes with special reference to cases of pancreatic lithiasis. *Surgery, Gynecology and Obstetrics*, vol. 31, 1920, pp. 437–48.

Bergerot, I., et al. Insulin B-chain reactive CD4+ regulatory T-cells induced by oral insulin treatment protect from type 1 diabetes by blocking the cytokine secretion and pancreatic infiltration of diabetogenic effector T-cells. *Diabetes*, vol. 48, no. 9, 1999, pp. 1720–29. doi: 10.2337/diabetes.48.9.1720.

Bernkop-Schnürch, A. Thiomers: A new generation of mucoadhesive polymers. *Advanced Drug Delivery Reviews*, vol. 57, no. 11, 2005, pp. 1569–82. doi: 10.1016/j.addr.2005.07.002.

Bliss, M. *The Discovery of Insulin: The Twenty-Fifth Anniversary Edition*. University of Toronto Press, 1982, JSTOR. www.jstor.org/stable/10.3138/j.ctt1wn0sjc.

Builders, P. F., et al. Preparation and evaluation of mucinated sodium alginate microparticles for oral delivery of insulin. *European Journal of Pharmaceutics and Biopharmaceutics*, vol. 70, no. 3, 2008, pp. 777–83. doi: 10.1016/j.ejpb.2008.06.021.

Carino, G. P. and Mathiowitz, E. Oral insulin delivery. *Advanced Drug Delivery Reviews*, vol. 35, 1999, pp. 249–257.

Casettari, L., et al. Effect of PEGylation on the toxicity and permeability enhancement of chitosan. *Biomacromolecules*, vol. 11, no. 11, 2010, pp. 2854–65. doi: 10.1021/bm100522c.

Centers for Disease Control and Prevention. National diabetes statistics report. US Department of Health and Human Services, 2017.

Cersosimo, E., et al. Pathogenesis of type 2 diabetes mellitus. In: *Endotext*, edited by K. R. Feingold et al., MDText.com, Inc., 2000. www.ncbi.nlm.nih.gov/books/NBK279115/.

Chaillous, L., et al. Oral insulin administration and residual (β-cell function in recent-onset type 1 diabetes: A multicentre randomised controlled trial. *The Lancet*, vol. 356, no. 9229, 2000, pp. 545–49. doi: 10.1016/S0140-6736(00)02579-4.

Cikrikci, S., et al. Development of PH sensitive alginate/gum tragacanth based hydrogels for oral insulin delivery. *Journal of Agricultural and Food Chemistry*, vol. 66, no. 44, 2018, pp. 11784–96. doi: 10.1021/acs.jafc.8b02525.

Clark, M., et al. Type 1 diabetes: A chronic anti-self-inflammatory response. *Frontiers in Immunology*, vol. 8, 2017, p. 1898. doi: 10.3389/fimmu.2017.01898.

Cornick, S., et al. Roles and regulation of the mucus barrier in the gut. *Tissue Barriers*, vol. 3, no. 1–2, 2015. doi: 10.4161/21688370.2014.982426.

Czuba, E., et al. Oral insulin delivery, the challenge to increase insulin bioavailability: Influence of surface charge in nanoparticle system. *International Journal of Pharmaceutics*, vol. 542, no. 1, 2018, pp. 47–55. doi: 10.1016/j.ijpharm.2018.02.045.

Date, A. A., et al. Nanoparticles for oral delivery: Design, evaluation and state-of-the-art. *Journal of Controlled Release : Official Journal of the Controlled Release Society*, vol. 240, 2016, pp. 504–26. doi: 10.1016/j.jconrel.2016.06.016.

Déat-Lainé, E., et al. Efficacy of mucoadhesive hydrogel microparticles of whey protein and alginate for oral insulin delivery. *Pharmaceutical Research*, vol. 30, no. 3, 2013, pp. 721–34. doi: 10.1007/s11095-012-0913-3.

De Meyts, P. The insulin receptor and its signal transduction network. In: *Endotext*, edited by K. R. Feingold et al., MDText.com, Inc., 2000. www.ncbi.nlm.nih.gov/books/NBK378978/.

Donner, T. Insulin: Pharmacology, therapeutic regimens and principles of intensive insulin therapy. In: *Endotext*, edited by K. R. Feingold et al., MDText.com, Inc., 2000. www.ncbi.nlm.nih.gov/books/NBK278938/.

Duckworth, W. C., et al. Insulin degradation: Progress and potential. *Endocrine Reviews*, vol. 19, no. 5, 1998, pp. 608–24. academic-oup-com.go.libproxy.wakehealth.edu, doi: 10.1210/edrv.19.5.0349.

Durham, T. B., et al. Dual exosite-binding inhibitors of insulin-degrading enzyme challenge its role as the primary mediator of insulin clearance in vivo. *The Journal of Biological Chemistry*, vol. 290, no. 33, 2015, pp. 20044–59. doi: 10.1074/jbc.M115.638205.

Ensign, L. M., et al. Oral drug delivery with polymeric nanoparticles: The gastrointestinal mucus barriers. *Advanced Drug Delivery Reviews*, vol. 64, no. 6, 2012, pp. 557–70. doi: 10.1016/j.addr.2011.12.009.

Fukuoka, Y., et al. Combination strategy with complexation hydrogels and cell-penetrating peptides for oral delivery of insulin. *Biological and Pharmaceutical Bulletin*, vol. 41, no. 5, 2018, pp. 811–14. doi: 10.1248/bpb.b17-00951.

Gedawy, A., et al. Oral insulin delivery: Existing barriers and current counter-strategies. *Journal of Pharmacy and Pharmacology*, vol. 70, no. 2, 2018, pp. 197–213. doi: 10.1111/jphp.12852.

Greimel, A., et al. Oral peptide delivery: In-vitro evaluation of thiolated alginate/poly(acrylic acid) microparticles. *Journal of Pharmacy and Pharmacology*, vol. 59, no. 9, 2007, pp. 1191–98. doi: 10.1211/jpp.59.9.0002.

He, P., et al. Poly(ester amide) blend microspheres for oral insulin delivery. *International Journal of Pharmaceutics*, vol. 455, no. 1, 2013, pp. 259–66. doi: 10.1016/j.ijpharm.2013.07.022.

Hinds, K. D. and S. W. Kim. Effects of PEG conjugation on insulin properties. *Advanced Drug Delivery Reviews*, vol. 54, no. 4, 2002, pp. 505–30. doi: 10.1016/S0169-409X(02)00025-X.

Holgado, M. A., et al. Protein-loaded PLGA microparticles engineered by flow focusing: Physicochemical characterization and protein detection by reversed-phase HPLC. *International Journal of Pharmaceutics*, vol. 380, no. 1, 2009, pp. 147–54. doi: 10.1016/j.ijpharm.2009.07.017.

Huang, X., et al. ZnO-based nanocarriers for drug delivery application: From passive to smart strategies. *International Journal of Pharmaceutics*, vol. 534, no. 1, 2017, pp. 190–94. doi: 10.1016/j.ijpharm.2017.10.008.

Huckaby, J. T. and S. K. Lai. PEGylation for enhancing nanoparticle diffusion in mucus. *Advanced Drug Delivery Reviews*, vol. 124, 2018, pp. 125–39. doi: 10.1016/j.addr.2017.08.010.

Hunter, A. C., et al. Polymeric particulate technologies for oral drug delivery and targeting: A pathophysiological perspective. *Nanomedicine: Nanotechnology, Biology and Medicine*, vol. 8, 2012, pp. S5–20. doi: 10.1016/j.nano.2012.07.005.

Jani, P. U., et al. Nanosphere and microsphere uptake via peyer's patches: Observation of the rate of uptake in the rat after a single oral dose. *International Journal of Pharmaceutics*, vol. 86, no. 2, 1992, pp. 239–46. doi: 10.1016/0378-5173(92)90202-D.

Jose, S., et al. Cross-linked chitosan microspheres for oral delivery of insulin: Taguchi design and in vivo testing. *Colloids and Surfaces B: Biointerfaces*, vol. 92, 2012, pp. 175–79. doi: 10.1016/j.colsurfb.2011.11.040.

Jose, S., et al. Predictive modeling of insulin release profile from cross-linked chitosan microspheres. *European Journal of Medicinal Chemistry*, vol. 60, 2013, pp. 249–53. doi: 10.1016/j.ejmech.2012.12.011.

Kalra, S., et al. Oral insulin. *Diabetology and Metabolic Syndrome*, vol. 2, no. 1, 2010, p. 66. doi: 10.1186/1758-5996-2-66.

Kenechukwu, F. C. and M. A. Momoh. Formulation, characterization and evaluation of the effect of polymer concentration on the release behavior of insulin-loaded Eudragit®-entrapped mucoadhesive microspheres. *International Journal of Pharmaceutical Investigation*, vol. 6, no. 2, 2016, p. 69. www.jpionline.org, doi: 10.4103/2230-973X.177806.

Khan, A. A., et al. Advanced drug delivery to the lymphatic system: Lipid-based nanoformulations. *International Journal of Nanomedicine*, vol. 8, 2013, pp. 2733–44. doi: 10.2147/IJN.S41521.

Kim, B.-Y., et al. Bioadhesive interaction and hypoglycemic effect of insulin-loaded lectin–microparticle conjugates in oral insulin delivery system. *Journal of Controlled Release*, vol. 102, no. 3, 2005, pp. 525–38. doi: 10.1016/j.jconrel.2004.10.032.

Kondiah, P. P. D., et al. Development of a gastric absorptive, immediate responsive, oral protein-loaded versatile polymeric delivery system. *AAPS PharmSciTech*, vol. 18, no. 7, 2017, pp. 2479–93. doi: 10.1208/s12249-017-0725-1.

Lee, J. H., et al. ZOT-derived peptide and chitosan functionalized nanocarrier for oral delivery of protein drug. *Biomaterials*, vol. 103, 2016, pp. 160–69. doi: 10.1016/j.biomaterials.2016.06.059.

Lopes, M. A., et al. Intestinal absorption of insulin nanoparticles: Contribution of M cells. *Nanomedicine: Nanotechnology, Biology and Medicine*, vol. 10, no. 6, 2014, pp. 1139–51. doi: 10.1016/j.nano.2014.02.014.

Ma, G. Microencapsulation of protein drugs for drug delivery: Strategy, preparation, and applications. *Journal of Controlled Release*, vol. 193, 2014, pp. 324–40. doi: 10.1016/j.jconrel.2014.09.003.

Ma, X. Y., et al. Preliminary study of oral polylactide microcapsulated insulin in vitro and in vivo. *Diabetes, Obesity and Metabolism*, vol. 2, no. 4, 2000, pp. 243–50. doi: 10.1046/j.1463-1326.2000.00080.x.

Madhav, M. Long-awaited dream of oral insulin: Where did we reach. *Asian Journal of Pharmaceutical and Clinical Research*, vol. 4, no. 2, 2011, pp. 15–20.

Marais, E., et al. Eudragit® L100/N-trimethylchitosan chloride microspheres for oral insulin delivery. *Molecules*, vol. 18, no. 6, 2013, pp. 6734–47. www.mdpi.com, doi: 10.3390/molecules18066734.

Marschütz, M. K. and A. Bernkop-Schnürch. Oral peptide drug delivery: Polymer-inhibitor conjugates protecting insulin from enzymatic degradation in vitro. *Biomaterials*, vol. 21, no. 14, 2000, pp. 1499–507.

Martins, S., et al. Insulin-loaded alginate microspheres for oral delivery: Effect of polysaccharide reinforcement on physicochemical properties and release profile. *Carbohydrate Polymers*, vol. 69, no. 4, 2007, pp. 725–31. doi: 10.1016/j.carbpol.2007.02.012.

Michels, A. and P. Gottlieb. Pathogenesis of type 1A diabetes. In: *Endotext*, edited by K. R. Feingold et al., MDText.com, Inc., 2000. www.ncbi.nlm.nih.gov/books/NBK279002/.

Mohy Eldin, M. S., et al. L-arginine grafted alginate hydrogel beads: A novel PH-sensitive system for specific protein delivery. *Arabian Journal of Chemistry*, vol. 8, no. 3, 2015, pp. 355–65. doi: 10.1016/j.arabjc.2014.01.007.

Momoh, M. A., et al. Influence of magnesium stearate on the physicochemical and pharmacodynamic characteristics of insulin-loaded eudragit entrapped mucoadhesive microspheres. *Drug Delivery*, vol. 22, no. 6, 2015, pp. 837–48. doi: 10.3109/10717544.2014.898108.

Morishita, M., et al. Novel oral insulin delivery systems based on complexation polymer hydrogels: Single and multiple administration studies in type 1 and 2 diabetic rats. *Journal of Controlled Release*, vol. 110, no. 3, 2006, pp. 587–94. doi: 10.1016/j.jconrel.2005.10.029.

Mundargi, R. C., et al. Poly(N-vinylcaprolactam-co-methacrylic acid) hydrogel microparticles for oral insulin delivery. *Journal of Microencapsulation*, vol. 28, no. 5, Aug. 2011, pp. 384–94. doi: 10.3109/02652048.2011.576782.

Naha, P. C., et al. Improved bioavailability of orally delivered insulin using eudragit-L30D coated PLGA microparticles. *Journal of Microencapsulation*, vol. 25, no. 4, 2008, pp. 248–56. doi: 10.1080/02652040801903843.

Niu, Mengmeng, et al. Hypoglycemic activity and oral bioavailability of insulin-loaded liposomes containing bile salts in rats: The effect of cholate type, particle size and administered dose. *European Journal of Pharmaceutics and Biopharmaceutics*, vol. 81, no. 2, 2012, pp. 265–72. doi: 10.1016/j.ejpb.2012.02.009.

Pavlović, N., et al. Bile acids and their derivatives as potential modifiers of drug release and pharmacokinetic profiles. *Frontiers in Pharmacology*, vol. 9, 2018. doi: 10.3389/fphar.2018.01283.

Pechenkin, M. A., et al. Use of protease inhibitors in composite polyelectrolyte microparticles in order to increase the bioavailability of perorally administered encapsulated proteins. *Pharmaceutical Chemistry Journal*, vol. 47, no. 1, 2013, pp. 62–69. doi: 10.1007/s11094-013-0898-1.

Pereira de Sousa, I., et al. Insulin loaded mucus permeating nanoparticles: Addressing the surface characteristics as feature to improve mucus permeation. *International Journal of Pharmaceutics*, vol. 500, no. 1–2, 2016, pp. 236–44. doi: 10.1016/j.ijpharm.2016.01.022.

Raguvaran, R., et al. Sodium alginate and gum acacia hydrogels of ZnO nanoparticles show wound healing effect on fibroblast cells. *International Journal of Biological Macromolecules*, vol. 96, 2017, pp. 185–91. doi: 10.1016/j.ijbiomac.2016.12.009.

Ramdas, M., et al. Alginate encapsulated bioadhesive chitosan microspheres for intestinal drug delivery. *Journal of Biomaterials Applications*, vol. 13, no. 4, 1999, pp. 290–96. doi: 10.1177/088532829901300402.

Rehmani, S. and J. E. Dixon. Oral delivery of anti-diabetes therapeutics using cell penetrating and transcytosing peptide strategies. *Peptides*, vol. 100, 2018, pp. 24–35. doi: 10.1016/j.peptides.2017.12.014.

Reis, C. P., et al. Alginate microparticles as novel carrier for oral insulin delivery. *Biotechnology and Bioengineering*, vol. 96, no. 5, 2007, pp. 977–89. doi: 10.1002/bit.21164.

Rekha, M. R. and C. P. Sharma. Synthesis and evaluation of lauryl succinyl chitosan particles towards oral insulin delivery and absorption. *Journal of Controlled Release*, vol. 135, no. 2, 2009, pp. 144–51. doi: 10.1016/j.jconrel.2009.01.011.

Renukuntla, J., et al. Approaches for enhancing oral bioavailability of peptides and proteins. *International Journal of Pharmaceutics*, vol. 447, no. 0, 2013, pp. 75–93. doi: 10.1016/j.ijpharm.2013.02.030.

Richardson, T. and D. Kerr. Skin-related complications of insulin therapy: Epidemiology and emerging management strategies. *American Journal of Clinical Dermatology*, vol. 4, no. 10, 2003, pp. 661–67. doi: 10.2165/00128071-200304100-00001.

Ru, G., et al. Effects of borneol on the pharmacokinetics of 9-nitrocamptothecin encapsulated in PLGA nanoparticles with different size via oral administration. *Drug Delivery*, vol. 23, no. 9, 2016, pp. 3417–23. doi: 10.1080/10717544.2016.1189466.

Sajeesh, S. and C. P. Sharma. Mucoadhesive hydrogel microparticles based on poly (methacrylic acid-vinyl pyrrolidone)-chitosan for oral drug delivery. *Drug Delivery*, vol. 18, no. 4, 2011, pp. 227–35. doi: 10.3109/10717544.2010.528067.

Sajeesh, S. and C. P. Sharma. Poly methacrylic acid-alginate semi-IPN microparticles for oral delivery of insulin: A preliminary investigation. *Journal of Biomaterials Applications*, vol. 19, no. 1, 2004, pp. 35–45. doi: 10.1177/0885328204042992.

Salama, N. N., et al. Tight junction modulation and its relationship to drug delivery. *Advanced Drug Delivery Reviews*, vol. 58, no. 1, 2006, pp. 15–28. doi: 10.1016/j.addr.2006.01.003.

Salatin, S. and A. Yari Khosroushahi. Overviews on the cellular uptake mechanism of polysaccharide colloidal nanoparticles. *Journal of Cellular and Molecular Medicine*, vol. 21, no. 9, 2017, pp. 1668–86. doi: 10.1111/jcmm.13110.

Sanger, F. Chemistry of insulin; determination of the structure of insulin opens the way to greater understanding of life processes. *Science (New York)*, vol. 129, no. 3359, 1959, pp. 1340–44.

Sezer, A. D. and J. Akbuğa. Release characteristics of chitosan treated alginate beads: I. sustained release of a macromolecular drug from chitosan treated alginate beads. *Journal of Microencapsulation*, vol. 16, no. 2, 1999, pp. 195–203. doi: 10.1080/026520499289176.

Sharma, S., et al. Preliminary studies on the development of IgA-loaded chitosan-dextran sulphate nanoparticles as a potential nasal delivery system for protein antigens. *Journal of Microencapsulation*, vol. 30, no. 3, 2013, pp. 283–94. doi: 10.3109/02652048.2012.726279.

Sheng, J., et al. Enhancing insulin oral absorption by using mucoadhesive nanoparticles loaded with LMWP-linked insulin conjugates. *Journal of Controlled Release*, vol. 233, 2016, pp. 181–90. doi: 10.1016/j.jconrel.2016.05.015.

Silva, C. M., et al. Insulin encapsulation in reinforced alginate microspheres prepared by internal gelation. *European Journal of Pharmaceutical Sciences*, vol. 29, no. 2, 2006, pp. 148–59. doi: 10.1016/j.ejps.2006.06.008.

Situ, W., et al. Preparation and characterization of glycoprotein-resistant starch complex as a coating material for oral bioadhesive microparticles for colon-targeted polypeptide delivery. *Journal of Agricultural and Food Chemistry*, vol. 63, no. 16, 2015, pp. 4138–47. doi: 10.1021/acs.jafc.5b00393.

Situ, W., et al. Resistant starch film-coated microparticles for an oral colon-specific polypeptide delivery system and its release behaviors. *Journal of Agricultural and Food Chemistry*, vol. 62, no. 16, Apr. 2014, pp. 3599–609. doi: 10.1021/jf500472b.

Škalko-Basnet, N. Biologics: The role of delivery systems in improved therapy. *Biologics : Targets and Therapy*, vol. 8, 2014, pp. 107–14. doi: 10.2147/BTT.S38387.

Smart, J. D. The basics and underlying mechanisms of mucoadhesion. *Advanced Drug Delivery Reviews*, vol. 57, no. 11, 2005, pp. 1556–68. doi: 10.1016/j.addr.2005.07.001.

Sonaje, K., et al. Biodistribution, pharmacodynamics and pharmacokinetics of insulin analogues in a rat model: Oral delivery using PH-responsive nanoparticles vs. subcutaneous injection. *Biomaterials*, vol. 31, no. 26, 2010, pp. 6849–58. doi: 10.1016/j.biomaterials.2010.05.042.

Sun, S., et al. PH-sensitive poly(lactide-co-glycolide) nanoparticle composite microcapsules for oral delivery of insulin. *International Journal of Nanomedicine*, 2015, doi: 10.2147/IJN.S81715.

Takeuchi, T. and S. Futaki. Current understanding of direct translocation of arginine-rich cell-penetrating peptides and its internalization mechanisms. *Chemical and Pharmaceutical Bulletin*, vol. 64, no. 10, 2016, pp. 1431–37. doi: 10.1248/cpb.c16-00505.

Thwala, L. N., et al. Protamine nanocapsules as carriers for oral peptide delivery. *Journal of Controlled Release: Official Journal of the Controlled Release Society*, vol. 291, 2018, pp. 157–68. doi: 10.1016/j. jconrel.2018.10.022.

Ubaidulla, U., et al. Chitosan phthalate microspheres for oral delivery of insulin: Preparation, characterization, and in vitro evaluation. *Drug Delivery*, vol. 14, no. 1, 2007a, pp. 19–23. doi: 10.1080/10717540600559478.

Ubaidulla, U., et al. Development and characterization of chitosan succinate microspheres for the improved oral bioavailability of insulin. *Journal of Pharmaceutical Sciences*, vol. 96, no. 11, 2007b, pp. 3010–23. doi: 10.1002/jps.20969.

Valainis, G., Thomas, D., Pankey, G. Penetration of ciprofloxacin into cerebrospinal fluid. *European Journal of Clinical Microbiology and Infectious Diseases*, vol. 5, no. 2, 1986, pp. 206–7.

Vanea, E., et al. Freeze-dried and spray-dried zinc-containing silica microparticles entrapping insulin. *Journal of Biomaterials Applications*, vol. 28, no. 8, 2014, pp. 1190–99. doi: 10.1177/0885328213501216.

Vinik, A., et al. Diabetic neuropathies. In: *Endotext*, edited by K. R. Feingold et al., MDText.com, Inc., 2000. www.ncbi.nlm.nih.gov/books/NBK279175/.

Wagner, A. M., et al. Designing the new generation of intelligent biocompatible carriers for protein and peptide delivery. *Acta Pharmaceutica Sinica B*, vol. 8, no. 2, 2018, pp. 147–64. doi: 10.1016/j.apsb.2018.01.013.

Wilcox, G. Insulin and insulin resistance. *Clinical Biochemist Reviews*, vol. 26, no. 2, 2005, pp. 19–39.

Williams, D. The relationship between biomaterials and nanotechnology. *Biomaterials*, vol. 29, no. 12, 2008, pp. 1737–38. doi: 10.1016/j.biomaterials.2008.01.003.

Williams, I. R. and R. L. Owen. Chapter 13- M cells: Specialized antigen sampling cells in the follicle-associated epithelium. In: *Mucosal Immunology (Fourth Edition)*, edited by J. Mestecky et al., Academic Press, 2015, pp. 211–29. doi: 10.1016/B978-0-12-415847-4.00013-6.

Wong, C. Y., et al. Recent advancements in oral administration of insulin-loaded liposomal drug delivery systems for diabetes mellitus. *International Journal of Pharmaceutics*, vol. 549, no. 1, 2018, pp. 201–17. doi: 10.1016/j.ijpharm.2018.07.041.

Zare-Akbari, Z., et al. PH-sensitive bionanocomposite hydrogel beads based on carboxymethyl cellulose/ZnO nanoparticle as drug carrier. *International Journal of Biological Macromolecules*, vol. 93, no. Pt A, 2016, pp. 1317–27. doi: 10.1016/j.ijbiomac.2016.09.110.

Zeng, Z., et al. Scalable production of therapeutic protein nanoparticles using flash nanoprecipitation. *Advanced Healthcare Materials*, 2018. onlinelibrary.wiley.com, doi: 10.1002/adhm.201801010.

Zhang, J., et al. Long-circulating heparin-functionalized magnetic nanoparticles for potential application as a protein drug delivery platform. *Molecular Pharmaceutics*, vol. 10, no. 10, 2013, pp. 3892–902. doi: 10.1021/mp400360q.

Zhang, M., et al. Preparation and characterization of monomethoxypoly(ethylene glycol)-insulin conjugates. *Die Pharmazie*, vol. 64, no. 3, 2009, pp. 190–96.

Zhang, P., et al. Goblet cell targeting nanoparticle containing drug-loaded micelle cores for oral delivery of insulin. *International Journal of Pharmaceutics*, vol. 496, no. 2, 2015, pp. 993–1005. doi: 10.1016/j. ijpharm.2015.10.078.

Zhu, S., et al. Enhanced oral bioavailability of insulin using PLGA nanoparticles co-modified with cell-penetrating peptides and engrailed secretion peptide (sec). *Drug Delivery*, vol. 23, no. 6, 2016, pp. 1980–91. doi: 10.3109/10717544.2015.1043472.

Zhu, Y.-J. and F. Chen. PH-responsive drug-delivery systems. *Chemistry: An Asian Journal*, vol. 10, no. 2, 2015, pp. 284–305. doi: 10.1002/asia.201402715.

Ziv, E. and M. Bendayan. Intestinal absorption of peptides through the enterocytes. *Microscopy Research and Technique*, vol. 49, no. 4, 2000, pp. 346–52. doi:10.1002/(SICI)1097-0029(20000515)49.

13 Insulin Delivery by a Bioartificial Pancreas

Kendall Jr WF
University of Florida

CONTENTS

13.1 INTRODUCTION

13.1.1 HISTORICAL PERSPECTIVES

13.1.1.1 Diabetes

Diabetes is a devastating disease that has been around for centuries. In ancient times, early humans were primarily hunters and gatherers and could often face periods of food shortage.[1] Although adequate food stores would help them to survive these challenging periods, obesity was relatively rare among them.[1] Then around 400 BC, sugarcane was discovered in the Ganges River Valley. It was then imported and grown in China in 100 AD, Persia in 500 AD, and then Egypt in 600 AD.[1] Sushruta was one of the first physicians to link obesity and diabetes with sugar intake.[1] Maimonides, a 12th century physician, noted that diabetes tended to occur more often in areas where sugar was a large part of the diet.[1]

Historically, the first mention of the disease that we now know as diabetes mellitus was made in the Ebers Papyrus, which was written around the 15th century BC, in which they mentioned a condition that caused abnormal polyuria.[2] Aulus Cornelius Celsus (30 BC–50 AD) thus provided an excellent clinical description of diabetes.[2] Galen (131–201 AD), a Greek philosopher and physician, described diabetes as a "weakness of the kidneys which cannot hold back water".[2] He noted that the disease was characterized by coincident thirst, and a voracious appetite, despite progressive emaciation ("wasting of the flesh"[2]). Chinese and Japanese providers noted that diabetic patients had large volumes of urine that attracted dogs because of its sweetness.[2] They also noted that some of these patients had furunculosis.[2] During the Brahman period of Hindu medicine (between 400 and 500 BC), which was dominated by three physicians: Charaka, Sushruta, and Vaghbata, the disease of "honey urine" was differentiated from 20 other varieties of polyuria.[2] It was described as a "disease of the rich and one that is brought about by the gluttonous overindulgence in oil, flour, and sugar".[2,3] At around the same period (~400 BC) "sweet urine disease" was mentioned in the oldest Chinese medical book that has been discovered: *The Yellow Emperor's Canon on the Traditional Chinese Medicine*.[3] Similar findings were noted in Arab medical texts from the 9th to the 11th century AD, including a medical encyclopedia written by Avicenna.[3]

The Arabian physician, Avicenna (980–1027 AD), recorded the features of diabetes in exquisite detail, including the fact that its etiology can be either primary or secondary.[2] The establishment of the diagnosis of diabetes based on an excessive amount of glucose was established based on observations by Thomas Willis in 1679 and then experiments by Matthew Dobson[2] in 1776. Dobson demonstrated for the first time that the "sweetness" found in the urine of diabetic patients contained a saccharine matter that fermented, and which was found to previously exist in the serum of the blood.[2] John Rollo, an Edinburgh-trained surgeon was the first to add the adjective mellitus (from the latin "honey") to diabetes.[3] Then during the first two decades of the 19th century, it was determined that the "sugar" that was excreted from diabetic subjects had characteristics of glucose rather than sucrose, including the discovery by the French chemist, Michael Chevreul, in 1815 that the sugar in diabetic urine was glucose.[2,3] Also during the 19th century, experiments by Claude Bernard and Pavy helped to elucidate the relationship of hyperglycemia, glycosuria, and the role of the liver in glycogen storage and glucose metabolism.[2,3] In 1857, Petter discovered acetone in diabetic urine. Kussmaul in 1874, then independently, Stadelman, Minkowski, and Naunyn, described findings such as the presence of beta-oxybutyric acid and "acidosis" that can be found in "diabetic coma".[2] The discovery of islets in the pancreatic gland occurred in 1869 by Langerhans.

In 1893, Gustave Edouard Laguesse, a French pathologist and histologist, after extensive studies, hypothesized that the islets of Langerhans produced the "internal secretions of the pancreas".[3,4] Von Mering and Minkowski, then demonstrated 20 years later that when dogs were totally pancreatectomized, they developed hyperglycemia, glycosuria, then finally died with ketosis in coma.[2] Vassale ligated the duct of Wirsung and noted that atrophy of the acinar tissue of the pancreas occurred without effect on the islets of Langerhans or development of hyperglycemia.[2] In 1900, Opie described hyaline degeneration of islets of Langerhans in cases of diabetes.[2] Ssobelow and Schulz in 1902 arrived at the same conclusion as Opie and proposed that development of an extract from islets of Langerhans would be effective in the treatment of diabetes.[2] The development of micromethods to assess glycemia, by the Norwegian physician Ivar Christian Bang in 1913, made the clinical and research measurement of blood glucose much more practical and easier.[3]

Moses Barron discovered that the islets of Langerhans were damaged while performing an autopsy on a patient with diabetes and suggested that damage to the islets was the cause of the diabetes and further deduced that the substance that was contained within the islets of Langerhans was the "antidiabetic treatment".[5] He later repeated the experiments that had been performed by Ssebelow and Schulz with similar results.[2]

13.1.1.2 Insulin

Several researchers worked on isolation of the active component of internal pancreatic secretion.[6] These included: John Rennie and Thomas Fraser (1902) extracted a substance from the endocrine pancreas of codfish and injected it into a dog, which presumably died from severe hypoglycemia.[6] Georg Ludwig Zuelzer (1907) collected a pancreatic extract which he injected into a dog after performing a total pancreatectomy.[6] The extract lowered the blood glucose and raised the pH.[6] He patented his extract with the name "acomatol"; however, he ran into problems with his product, when it was utilized on human patients, presumably due to complications from impurities and development of severe hypoglycemia.[6] The term "insuline" was first used by the Belgian clinician and physiologist Jean De Meyer, in 1909, to refer to the "internal secretions" of the pancreas.[3] Several other therapeutic approaches were also tried between 1910 and 1922.[7] These included: Henry Sewal (1911), who tried administering pancreatic extract orally.[7] W Groftor (1913) placed the pancreatic extract into acid-insoluble capsule for oral consumption.[7] In 1914, Guralin and Kramar placed extracts of pancreas and duodenal mucosa subcutaneously.[7]

Then after presenting four papers to the "Comptes rendus de la Societe de Biologie" between April and June 1921, on June 22, 1921, Nicolae Constantin Paulescu published work, in the European literature, extensively describing his experiments in detail, and naming the antidiabetic extract ("pancreine") that he had isolated.[8,9] Interestingly, his work went relatively unnoticed and he at the time received no credit for this discovery, although his work was referenced by Banting and Best, during their subsequent work.[8,9] Several months after Paulescu's publications, in collaboration with James Collip, a biochemist, who had earlier managed to extract a reasonably pure form of insulin from the pancreas of cattle, Banting and Best published work, showing that they were able to extract a relatively pure form of "isletin" (insulin), which, initially had failed after its administration on January 11, 1922 to a 14-year-old boy, Leonard Thompson with diabetes, with no clinical benefit. However, they were able to successfully repeat administration of an insulin extract, to the same patient, on January 23, 1922 and for 10 days, thereafter, with good response, including complete elimination of glycosuria and ketonuria, and significant gain of weight and strength.[2,3,5,6]

Purification and subsequent widespread usage of this extract (which they first called "isletin" then at Macleod's suggestion, they renamed it "insulin," reportedly unaware the name "insuline" had already been suggested by de Meyer), which significantly impacted the ability to more effectively treat diabetes and reduce the previously high incidence of ketosis and diabetic coma that was associated with several earlier modalities, such as the starvation diet, that were used to treat patient's suffering with diabetes prior to the isolation of insulin.[2,3] Other contributions such as the preparation of crystalline insulin in 1926 by Abel and the introduction of long-acting insulin preparations by Scott and Fisher, Hagedorn, and Hallas-Moller have increased the insulin regimens that are available for treating patients.[2] The recognition of insulin resistance and sensitivity, as well as the recognition of side effects such as lipodystrophies and allergies, occurred over time and helped to spur continued interest in pursuit of other treatment modalities.[2]

13.2 INSULIN DELIVERY BY AN ARTIFICIAL PANCREAS

The concept of an artificial pancreas was envisioned at least by the 1950s.[10] In 1959, Professor E Perry McCullagh demonstrated the concept of an implantable artificial endocrine pancreas.[10] This closed regulatory system included a glucose monitoring device, a transmitter, and an insulin syringe.[10] Development of this concept was pursued by many researchers, including Albisser et al in 1974 and Shichin et al in 1975.[10] Their devices included an autoanalyzer for blood glucose determination, a minicomputer system and a pump driving system.[10] The size of the system was then reduced, and a device called "Biostator" produced at Miles Laboratory in Elkhart IN and another device developed by the Osaka University group were produced.[10]

Technological advances such as the advent of continuous infusion insulin pumps in the 1970s, and then the development in the mid-2000s of the ability to continuously measure glucose and provide a feedback loop to the insulin pump, significantly impacted and advanced the viability of the concept.[11]

Various insulin pumps and continuous glucose monitoring (CGM) devices have been developed.[12] Some operate in manual mode as a traditional pump, or in automode as a closed-loop system with CGM utilization to alter basal insulin output.[12]

Several Predictive Low Glucose Systems have been developed.[13,14] These systems suspend insulin delivery if the 30 minutes predicted glucose is <80 mg/dL or if the observed glucose concentration falls below 70 mg/dL, and resumes insulin delivery the first time the system receives a CGM glucose reading higher than the previous reading.[13,14]

Overall, the systems have conceptually evolved from external devices to implantable devices.[10] Some studies have suggested that although closed-loop portal and peripheral venous insulin delivery systems seem equally effective regarding blood glucose control and insulin requirements, that portal insulin delivery is superior to peripheral delivery at maintaining more appropriate hepatic glucose handling and physiologic insulin profiles.[10]

Studies done in animal and human models have shown that insulin concentrations during steady-state conditions are typically two to fourfold higher in the portal vein than it is in the periphery after pulsating insulin delivery by the pancreas.[15] A positive portal to systemic insulin gradient is then thought to assist in balancing hepatic glucose output and peripheral glucose disposal, which then maintains glucose homeostasis in both postprandial and postabsorptive periods.[15] The glycemic control that is achieved by conventional subcutaneous insulin delivery is less physiologic than what is obtained with the positive portal to systemic gradient.[15] Subcutaneous insulin administration tends to result in higher than physiologic insulin concentrations at the peripheral tissue level.[15] Some theorize that the resultant overinsulinization that occurs with subcutaneous insulin administration shifts the primary site of insulin action away from the liver and towards the skeletal muscle, which then predisposes to hypoglycemia, at least in part due to the muscle being a larger glucose sink than the liver, which then contributes to decreased hepatic glucose uptake.[15] The use of intraperitoneal insulin delivery, wherein insulin is infused directly into the intraperitoneal space is thought to partially restore the positive portal to systemic insulin gradient, at least in part due to the intraperitoneal infused insulin being subsequently absorbed via the capillary of the visceral peritoneum into the portal vein.[15]

Artificial pancreas treatment, also referred to as "closed-loop glucose control," combines an insulin pump and CGM (in a "single hormone artificial pancreas system") with a control algorithm to deliver insulin in a glucose-responsive manner.[16]

This differs from conventional insulin pump therapy and threshold suspend technology in that it has a control algorithm that autonomously increases and decreases subcutaneous insulin delivery in response to real-time sensor glucose levels.[17]

In dual hormone artificial pancreas systems, glucagon can also be delivered in a similar glucose-responsive fashion.[16] In comparison to treatment options that utilize only insulin pumps or sensor augmented pumps, the artificial pancreas system can reduce the burden for patients by automatically adjusting the amount of insulin entering the body based on sensor glucose levels.[16]

A recent systematic review and meta-analysis has shown that artificial pancreas systems are an efficacious and safe treatment approach for people with type 1 diabetes, which leads to increased time in near normoglycemic range, and reduced time in hypoglycemia and hyperglycaemia.[14]

Despite advances, there continue to be several limitations with clinical application of the "artificial pancreas".[18] Since this subject is discussed elsewhere in this book, readers interested in the topic are referred to the relevant chapter. Suffice it to say that there are limitations associated with this insulin delivery systems.

13.2.1 LIMITATIONS OF EXOGENOUS INSULIN

After the initial discovery of insulin, its usage definitely saved numerous lives; however, the inability to replicate the exquisite glucose balance that pancreatic islets help to regulate has led to hyperglycemia-driven microvascular and macrovascular complication as well as "potentially fatal" episodes of hypoglycemia.[11] Banting appropriately noted in his Nobel lecture that "insulin is not a cure for diabetes; it is a treatment".[11]

The presence of excess insulin tends to predispose individuals to experience hypoglycemia.[19] It has been shown that in patients that self-reported severe hypoglycemia there is a 3.4-fold increase in mortality in contrast to individuals who reported mild hypoglycemia.[19]

Pancreatic islet biology is closely tied to gut and liver biology.[11] This, therefore, makes it extremely challenging for exogenously introduced insulin to mimic the dynamic patterns of normal insulin secretion.[11] The pancreas typically starts to secrete insulin onto the portal vein even prior to food being swallowed, then this is followed by rapid biphasic insulin release that returns to basal levels as the food is absorbed.[11] The normal kinetics of insulin release and the flow of insulin first to the liver and the complex interactions that normally occur cannot transpire with subcutaneous administration of insulin.[11] Insulin that is delivered subcutaneously has significant and variable delays (approximately 1 hour to peak levels) in entering the blood and limited liver passage.[29] Even with CGM, there is a variability in ongoing insulin needs.[29]

In some patients with type 1 diabetes, their overnight insulin needs were noted to vary from half up to threefold of the baseline amounts.[11] This variability is thought to be due to complex interactions between counterregulatory hormones and other physiologic interactions that occur with beta-islets.[11] The physiologic variability of the insulin requirements can leave patients being treated with exogenous insulin, even with usage of the artificial pancreas, with CGM, at risk for hypoglycemia, which can lead to coma and even death.[11]

13.3 CELL-BASED INSULIN DELIVERY SYSTEMS

13.3.1 PANCREAS TRANSPLANTATION

The pancreas became the fourth organ to be successfully transplanted in humans (following successful transplantation of kidney, liver, and heart).[20] On December 17, 1966, W Kelly and R Lillehei's team at University of Minnesota did a duct-ligated segmental pancreas transplant into 28-year-old uremic female patient.[21] The patient developed graft pancreatitis and the rejected kidney and pancreas ultimately had to be removed, and the patient died from pulmonary embolism, 13 days after the transplanted grafts were removed.[21] She did, however, have six insulin-free days after the transplant was performed.[21] Dr Felix Largiader, who was also at the University of Minnesota, in 1967, then successfully transplanted the whole pancreas with attached duodenal cuff in a canine model.[22] He connected the donor celiac artery to the host aorta, the donor portal vein to the vena cava, oversewed one end of the duodenum, and connected the other end of the duodenum to a roux-en-y jejunal segment.[22] Later that same year, Dr Lillehei successfully adopted the same technique to human transplants.[22] With evolution and refinement of surgical techniques, introduction of first cyclosporine and then other immunosuppressants, as well as better Human Leukocyte Antigen (HLA) matching techniques, the outcomes of pancreas transplants have significantly improved since the first 14 were performed at the University of Minnesota.[23]

Recent data show that the graft survival rate of whole pancreas transplant has improved to >95% at 1 year and >83% at 5 years' posttransplantation.[24] However, there are still some drawbacks to this form of treatment, including the need for major surgical intervention with associated mortality rate of up to 8% and potential associated morbidities which include graft thrombosis, pancreatic fistulae formation, and pseudocyst formation.[24] Also, patients that undergo pancreatic transplant must commit to and adhere to a "lifelong" (as long as the graft remains viable) immunosuppressive regimen that has potentially serious and life-altering side effects.[24] There have been attempts to overcome some of the associated morbidity and mortality that whole organ pancreas transplant treatment entails, by transplanting only the endocrine component of the pancreas (pancreatic islets of Langerhans).[24]

13.3.2 ISLET TRANSPLANTATION

13.3.2.1 Islet Isolation

In 1902, the idea of physically separating the endocrine tissue from the exocrine tissue prior to transplant was suggested by the Russian physician Leonid W Ssobolew.[3] In 1911, RR Bensley demonstration that islets could be stained with "neutral red" began to make this option potentially feasible.[3]

Partial pancreatic transplant was first attempted in 1924 by Pybus, who placed pieces of pancreatic tissue into the subcutaneous space of two patients, with reduction in glycosuria noted prior to rejection of the grafts.[25] Browning and Resnik, in 1951, showed that mouse fetal pancreatic tissue injected into the anterior chamber of the eye, survived longer than adult pancreatic pieces.[25] They also showed that in contrast, fetal and neonatal pieces that were implanted into the vitreous portion of the eye, the spleen, or subcutaneous tissue did not alter hyperglycemia and were also rapidly destroyed.[25] Then House, in 1958, showed that the hamster cheek pouch was an immunoprivileged site.[25] Studies by Coupland, in 1960, further demonstrated that the anterior chamber of the eye was an immune-privileged site with maintenance of and growth of islet tissue demonstrated after a year, in a rodent model.[25] Gonet in 1960 and 1965 similarly demonstrated that the testes were also an immune-privileged site.[25] As a result of these findings, the focus turned to using relatively pure fetal and neonatal endocrine islet tissue and placing it into immune-privileged sites such as the anterior chamber of the eye, testes, and the hamster cheek pouch.[25] These fetal and neonatal implant results demonstrated the potential of islet transplantation and that if placed in immune-privileged sites, they could be protected from immune destruction without immunosuppression.[25]

In 1964, Dr Hellestrom began the development of islet isolation techniques, by microscope microdissection of islets.[3] Although he had poor results regarding yield and quality, this technique continued until in Dr Moskalewski, in 1965, used a crude collagenase mixture to digest some islets out of a chopped guinea pig pancreas.[3,25] Then in 1967, Dr Paul E Lacy and Dr Mary Kostianovsky improved the current islet isolation techniques, utilizing intraductal injection of cold saline buffer to distend the pancreas to enhance collagenase release of islets, along with enzymatic digestion after harvesting and mincing the pancreas prior to final microscopic islet hand-picking.[3,25] Also, alternative purification procedures were aggressively pursued.[3] Density gradients utilizing sugar or albumin were developed.[3] Then Ficoll, a high molecular weight polymer of sucrose was introduced by Arnold Lindall at the University of Minnesota, in 1969.[3] Then after several other modifications were introduced, in 1985, Gotoh et al perfected the technique, introduced by Dr Paul E Lacy and Dr Mary in 1967, by utilizing an intraductal injection of collagenase instead of saline buffer.[3]

In 1972, Lacy and Ballinger observed an improvement, but not complete reversal of diabetes in rats that were transplanted with 400–600 islets intraperitoneally or intramuscularly.[3] Then in 1973, Reckard and Barker observed complete reversal of diabetes in rats that were transplanted with 800–1,200 islets.[3]

In 1973, the first study linking the choice of transplantation site with the outcome was performed by Charles Kemp, who demonstrated that when he transplanted 400–600 islets into the liver, he achieved complete reversal of diabetes in 24 hours.[3] However, in contrast, he had no success when he transplanted the islets into the peritoneal cavity or subcutaneously.[3] This observation significantly contributed to the liver being considered the "gold standard location for rodent as well as human islet transplant, although other sites have been evaluated.[3]

Camillo Ricordi introduced the Ricordi chamber, in 1988, which is a dissociation/filtration chamber that significantly improved the process and became the gold standard human and large animal pancreatic islet.[3] Then in 1989, Dr Lake et al reported a method that allowed large-scale purification of human islets, using the COBE 2991 processor.[3] This method remains the basis for techniques used to process human and large animal pancreatic tissue.[3]

13.3.2.2 Human Islet Allotransplantation

In 1990, Tzakis et al reported the first successful series of human islet allotransplants, using a steroid-free regimen, based on FK506.[26] This was the first study that showed long-term reversal of diabetes in humans with insulin independence.[26] This study encouraged many other centers to begin or renew their islet allotransplantation programs in places such as Edmonton, Milan, Miami, St Louis, and Minneapolis.[26] Then in 2000, the Edmonton group demonstrated long-term insulin independence in 7/7 patients.[26] Follow-up studies did show that some transplants failed to maintain long-term insulin dependence, with about one-quarter of the recipients requiring additional islet infusions by the second or third year posttransplant.[26]

However, this study stimulated greater interest in human pancreas transplant. After the first Edmonton report was released, several individual centers combined into larger multicenter groups, including: the Group Rhin-Rhone-Alpes-Geneve pour la Transplantation d'Ilots de Langerhans (GRAGIL) network in France and Switzerland, the Nordic Network for Clinical Islet Transplantation in the Scandinavian countries, and the Clinical Islet Transplant Consortium, which was international but concentrated in North America.[27] Such consortia allowed larger groups to collaborate and benefit from expertise at other experienced centers, facilitate sharing among members, and enabled streamlining of procurement, isolation, and transplantation procedures.[27]

The Immune Tolerance Network funded 10 centers around the world to participate in a multicenter trial of the Edmonton Protocol.[28] The National Institutes of Health (NIH) proposed six and later funded nine US centers to become "Islet Cell Resources" for the isolation, purification, and characterization of human pancreatic islet cells for transplantation into diabetic patients.[28] In addition, the Clinical Islet Transplant Consortium, also funded by the NIH, allocated $75 million to five centers to conduct a large-scale clinical trial of islet transplantation and to translate the practice of islet transplantation from clinical research to a clinical practice.[28]

Although dramatic progress has been made in islet transplantation, there remains difficulty in achieving consistent long-term graft function and insulin independence.[24] Also, the need for lifelong (at least for the life of the graft) immunosuppression to prevent islet rejection exposes the patients to potentially life altering, serious morbidities associated with chronic immunosuppression, such as development of renal dysfunction, increased susceptibility to infection, and increased risk of cancer.[24] In addition, nonimmunosuppressive as well as immunosuppressive factors may lead to graft failure.[24] These factors include poor islet quality, insufficient islet mass, poor vascularization, relative hypoxia of the transplanted islets, and instant blood-mediated inflammatory reaction.[24] It has also been discovered that various immunosuppressants, themselves, can have a deleterious effect on the pancreatic islets and lead to graft failure. Factors such as these have helped to continue to fuel the search for alternative solutions.[24]

In 1994, Soon Shiong transplanted an intraperitoneal infusion of pancreatic islets encapsulated in alginate polylysine alginate microcapsule.[24] He first infused 10,000 islet equivalents/kg, followed by another 5,000 islet equivalents/kg infusion 6 months later.[24] He reported that he achieved tight glycemic control for 9 months posttransplantation.[24]

Then in 2006, Calafiore intraperitoneally transplanted human islets microencapsulated within alginate Polyornithine Alginate (PLO) microcapsules into four nonimmunosuppressed patients.[24,29,30] All the patients were tested positive for C-peptide throughout 3 years of posttransplant follow-up.[24,29,30] Exogenous insulin needs were reduced in all four patients, with transient insulin independence noted in one patient.[24,29,30] No induction of HLA class 1 or class 2 antibodies was noted, and all the patients were tested negative for anti-GAD65 antibodies.[24,29,30] By 7 years post-transplant, however, all patients were again insulin-dependent on at least their original exogenous insulin regimen.[24,29,30]

Interestingly, one patient required an abdominal exploration for abdominal discomfort and was noted to have a cyst formation, with a fibrotic lump that contained mostly intact microcapsules with no viable islets.[24,30]

Other trials, such as "the seaweed diabetes trial," have looked at different microcapsule formations for human islet transplantation, with variable results.[24]

13.3.2.3 Islet Xenotransplantation

In 1994, CG Groth et al reported transplantation of fetal porcine islet-like cell clusters to 10 insulin-dependent diabetic kidney transplant patients.[27,28] In this study, the islets were transplanted into the portal vein of eight patients and under the kidney capsule in two patients.[28] All recipients were administered either antithymoglobulin or 15-deoxyspergualin for induction and then they were maintained on standard immunosuppressive regimens.[28] Four of the patients who received transplants in the portal vein secreted porcine c-peptide into the urine for 200–400 days.[28] Biopsy was performed on one of the patients who received islet-like cell clusters under the kidney capsule, and the sample was positive for insulin and glucagon immunostaining.[28] Unfortunately, none of the patients had a reduction in daily insulin dose during the study.[28] Despite any apparent lack of clinical benefit, this study suggested that porcine pancreatic endocrine tissue could survive in humans.[28]

In 2005, a report was published from Mexico in which 12 adolescents with type 1 diabetes were implanted with macroencapsulated neonatal porcine islets and sertoli cells.[28,31] Each patient had two devices implanted in the subcutaneous layer of their upper anterior abdominal wall, which was left in place for 2 months to allow the formation of vascularized collagen tissue.[31] Then the rod portion of the devices was removed and 250,000 islets with 30–100 sertoli cells were then transplanted into the devices of each patient.[31] Eleven patients then required a second transplant 6–9 months later.[31] Daily insulin doses decreased in six patients and was increased in six patients.[28] Two patients achieved insulin independence.[31] The mean glycated Hemoglobin (HgbA1C) went from being >10% pretransplant, to being <10% posttransplant.[31] After the initial trial, additional subjects were added. There were 21 total patients included in the study.[31] Urinary porcine c-peptide was detectable for several years posttransplant, and the overall incidence of diabetic complications was much lower than expected.[31,32]

In 2007, Living Cells Technology reported on the outcome of a trial that they had initiated in 1996.[24] In this study they transplanted porcine islets encapsulated in alginate–PLO microcapsules, intraperitoneally into a 41-year-old Caucasian male with type 1 diabetes, utilizing a 15,000-islet equivalent/kg aliquot.[24] By 90 days posttransplant, his exogenous insulin requirements had reduced by 30%, and his HgbA1C reflected improved glycemic control.[24] His C-peptide levels peaked at 4 months and remained detectable at 11 months.[24] By 11 months, however, his graft became nonfunctional and his exogenous insulin dose returned to at least pretransplant level.[24] He underwent a laparoscopy that revealed opaque nodules throughout the omentum and mesentery.[24] Interestingly, there were no signs of peritoneal reaction or fibrosis.[24] Biopsies of the nodules showed opaque microcapsules with intact live cell clusters that stained sparsely for insulin and glucagon and produced small amounts of insulin in response to in vitro glucose challenge.[24] He was monitored long-term and showed no evidence of porcine viral or retroviral infection.[24]

In 2007, a report was published from New Zealand, of neonatal porcine islets encapsulated in alginate–polylysine–alginate with sustained response of the islets.[28] By 12 weeks posttransplant, the average daily insulin dose had been reduced by about 30%, but then returned to pretransplant levels by 49 weeks posttransplant.[28] Urinary porcine c-peptide was detected up to 11 months posttransplant.[28] The HgbA1c decreased from a pretransplant level of 9.3%–7.8% at 14 months posttransplant.[28] Also, at 5 years posttransplant a biopsy sample was still immunohistochemically positive for insulin and glucagon.[28] In 2009, the islet group in Pittsburgh demonstrated long-term islet graft function, for up to 1 year, in streptozocin-induced diabetic nonhuman primates transplanted with pig islets genetically modified to express a human complementary-regulatory protein (hCD46).[27] The expression of hCD46 was designed to limit antibody-mediated rejection and allow for reduction in immunosuppression.[27] It did not, however, reduce initial islet loss.[27] In 2014, they achieved comparable success with a multitransgenic pig that had four modified genes: GTKO; hCD46; human tissue factor pathway inhibitor, for antithrombosis and anti-inflammatory effects; and CTL4-Ig, to inhibit cellular immune response.[27] They again successfully maintained islet engraftment and function for up to 1 year.[27]

At the Seoul National University in Korea, CG Park and colleagues successfully maintained normoglycemia in diabetic primates after porcine islet transplantation for >600 days.[27] Both the Pittsburgh and Seoul studies utilized anti-CD154 monoclonal antibody-based immunosuppression to prevent rejection.[27] This agent, however, has unfortunately been associated with thromboembolic complications in humans, and so this study is not clinically translatable to humans.[27] In 2012, a phase 1 & 2 trial was conducted in Russia, during which neonatal porcine islets encapsulated in alginate–poly L ornithine–alginate were transplanted into seven patients with type 1 diabetes, with each patient receiving one to three rounds of transplants.[28] No marked adverse events were reported.[28] Five patients had improvement in blood glucose; and two patients achieved insulin independence for up to 32 weeks.[28]

A 2012 report of a phase 1/2 trial was conducted by Diabecell in New Zealand and Russia, involving transplantation of encapsulated porcine islets into 14 type 1 diabetic patients.[24] In this study, they transplanted the first 4 patients with 10,000 islet equivalents (IEQ)/kg and achieved 76% reduction in hypoglycemic awareness after 7–12 months follow-up posttransplant.[24] Another four patients were transplanted with 15,000 IEQ/kg, and four other patients were transplanted with 20,000 IEQ/kg, and the last two patients were transplanted with 5,000 IEQ/kg.[24] Reportedly the level of HgbA1C has been <7% for more than 600 days, with a significant reduction of hypoglycemic events.[24]

There is major concern about transmission of porcine pathogenic microorganisms and porcine endogenous retroviruses (PERV).[28] Despite this concern, reviews of humans that have received porcine xenotransplant products have revealed no PERV infections by Polymerase Chain Reaction analysis.[28,33] Also, techniques whereby some PERV genes can be inactivated by CRISPR-CAS9 technology has been developed.[28,34]

The International Transplantation Association published an islet xenotransplantation consensus statement regarding the conditions for undertaking clinical trials of porcine islet products. This consensus statement covered several major areas of concern, and had a strong focus on safety.[28,35] A study following these new guidelines was undertaken in New Zealand and reported in 2014.[28] This study concluded that encapsulated neonatal porcine islets xenotransplantation was safe and resulted in reduced episodes of unaware hypoglycemia in unstable type 1 diabetic patients.[28] They noted in this study that tests for PERV DNA and RNA were negative in the blood of all patients and that the number of unaware hypoglycemic episodes were reduced after 1-year posttransplant.[28]

Phase I, IIA, and IIb clinical trials of porcine islet xenotransplantation (diabecell) were also performed in Argentina from 2012 to 2014, and during this study, treated patients were maintained at HgbA1c <7 for >600 days.[28,36,37]

13.4 BIOARTIFICIAL PANCREAS SYSTEMS

13.4.1 Immunoisolation

These limitations helped to fuel the ongoing quest for development of a bioartificial pancreas. Glycemic variability has been shown to improve with islet transplantation.

There have been several studies that have shown high levels of insulin independence, and good control of hypoglycemia can be obtained in the short term with islet transplantation, with other studies showing improvements in medium- to long-term outcomes.[19]

There have been four main structural approaches towards this end: (i) microdevices that encapsulate individual islets or small groups of islets within spherically shaped capsules that provide the permselective function, (ii) conformal coatings placing a thin covering around individual islets that is permselective, (iii) nanoencapsulation and layer-by-layer coatings, which place a thin film of protection on each islet, and (iv) macrodevices that hold the islets within a major structure with selective permeability component on the perimeter of the device.[25,38]

13.4.2 MICROENCAPSULATION

Microcapsule formation was used for many industrial applications in the 1930s.[17] Thomas MS Chang perfected the world's first artificial cell.[25] He encapsulated hemoglobin in a semipermeable plastic bag that functioned nearly as well as a red cell.[25] He coined the term "microencapsulation".[39]

Biscegli was the first researcher to pioneer the transplantation of encapsulated tissue when he placed mouse tumor cells in a polymer matrix, which he then transplanted into the abdomen of a guinea pig, after which he was able to maintain the host's survival without rejection.[40] Then in 1980, Lim and Sun published studies showing successful encapsulation of pancreatic islets.[25] This led to widespread pursuit of islet encapsulation as a treatment for diabetes.[25]

Microcapsule droplets are typically made after suspending the islets in a solution, then generating droplets from this solution by various methods including air jet spray method, electrostatic generators, internal gelation emulsion, submerged oscillating coaxial extrusion nozzles, conformal coatings, or spinning disk atomization.[41] In our work, the approach that we had adopted in islet microencapsulation involves the generation of alginate microbeads embedded with islets followed by permselective coating with PLO tissue with a final coating with alginate, to enhance tissue biocompatibility with the construct after implantation, as illustrated in Figure 13.1.[42–45] Figure 13.2 shows the insulin response to changes in glucose concentrations in a dynamic perfusion system of encapsulated rat islets from our lab.

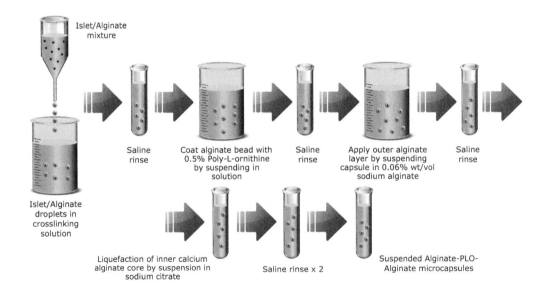

FIGURE 13.1 Brief description of our initial islet microencapsulation process, which has since been modified: (a) Suspend islets in alginate solution; (b) Remove excess solution, rinse with saline, remove excess saline; (c) Suspend in poly-L-ornithine solution; (d) Remove excess solution, rinse with saline, remove excess saline; (e) Suspend in alginate solution; (f) Remove excess alginate solution, rinse with saline, remove excess saline; (g) Suspend in sodium citrate solution; (h) Remove excess sodium citrate solution, rinse with saline twice; (i) Additional treatments can be done at this point, as desired/warranted.

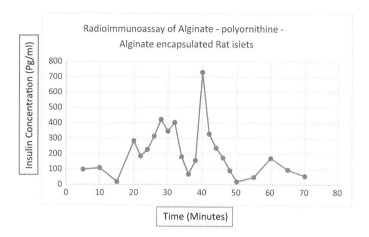

FIGURE 13.2 Rat islets encapsulated in Alginate–polyornithine–alginate microcapsules: Encapsulated islets were exposed to a 3.3 mM glucose solution and perfused for 20 minutes, they were then exposed to a 16.7 mM glucose solution and perfused for 30 minutes. They were then exposed to a 3.3 mM glucose solution and perfused for another 20 minutes. Samples were collected every 5 minutes for the first 20 minutes, then every 2 minutes for the next 30 minutes, and then every 5 minutes for the last 20 minutes. Radioimmunoassay of each sample was subsequently performed, with results as shown.

One major challenge that significantly impacts the applicability of microencapsulation for islet transplantation is the biocompatibility of the materials used for encapsulation.[46] Conceptually an ideally biocompatible microcapsule would be immunologically inert and would be free from immunologic responses such as fibrotic overgrowth, which would encourage long-term islet cell survival.[46]

As part of the quest to find the ideal material, various natural and synthetic materials have been investigated for use in islet encapsulation. They have included: alginate, chitosan, agarose, cellulose, copolymers of acrylonitrile, xanthan, polyethylene glycol (PEG), polyvinyl alcohol, polyurethane, poly (ether) sulfone, polypropylene, sodium polystyrene sulfate, Alginate/aminopropyl-silicate, electrospun nylon, polyacrylates (such as poly-hydroxyethylmetacrylate-methyl methacrylate, dimethylaminoethyl methacrylate, polyacrilonitrile, and polyacrylamide), polyepoxides, polyamides, polyphosphazenes, biodritin, amino-propyl silicate, saccharide-peptide hydrogel, and AN69.[41,46–63]

13.4.2.1 Alginate-Based Microcapsules

Alginate is an unbranched binary copolymer of 1-4 linked β-D-mannuronic and α-L-guluronic acid that can be isolated from algae species, including *Laminaria hyperborea*, *Macrocystis pyrifera*, *Ascophyllum nodosum*, *Laminaria digitata*, *Ascophyllum nodosum*, *Laminaria japonica*, *Eclonia maxima*, *Lessonia nigrescens*, *Durvillea antarctica*, and *Sargassum* spp,[62] can also be found as a polysaccharide in bacteria such as *Azotobacter vinelandii* and *Pseudomonades*.[62]

The alginate is typically extracted by treating the algae with aqueous alkali solutions, commonly with sodium hydroxide (NaOH).[58] Then either sodium or calcium chloride is added to the filtrate to precipitate the alginate.[64] The alginate salt can then be transformed into alginic acid by treatment with dilute hydrodrochloric acid (HCl).[64] After further purification and conversion, water-soluble sodium-alginate powder can be produced.[64]

The two major amino acid polymers that are typically utilized in forming alginate microcapsules are poly-L-lysine (PLL) and poly-L ornithine (PLO).[65] PLO is thought by some researchers to have better performance, regarding preventing the infiltration of the immune system into the microcapsule.[65] It also seems to show more resistance against mechanical stresses, such as changes in osmotic pressure.[65] Conversely, some researchers have suggested that PLL is less immunogenic than PLO.[66]

Several studies have evaluated the use of barium, rather than PLL or PLO to form barium alginate microcapsules.[24] While some studies have suggested that high G barium alginate microcapsules produced higher strength, more stable microcapsules, with less permeability compared to IgG.[24] Further studies, however, revealed that the pericapsular fibrotic overgrowth directed towards the alginate microcapsules seemed to be species specific with no or very little response noted in small animals, like rodents, but a strong response when transplanted into larger animals like pigs and baboons.[24]

It has also been suggested that microcapsules made from high G alginate are stronger, more stable, and undergo less swelling than microcapsules made from high M alginate.[24] This is thought to occur because it is thought that divalent cations that are used in the capsule formation process are thought to bind more strongly to the G residues than they do to the M residues.[24]

Efforts to attempt to decrease the immunogenicity and reduce the immune reaction have included modification of the surface chemistry of alginate microcapsules.[24] Some studies have shown that coating alginate–chitosan microcapsules with methoxy poly (ethylene glycol) (MPEG) can create a more biocompatible and protein-repellent surface that prevents gamma globulin (IgG) and fibrinogen protein adsorption, which are key components of pericapsular fibrotic overgrowth (PFO) formation.[24] In another study empty (no islets) genipin-modified alginate PLO alginate microcapsules exhibited improved hydrophilicity and biocompatibility with less observed PFO, upon transplantation into the peritoneal cavity of mice.[24] Unfortunately, when islets were encapsulated in the same formulation, however, the biocompatibility was significantly reduced.[24]

It has been noted that in the posttransplantation period the host response often starts with nonspecific protein adsorption, which subsequently leads to adhesion of immune cells and fibroblasts unto the capsule surface.[63] This process has been termed "biofouling"; several studies have focused on trying to find ways to modify the outer layer of the transplanted microcapsules in order to abrogate this process (a process called "antibiofouling").[63] PEG is one of the most commonly applied molecules utilized to try to prevent or decrease this process.[63] It has been noted that the efficacy of the PEG molecules depends on variables such as chain density, length, and conformation of the utilized molecules, with the protein resistance of a PEG surface proportionally increasing with higher polymerization degrees and denser brush bristles on the surface.[63] PEG has been applied to coat alginate capsules in an effort to lower permeability and enhance mechanical stability but also to serve as an antibiofouling layer.[63] Several other agents are being evaluated with varying results.[24]

Other attempts to decrease PFO include coencapsulation of islets with immunomodulatory companions or bioengineered cells.[24] Various materials and substances such as Sertoli cells, mesenchymal stem cells, and genetically modified cells have been studied with some favorable results.[24]

Short-term use of immunosuppressants, for 10–30 days, in order to decrease or prevent the development of PFO, has also been evaluated.[24] Some researchers, however, think that this would defeat the ultimate goal of the encapsulation strategy, so not many research groups are pursuing this strategy.[24]

13.4.2.2 Nanoencapsulation

Conformal coatings or layer-by-layer coatings involve the application of hydrogels to the surface of islets or other cell aggregates to form nanoliter droplet crosslinked coatings. This allows "shrink wrap type coating" of islet cell clusters.[24,25,67]

Unfortunately, although transplantation of conformally coated porcine islets led to normalization of blood sugar after transplantation into nonimmunosuppressed diabetic rodents, similar success was not obtained when similar microencapsulated islets were transplanted into larger animals.[24] This was thought to at least be in part due to a strong immune response against the PEG coatings that occurred in larger animal models.[24] Modification of the PEG component, so as to improve binding to photoinitiators and accelerate crosslinking to make them less reactive in large animals, led to decreased hypoglycemic episodes in a subsequent study involving two type 1 diabetic patients; however, none of the patients achieved insulin independence, and their C-peptide levels were lower than expected.[24]

The layer-by-layer technique allows for polyelectrolyte layers to be made by alternate deposition of oppositely charged polyions onto charged substrates using self-assembly processes of polymers involving electrostatic interactions.[68]

This method significantly reduces the capsule thickness, which is thought to improve the insulin release kinetics, and to promote diffusion of metabolites and waste products.[24]

Various materials have been used to form the layers including PEG (which is the most commonly used polymer), polystyrene sulfonate, polyallylamine, polyvinyl alcohol, hyaluronic acid, and PLL.[24,68]

13.4.3 MACROENCAPSULATION

Macrocapsules are typically larger devices that tend to possess a planar or cylindrical geometry and a smaller surface-to-volume ratio.[69]

There are three major types of macroencapsulation devices, which include (i) extravascular diffusion devices. These macrocapsule devices are typically placed outside of the vasculature, in locations such as the peritoneal cavity, the subcutaneous tissue, or an omental pocket; (ii) intravascular diffusion devices. Such devices are connected to vasculature in such a way that the functional part of the devices is located within an artery and (iii) intravascular ultrafiltration devices, which are connected to an artery, but also have a connection that allows for delivery of insulin into a vein.[25]

13.4.4 EXTRAVASCULAR DIFFUSION DEVICES

Extravascular diffusion devices depend on diffusive transport.[70]

In 1933, Bisceglie published the results of implanted insulinoma cells in a permselective membrane to determine the effect of loss of vasculature on survival of implanted tissues.[25] Several types of diffusion devices were designed, including devices made by the Millipore Corporation, Amicon, and Cytotherapeutics.[25] The use of hydrogels, such as AN69 (which is a copolymer of acrylonitrile and sodium methallyl sulfonate), polyvinyl alcohol and agarose have been studied over the last few decades as a means to achieve greater biocompatibility for microencapsulation, with variable degrees of success.[70]

Baxter Healthcare then introduced a "pouch-like" device in the 1990s, which was a planar device of two composite membranes sealed at all sides with a loading port or ports.[25,70] The outside of the device was designed to encourage capillary ingrowth in one section and also had a semipermeable hydrogel membrane for allograft immune protection.[25,70] This device eventually became the theracyte device.[25,70]

Qi et al introduced a sheet-type macroencapsulation device using polyvinyl alcohol hydrogel in 2004.[68] Dufrane et al created a monolayer cellular device in 2010.[64] Both of these devices showed a decrease in hyperglycemia during animal studies.[70]

Islets were seeded as a monolayer on an acellular collagen matrix.[68] This configuration seemed to enhance their interaction with a biologic membrane and increased islet concentration per surface area.[70]

Toleikis et al created a pouch which consisted of a multichannel sheet inserted with an array of rods in 2010.[68] The device was placed under the skin for a month to create better vascular integration, then the rods were removed to expose channels that allowed the infusion of transplanted islets into the device.[70]

β Air devices focused on creating devices that contained an empty portion of the device connected to tubing that allows for daily replacement of oxygen through external tubing and then an islet containing chamber.[63,71,72]

At least two different prototypes were developed.[73] They differed in the surface area of the islet containing slab, method of gas chamber ventilation, and the composition of the infused gas mixture.[73]

One of the most serious drawbacks noted during the pursuit of this technology has been loss of viability of the transplanted islets due to central necrosis of the tissue clusters.[70] In addition, immunologic rejection of the pancreatic cells tends to occur, due to various factors such as mechanical rupture of the membranes, biochemical instability, islet cell heterogeneity, and the broad distribution of pore sizes in the encapsulation materials (which affects the ability of antibodies and cytokines to be sufficiently excluded in many hydrogel macrocapsules).[70]

13.4.5 POLYMER SCAFFOLDS

Scaffolds have been explored as a means of recreating and mimicking the pancreatic environment.[74] Both natural and synthetic polymers have been utilized in these efforts.[74]

Several studies have focused on creating pancreatic scaffolds that try to provide a microenvironmental niche that is similar to the complex extracellular matrix (ECM) environment that pancreatic islets are normally exposed to in vivo.[74–81]

Several synthetic and/or microfabricated materials have been utilized, such as silk-based hydrogels, poly (lactide-co-glycolide) (PLG) scaffolds, chitosan/poly(lactic-co-glycolic acid) (PLGA), scaffolds, collagen-based scaffolds with incorporated oxygen generating and/or vessel generating compounds, nonwoven/sponge fabrics in a hyaluronan-based scaffold, and an injectable saccharide-peptide gel.[70, 74–82]

Some researchers have experimented with the addition of ECM components such as fibrin and fibronectin, as well as modifications of the configuration of the scaffold.[74–81]

In addition, utilization of biologic materials such as decellularized pancreatic tissue and decellularized pericardium have been studied.[75–79]

13.4.6 INTRAVASCULAR DIFFUSION DEVICES

In 1972, Knazek demonstrated, in vitro, that multiple fiber devices with islets implanted in the walls of the hollow fibers and perfused with culture medium were able to maintain viable islets.[25] This led to the development of similar devices that were then developed and anastomosed intravascularly.[25]

There were issues with bleeding and/or clotting, with both intravascular diffusion chambers and intravascular ultrafiltration chambers. This led to various modifications of the original designs.[25,39]

One such design leads to successful insulin independence in a large animal xenograft model for many months.[25] However, one of the last surviving dogs died of acute blood loss due to breakdown of the arterial device connection, just as the Food and Drug Administration (FDA) approval process was proceeding.[25] This caused the clinical trial to be denied and subsequent funding withdrawn.[25]

Other studies, including a pilot study utilizing a device that contained a silicon nanopore membrane with xeno-transplanted pancreatic islets, were anastomosed to the internal carotid artery and the external jugular vein in a pig model.[83] The results were reportedly promising. There was high islet viability posttransplant (>85%) along with C-peptide concentration of 144 pM noted in the outflow ultrafiltrate.[83]

13.5 CONCLUSION

Diabetes continues to be a scourge on our society, with individuals that are afflicted with this disease, being subjected to a dramatic life-changing process. They are subjected to the continuous need for serial glucose monitoring. Without the intervention of a pancreas or pancreatic islet transplant, they ultimately require either oral diabetic medications or administration of insulin, depending on the type of diabetes that they are afflicted with. The usage of implantable devices, such as the insulin pump or variations of the artificial pancreas, has had some success in controlling the associated hyperglycemia. As discussed above, the various exogenous insulin treatment modalities, including the insulin pump and the artificial pancreas are all fraught with potential complications, such as the potential for life-threatening hypoglycemia. Successful development of a reproducible and reliable bioartificial pancreas should provide a better treatment modality that should have less morbidity, as it should more closely mimic the physiologic responses of endogenous insulin and be able to avoid the need for immunosuppressive medications and their associated potential comorbidities. With continued efforts, we hope to successfully solve this challenging conundrum one day. Such work continues in the lab of my mentor Dr Emmanuel Opara and other laboratories around the world.

REFERENCES

1. Johnson RJ, Sanchez-Lozada LG, Andrews P, Lanaspa MA. Perspective: A historical and scientific perspective of sugar and its relation with obesity and diabetes. *Adv. Nutr.* 2017. 8: 412–422.
2. Notelovitz M. Milestones in the history of diabetes – A brief survey. *SA Med. J.* 1970 Oct 10. 44(40): 1158–1161.
3. Ramirez-Dominguez M. Historical background of pancreatic islet isolation. Advances in Experimental Medicine and Biology. *Springer* September 2016. 938 1–9. doi:10.1007/978-3-319-30924-2_1.
4. Hoet JP. Gustave edouard laguesse: His demonstration of the significance of the islands of Langerhans. *Diabetes* 1953 July–Aug. 2(4): 322–324.
5. King KM, Rubin G. A history of diabetes: From antiquity to discovering insulin. *Brit. J. Nurs.* 2002 Oct-Oct 22. 12(18): 1091–1095.
6. Zajac J, Shrestha A, Patel P, Poretsky L. The main events in the history of diabetes mellitus. (In Poretsky L, Eds) *Princ. Diabetes Mellitus.* 3–16. doi:10.1007/978-0-387-09841-8_1.
7. Ahmed AM. History of diabetes mellitus. *Saudi Med. J.* 2002. 23(4): 373–378.
8. Ionescu-Tirgoviste C, Buda O. Nicolae constantin paulescu: The first explicit description of the internal secretion of the pancreas. *Act. Med. Hist. Adriat.* 2017 Dec. 15(2): 303–322.
9. Sonksen PH. The evolution of insulin treatment. *Clin. Endocrinol. Metab.* 1977. 6(2): 481–497.
10. Nishida K, Shimoda S, Ichinose K, Araki E, Shichiri M. What is artificial endocrine pancreas? Mechanism and history. *World J Gastroenterol.* 2009 Sept 7. 15(33): 4105–4110.
11. Latres E, Finan DA, Greenstein JL, Kowalski A, Kieffer TJ. Navigating two roads to glucose normalization in diabetes: Automated insulin delivery devices and cell therapy. *Cell Metab.* 2019. 29(3): 545–563. doi:10.1016/j.cmet.2019.02.007.
12. Allen N, Gupta A. Current diabetes technology: Striving for the artificial pancreas. *Diagnostics* 2019. 9: 31. doi:10.3390/diagnostics9010031.
13. Dadlani V, Pinsker JE, Dassau E, Kudva YC. Advances in closed-loop insulin delivery systems in patients with type 1 diabetes. *Curr. Diabetes Rep.* 2018. 18: 88. doi:10.1007/s11892-018-1051-z.
14. Kovatchev B. A century of diabetes technology: Signals, models, and artificial pancreas control. *Trends Endocrin. Metab.* 2019 July. 30(7): doi:10.1016/j.tem.2019.04.008.
15. Bally L, Thabit H, Hovorka R. Finding the right route for insulin delivery – An overview of implantable pump therapy. *Expert Opin. Drug Deliv.* 2017 Sept. 14(9): 1103–1111. doi:10.1080/17425247.2017.1267138.
16. Bekiari E, Kitsios K, Thabit H, Tauschmann M, Athanasiadou E, Karagiannis T, Haidich AB, Hovorka R, Tsapas A. Artificial pancreas treatment for outpatients with type 1 diabetes: Systematic review and meta-analysis. *BMJ* 2018. 361: k1310. doi:10.1136/bmj.k1310.
17. Bally L, Thabit H, Kojzar H, Mader JK, Qerimi-Hyseni J, Hartnell S, Tauschmann M, Allen JM, Wilinska ME, Pieber TR, Evans ML, Hovorka R. Day-and-night glycaemic control with closed-loop insulin delivery versus conventional insulin pump therapy in free-living adults with well controlled type 1 diabetes: An open-label, randomised, crossover study. Lancet Diabetes Endocrinol. 2017 April. 5(4): 261–270. www.thelancet.com/diabetes-endocrinology.
18. Nijhoff MF, de Koning EJP. Artificial pancreas or novel beta-cell replacement therapies: A race for optimal glycemic control? *Curr. Diab. Rep.* 2018. 18: 110. doi:10.1007/s11892-018-1073-6.
19. Holmes-Walker DJ, Gunton JE, Hawthorne W, Payk M, Anderson P, Donath S, Lloudovaris T, Ward GW, Kay TWH, O'Connell PJ. Islet transplantation provides superior glycemic control with less hypoglycemia compared with continuous subcutaneous insulin infusion or multiple daily insulin injections. *Transplantation* 2017. 101: 1268–1275.
20. Starzl TE, Thai N, Shapiro R. The history of pancreas transplantation. In *Pancreatic Transplantation.* 1st Ed. 2006. doi:10.3109/9781420016666.
21. Squifflet JP. *Kidney and Pancreas Transplantation: The History of Surgical Techniques and Immunosuppression.* Intech open. Current Issues and future direction in kidney transplantation. 2013. doi:10.5772/55347.

22. Busnardo AC, Didio LJA, Tidrick RT, Thomford NR. History of the pancreas. *Am. J. Surg.* 1983. 146: 539–550.
23. Sutherland DER, Gores PF, Farney AC, Wahoff DC, Matas AJ, Dunn DL, Gruessner RWG, Najarian JS. Evolution of kidney, pancreas, and islet transplantation for patients with diabetes at the University of Minnesota. 1993. *Am. J. Surg.* 166: 456–490.
24. Vaithilingham V, Bal S, Touch BE. Encapsulated islet transplantation: Where do we stand? *Rev. Diab. Stud.* 2017. 14(1): 51–78. doi:10.1900/RDS.2016.14.51.
25. Scharp DW, Marchetti P. Encapsulated islets for diabetes therapy: History, current progress, and critical issues requiring solution. *Adv. Drug Deliv. Rev.* 2014 Apr. 67–68: 35–73. doi:10.1016/j.addr.2013.07.018. Epub 2013 Aug 1.
26. Ricordi C, Strom TB. Clinical islet transplantation: Advances and immunological challenges. *Nat. Rev. Immunol.* 2004 Apr. 4: 259–268.
27. Bottino R, Knoll MF, Knoll CA, Bertera S, Trucco MM. The future of islet transplantation is now. *Front Med (Lausanne)* 2018 Jul 13. 5: 202. doi:10.3389/fmed.2018.00202. eCollection 2018.
28. Matsumoto S, Tomiya M, Sawamoto O. Current status and future of clinical islet xenotransplantation. *J. Diabetes.* 2016 Jul. 8(4): 483–493. doi:10.1111/1753-0407.12395.
29. Calafiore R, Basta G, Luca G, Lemmi A, Montanucci MP, Calabrese G, Racanicchi L, Mancuso F, Paolo BP. Microencapsulated pancreatic islet allografts into nonimmunosuppressed patients with type 1 diabetes. *Diab. Care* 2006. 29(1): 137–138.
30. Basta G, Montanucci P, Luca G, Boselli C, Noya G, Barbaro B, Qi M, Kinzer KP, Oberholzer J, Calafiore R. Long-term metabolic and immunological follow-up of nonimmunosuppressed patients with type 1 diabetes treated with microencapsulated islet allografts. *Diab. Care* 2011. 34: 2406–2409.
31. Valdes-Gonzalez R, Rodriguez-Ventura AL, White DJ, Bracho-Blanchet E, Castillo A, Ramírez-González B, López-Santos MG, León-Mancilla BH, Dorantes LM. Long-term follow-up of patients with type 1 diabetes transplanted with neonatal pig islets. *Clin. Exp. Immunol.* 2010 Dec. 162(3): 537–542. doi:10.1111/j.1365-2249.2010.04273.x. Epub 2010 Oct 21.
32. Berney T, Ricordi C. Islet cell transplantation: The future? *Langenbeck Arch. Surg.* 2000. 385: 373–378.
33. Denner J, Scobie L, Schuurman HJ. Is it currently possible to evaluate the risk posed by PERVs for clinical xenotransplantation? *Xenotransplantation* 2018 Jul. 25(4): e12403. doi:10.1111/xen.12403. Epub 2018 May 13.
34. Scobie L, Denner J, Schuurman HJ. Inactivation of porcine endogenous retrovirus in pigs using CRISPR-Cas9, editorial commentary. *Xenotransplantation* 2017 Nov. 24(6): doi:10.1111/xen.12363. Epub 2017 Nov 12.
35. Hering BJ, O'Connell PJ. First update of the international xenotransplantation association consensus statement on conditions for undertaking clinical trials of porcine islet products in type 1 diabetes-Chapter 6: Patient selection for pilot clinical trials of islet xenotransplantation. *Xenotransplantation* 2016 Jan–Feb. 23(1): 60–76. doi:10.1111/xen.12228. Epub 2016 Feb 26.
36. Aghazadeh Y, Nostro MC. Cell therapy for type 1 diabetes: Current and future strategies. *Curr. Diab. Rep.* 2017 Jun. 17(6): 37. doi:10.1007/s11892-017-0863-6.
37. Matsumoto S, Abalovich A, Wechsler C, Wynyard S, Elliott RB. Clinical benefit of islet xenotransplantation for the treatment of type 1 diabetes mellitus. *EBioMedicine* 2016. 12: 255–262. Elsevier. EBiomedicine.com. (http://creativecommons.org/licenses/by-nc-nd/4.0/).
38. O'Sullivan ES, Vegas A, Anderson DG, Weir GC. Islets transplanted in immunoisolation devices: A review of the progress and the challenges that remain. *Endocr. Rev.* 2011 Dec. 32(6): 827–844. doi:10.1210/er.2010-0026. Epub 2011 Sep 27.
39. Schweicher J, Nyitray C, Desai TA. Membranes to achieve immunoprotection of transplanted islets. *Front Biosci. (Landmark Ed.)* 2014 Jan. 1(19): 49–76.
40. Lee S, Sathialingam M, Alexander M, Lakey J. Physical protection of pancreatic islets for transplantation. In *Biomaterials-Physics and Chemistry-New Edition.* 2017. IntechOpen. doi:10.5772/Intechopen.71285.
41. Pareta R, Sanders B, Babbar P, Soker T, Booth C, McQuilling J, Sivanandane S, Stratta RJ, Orlando G, Opara EC. Immunoisolation: Where regenerative medicine meets solid organ transplantation. *Expert Rev. Clin. Immunol.* 2012 Sep. 8(7): 685–692. doi:10.1586/eci.12.64.
42. McQuilling JP, Opara EC. Methods for incorporating oxygen-generating biomaterials into cell culture and microcapsule systems. In: Opara E. (ed) *Cell Microencapsulation. Methods in Molecular Biology.* 2017, vol 1479. Humana Press, New York, NY.
43. Opara EC, Mirmalek-Sani SH, Khanna O, Moya ML, Brey EM. Design of a bioartificial pancreas. *J. Investig. Med.* 2010 Oct. 58(7): 831–837. doi:10.231/JIM.0b013e3181ed3807.

44. Khanna O, Moya ML, Opara EC, Brey EM. Synthesis of multilayered alginate microcapsules for the sustained release of fibroblast growth factor-1. *J. BioMed. Mat. Res.* 2010 19 August. 95(2): 632–640. doi:10.1002/jbm.a.32883.

45. Opara EC. Applications of cell microencapsulation. In: Opara E. (ed) *Cell Microencapsulation. Methods in Molecular Biology.* 2017, vol 1479. Humana Press, New York, NY.

46. Omami M, McGarrigle JJ, Reedy M, Isa D, Ghani S, Marchese E, Bochenek MA, Longi M, Xing Y, Joshi I, Wang Y, Oberholzer J. Islet microencapsulation: Strategies and clinical status in diabetes. *Curr. Diab. Rep.* 2017. 17: 47. doi:10.1007/s11892-017-0877-0.

47. Risbud M, Hardikar A, Bhonde R. Chitosan-polyvinyl pyrrolidone hydrogels as candidate for islet immunoisolation: In vitro biocompatibility evaluation. *Cell Transplant.* 2000 Jan–Feb. 9(1): 25–31.

48. de Vos P, Lazarjani HA, Poncelet D, Faas MM. Polymers in cell encapsulation from an enveloped cell perspective. *Adv. Drug Deliv. Rev.* 2014 Apr. 67–68: 15–34. doi:10.1016/j.addr.2013.11.005. Epub 2013 Nov 22.

49. Orive G, Santos E, Poncelet D, Hernández RM, Pedraz JL, Wahlberg LU, De Vos P, Emerich D. Cell encapsulation: Technical and clinical advances. *Trends Pharmacol. Sci.* 2015 Aug. 36(8): 537–546. doi:10.1016/j.tips.2015.05.003. Epub 2015 Jun 8.

50. Maria-Engler SS, Mares-Guia M, Correa ML, Oliveira EM, Aita CA, Krogh K, Genzini T, Miranda MP, Ribeiro M, Vilela L, Noronha IL, Eliaschewitz FG, Sogayar MC. Microencapsulation and tissue engineering as an alternative treatment of diabetes. *Braz. J. Med. Biol. Res.* 2001 Jun. 34(6): 691–697.

51. Liao SW, Rawson J, Omori K, Ishiyama K, Mozhdehi D, Oancea AR, Ito T, Guan Z, Mullen Y. Maintaining functional islets through encapsulation in an injectable saccharide-peptide hydrogel. *Biomaterials* 2013 May. 34(16): 3984–3991. doi:10.1016/j.biomaterials.2013.02.007. Epub 2013 Mar 7.

52. Risbud MV, Bhargava S, Bhonde RR. In vivo biocompatibility evaluation of cellulose macrocapsules for islet immunoisolation: Implications of low molecular weight cut-off. *J. Biomed. Mater. Res. A.* 2003 Jul 1. 66(1): 86–92.

53. Qi Z, Yamamoto C, Imori N, Kinukawa A, Yang KC, Yanai G, Ikenoue E, Shen Y, Shirouzu Y, Hiura A, Inoue K, Sumi S. Immunoisolation effect of polyvinyl alcohol (PVA) macroencapsulated islets in type 1 diabetes therapy. *Cell Transplant.* 2012. 21(2–3): 525–534. doi: 10.3727/096368911X605448.

54. Sakai S, Ono T, Ijima H, Kawakami K. Newly developed aminopropyl-silicate immunoisolation membrane for a microcapsule-shaped bioartificial pancreas. *Ann. N. Y. Acad. Sci.* 2001 Nov. 944: 277–283.

55. Schaffellner S, Stadlbauer V, Stiegler P, Hauser O, Halwachs G, Lackner C, Iberer F, Tscheliessnigg KH. Porcine islet cells microencapsulated in sodium cellulose sulfate. *Transplant Proc.* 2005 Jan–Feb. 37(1): 248–252.

56. Zheng G, Liu X, Wang X, Chen L, Xie H, Wang F, Zheng H, Yu W, Ma X. Improving stability and biocompatibility of alginate/chitosan microcapsule by fabricating bi-functional membrane. *Macromol. Biosci.* 2014 May. 14(5): 655–666. doi:10.1002/mabi.201300474. Epub 2014 Jan 17.

57. Sakai S, Ono T, Ijima H, Kawakami K. Alginate/aminopropyl-silicate/alginate membrane immunoisolatability and insulin secretion of encapsulated islets. *Biotechnol. Prog.* 2002 Mar–Apr. 18(2): 401–403.

58. Krishnan L, Clayton LR, Boland ED, Reed RM, Hoying JB, Williams SK. Cellular immunoisolation for islet transplantation by a novel dual porosity electrospun membrane. *Transplant Proc.* 2011 Nov. 43(9): 3256–3261. doi:10.1016/j.transproceed.2011.10.031.

59. Olabisi RM. Cell microencapsulation with synthetic polymers. *J. Biomed. Mater. Res. A* 2015 Feb. 103(2): 846–859. doi:10.1002/jbm.a.35205. Epub 2014 Aug 18.

60. Campos-Lisbôa AC, Mares-Guia TR, Grazioli G, Goldberg AC, Sogayar MC. Biodritin microencapsulated human islets of Langerhans and their potential for type 1 diabetes mellitus therapy. *Transplant Proc.* 2008 Mar. 40(2): 433–435. doi:10.1016/j.transproceed.2008.01.057.

61. Campanha-Rodrigues AL, Grazioli G, Oliveira TC, Campos-Lisbôa AC, Mares-Guia TR, Sogayar MC. Therapeutic potential of laminin-biodritin microcapsules for type 1 diabetes mellitus. *Cell Transplant.* 2015. 24(2): 247–261. doi:10.3727/096368913X675160. Epub 2013 Nov 20.

62. Paredes Juárez GA, Spasojevic M, Faas MM, de Vos P. Immunological and technical considerations in application of alginate-based microencapsulation systems. *Front Bioeng. Biotechnol.* 2014 Aug 6. 2: 26. doi:10.3389/fbioe.2014.00026. eCollection 2014.

63. Hu S, deVos P. Polymeric approaches to reduce tissue responses against devices applied for islet-cell encapsulation. *Front Bioeng. Biotech.* 2019. 7: 134. doi:10.3389/fbioe.2019.00134.

64. Lee KY, Mooney DJ. Alginate: Properties and biomedical applications. *Prog. Polym. Sci.* 2012 Jan. 37(1): 106–126.

65. Ebrahimi A, Rahim F. Recent immunomodulatory strategies in transplantation. *Immunol. Invest.* 2014. 43(8): 829–837. doi:10.3109/08820139.2014.915414.

66. Ponce S, Orive G, Hernández R, Gascón AR, Pedraz JL, de Haan BJ, Faas MM, Mathieu HJ, de Vos P. Chemistry and the biological response against immunoisolating alginate-polycation capsules of different composition. *Biomaterials* 2006 Oct. 27(28): 4831–4839.

67. Tomei AA, Manzoli V, Fraker CA, Giraldo J, Velluto D, Najjar M, Pileggi A, Molano RD, Ricordi C, Stabler CL, Hubbell JA. Device design and materials optimization of conformal coating for islets of Langerhans. *Proc. Natl. Acad. Sci. U S A.* 2014 Jul 22. 111(29): 10514–10519. doi:10.1073/pnas.1402216111. Epub 2014 Jun 30.

68. Zhang J, Zhu Y, Song J, Yang J, Pan C, Xu T, Zhang L. Novel balanced charged alginate/PEI polyelectrolyte hydrogel that resists foreign-body reaction. *ACS Appl. Mater. Interfaces* 2018 Feb 28. 10(8): 6879–6886. doi:10.1021/acsami.7b17670. Epub 2018 Feb 14.

69. Uludag H, De Vos P, Tresco PA. Technology of mammalian cell encapsulation. *Adv. Drug Del. Rev.* 2000. 42: 29–64.

70. Song S, Roy S. Progress and challenges in macroencapsulation approaches for type 1 diabetes (T1D) treatment: Cells, biomaterials, and devices. *Biotechnol. Bioeng.* 2016 Jul. 113(7): 1381–1402. doi:10.1002/bit.25895. Epub 2016 Jan 4.

71. Orive G, Emerich D, Khademhosseini A, Matsumoto S, Hernández RM, Pedraz JL, Desai T, Calafiore R, de Vos P. Engineering a clinically translatable bioartificial pancreas to treat type I diabetes. *Trends Biotechnol.* 2018 Apr. 36(4): 445–456. doi:10.1016/j.tibtech.2018.01.007. Epub 2018 Feb 15

72. Evron Y, Colton CK, Ludwig B, Weir GC, Zimermann B, Maimon S, Neufeld T, Shalev N, Goldman T, Leon A, Yavriyants K, Shabtay N, Rozenshtein T, Azarov D, DiIenno AR, Steffen A, de Vos P, Bornstein SR, Barkai U, Rotem A. Long-term viability and function of transplanted islets macroencapsulated at high density are achieved by enhanced oxygen supply. *Sci. Rep.* 2018 Apr 25. 8(1): 6508. doi:10.1038/s41598-018-23862-w.

73. Barkai U, Weir GC, Colton CK, Ludwig B, Bornstein SR, Brendel MD, Neufeld T, Bremer C, Leon A, Evron Y, Yavriyants K, Azarov D, Zimermann B, Maimon S, Shabtay N, Balyura M, Rozenshtein T, Vardi P, Bloch K, de Vos P, Rotem A. Enhanced oxygen supply improves islet viability in a new bioartificial pancreas. *Cell Transplant.* 2013. 22(8): 1463–1476. doi:10.3727/096368912X657341. Epub 2012 Oct 3.

74. Smink AM, de Haan BJ, Lakey JRT, de Vos P. Polymer scaffolds for pancreatic islet transplantation - Progress and challenges. *Am. J. Transplant.* 2018 Sep. 18(9): 2113–2119. doi:10.1111/ajt.14942. Epub 2018 Jun 13.

75. Xi w, Wang K, Zhang W, Qiang M, Luo Y. A bilaminated decellularized scaffold for islet transplantation: Structure, properties and functions in diabetic mice. *Biomaterials* 2017. 138: 80–90.

76. Katsuke Y, Yagi H, Okkitsu T, Kitago M, Tajima K, Kadota Y, Hibi T, Abe Y, Shinoda M, Itano O, Takeuchi S, Kitagawa Y. Endocrine pancreas engineered using porcine islets and partial pancreatic scaffolds. *Pancreat* 2016. 16: 922–930.

77. Davis NE, Beenken-Ruthkopf LN, Mirsoian A, Kojic N, Kaplan DL, Barron AE, Fontaine MJ. Enhanced function of pancreatic islets co-encapsulated with ECM proteins and mesenchymal stromal cells in a silk hydrogel. *Biomaterials* 2012. 33: 6691–6697.

78. Zhu M, Wang K, Mei J, Li C, Zhang J, Zheng W, An D, Xiao N, Zhao Q, Kong D, Wang L. Fabrication of highly interconnected porous silk fibroin scaffolds for potential use as vascular grafts. *Acta Biomat.* 2014. 10: 2014–2023.

79. Montazeri L, Hojjati-Emami S, Bonakdar S, Tahamtani Y, Hajizadeh-Saffar E, Noori-Keshtkar M, Najar-Asl M, Ashtiana MK, Baharvand H. Improvement of islet engrafts by enhanced angiogenesis and microparticle-mediated oxygenation. *Biomaterials* 2016. 89: 157–165.

80. Daoud JT, Petropavlovskaia MS, Patapas JM, Degrandpre CE, Diraddo RW, Rosenberg L, Tabrizian M. Long-term in vitro human pancreatic islet culture using three-dimensional microfabricated scaffolds. *Biomaterials* 2011. 32: 1536–1542.

81. Shalaly ND, Ria M, Johansson U, Avall K, Berggren PO, Hedhammar M. Silk matrices promote formation of insulin-secreting islet-like clusters. *Biomaterials* 2016. 90: 50–61.

82. Gibly RF, Zhang X, Lowe Jr. WL, Shea LD. Porous scaffolds support extrahepatic human islet transplantation, engraftment and function in mice. *Cell Transpl.* 2013. 22(5): 811–819. doi:10.3727/096368912X636966.

83. Song S, Blaha C, Moses W, Park J, Wright N, Groszek J, Fissell W, VArtanian S, Posselt AM, Roy S. An intravascular bioartificial pancreas device (iBAP) with silicon nanopore membranes (SNM) for islet encapsulation under convective mass transport. *Lab Chip* 2017. May 16. 17(10): 1778–1792. doi:10.1039/c7lc00096k.

14 Transdermal Drug Delivery

Brahmeshwar Mishra
Indian Institute of Technology (Banaras Hindu University), India

Gunjan Vasant Bonde
University of Petroleum and Energy Studies, India
Indian Institute of Technology (Banaras Hindu University), India

CONTENTS

14.1   INTRODUCTION

Over the years, many drugs have been discovered that are preferably administered by either oral or parenteral route (Chaudhri et al. 2010). However, most therapeutic drugs undergoing enzymatic degradation and first-pass metabolism like peptides, and also acid labile drugs, those cannot be given orally. On the other hand, pain associated with injections, needle phobias, and requirement of a medical practitioner are some severe limitations of the parenteral route of administration (Sivamani, Liepmann, and Maibach 2007). Optimum therapeutic results call upon not only efficient drug delivery but also proper selection of drugs. Thus, the quest to overcome these setbacks promotes the research for novel strategies and put forth the innovative approach of drug delivery via skin. Transdermal drug delivery systems (TDDS) employ the skin, a readily available large surface, for administration and transport of drug (Santos et al. 2018). The patches or TDDS are the devices that deliver drug painlessly and at a controlled rate on application to the intact skin, either for local treatment of skin tissues or for systemic therapy for a prolonged period (Uchechi, Ogbonna, and Attama 2014). Therefore, TDDS has become, indeed, more appealing to patients due to advantages, superseding that of other conventional routes, over the years.

The transdermal delivery has been utilized from a longback (Prausnitz and Langer 2008) and is evidenced by specific reports that mention the use of belladonna plasters for analgesia and mustard plasters for treating chest congestion (Uchechi, Ogbonna, and Attama 2014, Pastore et al. 2015). Rein, in 1924, postulated that barrier for transdermal diffusions is exhibited by the junction of stratum corneum (SC) and epidermis (Rein 1924). The fact of enhanced rate of water loss from the skin by removing the SC was put forth by Blank (Blank 1964), whereas Scheuplein and his team confirmed that the SC is the limiting factor for passive transdermal permeation (Scheuplein 1965). However, Michaels and colleagues then, by using model drugs, evaluated apparent diffusion coefficients in the SC and demonstrated that some of them have good permeability across the SC even in the presence of intact skin barrier (Michaels, Chandrasekaran, and Shaw 1975). This evolution boosted the research in TDDS and came up with the first patch in 1970, which was then approved in 1979 by United States Food and Drug Administration (USFDA). The first TDDS was a scopolamine-loaded patch delivering the drug for 3 days and used to treat motion sickness (Mali 2015). And further, the advents in newer and novel approaches lead to the development of numerous with a wide variety of patches formulated till date for broader applications (Prausnitz, Mitragotri, and Langer 2004). The commercially available TDDS are enlisted in Table 14.1.

14.1.1 Advantages

- It is the better alternative to avoid the first-pass metabolism after absorption from gastro-intestinal tract (GIT), e.g., Transdermal Nitroglycerin (Mali 2015, Escobar-Chávez 2012, Sidat et al. 2019).
- They can provide protection of drug against gastrointestinal problems such as enzymatic degradation (e.g., fentanyl, estradiol) in stomach, gastro-intestinal pH interactions, gastric emptying, and drug interaction with orally taken drugs or ingested food (Brown et al. 2006, Singh et al. 2015, Bruno, Miller, and Lim 2013, Van Gele et al. 2011).
- In the circumstances, where unconscious, uncooperative or nauseated patients cannot be administered orally, TDDS can serve as a suitable alternative.
- It can provide a prolonged and controlled delivery over an extended period.
- The extended release can minimize the systemic toxicities caused by peaks and valleys of drug concentration in blood following multidose administration by oral or parenteral route (Alexander et al. 2012, Singh et al. 2015).
- It can provide better patient compliance due to convenient, noninvasive, and painless drug delivery.
- The prolonged activity of drugs with narrow therapeutic window or short half-life can be achieved through its controlled transdermal release from drug reservoir applied as a patch.
- Target or diseased site can directly be accessed, e.g., treatment of skin disorders such as fungal infections, eczema, and psoriasis.
- In contrast to parenteral dosage forms, no need of a medical practitioner to administer, avoid the risk of spread of diseases via reuse of hypodermic needles, particularly in developing countries, while self-administration and termination of dose in any adverse event have been made possible by TDDS (Prausnitz and Langer 2008, Miller and Pisani 1999).
- Enhancement of therapeutic efficacy by dose reduction, in turn, reduction in systemic side effects, can overall reduce healthcare treatment costs (Uchechi, Ogbonna, and Attama 2014, Prausnitz, Mitragotri, and Langer 2004).
- The latest programmable systems employed to transdermal patch can be adopted to achieve variable-rate or on–off drug delivery (Uchechi, Ogbonna, and Attama 2014, Wu et al. 2010).

TABLE 14.1
List of USFDA-Approved Transdermal Therapeutic Systems

Approved	Name of TDDS	Name of the Drug	Indication	Design	Period
1981	Transderm-scop®	Scopolamine	Motion sickness	DIA[c]	3 d[d]
1984	Catapres-TTS®	Clonidine	Hypertension	Reservoir	7 d
1984	Climara®	Estradiol	FHRT[a]	DIA	7 d
1986	Estraderm®	Estradiol	FHRT	Reservoir	3–4 d
1990	Duragesic®	Fentanyl	Chronic pain	DIA	3 d
1994	Vivelle®	Estradiol	FHRT	DIA	3–4 d
1995	Androderm®	Testosterone	Hypogonadism	Reservoir	24 hours
1995	Nitro-Dur®	Nitroglycerine	Angina pectoris	DIA	12–14 hours
1996	Alora®	Estradiol	FHRT	DIA	3–4 d
1996	Nicoderm®	Nicotine	Smoking cessation	Reservoir	24 hours
1996	Nicotrol®	Nicotine	Smoking cessation		24 hours
1996	Transderm-Nitro®	Nitroglycerine	Angina pectoris	Reservoir	7–10 hours
1996	Minitran®	Nitroglycerine	Angina pectoris		24 hours
1997	Testoderm-AT®	Testosterone	Hypogonadism	Reservoir	24 hours
1998	CombiPatch®	Estradiol/ Norehindroneacetate	FHRT	DIA	3–4 d
1998	Prostep®	Nicotine	Smoking cessation	Reservoir	24 hours
1999	Vivelle-Dot®	Estradiol	FHRT	DIA	3–4 d
1999	Lidoderm®	Lidocaine	Post-herpetic neuralgia pain	DIA	12 hours
1999	Habitrol®	Nicotine	Smoking cessation	Matrix	24 hours
2001	Ortho-Evra®	EthinylEstradiol/ Norelegestromin	Female contraception	DIA	7 d
2003	Climara-Pro®	Estradiol/Levonorgestrel	FHRT[a]	DIA	7 d
2003	Oxytrol®	Oxybutynin	Overactive bladder	DIA	3–4 d
2004	Menostar®	Estradiol	FHRT[a]	DIA	7 d
2004	Lidopro®	Lidocaine hydrochloride and epinephrine	Topical analgesic		12 hours
2006	Daytrana®	Methylphenidate	ADHD[b]	DIA	9 hours
2006	Emsam®	Selegiline	Depressive disorder	Reservoir	24 hours
2007	Flector®	Diclofenac epolamine	Acute pain	DIA	12 hours
2007	Exelon®	Rivastigmine	Alzheimer's and Parkinson's	Matrix	24 hours
2007	Neupro®	Rotigotine	restless leg syndrome	DIA	24 hours
2008	Sancuso®	Granisetron	Chemotherapy	DIA	7 d
2008	Salonpas®	Methyl salicylate and methanol	Muscles and joints pain	DIA	8–12 hours
2009	Qutenza®	Capsaicin	Neuropathic pain	DIA	1 hour
2010	Butrans®	Buprenorphine	Chronic pain	DIA	7 d
2012	Minivelle®	Estradiol	FHRT	DIA	3–4 d

Source: (Banerjee et al. 2014, Santos et al. 2018, Kandavilli, Nair, and Panchagnula 2002, USFDA, Brown et al. 2006, Watkinson et al. 2016).

[a] FHRT = Female hormone replacement therapy
[b] ADHD = Attention deficit hyperactivity disorder
[c] DIA = drug in adhesive
[d] d = days

14.1.2 Disadvantages

- Very few drugs can be used through TDDS as specific characteristics must be possessed by the drug to traverse through skin layers (Bos and Meinardi 2000, Brown et al. 2006).
- Since the composition of skin (lipids and protein) gets altered in geriatric patients, TDDS may not be very helpful for them (Kaur et al. 2016).
- The peptidases and esterases can metabolize the drug even before reaching the systemic circulation during their passage through the skin (Alexander et al. 2012, Kaur et al. 2014).
- The local higher concentration of drug in underlying tissue may cause local complications such as erythema, contact dermatitis, sensitization, or irritation, necessitating discontinuation (Kaur et al. 2015).
- TDDS are unsuitable for drugs requiring higher blood concentration to elicit pharmacological action.
- TDDS cannot be employed in case of the drug or a clinical event where the quick onset of action is intended, due to occurrence of lag time between patch administration and the onset of action.
- Some applications of the patch are uncomfortable, e.g., patch of scopolamine to be applied behind the ear.
- The turnover of SC cells can limit the period for patch application on the skin.

14.1.3 Criteria to Be Considered

14.1.3.1 Requirements for Transdermal Drug Candidates

- Very few drugs (molecular weight <500 Da) are suitable for TDDS as the diffusivity through SC is inversely proportional to molecular mass (Ruan et al. 2016).
- The drug candidate must possess not only high permeability and adequate lipophilicity (log P between 1 and 3) to follow the intracellular route of absorption but also sufficient hydrophilicity to solubilize in the blood and achieve systemic concentration easily (Roberts et al. 2017, Larraneta et al. 2016).
- TDDS can be adopted for only potent drugs requiring dose less than 10 mg and must be well tolerated by the skin (Jassim, Sulaiman, and Jabir 2018).
- The drug should have short half-life (Gaikwad 2013).
- Drugs with low melting point (<200°C) are suitable candidates for TDDS (Khan et al. 2015).
- The drug candidate must have appropriate solubility parameter (estimate of cohesion energy of the unionized form) (ideally about 18–22 MPa) (Wolff 2014).
- The pH of the saturated solution of drug candidate should fall in between 5 and 9 (Jain 1997).

14.1.3.2 Requirements for Transdermal Formulations

- The pharmaceutical excipients used for the preparation of the device/patch must have compatibility within them and should not be skin irritant.
- Formulation factors such as drug particle size, chemical potential of the drug, codelivery of penetration enhancers (PE), selection of drug carrier systems (like micro- or nanoemulsions, liposomes, transferosomes, etc.) can significantly influence the rate of diffusion and drug delivery.
- The excipient must not interfere with the absorption of drug (Otberg et al. 2008).
- The formulation must be capable of providing constant outflow of the drug by maintaining the concentration gradient of the drug across the skin (Tiwari et al. 2013).

- The adhesives exploited for the formulation of patches should have sufficient adhesive properties so that it can maintain skin contact over an intended period. At the same time, the adhesive must have optimum cohesive properties to avoid any residues on skin or clothes after removal of the patch (Cilurzo, Gennari, and Minghetti 2012).

14.2 STRUCTURE OF THE SKIN

The skin is the body's largest organ and accounts for approximately 16% of human body weight and covers about $2\,m^2$ surface area in adults (Abd et al. 2016, Goyal et al. 2016). It is in direct contact with the environment and is responsible for providing first-line defense against invading microorganisms, protection against heat and ultraviolet radiation, regulates homeostasis, and acts as a physical barrier to the environment (Van Gele et al. 2011, Baroni et al. 2012). The structure (illustrated in Figure 14.1a) and thickness of human skin can vary widely but generally is about 1.5 mm in thickness and consist of three layers.

14.2.1 SC AND EPIDERMIS

It is the outermost layer of skin comprising an outer SC and viable inner epidermis. The thickness of SC varies between 10 and 20 µm depending on the anatomical site and is indeed responsible for its barrier function. The SC is made up of dead and anucleated corneocytes forming matrix-type structure with multilamellar lipids (5%–15%). These lipids are ceramides, cholesterol sulfate, cholesterol, and free fatty acids (Marwah et al. 2016). The SC is generally referred as a "brick-and-mortar" architecture due to the arrangement of long, flat, tile-like shape of the corneocytes (Menon, Cleary, and Lane 2012).

Immediately underlying to the SC, the viable epidermis is 0.06–0.8 µm thick and composed of dermal fibroblasts and keratinocytes (which further differentiated as corneocytes) arranged in 4–5 layers, as shown in Figure 14.1b (stratum lucidum, stratum granulosum, stratum spinosum, and stratum basale) (Goyal et al. 2016). It is associated with some metabolic activities, drug binding, active transport, and surveillance; but avascular structure (Van Gele et al. 2011, Baroni et al. 2012).

14.2.2 DERMIS

Below the epidermis is the 3–5 mm thick dermis. It is a highly vascular structure consisting of connective tissues with collagen and elastin fibers as the extracellular matrix, lymphatic vessels, and nerve endings. It hosts various skin appendages such as sebaceous and sweats glands as well as hair follicles, etc. (Montenegro et al. 2016). Also, it is associated with homeostasis functions regulating body temperature, nutrients, and oxygen supply to the skin and excreting toxic waste. The fibroblasts and macrophages also reside in the dermis and are responsible for the synthesis as well as the renewal of extracellular matrix and immune defense against invading foreign material, respectively. The extensive blood capillary beds serve as the first site of systemic access to drug molecules (Wong 2014, Abd et al. 2016).

14.2.3 HYPODERMIS

The hypodermis or subcutaneous tissue is the innermost skin layer (Van Gele et al. 2011). It is about 3 mm thick and consists of loose connective tissue and fat (50% of the body fat). It acts as a fat storing zone and also serves as a supporting membrane for an epidermal and dermal layer of skin. Being a fatty structure, it acts as a mechanical shock-absorbing and insulation material against adverse environment (Baroni et al. 2012).

The SC and viable epidermis alternatively serve as a permeation barrier for drug molecule as removal of SC did not increase the delivery. However, drug delivery was reported to increase

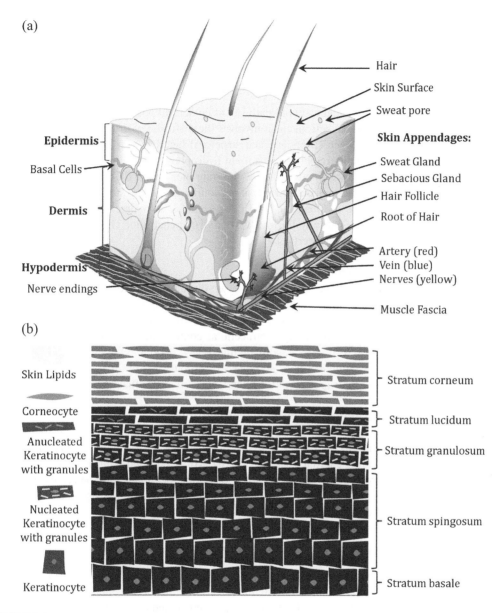

FIGURE 14.1 Schematic presentation of organization of (a) skin layers and (b) epidermis. (Based on Carter, Narasimhan, and Wang 2019, Polat, Blankschtein, and Langer 2010.)

significantly upon removal of both SC and viable epidermis when compared with removal of SC alone (Schoellhammer, Blankschtein, and Langer 2014, Andrews, Jeong, and Prausnitz 2013). Hence, the whole epidermis poised the barrier for TDD, whereas the dermis and hypodermis constitute the practical skin barriers against traumatic and thermal shocks.

14.3 DRUG PENETRATION PATHWAYS THROUGH THE SKIN

Based on the path that the drug traversed to permeate through the skin, the pathways can be identified as either transepidermal pathway, i.e., through the epidermis or the appendageal/shunt pathway, i.e., through hair follicles and sweat glands.

14.3.1 TRANSEPIDERMAL PATHWAY

The transepidermal pathway involves drug substances that are permeated directly through the SC can be accomplished in two ways:

14.3.1.1 Intercellular Pathway

It is supposed to be the primary and essential pathway of epidermal penetration. Drug diffusion in intercellular channels is highly anisotropic as it involves the diffusion of drug molecules along the tortuous routes present in between successive and structural heterogenous lipid lamellae around the corneocytes. The interlamellar region is made up of hydrophobic chains having more flexibility and less ordered lipids, and hence lipophilic drugs migrate along with these comparatively fluid lipid tails. However, hydrophilic molecules traverse predominantly along surfaces of a few water-containing interlamellar spaces or along the lipid polar heads. The intercellular route, therefore, forms the essential and feasible pathway for transdermal drug penetration (Escobar-Chávez 2012, Alexander et al. 2012, Wong 2014, Roberts et al. 2017).

14.3.1.2 The Transcellular Route

The transcellular route involves the migration of drug through the cytoplasm of corneocytes, which have low lipid contents, and also through the intercellular lipid matrix, consisting mainly of fatty acids, ceramides, and cholesterol. As the drug has to traverse via the variety of lipophilic (extracellular compartment) and hydrophilic (intracellular compartment) portions this pathway is highly resistant to permeation (Carter, Narasimhan, and Wang 2019). On the other hand, the skin anatomy, where corneocytes cellular groups show less or no lateral overlap, e.g., wrinkles of the skin, provides less resistance to drug permeation (Van Gele et al. 2011, Jhawat et al. 2013).

14.3.1.3 Transappendageal/Shunt/Transfollicular Pathway

The skin structure is pierced by plentiful appendages like sweat ducts and hair follicles (covering about 0.1% of skin surface area) creating direct assessable channels across the SC and epidermis to reach the dermis and underlying capillary beds (Prausnitz, Mitragotri, and Langer 2004). Indeed, it is considered as the preferred pathway for hydrophilic drugs and documented to be critical for iontophoresis approach for drug penetration enhancement (Khan et al. 2015). It has also been suggested as the vital route in both passive and active transdermal diffusion of drugs.

14.4 APPROACHES FOR PERMEATION IMPROVEMENT

The transdermal route has become an indispensable route for the delivery of drugs over time, by virtue of its advantages, when topical, local, or systemic effects are intended. Although various natural ways of transdermal drug diffusion have been extensively studied and reported by the pharmaceutical fraternity, it becomes, indeed, necessary to explore through multiple strategies to potentiate the drug diffusion (of both hydrophobic and hydrophilic drugs) and to enhance the drug flux across the SC and epidermis. The extensive research in the area brought forward numerous techniques, and they were classified as passive and active techniques of penetration enhancement.

The techniques which promote either the driving force of drug diffusion, i.e., thermodynamics of drug molecule or increase the permeability of the skin, are known as passive techniques of penetration enhancement. This approach is accomplished by adding PE, taking advantage of nanoformulations or vesicles, and employing a prodrug/metabolic approach. Primarily numerous natural agents were used to aid in skin penetration, then followed by the various chemical entities were identified as potential PEs; which manipulate passive pathways of drug permeation. Despite the higher success and wider acceptance due to better dose control and patient compliance of passive techniques, these techniques are still limited to a small number of drugs due to inability to deliver a large dose and hydrophilic drugs like proteins and peptides, etc. These setbacks boosted the surge of research through the novel techniques which exploit external energy sources serving as a driving force or aid in disrupting the skin barrier and identified as active techniques of drug penetration. The approach involves the use of electric (iontophoresis (Banerjee et al. 2019, Fernández-Cuadros et al. 2019, Panzade 2012), electroporation (Anirudhan and Nair 2019, Yang, Zhang, and Gu 2018, Hartmann et al. 2018)), sound waves (sonophoresis (Mitragotri 2017, Polat, Blankschtein, and Langer 2010)), or mechanical (microneedles (MN) (Jin et al. 2019, Yao et al. 2019, Luzuriaga et al. 2018)), etc. as a way to achieve drug permeation across the skin (Ghosh et al. 2015, Santos et al. 2018).

Extensive studies of various PEs elucidated the possible mechanisms of penetration enhancement. Barry gave the lipid–protein partitioning theory. In consonance with this theory, the principal mechanisms were identified as (i) the fluidity of skin structure improved by interactions with the intracellular keratin; (ii) interactions with the intercellular lipids or extraction of skin lipids to some extent; (iii) cosolvency effect of absorbed enhancer in the skin, in other words, modify the drug partitioning characteristics of the skin which locally improves dissolving capacity of the barrier for drugs (Alexander et al. 2012). All these mechanisms increase the fluidity of the skin layers that promote drug diffusion in deeper layers of skin. Another mechanism involves change of the thermodynamic activity of the drug by the PE-like methanol (Escobar-Chavez, Rodriguez-Cruz, and Dominguez-Delgado 2012). Newer physical strategies are based on the principal of either physical disruption of the SC to increase the diffusion flux of drug across the skin (e.g., electroporation, sonophoresis, etc.) or bypassing the SC (e.g., MNs) (Yang, Bugno, and Hong 2013). Additionally, physical insult can activate the immune system at that site, an essential feature for vaccination (Schoellhammer, Blankschtein, and Langer 2014).

14.5 PENETRATION ENHANCERS (PE)

The PE seems to alter the obstructive function of the SC reversibly with no damage to the viable cell. Albeit numerous chemicals have been investigated for their potential as PEs in animal or human skins, to date, none of them were reported to have ideal properties (Kress 2009, Marwah et al. 2016). Some of the attributes supposed to be owned by ideal PE are as follows:

- They must be nonallergenic, nonirritating, and nontoxic and should not possess any pharmacological activity.
- The effect produced by PE must be rapid and reversible.
- On removal, it should be easily removed from the location and allow to maintain healthy skin physiology and anatomy rapidly.
- They must be cosmetically acceptable with suitable skin aesthetics.
- They should be compatible with most commonly used pharmaceutical excipients as well as drugs, by formulation point of view.

14.5.1 Chemical Approaches

The plentiful of chemical entities were extensively evaluated throughout the past decades, and are recommended as PEs. This comprehensive list involves numerous classes of chemical substances such as water, natural compounds, synthetic chemicals, surfactants, and some novel PEs. Natural PE includes essential oils, terpenes, terpenoids, lipids, etc. (Saini, Baghel, and Chauhan 2014, Das and Ahmed 2017, Gao et al. 2014), whereas other chemicals employed as PEs are hydrocarbons alcohols, azones, acids amines, amides, esters, biodegradable polymers, and ionic liquids (Yang, Bugno, and Hong 2013, Sidat et al. 2019). Recently, some research groups were getting interested in the synthesis of some novel PEs via chemical synthesis or derivatization of natural moieties and explored their skin penetration potential by *in silico* studies (Gao et al. 2014, Marepally et al. 2013, Gupta et al. 2019). Table 14.2 enlists the chemical PEs widely used in TDDS.

TABLE 14.2
List of Chemicals and Some Miscellaneous PEs Widely Used in TDDS with Their Respective Mechanism of Action

Chemical PEs		
Type of enhancer	Example	Mechanism of Action
Terpenes, Terpenes along with 80% propylene glycol (PG), Unsaturated sesquiterpene (Chen et al. 2016, Das and Ahmed 2017)	L-Menthol, 1,8-cineole, menthone, limonene, nerolidol, alpha-bisabolol	Form eutectic mixture with drug and enhance its solubility. Alters the barrier properties of SC. Increases lipid destruction in the SC due to terpenes. Increases partition due to high PG content. Increases lipid fluidity of SC.
Essential oils (Sinha and Kaur 2000, Williams and Barry 2012)	Eucalyptus, peppermint, turpentine oil	Combined process of partition and diffusion
Pyrrolidones (Mathur, Satrawala, and Rajput 2014)	N-methyl-2-pyrrolidone (NMP), N-dodecyl-2-pyrrolidone	Enhances transdermal permeation through polar routes of skin, perturbation of SC lipid lamellae.
Azone (Pathan and Setty 2009)	Azone in combination with PG, 1-geranylazacycloheptan-2-one (GAH), 1-farnesylazacycloheptan-2-one (FAH)	Facilitates drug permeation through its lipid-fluidizing ability by disruption of lipid bilayer, Increases moisture content in SC, PG promotes intracellular transport
Fatty acids and esters (Saini, Baghel, and Chauhan 2014, Mathur, Satrawala, and Rajput 2014, Sinha and Kaur 2000)	Oleic acid, capric acid, myristic acid, lauric acid	Increases partition coefficient and diffusivity, increases solvent penetration, disruption of lipid bilayer
Sulfoxides (Pathan and Setty 2009)	Dimethyl sulfoxide (DMSO), decylmethylsulfoxide (DCMS) + ethanol	Changes the conformation of SC alpha helix to beta sheet, interacts with the lipids and proteins causing protein denaturation in SC
Compounds similar to sulfoxides (Sinha and Kaur 2000)	N,N-dimethylamides, dimethylacetamide (DMA)	Promotes absorption through polar route by increasing the diffusion and portioning of the drug.
Alcohols (Mathur, Satrawala, and Rajput 2014)	Ethanol	Extracts large amounts of lipids from the SC
	N-alkanols	Increases the number of free sulfhydryl groups of keratin in SC proteins
	PG	PG solvates the SC, occupying hydrogen bonding sites
Short chain glycerides (Okumura et al. 1991)	Tricaprylin (TCP) glyceryltricaprylate	Increases fluidity of lipoidal membrane of SC
Phospholipids (Mathur, Satrawala, and Rajput 2014)	Phosphatidyl glycerol derivative, phosphatidyl choline derivatives, phosphatidyl ethanolamine derivatives	Enhances the penetration of topically applied drugs
Lipid synthesis inhibitors (Tsai et al. 1996)	5-(Tetradecyloxy)-2-furancarboxylic acid (TOFA), fluvastatin (FLU), and cholesterol sulfate (CS)	TOFA is a fatty acid synthesis inhibitor, FLU and CS are cholesterol synthesis inhibitors. These agents delay the recovery of barrier damage produced by prior application of DMSO or acetone
Amino acid derivatives (Büyüktimkin, Büyüktimkin, and Rytting 1996)	N-Dodecyl-l-amino acid methyl ester, N-pentyl-N-acetyl prolinate	Hydrogen bonding and dipole–dipole interactions

(Continued)

TABLE 14.2 (*Continued*)
List of Chemicals and Some Miscellaneous PEs Widely Used in TDDS with Their Respective Mechanism of Action

Chemical PEs		
Type of enhancer	**Example**	**Mechanism of Action**
Surfactants (Ghafourian, Nokhodchi, and Kaialy 2015, Pandey et al. 2014)	Dodecyl-N,N-dimethylamino acetate	Causes the disruption of the lipoidal bilayer and induces changes in the lipid structure of SC
	Sodium lauryl sulfate (SLS)	At 1% SLS disrupts lipid and protein components reversibly. Increased hydration of SC
Urea (Pathan and Setty 2009)	Cyclic urea	Facilitates hydration of SC and forms hydrophilic diffusion channels
Oxazolidinone (Mathur, Satrawala, and Rajput 2014, (Pathan and Setty 2009)	4-decyloxazolidin-2-one	Ability to localize coadministered drug in skin layers owing to their closely related structure to sphingosine and ceramide lipids; skin components
Miscellaneous PEs		
Enzymes (Patil et al. 1996)	Phosphatidyl choline-dependent enzyme phospholipase C, triacylglycerol hydrolase [TGH], acid phosphatase, phospholipase A2	Causes metabolism of phosphatidyl choline in the barrier lipids
Prodrugs (Morrow et al. 2007)	5-Fluoro uracil, naproxen, diclofenac, theophylline	Designed to have more lipophilicity than the active drug and hence skin partition will be increased
Ion pairs (Morrow et al. 2007)	Ibuprofen and triethylamine, salicylic acid and alkylamines	The ionic drugs are combined with the oppositely charged ions so that they form a neutral molecule which diffuses through SC and gets separated in the dermis layer of the skin.

14.5.2 PHYSICAL APPROACHES

Innovative ideas in the TDDS approaches were developed to achieve SC penetration by numerous physical mechanisms. The surge in the interest of physical strategies come up with some novel techniques that exploit physical forces as a driving force for drug penetration through the SC. Therefore, these approaches are also known as active penetration pathways. These consisted of the application of eclectic current, ultrasound waves, radiofrequency, LASER radiations, high temperature, magnetism, etc. However, other approaches depending on the direct disruption of the SC and/or epidermis, as reported in the literature, practiced in skin abrasion, suction ablation, or MNs (see Section 15.9.3.1 for detailed discussion). The review on principal mechanisms and their applications is presented in Table 14.3.

14.5.3 FORMULATION APPROACHES

The modern pharmaceutical era is dealing with the evolution of development and applications of novel nanocarrier dosage forms. A search through literature brings to notice that various research groups employed nanovesicles, nanoparticles, polymeric micelles, liposomes, solid lipid nanoparticles (SLN), etc.; the comprehensive discussion thereof is given in points 15.9.1 and 15.9.2.

TABLE 14.3

The Review on Principal Mechanisms and Their Applications of Various Physical Approaches Used for Drug Permeation Across the Skin

Methods	Technique	Drug Properties	Mechanism of Action	Side Effects	Limitation in Practice
Iontophoresis/electromigration/electrorepulsion/electroosmosis (Escobar-Chavez, Rodriguez-Cruz, and Dominguez-Delgado 2012, Kalluri and Banga 2011, Prausnitz and Langer 2008)	Electrical current 0.5 mA/cm² for minutes or hours	Low and high molecular weight drugs particularly 10–15 kDa	Electrode is placed on the skin along with the drug solution having the same charge and a current of 0.5 mA is applied, the drug molecule is repelled by electrode because of the same charge through the skin to the opposite charge electrode and delivers the drug at a faster rate.	Due to the reversal of polarity, alternating current causes fewer skin burns, which is due to hydrogen and hydroxyl ions produced in the alternate cycle to neutralize ions produced in the previous cycle.	The narrow range of electric field parameter.
Sonophoresis/phonophoresis (Polat et al. 2011, Azagury et al. 2014, Schoellhammer, Blankschtein, and Langer 2014)	Low frequency 20–100 kHz for the order of tens of minutes	Low and high molecular weight drugs	Ultrasound cavitation induces lipid bilayer defects in SC. It results in water migration into the disordered lipid regions and leads to the formation of aqueous channels. Noncavitational mechanisms are possible and include convection with acoustic streaming and reduced boundary layers, thermal effects, mechanical or radiation pressure effects, and lipid extraction.	The use of high ultrasound amplitudes can bring discomfort, slight and transient erythema, dermal necrosis, or burn and tinnitus. In comparison to high-frequency sonophoresis, low-frequency sonophoresis lacks the safety records from the perspective that it is a more permeating tool.	Ultrasound energy emitted can be poorly calibrated.
Electroporation (Brown et al. 2006, A Charoo et al. 2010, Wong 2014, Prausnitz, Mitragotri, and Langer 2004)	Electrical voltage 50–1,500 V for micro to milliseconds and a few seconds to a minute gap between pulses	Small molecules, proteins, peptides and oligonucleotides (>7 kDa)	Electroporation results in heat-induced lipid fluidization, and temporary new aqueous pores are formed within the SC followed by electrophoresis and diffusion.	The level of sensation, such as muscle contraction, itching, tingling, pricking, and pain, could rise with an increase in pulse rate, duration, and voltage.	More skin damage than iontophoresis.
Magnetophoresis (Brown et al. 2006, Wong 2014)	Magnetic field 5–300 mT throughout drug treatment	Low molecular weight drug with diamagnetic properties.	The improved drug partition is attributed to the repulsion of diamagnetic substances across the skin by the magnetic field and less dependent on changing the barrier property of SC.	–	The low energy of action.

(Continued)

TABLE 14.3 (*Continued*)

The Review on Principal Mechanisms and Their Applications of Various Physical Approaches Used for Drug Permeation Across the Skin

Methods	Technique	Drug Properties	Mechanism of Action	Side Effects	Limitation in Practice
Laser ablation (Kalluri and Banga 2011, Wong 2014)	Photomechanical waves in the hundreds of atmospheres (300–1,000 bar) for 100 ns–10 μs	Low and high molecular weight drugs	A photomechanical wave causes vibrational heating within the irradiated area, which results in vaporization of the skin components and pore formation in the SC.	There is no observable injury to keratinocytes with a single application of pressure wave, and only minor erythema is developed with 1 μs pressure wave. Multiple doses of pressure waves may, however, cause cell injury.	Risk of cell injury is high.
Needleless injection (Kamboj et al. 2013, Marwah et al. 2016)	Use of pressurized inert gas to propel drug particle across skin	drugs that do not require frequent dosing, e.g., vaccines	Some of the methods are as follows: Intrajet: In this technique, pressurized nitrogen gas is used to propel the liquid drug solution into small pores of the skin. Implajet: Here a minute pore is created by pushing a tiny tip through the skin, and then the drug is introduced through this pore. Jet-syringe: A jet-syringe is suitable for short-term injection therapy. It can inject up to 0.5 mL drug solution by using a prefilled or adjustable ampoule. Iject is used for subcutaneous or intramuscular injection. It is a hand operated, lightweight device capable of delivering 0.1 mL to 1 mL drug solution.	Long-term effects of repeated application and bombarding of particles on skin surface is still not known.	Its use is restricted to solid particulates and high cost and nonprogrammable for individualization of dose.

(Continued)

TABLE 14.3 (*Continued*)
The Review on Principal Mechanisms and Their Applications of Various Physical Approaches Used for Drug Permeation Across the Skin

Methods	Technique	Drug Properties	Mechanism of Action	Side Effects	Limitation in Practice
Tape stripping (Morrow et al. 2007)	Repeated application and removal of adhesive	Molecular weight less than 986 Da	Removal of the layers of SC by repeated application and removal of adhesive to the skin surface.	Various factors like type of adhesive, pressure of removal of tape, and anatomical site influence the process.	Process parameters vary for individuals
Suction ablation (Brown et al. 2006)	Application of a vacuum or negative pressure	—	Suction blister formed by the removal of layers of SC, while leaving the basal membrane intact, thus facilitates the permeation of drugs. Epidermatome is used to remove the upper surface of the blister	Prolonged length of time required to achieve a blister	—
Thermal ablation (Morrow et al. 2007)	Alternating current at radiofrequency (100 kHz) electrodes, inserted into the skin	—	Ions within the skin attempt to follow the change in the direction of the alternating current, resulting in frictional heating and subsequent cell ablation. This creates microchannels facilitating drug transport.	Two-step process involving first step of thermal treatment followed by application dosage form.	Integrated systems are required to perform two-step process.
Microscissoring (Morrow et al. 2007)	Sharp particles of aluminum oxide accelerated by pressurized nitrogen stream	—	Accelerated sharp particles of aluminum oxide disrupt the SC producing microcuts on skin surface that helps in drug permeation.	Requires pretreatment of the skin making less favorable for routine use.	Accidental deposition of metal particle in skin causes infection.

14.6   DIFFUSION KINETICS INVOLVED IN TDDS

For TDDS development, it becomes indeed necessary to interpret the permeation kinetics of the drug. The drug absorption kinetics and its diffusion across the skin can be better understood by taking various steps, that drug seems to undergo during its absorption, into consideration. The drug traverses from patch to the skin in the following steps:

- The drug diffuses within the delivery system and partitioned from reservoir to either adhesive layer or then into rate-controlling membrane (if available in some patches), i.e., to the patch–SC interface
- Then its sorption to the skin surface and then partition into the SC
- Permeation and diffusion across the epidermis
- Partitioned into dermis
- Then encounters capillary bed where it diffuses into the blood for its systemic circulation.

The mechanism is sought to be the passive diffusion of the drug, and it takes down the concentration gradient from the higher concentration region (from patch reservoir and the skin surface) to the lower concentration region (to the skin and then deeper tissues). The fact of passive diffusion can be better understood by Fick's first law of diffusion and is presented as

$$J = -AD\left(\frac{dc}{dx}\right) \tag{14.1}$$

where J is the flux of the drug across the skin per unit skin surface area, A. The concentration gradient across the thickness of skin is represented as $\frac{dc}{dx}$ and D stands for the coefficient of diffusion of the drug (Prakash et al. 2016, Alkilani, McCrudden, and Donnelly 2015). The negative sign indicates that the diffusion process is opposite to the direction of concentration. The above equation can be rewritten using Fick's second law for steady-state diffusion kinetics:

$$J_{ss} = \frac{AD_{ss}K_{ss}C}{L_{ss}} \tag{14.2}$$

where K_{ss} is the partition coefficient of the drug in the medium of doner to receiver compartment, and L_{ss} is the diffusion path length after steady-state establishment (Goyal et al. 2016, Barry 2002). Unless the patch remains firmly attached to the skin, the A is never going to change and hence by considering C_d and C_r as the concentration in doner (skin surface) and receiver (skin inner layers or blood in dermal capillary) compartment, above equation can be rewritten as

$$J_{ss} = P_{ss}(C_d - C_r) \tag{14.3}$$

where P_{ss} is the overall permeability constant and is given by the following equation:

$$P_{ss} = \frac{D_{ss}K_{ss}}{L_{ss}} \tag{14.4}$$

Under certain conditions, permeability seems to be constant, and therefore, the flux or the amount of drug penetration through the skin surface depends upon the concentration gradient established across the skin surface (Kathe and Kathpalia 2017). Until and unless the drug concentration on the skin surface remains high and constant than underneath tissues, the drug diffuses at a constant rate (R_a, drug absorption rate). This could be accomplished by maintaining the drug release rate (R_r) from the patch higher than drug absorption rate, i.e., $R_r > R_a$ (Tiwari et al. 2013). Conclusively, the rate and amount of drug delivered to skin or the systemic circulation depend on rate of drug release from patch and drug concentration on the skin surface, ideally, as the C_r always remains less due to metabolism and drug-sweeping by blood. Therefore, the patches or TDDS are considered as controlled drug delivery systems that can indeed deliver the constant amount of drug dose over the period and also the rate can be managed by manipulating the formulation design.

14.7 FORMULATION CONSIDERATIONS AND COMPONENTS OF TDDS

14.7.1 POLYMERS

With conventional polymers, advent in polymer science had come up with various sophisticated polymers that are employed for the preparation of TDDS for multiple purposes. Polymers provide rigidity to the final dosage form and strengthen the foundation of TDDS. They can be used as a matrix-forming component, adhesives, rate limiting membranes, liners, and a backing layer, etc. (Prausnitz, Mitragotri, and Langer 2004). However, polymers should possess some essential characteristics, indeed, to be used as a component of TDDS. Those involve stability, nonreactivity with other excipients, ease to manufacture/fabricate, and acts as an inert drug carrier. Having biocompatibility and chemical compatibility is obvious. Physical and chemical properties of polymer should be such that they do not alter the diffusion of the drug as well as deteriorate throughout the period of application.

14.7.2 ADHESIVES

The adhesive, a crucial constituent, ensures an intimate contact between delivery device and the skin. At the same time, the drug has to pass through the diffusion-controlled membrane and then adhesive layer to get to the skin surface after application of the transdermal patch. Therefore, the adhesives and their adhesion property are vital for the quality, efficacy, and safety of TDDS (Wokovich et al. 2006).

The excellent adhesive should be a biocompatible, nonirritant, and nonsensitizing polymer. It should be water and humidity resistant and should form good adhesive bonds irrespective of skin structure like oily, hairy, or wrinkled skin. They should possess optimum adhesive properties so that they can establish and maintain bonds with the skin for an intended period while must be a cohesive material so that they can easily be removed from skin without retaining residues on the skin or any skin damage (Cilurzo, Gennari, and Minghetti 2012). Hence, the quality of TDDS depends on the nature of the bond formed between skin and patch, which reflects the consistency of drug delivered (Gutschke et al. 2010). Improper adhesion leads to reduction in the surface area of contact, falling off, or patch lift that eventually resulted in incorrect dosing of patients.

Commonly used pressure-sensitive adhesives are Silicone, Polyisobutylene, Eudragit NE, Eudragit E100, Eudragit L100, and Polyacrylate, which are either applied as a layer or layered at the periphery of the face of TDDS (Banerjee et al. 2014). However, a natural sticky polymer, karaya gum, is also utilized as adhesive in some TDDS. Some new adhesives include either utilization of hydrogel-forming hydrophilic polymers, and polyurethanes (Gansen and Dittgen 2012, Santos et al. 2018) or the chemical modification by grafting or incorporation of some monomers or additional functionalities to the existing adhesive polymers (Zhao et al. 2019).

14.7.3 RATE-CONTROLLING MEMBRANE

The membrane acts as a gateway for the drug to pass through at a specific diffusion rate and also holds a reservoir rigid in place. Primarily drug was blended with polymers, and their ratio governs the rate of diffusion from the face of TDDS to the skin surface. Some TDDS employ semipermeable membranes to control the rate of drug diffusion from the reservoir. These are synthesized by a combination of three different monomers (sec-butyl tiglate, 4-hydroxybutyl acrylates, 2-hydroxy-3-phenoxypropylacrylate) (Zhan et al. 2006). Ethylene vinyl acetate is also a commonly used material for rate-controlling membrane (Banerjee et al. 2014). Addition of a hydrophilic polymer can help to modify the drug release rate from patch. Thus, the availability of drug at the skin surface is ensured with the help of the rate-controlling membrane (Ajazuddin et al. 2013).

14.7.4 RELEASE LINERS

The release liner is the component of TDDS, which is in intimate contact with the adhesive layer during storage and transportation that is peeled off and discarded before the application. The liner is made up of a chemically inert material. Polyester foils and other metalized laminates can also be utilized for the purpose. The base of release liner is fabricated from nonocclusive (e.g., paper fabric) or occlusive (e.g., polyvinylchloride, polyethylene) material, whereas a release coating layer is prepared from silicon or Teflon (Alexander et al. 2012, Kandavilli, Nair, and Panchagnula 2002).

14.7.5 BACKING LAYER

The backing layer protects the environment and holds the whole TDDS as a single unit. These also serve for esthetic purpose. The backing layer must be selected so that the drug should not leach or permeate to the backing layer. Backing layers are films usually made up of polyethylene (CoTran 9720 and CoTran 9722), polyurethane (CoTran 9701), polyester (Scotchpak 9723), ethyl vinyl acetate (CoTran 9702 and CoTran 9706), polyolefin film, and aluminum vapor-coated layer (Gaikwad 2013, Kandavilli, Nair, and Panchagnula 2002, Banerjee et al. 2014).

14.7.6 PLASTICIZERS

Along with the other essential excipients, plasticizers are added to modify the property of films such as brittleness, ductility, flexibility, and also to aid in adhesiveness of films. Plasticizers are usually solids of low melting point and nonvolatile liquids which on addition to polymers can change some particular mechanical and physical properties of the material. Generally utilized plasticizers for TDDS are phthalate esters, phosphate, glycerol or sorbitol, fatty acid esters, PEG 200, and PEG 400, from 5% to 20% w/w (dry weight). The mechanical properties of TDDS and the permeability of drugs are greatly influenced by the proper selection of a suitable plasticizer and its concentration, as reported in the literature (Amnuaikit et al. 2005, Alexander et al. 2012, Malvey, Rao, and Arumugam 2019, Kathe and Kathpalia 2017).

14.8 DESIGN OF TDDS

The design of TDDS or patches involves the compilation of all the above-discussed component/s as a compact device to deliver the drug. The available patches can be classified into the following four types based on their compilation.

14.8.1 RESERVOIR SYSTEMS

As the name suggests, these patch types consist of a drug reservoir built between a rate-controlling membrane and an impermeable back layer with liner as a face front. The rate-controlling membrane governs the drug release rate. The drug reservoir can be formulated as a suspension, solution, gel, or a solid polymer matrix containing the uniformly dispersed drug. A biocompatible adhesive polymer layer is applied either entirely or as a periphery to aid the attachment to the skin. These type of patches offer better control over the flexibility in design and control over delivery rates and, however, possess intricate design (Kandavilli, Nair, and Panchagnula 2002). Based on these principals, Pichayakron et al. fabricated nicotine-loaded patch, where a concentrated solution of nicotine served as a reservoir and deproteinized natural rubber film acts as a rate-controlling membrane (Pichayakorn et al. 2013). Another example of reservoir-patch is demonstrated by Weimann et al., which consisted of a gel reservoir housing a mixture of cannabinoid, a polar liquid, and a gelling agent (Weimann 2018).

14.8.2 DRUG-IN-ADHESIVE SYSTEM

The drug is dispersed evenly in the adhesive polymer, and the patch is fabricated by either hot-melting the medicated adhesive on an impermeable back layer or solvent casting method. The reservoir is then applied with an unmedicated adhesive polymer on the top face, and this acts as a patch–skin interface. By contrast to reservoir patches, these patches offer limited flexibility in their design whilst their ease of manufacture. The skin permeability determines and governs the rate of drug delivery in matrix type of patches (Alexander et al. 2012). Ganti et al. successfully developed the drug-in-adhesive matrix-type transdermal patch containing 4-benzylpiperidine, where they employed silicon-based adhesive as a matrix-forming polymer (Ganti et al. 2018). On the same basis, Jain et al. fabricated the patch for the delivery of donepezil (Jain, Lee, and Singh 2018).

14.8.3 MATRIX-DISPERSION SYSTEM

In such systems, the drug reservoir is prepared by dispersion of the drug into the nonadhesive polymer (lipophilic or hydrophilic). The matrix-containing drug is fabricated as a disc which is attached to an occlusive base and positioned in a chamber made of a backing layer. The adhesive is then spread on the medicated disc's circumference so that skin comes in direct contact to medicated disc surface except for the adhesive rim. So, the drug directly diffuses from the matrix to the patch–skin interface. Pichayakron et al. fabricated the matrix type of patch of nicotine by the using deproteinized rubber and hydroxypropylmethyl cellulose as a matrix-forming polymer (Pichayakorn et al. 2012), whereas Suksaeree et al. prepared nicotine patch with pectin for matrix (Suksaeree et al. 2018).

14.8.4 MICRORESERVOIR SYSTEMS

This type of system exploits the principal of both matrix and reservoir systems. The fabrication is carried out in two phases: the first phase involves the formation of drug suspension in an aqueous hydrophilic polymer solution. Then, it is dispersed in homogeneous lipophilic polymer solution which was immediately stabilized by *in situ* crosslinking of lipophilic polymer, which results in entrapment of numerous unleachable microspheres of drug reservoirs. Such an approach was employed by Dsa et al. to deliver insulin where insulin niosomes act as a microreservior (Dsa et al. 2018). Another attempt was carried out by Wolff et al., where the patch contained the microreservior, in the form of solid dispersion of rotigotine and polyvinylpyrrolidone, distributed in dispersing agent (Wolff et al. 2018).

14.9 INNOVATIVE STRATEGIES FOR TDDS

14.9.1 VESICULAR SYSTEM BASED TDDS

A search through the literature evidenced that vesicles could not only act as a successful drug carrier for the transdermal delivery and facilitate the sustained release of loaded drug acting as a depot but also serve as a PE facilitating drug penetration across the skin owing to their unique structure; Figure 14.2 demonstrates various ways followed by vesicular systems to achieve transdermal

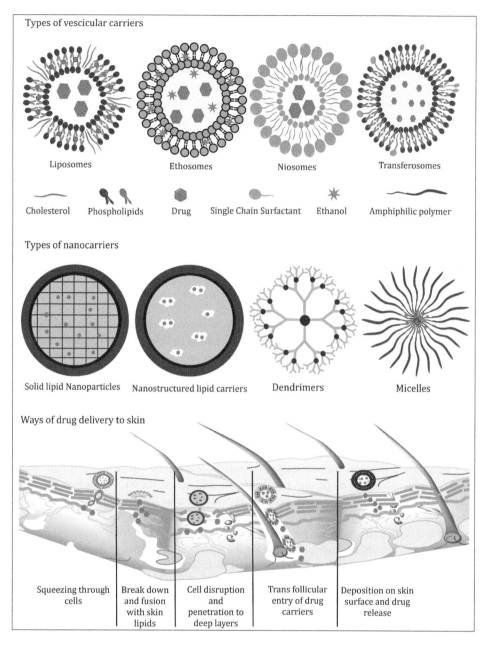

FIGURE 14.2 A schematic illustration of the structural construction of various types of vesicles and nano-carriers that are employed for TDD and the pathways they follow to transport the drug to deeper layers of skin. (Based on Roberts et al. 2017, Carter, Narasimhan, and Wang 2019, Bonde et al. 2018.)

delivery (Singh et al. 2015). Moreover, these vesicles are used as a membrane-limiting barrier to modulate systemic absorption in transdermal formulations. Vesicular lipid carriers include liposomes, transferosomes, niosomes, ethosomes, spingosomes, aquasomes, pharmacosomes; schematic structures of them are shown in Figure 14.2 (Pîrvu et al. 2010, Singh et al. 2015, Carter, Narasimhan, and Wang 2019). However, some vesicular systems like spingosomes, aquasomes, and pharmacosomes did not receive much consideration for transdermal delivery.

14.9.1.1 Liposomes

Liposomes are microscopic and thermodynamically stable vesicles of colloidal dimensions. They comprised of one or more lipid bilayers arranged in a concentric fashion. The core liposomes can house hydrophilic drugs, whereas lipophilic drugs get entrapped in between the lipid bilayers. Hydrophilic drug cannot readily pass through the lipid bilayers (Uchechi, Ogbonna, and Attama 2014, Ahmed, Shan, et al. 2019). Lipids of liposome interact with the biological membrane and can modify the structure of upper skin that facilitates the transport of both hydrophobic and hydrophilic drugs at the site of action. The nature of liposomes makes them extremely promising in TDD by facilitating drug penetration, reducing side effects, improving pharmacological effects, providing controlled drug release, and protecting drug from *in situ* metabolism (Pierre and Costa 2011, Cristiano et al. 2018).

Based on the concept of liposomes, Mezei and Gulasekharam compared an ointment and a liposomal lotion containing an equal concentration of triamcinolone acetonide. They conclude that the liposomal system was preferentially able to deliver 4–5 folds more steroid to the dermis and epidermis as compared to ointment, while a least amount of drug got absorbed systemically. Similarly, several attempts have been made to enhance percutaneous absorption of diclofenac, β-histidine, tetracaine, and triamcinolone through liposomes by numerous research groups (Cristiano et al. 2018, Mezei and Gulasekharam 1982).

14.9.1.2 Transferosomes

Transferosomes are ultradeformable liposomes with bilayered architecture prepared from lipids (e.g., soya phosphatidyl choline). An edge activator is added to lipids to convey deformability and elasticity to the bilayer by lowering its interfacial tension and destabilizing the lipid bilayer of the vesicles (Benson 2006, Singh et al. 2015). Like liposome, transferosomes are also primarily composed of phospholipids in addition to edge activators such as Span 80, deoxycholate, dipotassium glycyrrhizinate, sodium cholate, or Tween 80 (Cristiano et al. 2018). Unlike to liposome transferosomes are more hydrophilic which enables transferosomal membrane to swell more as compared to bilayers of conventional lipid vesicle and, thus, exploits the hydrophilic pathways or pores to access the entry through the SC (Singh et al. 2015, Benson 2006). The edge activator promotes rapid vesicular penetration through the intercellular lipids of the SC by squeezing through epidermal pores and facilitates the drug molecules penetration in and across the SC. Therefore, the structure and mechanism of their interaction with skin can provide the clue for their utilization in TDDS.

Transferosome is a versatile carrier for systemic as well as local delivery of macromolecules such as hydrophilic macromolecules, proteins and peptides (insulin), steroids (corticosteroid), other drugs (ketoprofen, anticancer drugs), and also for the transport of genetic material. These nanocarriers seem to be more effective than liposomes, and their flexibility allows for the development of transdermal vaccine (Benson 2006, Pierre and Costa 2011, Khan et al. 2015).

For the purpose, Jiang *et al.* developed paintable oligopeptide hydrogel-containing paclitaxel (PTX)-encapsulated and cell-penetrating peptide-loaded transferosome and aimed to improve PTX delivery transdermally for the treatment of topical melanoma. This modified transferosome formulation plastered over the skin above the melanoma tumor. They found that transferosomes provided extended retention on the skin and slowed down the tumor growth. Further, fictionalization of PTX transferosomes with cell-penetrating-peptide improved the transportation and accumulation into the tumor. The combination of topical application of prepared drug-loaded transferosome and the systemic chemotherapy using Taxol, a marketed PTX dosage form, resulted in higher antitumor efficiency as observed in xenograft B10F16 melanoma mouse model (Jiang et al. 2018).

14.9.1.3 Niosomes

Niosomes are the vesicles prepared from nonionic surfactants and formed by their self-assembly in an aqueous medium. Based on the method of preparation and their internal structure, they may be unilamellar or multilamellar (Morrow et al. 2007). During the formation of niosomes, the nonionic surfactants self-assemble themselves in bilayer structure; meanwhile hydrophobic drugs are incorporated within the bilayer whereas hydrophilic drugs are confined within the vesicle's inner space. The formation and drug encapsulation efficiency of niosomes are dependent on surfactant's hydrophilic–lipophilic balance (HLB) value, and it has been usually observed that the highest drug entrapment efficiency can be obtained with a surfactant of HLB value 8.6 (Carter, Narasimhan, and Wang 2019, Khan et al. 2015).

Many researchers explored the use of niosomes in systemic and topical products and utilized to encapsulate various drugs like anti-inflammatory drugs, estradiol, lidocaine, anticancer substances, peptide drugs, noninvasive vaccines and anti-infective agents (Escobar-Chávez 2012). Zhang et al. investigated the internalization of Span-40 based salidroside-loaded niosomes for cutaneous absorption of salidroside on human cellosaurus embryonic skin fibroblasts (CCC-ESF), and human epidermal immortal keratinocytes (HaCaT). The transdermal flux of the niosomal preparation was notably higher than its aqueous solution. Further, they investigated the internalization of niosomes and found that the pinocytotic vesicles and macropinocytosis were primary mechanisms of internalization by HaCaT cells, whereas CCC-ESF cells internalized niosomes via pinocytotic vesicles and lysosomes mediated endocytosis. Thus, the niosomal formulations could improve, as reported here, the dermal and transdermal salidroside delivery (Zhang et al. 2015).

14.9.1.4 Ethosomes

Ethosomes are soft, malleable, homogeneous multilamellar vesicles of lipid, ethanol (in relatively high concentrations (20%–50%), and water (Khan et al. 2015). The high level of ethanol (an ideal PE) provides vesicles with soft, flexible, and elastic properties, which enhances its fluidity of SC by disturbing the organization of lipid bilayer barrier of the SC. The incorporation of ethanol and cholesterol can enhance the elasticity and stability of ethosomes by altering its phase transition temperature on interaction with phosphatidylcholine. They can provide efficient drug delivery under both occlusive and nonocclusive conditions which fundamentally differentiates ethosomes from liposomes and transferosomes (Cristiano et al. 2018, Singh et al. 2015, Uchechi, Ogbonna, and Attama 2014). For these reasons, they are considered safe and efficient drug delivery systems and have wide future applications. Ethosomes can deliver cationic drugs like trihexyphenidyl and propranolol and highly lipophilic molecules such as minoxidil and testosterone, as well (Morrow et al. 2007). Ethosomes exhibit negative zeta potential and both hydrophobic and hydrophilic drugs can be loaded in them with higher entrapment efficiency. These peculiar properties demonstrate their superiority over conventional liposomes for TDD (Cristiano et al. 2018, Uchechi, Ogbonna, and Attama 2014).

In recent studies, many researchers compared the potential of liposomes and ethosomes for their transdermal delivery. Zhang et al. prepared novel psoralen-loaded ethosomes and investigated their transdermal delivery. They estimated transdermal flux and skin deposition of drug in the form of niosomes and liposomes separately and inferred that the transdermal fluxes of ethosomal psoralen were approximately ten fold higher than that of liposomal psoralen. Further, they concluded that ethosomes exhibit more biocompatibility with human ESFs than an equivalent ethanol solution (Zhang et al. 2014).

Similarly, Ma et al. developed paeonol-loaded ethosomes to improve oral bioavailability, poor stability, aqueous solubility of paeonol, and intended for transdermal administration. The optimized paeonol-loaded ethosomes showed increased encapsulation efficiency, *in vitro* transdermal absorption, and skin retention. They proved that the deposition and cumulative penetration of paeonol in the form of ethosomes were notably greater than its hydroethanolic (25%) solution. It indicates that ethosomes not only improved transdermal absorption but also enhanced accumulation in skin tissues. The safety of the prepared ethosomes was confirmed by histopathological studies (Ma et al. 2018).

14.9.1.5 Nanoemulsions

Nanoemulsions are a metastable, isotropic, immiscible, and translucent liquid dispersed system of water and oil in which the interfacial tension is significantly reduced. The interfacial tension is reduced by an interfacial film of added surfactants and/or cosurfactant that forms thermodynamically stable droplets of less than 100 nm size (Khan et al. 2015, Uchechi, Ogbonna, and Attama 2014). Nanoemulsions consist of either oil-in-water (oil droplets dispersed in a continuous aqueous system) or water-in-oil (aqueous droplets dispersed in a continuous oil system) forming droplets/dispersed phase in nanometric sizes. The oil-in-water nanoemulsions are best to deliver lipophilic drugs while the hydrophilic drugs are formulated using water-in-oil nanoemulsion (Escobar-Chávez 2012, Khan et al. 2015). Thus, the nature of drug governs the selection of type of nanoemulsion where drug is always dissolved in respective internal dispersed medium. In other words, hydrophobic drug is dissolved in oil phase and formulated as oil-in-water nanoemulsion while vice versa is true for hydrophilic drugs.

The nanoemulsions have gained considerable interest in TDD owing to additional benefits of the oil and surfactant content which may aid the transdermal drug permeation. They can act as a permeation enhancer through interacting with protective lipid layers of the skin and modify barrier function of the skin. Nanoemulsions have widespread application for transdermal delivery of nimesulide, gamma tocopherol, methyl salicylate, caffeine, insulin, aspirin, and plasmid DNA (Uchechi, Ogbonna, and Attama 2014).

14.9.2 Nanocarriers Based TDDS

Recently, the development in the nanotechnology opens a novel avenue for the drug delivery systems. The scientists have prepared and investigated a plethora of nanocarriers for their potential to deliver and improve the transportation of drugs to the skin and identified them as a successful vehicle to deliver many molecules like DNA, peptides, proteins, drugs, etc. Some of them are discussed over here in the focus of their application for TDDS. It has been observed that drug-loaded nanocarriers often collocate in hair follicles and thereby traverse through the superficial layers of the SC; subsequently caused the release of drugs into the deeper layers of the skin. The most commonly used nanocarriers for TDDS are dendrimers, SLNs, micelles, metal nanoparticles, nanostructured lipid carriers (NLCs), and polymeric nanoparticles, and their structural construction can be depicted in Figure 14.2 (Goyal et al. 2016).

14.9.2.1 Nanoparticles

Nanoparticles (NPs) are particles of solid core with nanoscale size (1–1,000 nm), which forms a distinct phase in aqueous suspension (Husseini and Pitt 2008, Roberts et al. 2017). However, NPs with 50–500 nm are of importance in light of TDDS (Carter, Narasimhan, and Wang 2019). Several categories of solid nanoparticles have been developed to date. Polymeric nanoparticles have a solid core consisting of a matrix of drug and nonsoluble or biodegradable polymers. Thus, the drug release can be either by degradation/erosion of matrix or the diffusion of the drug from the matrix core. Another approach involves the principal of prodrug where the drug is linked to the polymer, which on contact with tissue fluid breaks down to release the free drug. Various synthetic and natural polymers like poly(lactic-co-glycolic acid) (PLGA), polylactic acid (PLA), polysaccharides, and metals like gold or silver are utilized for their preparation (Vogt et al. 2016, Carter, Narasimhan, and Wang 2019, Khan et al. 2015). NPs can also encourage immunomodulation since they can even move to the lymph nodes from layers of skin. (Escobar-Chávez 2012). Moreover, the gold NPs were found to promote the percutaneous absorption of codelivered proteins and also avoid the tedious step of drug loading into the nanoparticulate system (Huang et al. 2010). The search through literature demonstrates the successful application of NPs for the transdermal delivery of the plethora of drugs such as minoxidil, triptolide, DNA, cyclosporin A, flufenamic acid, testosterone, caffeine, 5-fluorouracil, celecoxib, and coenzyme Q. (Escobar-Chávez 2012). More recently, the solid NPs made up of silk fibroin having 40 nm volume diameter were prepared and found that they successfully reached to the dermis to facilitate transdermal delivery (Takeuchi et al. 2019).

14.9.2.2 Solid Lipid Nanoparticles

SLNs composed of a solid lipid core and have three primary components: lipids, surfactants, and water. However, a steric/charged surfactant or polymer can usually be added to stabilize the SLNs dispersion. The structural makeup of SLNs may be either a drug-enriched core, homogenous matrix, or drug-enriched shell. These proved to be suitable carrier for hydrophobic drugs (Goyal et al. 2016). Owing to its lipid nature and occlusive properties they can form a film over the skin and can facilitate the skin hydration and protection (Roberts et al. 2017). By considering their characteristics, Jeon et al. synthesized retinyl palmitate-loaded surface-modified SLNs. The investigation indicated that the cutaneous distribution of retinyl palmitate improved by 4.8 times to that of neutral SLNs, owing to the negatively charged SLNs (Jeon et al. 2013).

14.9.2.3 Nanostructured Lipid Carriers

NLCs are a dispersion of a liquid lipid phase into a bulk of solid lipid matrix. NLCs are reported to have a higher potential for drug loading and possess better stability when compared with SLNs (Roberts et al. 2017, Montenegro et al. 2016). Owing to their lipid nature, NLCs are anticipated to have higher efficiency to permeate the skin layers and can find their application as TDDS. The attempt to employ NLCs for TDDS was carried out by Yue et al., where they synthesized a novel polymer, hyaluronic acid, and linoleic acid conjugated propylene glycol. The NLCs were prepared from the polymer and loaded with bupivacaine, a local anesthetic. The findings of *in vitro* and *in vivo* investigations not only showed higher efficiency of NLCs as nanocarriers for dermal drug delivery but also served as a sustained drug delivery by prolonging the anesthetic action of bupivacaine (Yue, Zhao, and Yin 2018).

Meanwhile, Gu et al. employed NLCs loaded with triptolide for their transdermal delivery. They showed that NLCs not only effectively penetrate the skin but also effectively partitioned into skin tissues than blood; as intended for local action. Thus, tripolide-loaded NLCs can be used to target skin tissues locally, since they effectively inhibited knee edema associated with rheumatoid arthritis (Gu et al. 2019). Likewise, several attempts were done to deliver the drug transdermally for either local or systemic effects (Montenegro et al. 2016).

14.9.2.4 Dendrimer

Dendrimers are an eminent class of macromolecules having highly branched, monodispersed structure and synthetically made of numerous small molecules to form a 3-D architecture macromolecule; thus can form particles of nanoscale (<15 nm) size (Vogt et al. 2016, Escobar-Chávez 2012, Dianzani et al. 2014). The loading of the drug can be done by both ways; attaching the drug to the free ends of numerous branches of dendrimer and can be sequestered inside the dendrimer. Thus, the drug release is expected by the diffusion mechanism (Husseini and Pitt 2008). Poly(2,2-bis (hydroxymethyl)propionic acid) scaffold, polyamidoamines, polypropylimines, poly(L-lysine) scaffold, polyesters (PGLSA-OH), and aminobis(methylenephosphonic acid) scaffold are examples of most commonly used dendrimers (Sun et al. 2012). Dendrimer-based nanocarrier system is found to be of interest due to their multidisciplinary applications and is proved as a good alternative for drug delivery systems in TDDS owing to their nanosize. Pentek et al. attempted the delivery of resveratrol by complexing it with polyamidoamine (PAMAM) dendrimer and found that the dendrimer not only improved the solubility and stability of the drug in aqueous medium but also facilitated skin penetration of resveratrol (Pentek et al. 2017). Another attempt to improve transdermal delivery of silibinin and epigallocatechin-3-gallate (EGCG) was carried out by Shetty et al. and demonstrated 3.96- and 9.82-fold increase in the skin penetration of both drugs complexed with dendrimer by using excised rat skin permeation studies (Shetty et al. 2017).

14.9.2.5 Micelles

Micelles are core–shell structures having a hydrophobic core and hydrophilic shell formed instantly by self-assembly of amphiphiles in an aqueous environment (Bonde et al. 2018). These are spherical nanovesicles prepared by using di/triblock polymers such as Pluronic, Soluplus, and Solutol. (Husseini and Pitt 2008). Owing to core–shell structure, micelles are specially employed to improve the drug delivery and loading of hydrophobic drugs sequestering them inside the core (Singh et al. 2018), whereas the outer hydrophilic corona facilitates their travel and stability in an aqueous environment; a prerequisite for the transcellular route in TDD. Thus, Ahmed et al. investigated the use of Vinpocetine-loaded micelle prepared from D-α-tocopherol polyethylene glycol 1000 succinate-α lipoic acid for transdermal delivery and reported their higher localization in skin tissues (Ahmed, El-Say, et al. 2019). On the other hand, Wang et al. prepared and evaluated glycyrrhizic acid micelle of approx. 10 nm size and loaded with podophyllotoxin. They observed the accumulation of micelles preferably in the epidermis and retention for further 12 h (Wang et al. 2016).

14.9.3 Physical Approach Based TDDS

14.9.3.1 MN-Based TDDS

In last two decades, MNs have been made possible to develop due to the advent in technologies and were introduced as an efficient, self-applied, painless, and minimally invasive technique (Zhu, Wang, et al. 2016, Cheung and Das 2016). MNs are tiny small micron-sized projections on one side of the transdermal patch, which on application to the skin pierces through the skin thereby breaches the SC, forming microchannels and facilitating drug delivery. MNs arranged as an array of tiny needles of approximately 10–900 μm in length with 10–50 μm width. These are fabricated from various materials like silicon, ceramics, metals, glass, polymers, carbohydrates, etc. (Ye et al. 2018) and with multiple geometries (e.g., conical (Zhu, Wang, et al. 2016), cylindrical (Chiappini 2018), pyramidal (Falo, Erdos, and Ozdoganlar 2018, Narayanan and Raghavan 2018), arrowhead (Chu and Prausnitz 2011)). The microchannels are so tiny that the patient feels no pain but large enough to deliver macromolecules (Larraneta et al. 2016). The advents in MNs formulation put forth some novel modes of drug delivery, which includes the following approaches and are illustrated schematically in Figure 14.3.

a. **Coated MNs ("Coat and poke" approach);** where drug is coated over the surface of MNs, which on the insertion into the skin dissolve in contact with tissues to release the drug.

b. **Solid MNs with two-step process ("Poke and patch" approach);** where solid MNs gently pressed against skin to create microchannels first, followed by drug patch or formulation application to the pretreated site. Employing the above two approaches, Narayanan *et al.* prepared silicon solid MNs and coated them with gold (Narayanan and Raghavan 2018). This approach is particularly suitable for macromolecules and water-insoluble drugs and was demonstrated by Qiu et al.; they pretreated the skin surface with MN array with 484 octagonal, pyramidal, and micron-sized MNs (150 μm height and 100 μm length). Then, elastic liposome docetaxel was applied over that surface to achieve transdermal delivery. The findings of investigations revealed that the transdermal flux of Docetaxel (1.3–1.4 μg/cm^2/h) was markedly enhanced with lowering lag time (approximately 70%) in comparison to traditional liposomes, when the site was pretreated with MNs (Qiu et al. 2008).

c. **Soluble and separating MNs ("Poke and release" approach);** where drug and biodegradable polymer fabricated as soluble and biodegradable MNs which on application to skin gets separated from patch and remains in the skin and controlled drug release (Luo et al. 2019, Ita 2017). These are preferred due to safety, low cost, and high loading capacity, batch-to-batch reproducibility, and ease of fabrication (Chen et al. 2015). Zhu et al. fabricated rapidly separating MNs from polylactic acid that was coated with

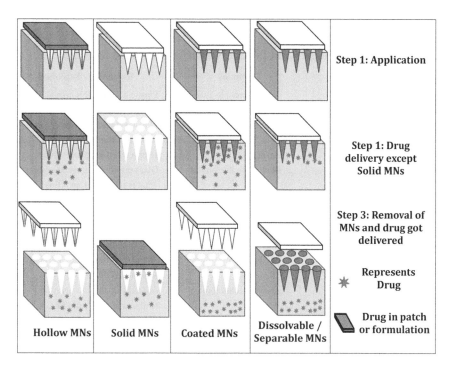

FIGURE 14.3 A schematic illustration of the types of MNs and their mechanisms for drug delivery. (Based on Larraneta et al. 2016.)

polyvinyl alcohol/sucrose gel (Zhu, Wang, et al. 2016), whereas dissolvable patchless MNs were fabricated and applied to skin by a device called Microlancer, which is compatible to deliver any macromolecule like insulin and vaccines and is invented by Lahiji et al. (Lahiji, Dangol, and Jung 2015).

d. **Hollow MNs ("Poke and flow" approach);** which acts as tiny hollow structures through which drug can be injected. K. van der Maaden et al. prepared hollow MNs to deliver the liposomal Human Papilloma Virus E7$_{43-63}$ synthetic long peptide vaccine to induce response from T-helper and cytotoxicity (van der Maaden et al. 2018).

e. **Bioresponsive MNs;** where MNs fabricated to respond to any physiological change (e.g., pH, glucose, reactive oxygen species, and enzymes) that acts as a trigger to deliver the drug and can serve as an on-demand delivery (Yu et al. 2015).

The MNs thus found numerous applications by virtue of their advantages especially the delivery of macromolecules such as proteins and peptides, vaccines for hepatitis B, insulin, oligonucleotides, Polymixin B and Japanese encephalitis and antirheumatic drugs, and plasmid DNA (Schoellhammer, Blankschtein, and Langer 2014, Economidou, Lamprou, and Douroumis 2018, Ye et al. 2018, Cole et al. 2018).

A recent application of light-responsive MNs where Chen et al. formulated the on-demand polycaprolactone MNs containing drug and silica-coated lanthanum hexaboride, which when irradiated with near-IR radiation to elevate the temperature leads to drug delivery by melting at 50°C (Chen et al. 2015). Another example of on-demand delivery is the bioresponsive MNs fabricated by Yu et al. to deliver insulin from crosslinked-hyaluronic acid matrix consisting of glucose-responsive vesicles triggered by the local tissue hypoxia. Hypoxia is generated due to the consumption of oxygen in body fluids when glucose oxidase (GOx) catalyzes glucose oxidation when glucose levels go high (Yu et al. 2015). Another example of stimulus-responsive is a hydrogel-forming MN arrays, developed

TABLE 14.4

Commercial Technologies and Products That Employ MNs for TDD

Name of TDDS	Company	Technology Exploited
Hollow microstructured transdermal system (hMTS)	3M pharmaceuticals	Plastic hollow MNs coated with drug solution
Solid microstructured transdermal system (sMTS)	3M pharmaceuticals	Plastic solid MNs coated with drug solution
MacroFlux®	Zosano	Drug-coated titanium MN arrays
BD Soluvia™	Becton Dickinson	Glass prefillable syringe system that is integrated with tiny MNs
MicroCor®	Corium	Rapidly dissolving MNs
DermaRoller®	DermaRoller	Titanium solid MNs
Soluble MNs	Elegaphy	Saccharide soluble MNs
MicronJet™	NanoPass and silex microsystems	Hollow micropyramidal MNs fabricated from silicon crystals
TheraJectMAT and VaxMAT	TheraJect	Rapidly dissolving MNs
PyraDerm™	Apogee technology	Coated silicon MNs array
Micro-Trans™	Valeritas	Hollow metal or solid PLGA MNs

by Hardy et al., which enable the delivery of ibuprofen in response to light. MN arrays were fabricated by a combination of polymers, ethylene glycol dimethacrylate, and 2-hydroxyethyl methacrylate (Hardy et al. 2016). The modern technology of 3-D printing also exploited to fabricate MNs as intended (Luzuriaga et al. 2018, Economidou, Lamprou, and Douroumis 2018). The paradigm shift from MNs to nanoneedle development can also be observed in the MNs (Zhao et al. 2018, Peng et al. 2018, Kavaldzhiev et al. 2018, Zhu, Yuen, et al. 2016). Various companies indulged in the fabrication of MNs developed as well as commercialized them; some examples are given in Table 14.4.

Despite higher success in the development of numerous types of MN-based TDDS and having shown promising results in animal models, their commercial application is limited due to some setbacks. MNs have limited surface for either drug loading or coating restricting their use in the case of potent drugs. On the other hand, the control over dose accuracy is compromised as compared to hypodermic needles. Interpersonal variation in dosing was observed due to the thickness of SC varies between individuals. Another significant concern may arise when either the tip of metal MNs breaks and remains in the skin or the inner lumen of hollow MNs is hindered by compressed tissues (Bariya et al. 2012).

14.9.3.2 Miscellaneous TDDS

Besides MNs, numerous ways for TDD have been identified by exploring and using physical methods to cross the SC. These methods are also known as active transport pathways for drug penetration as these methods exploit different physical forces to expel the drug in deeper layers of skin. The techniques, side effects, and limitations of these methods are discussed in Table 14.3.

14.10   QUALITY CONTROL OF TDDS

14.10.1   Physical Characterization

14.10.1.1   Thickness of the Patch

Vernier caliper, screw gauze, or digital micrometer is used to measure the thickness of the transdermal patch at various points, and the average thickness is calculated to verify whether the thickness of the fabricated patch is within the intended limit (Jassim, Sulaiman, and Jabir 2018,

Nair et al. 2013, Laffleur et al. 2018). The thickness is a rough estimate of drug content uniformity all over the patch surface and matrix.

14.10.1.2   Weight Uniformity

Before weighing, the patches were dried to a constant weight at 60°C for a fixed period. Specified areas having the same surface area are cut and weighed from various parts of the patch. The average weight is to be estimated as a weight uniformity measure with their standard deviation.

14.10.1.3   Folding Endurance

The folding endurance is the measure of flexibility of the dried films and is determined as the number of times that the patch of the specified area can be folded at the same location without breaking (Akram et al. 2018).

14.10.1.4   Tensile Strength

Tensile strength of patches is determined by clamping a patch in between two clamps that are pulled apart. The force required for breaking the patch or nicking of the patch was measured and is corresponded to the tensile strength of patch.

$$\text{Tensile strength} \left[\frac{N}{mm^2} \right] = \frac{\left(\text{required weight for rupture} \left[kg \right] \times 9.81 \left[\frac{m}{s} \right] \right)}{\left(\text{cross sectional area} \left[mm \right] \times \text{thickness of patch} \left[mm \right] \right)} \quad (14.5)$$

14.10.1.5   Percentage Moisture Content

The pieces of a specific size from the patch are cut. After noting down the initial weight of each piece, they are allowed to dry individually in desiccators containing activated silica or fused calcium chloride at ambient or slightly elevated temperature. The pieces are weighed intermittently to observe a loss in weight till constant weight is achieved. The loss of weight in percentage seems to be corresponding to the moisture content and is determined as

$$\text{Percentage} \left(\% \right) \text{of moisture content} = \frac{\text{Initial weight} - \text{Final constant weight}}{\text{Initial weight}} \times 100 \quad (14.6)$$

14.10.1.6   Content Uniformity Test

The test is performed by randomly selecting 10 patches and the content of each patch is solubilized in the specific media to extract out the drug completely. Sophisticated and validated methods like high performance liquid chromatography (HPLC) are used to quantify the content of each patch. If the content of 9 out of 10 patches is between 85% and 115% of the specified value and the remaining patch has content from 75% to 125% of the specified value, then transdermal patches seem to pass the test of content uniformity. However, additional 20 patches have to be tested if drug content of 3 patches is in the range of 75%–125%. The transdermal patches are said to pass the test if these 20 patches ranged from 85% to 115%.

14.10.1.7   Drug Content

The content of the patch is determined by dissolving a specified area of patch in a specified volume of a suitable solvent. Then the solution is analyzed by HPLC to determine the drug contents.

14.10.1.8   Water Vapor Transmission Studies (WVT)

The test is carried out to measure the tendency of the patch to hold or transmit the water vapors and performed in two ways. The patch piece of the specified surface area is sticked to the surface of vials, and the vials are placed in desiccators containing 200 mL of saturated potassium chloride and saturated sodium bromide solution. The desiccators were firmly closed and humidity was noted inside the desiccators. The vials after specified time are weighed.

In another method, 1 g of calcium chloride is weighed and placed in vials containing a piece of the patch. After weighing the vials, they are kept in the humidity chamber maintained at 68% RH. At the end of specified time intervals, the vials are weighed, and the weight increase is referred as a quantity of the moisture transmitted by the patch (Gaikwad 2013).

14.10.1.9 Stability Studies

Stability studies can be performed in accordance with the International Council of Harmonization (ICH) guidelines by storing the TDDS samples for 6 months at 40°C ± 0.5°C and 75%RH ± 5%RH. The samples are removed at 0, 30, 60, 90, and 180 days and the drug content is analyzed appropriately.

14.10.2 Release Performance of TDDS

14.10.2.1 *In Vitro* Drug Release Studies

The test provides the estimate of drug that is released from the patch within a specific time and under controlled conditions. For the purpose, the United States Pharmacopoeia (USP) dissolution apparatus V, i.e., Paddle over disks apparatus is used to determine the release of drugs from patches. The patches' definite thickness and shape are weighed, and sticked to the glass plate; that is then submerged in a dissolution medium. The paddle is positioned over the disk at a distance of 2.5 cm and rotated at a predetermined speed. The aliquots can be removed at appropriate time intervals and analyzed by either UV spectrophotometer or HPLC (Akram et al. 2018, Shabbir et al. 2018).

14.10.2.2 *Ex Vivo* Skin Permeation Studies

The skin permeation is simulated in the *ex vivo* skin permeation evaluation using diffusion cell. The Franz diffusion cell has a donor compartment (housed a formulation under test) and receiver (containing dissolution media) compartment, and in between them an excised and cleaned full-length rat skin (or human cadaver skin if available) is placed facing its dermal face to the donor compartment. The whole assembly is then maintained at specified conditions and the dissolution medium is stirred continuously with a magnetic stirrer. Then the aliquot is withdrawn as treated similar to *in vitro* release studies for analysis. The permeation flux of drug across the skin is then calculated by considering the total amount of drug released in a specific period through per unit surface area of skin. The flux is referred as the estimate of the exact quantity of drug that permeates through the skin and to the systemic circulation, not taking skin metabolism into consideration. Recently, artificially developed skin models can be exploited to determine the dermal penetration of the drug (Abd et al. 2016, Van Gele et al. 2011, Ganti et al. 2018).

14.10.3 Skin Irritation Study

Healthy rabbits were employed as test subjects for studying skin irritation possibly caused by patch application to the skin. The rabbit's dorsal surface is dehaired and cleaned thoroughly followed by application of the representative formulations or patches. A day later, the patches are removed and examined for any evidence of skin irritation and assigned grades from 1 to 5 based on the severity of skin injury, viz. erythema or edema (Nair et al. 2013).

14.10.4 Evaluation of Adhesive Properties of TDDS

The adhesive performance of TDDS is a crucial factor that determines the form of contact and interface formed with skin and hence safety as well as the efficacy of TDDS. The adhesive is characterized by its three properties, viz. peel (the force needed to remove a patch from the surface), shear (the flow resistance of the matrix), and tack (the ability to bind the surface of another material on short contact and under light pressure). Therefore, it becomes necessary to evaluate these characteristics of adhesive in its final TDDS form. For the purpose, the adhesive performance was monitored using several *in vitro* techniques in terms of shear strength, tack, and peel adhesion (Minghetti, Cilurzo, and Casiraghi 2004).

14.10.4.1 Peel Adhesion Test

The force needed to peel an adhesive off the surface where it is attached is referred to as the peel adhesion force. Most commonly employed test for peel adhesion consists of a substrate of stainless steel and peel angles of 90° or 180°. An exact width of a test sample is cut and attached to the stainless steel surface for 1 minute, and it is peeled off at the speed of 300 mm/min. The peel adhesion force is taken as the force required to peel off the adhesive off the substrate and is presented as force per unit of width (e.g., N/m). Peel adhesion force is the estimate of the adhesive strength of the adhesive since the force is intentionally employed to break the adhesive bonds formed between the adhesive and substrate. The peel adhesion depends not only on formulation parameters like the type and amount of additives, the molecular weight of the adhesive polymer, the TDDS backing, and adhesive thickness but also on the experimental parameters such as peel angle, substrate, dwell time, and peel speed. The peel adhesion value depends on the sample width but not on its length (Banerjee et al. 2014, Wokovich et al. 2006, Audett and Won 2018).

14.10.4.2 Thumb/Probe Tack Test

Previously, it is performed by slightly touching the adhesive surface with the thumb for a short time, and the force needed to break the bond was sensed. Therefore the test was referred to as thumb tack test. However, the test is highly subjective depending on the evaluator, and no absolute value of force was measured. Therefore, another test, probe tack test, was developed. For a probe tack test, a probe of the specific surface area was allowed to touch the adhesive surface by applying slight pressure for a short while, and the force required to break the bond was measured. The instruments like Texture Analyzer can measure tack in terms of not only the peak force but also the tack energy (Satas 1989, Wokovich et al. 2006, Quaroni et al. 2018).

14.10.4.3 Rolling Ball Tack Test

The rolling ball tack test is the measure of a combination of bond making and breaking processes. In this procedure, an 11-mm-diameter stainless steel ball weighing 5.6 mg is rolled down an inclined track (21°, 30°) to come in to contact at the bottom with horizontal upward-facing adhesive. Adhesive patches are cut in strips and conditioned for 24 hours at 75% RH. The running of the ball on the track is 5.5 mm. The distance the ball traveled out along the tape is taken as the measure of tack. The distance the ball rolled gives an inverse compressed scale of tack; the higher the distance, the less tacky the adhesive, but not in proportion to the ratio of distance. The reciprocal of rollout distance was taken as the tack value. When the rolling of the ball on the adhesive tape was superior to 25 cm, the tack value was considered zero. The results were the average of five determinations and were expressed as the reciprocal of running off the ball on the adhesive tape (Laffleur et al. 2018).

14.10.4.4 Shear Adhesion/Creep Compliance Test

The cohesive strength is the viscoelastic property of an adhesive and can be related to its performance when applied to skin. Low cohesion is indicated by high creep compliance of adhesive polymer and is influenced by the molecular weight, the composition of the polymer, type and the amount of tackifier added, and the degree of crosslinking. The test involves applying an adhesive-coated tape to the stainless steel surface, and the hook is mounted to the tape end. Then, a specified weight has hung the hook to pull it in a parallel direction to the surface. Shear adhesion strength is determined by the time the adhesive tape takes to remove from the plate. The longer the time taken for removal signifies the greater shear strength of the material and less creepiness of an adhesive (Cilurzo, Gennari, and Minghetti 2012, Ganti et al. 2018).

14.11 CONCLUSION AND FUTURE PROSPECTS

Over the years, TDDS are fetching significant attention for the development of newer strategies to achieve drug penetration across the skin followed by their commercialization for application in clinical practice. These systems are proved to be promising delivery systems and enhanced the therapeutic potential of drugs that undergo degradation, metabolism in stomach and hepatic portal system before reaching to the systemic circulation, especially in case of protein and peptides drugs. In addition to this, TDDS had also been employed for delivery of vaccines, non-steroidal anti-inflammataory Drugs (NSAIDS), and even for genetic materials. Besides conventional TDDS, newer techniques like iontophoresis and sonophoresis have been used to deliver hydrophilic drugs. Owing to their ability to provide controlled release, these were especially explored for insulin delivery, while their combinations with smarter biosensing techniques are capable of delivering on-demand insulin. Further, their use for sustained delivery of drugs like local anesthetic, antibacterial agents for local action, promisingly avoids requirement of larger drug doses and unnecessary exposure to other body parts. Conclusively, TDDS serve as a better and promising alternative drug delivery. However, challenges exist due to the intersubject variation in response and the absence of powerful animal models to assess the long-term safety concerns. Thus, such challenges need to be addressed through further research and development as well as via combination of existing and newer strategies.

REFERENCES

A Charoo, Naseem, Ziyaur Rahman, Michael A Repka, and S N Murthy. 2010. "Electroporation: An avenue for transdermal drug delivery." *Current Drug Delivery* 7 (2):125–136.

Abd, Eman, Shereen A Yousef, Michael N Pastore, Krishna Telaprolu, Yousuf H Mohammed, Sarika Namjoshi, Jeffrey E Grice, and Michael S Roberts. 2016. "Skin models for the testing of transdermal drugs." *Clinical Pharmacology: Advances and Applications* 8:163.

Ahmed, Kamel S, Xiaotian Shan, Jing Mao, Lipeng Qiu, and Jinghua Chen. 2019. "Derma roller® microneedles-mediated transdermal delivery of doxorubicin and celecoxib co-loaded liposomes for enhancing the anticancer effect." *Materials Science and Engineering: C* 99:1448–1458.

Ahmed, Osama AA, Khalid M El-Say, Bader M Aljaeid, Shaimaa M Badr-Eldin, and Tarek A Ahmed. 2019. "Optimized vinpocetine-loaded vitamin e D-α-tocopherol polyethylene glycol 1000 succinate-alpha lipoic acid micelles as a potential transdermal drug delivery system: in vitro and ex vivo studies." *International Journal of Nanomedicine* 14:33.

Ajazuddin, Amit Alexander, Basant Amarji, and Parijat Kanaujia. 2013. "Synthesis, characterization and in vitro studies of pegylated melphalan conjugates." *Drug Development and Industrial Pharmacy* 39 (7):1053–1062.

Akram, Muhammad Rouf, Mahmood Ahmad, Asad Abrar, Rai Muhammad Sarfraz, and Asif Mahmood. 2018. "Formulation design and development of matrix diffusion controlled transdermal drug delivery of glimepiride." *Drug Design, Development and Therapy* 12:349.

Alexander, Amit, Shubhangi Dwivedi, Tapan K Giri, Swarnlata Saraf, Shailendra Saraf, and Dulal Krishna Tripathi. 2012. "Approaches for breaking the barriers of drug permeation through transdermal drug delivery." *Journal of Controlled Release* 164 (1):26–40.

Alkilani, Ahlam, Maelíosa T McCrudden, and Ryan Donnelly. 2015. "Transdermal drug delivery: Innovative pharmaceutical developments based on disruption of the barrier properties of the stratum corneum." *Pharmaceutics* 7 (4):438–470.

Amnuaikit, Chomchan, Itsue Ikeuchi, Ken-ichi Ogawara, Kazutaka Higaki, and Toshikiro Kimura. 2005. "Skin permeation of propranolol from polymeric film containing terpene enhancers for transdermal use." *International Journal of Pharmaceutics* 289 (1–2):167–178.

Andrews, Samantha N, Eunhye Jeong, and Mark R Prausnitz. 2013. "Transdermal delivery of molecules is limited by full epidermis, not just stratum corneum." *Pharmaceutical Research* 30 (4):1099–1109.

Anirudhan, TS, and Syam S Nair. 2019. "Development of voltage gated transdermal drug delivery platform to impose synergistic enhancement in skin permeation using electroporation and gold nanoparticle." *Materials Science and Engineering: C* 102:437–446.

Audett, Jay, and Chee Youb Won. 2018. Fentanyl transdermal delivery system. Google Patents.

Azagury, Aharon, Luai Khoury, Giora Enden, and Joseph Kost. 2014. "Ultrasound mediated transdermal drug delivery." *Advanced Drug Delivery Reviews* 72:127–143.

Banerjee, Amrita, Renwei Chen, Shamsul Arafin, and Samir Mitragotri. 2019. "Intestinal iontophoresis from mucoadhesive patches: A strategy for oral delivery." *Journal of Controlled Release* 297:71–78.

Banerjee, Subham, Pronobesh Chattopadhyay, Animesh Ghosh, Pinaki Datta, and Vijay Veer. 2014. "Aspect of adhesives in transdermal drug delivery systems." *International Journal of Adhesion and Adhesives* 50:70–84.

Bariya, Shital H, Mukesh C Gohel, Tejal A Mehta, and Om Prakash Sharma. 2012. "Microneedles: An emerging transdermal drug delivery system." *Journal of Pharmacy and Pharmacology* 64 (1):11–29.

Baroni, Adone, Elisabetta Buommino, Vincenza De Gregorio, Eleonora Ruocco, Vincenzo Ruocco, and Ronni Wolf. 2012. "Structure and function of the epidermis related to barrier properties." *Clinics in Dermatology* 30 (3):257–262.

Barry, BW. 2002. "Drug delivery routes in skin: A novel approach." *Advanced Drug Delivery Reviews* 54:S31–S40.

Benson, Heather AE. 2006. "Transfersomes for transdermal drug delivery." *Expert Opinion on Drug Delivery* 3 (6):727–737.

Blank, Irvin H. 1964. "Penetration of low-molecular-weight alcohols into skin. I. Effect of concentration of alcohol and type of vehicle." *The Journal of Investigative Dermatology* 43:415–420.

Bonde, Gunjan Vasant, Sarita Kumari Yadav, Sheetal Chauhan, Pooja Mittal, Gufran Ajmal, Sathish Thokala, and Brahmeshwar Mishra. 2018. "Lapatinib nano-delivery systems: A promising future for breast cancer treatment." *Expert Opinion on Drug Delivery* 15 (5):495–507.

Bos, Jan D, and Marcus MHM Meinardi. 2000. "The 500 Dalton rule for the skin penetration of chemical compounds and drugs." *Experimental Dermatology* 9 (3):165–169.

Brown, Marc B, Gary P Martin, Stuart A Jones, and Franklin K Akomeah. 2006. "Dermal and transdermal drug delivery systems: Current and future prospects." *Drug Delivery* 13 (3):175–187.

Bruno, Benjamin J, Geoffrey D Miller, and Carol S Lim. 2013. "Basics and recent advances in peptide and protein drug delivery." *Therapeutic Delivery* 4 (11):1443–1467.

Büyüktimkin, Servet, Nadir Büyüktimkin, and J Howard Rytting. 1996. "Interaction of indomethacin with a new penetration enhancer, dodecyl 2-(NN-dimethylamino) propionate (DDAIP): its effect on transdermal delivery." *International Journal of Pharmaceutics* 127 (2):245–253.

Carter, Prerana, Balaji Narasimhan, and Qun Wang. 2019. "Biocompatible nanoparticles and vesicular systems in transdermal drug delivery for various skin diseases." *International Journal of Pharmaceutics* 555:49–62.

Chaudhri, Buddhadev Paul, Frederik Ceyssens, Piet De Moor, Chris Van Hoof, and Robert Puers. 2010. "A high aspect ratio SU-8 fabrication technique for hollow microneedles for transdermal drug delivery and blood extraction." *Journal of Micromechanics and Microengineering* 20 (6):064006.

Chen, Jun, Qiu-Dong Jiang, Ya-Ping Chai, Hui Zhang, Pei Peng, and Xi-Xiong Yang. 2016. "Natural terpenes as penetration enhancers for transdermal drug delivery." *Molecules* 21 (12):1709.

Chen, Mei-Chin, Ming-Hung Ling, Kuan-Wen Wang, Zhi-Wei Lin, Bo-Hung Lai, and Dong-Hwang Chen. 2015. "Near-infrared light-responsive composite microneedles for on-demand transdermal drug delivery." *Biomacromolecules* 16 (5):1598–1607.

Cheung, Karmen, and Diganta B Das. 2016. "Microneedles for drug delivery: trends and progress." *Drug Delivery* 23 (7):2338–2354.

Chiappini, Ciro. 2018. "Porous silicon microneedles and nanoneedles." In *Handbook of Porous Silicon*:185–201.

Chu, Leonard Y, and Mark R Prausnitz. 2011. "Separable arrowhead microneedles." *Journal of Controlled Release* 149 (3):242–249.

Cilurzo, Francesco, Chiara GM Gennari, and Paola Minghetti. 2012. "Adhesive properties: A critical issue in transdermal patch development." *Expert Opinion on Drug Delivery* 9 (1):33–45.

Cole, Grace, Ahlam A Ali, Cian M McCrudden, John W McBride, Joanne McCaffrey, Tracy Robson, Vicky L Kett, Nicholas J Dunne, Ryan F Donnelly, and Helen O McCarthy. 2018. "DNA vaccination for cervical cancer: Strategic optimisation of RALA mediated gene delivery from a biodegradable microneedle system." *European Journal of Pharmaceutics and Biopharmaceutics* 127:288–297.

Cristiano, Maria C, Felisa Cilurzo, Maria Carafa, and Donatella Paolino. 2018. "Innovative vesicles for dermal and transdermal drug delivery." In A.M. Grumezescu (Ed.), *Lipid Nanocarriers for Drug Targeting.* William Andrew Publishing: Norwich, New York, 175–197.

Das, Asha, and Abdul Baquee Ahmed. 2017. "Natural permeation enhancer for transdermal drug delivery system and permeation evaluation: A review." *Asian Journal of Pharmaceutical and Clinical Research* 10:5–7.

Dianzani, Chiara, Gian Paolo Zara, Giovanni Maina, Piergiorgio Pettazzoni, Stefania Pizzimenti, Federica Rossi, Casimiro Luca Gigliotti, Eric Stefano Ciamporcero, Martina Daga, and Giuseppina Barrera. 2014. "Drug delivery nanoparticles in skin cancers." *BioMed Research International*:1–13.

Dsa, Joyline, Manish Goswami, BR Singh, Nidhi Bhatt, Pankaj Sharma, and Meenakshi K Chauhan. 2018. "Design and fabrication of a magnetically actuated non-invasive reusable drug delivery device." *Drug Development and Industrial Pharmacy* 44 (7):1070–1077.

Economidou, Sophia N, Dimitrios A Lamprou, and Dennis Douroumis. 2018. "3D printing applications for transdermal drug delivery." *International Journal of Pharmaceutics* 544 (2):415–424.

Escobar-Chavez, Jose Juan, Isabel Marlen Rodriguez-Cruz, and Clara Luisa Dominguez-Delgado. 2012. "Chemical and physical enhancers for transdermal drug delivery." In Pharmacology. IntechOpen.

Escobar-Chávez, José Juan. 2012. "Nanocarriers for transdermal drug delivery." *Skin* 19:22.

Falo Jr, Louis D, Geza Erdos, and O Burak Ozdoganlar. 2018. Tip-loaded microneedle arrays for transdermal insertion. Google Patents.

Fernández-Cuadros, Marcos E, Ogla S Pérez-Moro, Maria Jesus Albaladejo-Florin, Ruben Algarra-López, and Luz Casique-Bo-canegra. 2019. "Calcifying tendonitis of the ankle, effectivenness of 5% acetic acid iontophoresis and ultrasound over achiles tendon: A prospective case series." *International Journal of Foot and Ankle* 3:023.

Gaikwad, Archana K. 2013. "Transdermal drug delivery system: Formulation aspects and evaluation." *Comprehensive Journal of Pharmaceutical Sciences* 1 (1):1–10.

Gansen, P, and M Dittgen. 2012. "Polyurethanes as self adhesive matrix for the transdermal drug delivery of testosterone." *Drug Development and Industrial Pharmacy* 38 (5):597–602.

Ganti, Sindhu S, Sonalika A Bhattaccharjee, Kevin S Murnane, Bruce E Blough, and Ajay K Banga. 2018. "Formulation and evaluation of 4-benzylpiperidine drug-in-adhesive matrix type transdermal patch." *International Journal of Pharmaceutics* 550 (1–2):71–78.

Gao, Huile, Yuchen Wang, Chen Chen, Jun Chen, Yan Wei, Shilei Cao, and Xinguo Jiang. 2014. "Incorporation of lapatinib into core–shell nanoparticles improves both the solubility and anti-glioma effects of the drug." *International Journal of Pharmaceutics* 461 (1):478–488.

Ghafourian, Taravat, Ali Nokhodchi, and Waseem Kaialy. 2015. "Surfactants as penetration enhancers for dermal and transdermal drug delivery." In *Percutaneous Penetration Enhancers Chemical Methods in Penetration Enhancement*. Springer:207–230.

Ghosh, Animesh, Subham Banerjee, Santanu Kaity, and Tin W Wong. 2015. "Current pharmaceutical design on adhesive based transdermal drug delivery systems." *Current Pharmaceutical Design* 21 (20):2771–2783.

Goyal, Ritu, Lauren K Macri, Hilton M Kaplan, and Joachim Kohn. 2016. "Nanoparticles and nanofibers for topical drug delivery." *Journal of Controlled Release* 240:77–92.

Gu, Yongwei, Xiaomeng Tang, Meng Yang, Dishun Yang, and Jiyong Liu. 2019. "Transdermal drug delivery of triptolide-loaded nanostructured lipid carriers: Preparation, pharmacokinetic, and evaluation for rheumatoid arthritis." *International Journal of Pharmaceutics* 554:235–244.

Gupta, Rakesh, Balarama Sridhar Dwadasi, Beena Rai, and Samir Mitragotri. 2019. "Effect of chemical permeation enhancers on skin permeability: In silico screening using molecular dynamics simulations." *Scientific Reports* 9 (1):1456.

Gutschke, Eva, Stefan Bracht, Stefan Nagel, and Werner Weitschies. 2010. "Adhesion testing of transdermal matrix patches with a probe tack test–In vitro and in vivo evaluation." *European Journal of Pharmaceutics and Biopharmaceutics* 75 (3):399–404.

Hardy, John G, Eneko Larrañeta, Ryan F Donnelly, Niamh McGoldrick, Katarzyna Migalska, Maelíosa TC McCrudden, Nicola J Irwin, Louise Donnelly, and Colin P McCoy. 2016. "Hydrogel-forming microneedle arrays made from light-responsive materials for on-demand transdermal drug delivery." *Molecular Pharmaceutics* 13 (3):907–914.

Hartmann, Petra, Edina Butt, Ágnes Fehér, Ágnes Lilla Szilágyi, Kurszán Dávid Jász, Boglárka Balázs, Mónika Bakonyi, Szilvia Berkó, Gábor Erős, and Mihály Boros. 2018. "Electroporation-enhanced transdermal diclofenac sodium delivery into the knee joint in a rat model of acute arthritis." *Drug Design, Development and Therapy* 12:1917.

Huang, Yongzhuo, Faquan Yu, Yoon-Shin Park, Jianxin Wang, Meong-Cheol Shin, Hee Sun Chung, and Victor C Yang. 2010. "Co-administration of protein drugs with gold nanoparticles to enable percutaneous delivery." *Biomaterials* 31 (34):9086–9091.

Husseini, Ghaleb A, and William G Pitt. 2008. "Micelles and nanoparticles for ultrasonic drug and gene delivery." *Advanced Drug Delivery Reviews* 60 (10):1137–1152.

Ita, Kevin. 2017. "Dissolving microneedles for transdermal drug delivery: Advances and challenges." *Biomedicine & Pharmacotherapy* 93:1116–1127.

Jain, Amit K, Eun Soo Lee, and Parminder Singh. 2018. Transdermal Adhesive Composition Comprising a Poorly Soluble Therapeutic Agent. Google Patents.

Jain, Narendra Kumar. 1997. Controlled and Novel Drug Delivery. CBS Publishers & Distributors: Delhi, India.

Jassim, Zainab E, Halah Talal Sulaiman, and Saba Abdul Hadi Jabir. 2018. "Transdermal drug delivery system: A review." *Journal of Pharmacy Research* 12 (5):802.

Jeon, Ho Seong, Jo Eun Seo, Min Soo Kim, Mean Hyung Kang, Dong Ho Oh, Sang Ok Jeon, Seong Hoon Jeong, Young Wook Choi, and Sangkil Lee. 2013. "A retinyl palmitate-loaded solid lipid nanoparticle system: Effect of surface modification with dicetyl phosphate on skin permeation in vitro and anti-wrinkle effect in vivo." *International Journal of Pharmaceutics* 452 (1–2):311–320.

Jhawat, Vikas Chander, Vipin Saini, Sunil Kamboj, and Nancy Maggon. 2013. "Transdermal drug delivery systems: Approaches and advancements in drug absorption through skin." *International Journal of Pharmaceutical Sciences Review Research* 20 (1):47–56.

Jiang, Tianyue, Tong Wang, Teng Li, Yudi Ma, Shiyang Shen, Bingfang He, and Ran Mo. 2018. "Enhanced transdermal drug delivery by transfersome-embedded oligopeptide hydrogel for topical chemotherapy of melanoma." *ACS Nano* 12 (10):9693–9701.

Jin, Quanchang, Hui-Jiuan Chen, Xiangling Li, Xinshuo Huang, Qianni Wu, Gen He, Tian Hang, Chengduan Yang, Zhen Jiang, and Enlai Li. 2019. "Reduced graphene oxide nanohybrid–Assembled microneedles as mini-invasive electrodes for real-time transdermal biosensing." *Small* 15 (6):1804298.

Kalluri, Haripriya, and Ajay K Banga. 2011. "Transdermal delivery of proteins." *Aaps Pharmscitech* 12 (1):431–441.

Kamboj, Sunil, Vikas Jhawat, Vipin Saini, and Suman Bala. 2013. "Recent advances in permeation enhancement techniques for transdermal drug delivery systems: A review." *Current Drug Therapy* 8 (3):181–188.

Kandavilli, Sateesh, Vinod Nair, and Ramesh Panchagnula. 2002. "Polymers in transdermal drug delivery systems." *Pharmaceutical Technology* 26 (5):62–81.

Kathe, Kashmira, and Harsha Kathpalia. 2017. "Film forming systems for topical and transdermal drug delivery." *Asian Journal of Pharmaceutical Sciences* 12 (6):487–497.

Kaur, Mandeep, Basant Malik, Tarun Garg, Goutam Rath, and Amit K Goyal. 2015. "Development and characterization of guar gum nanoparticles for oral immunization against tuberculosis." *Drug Delivery* 22 (3):328–334.

Kaur, Mandeep, Tarun Garg, Goutam Rath, and Amit Kumar Goyal. 2014. "Current nanotechnological strategies for effective delivery of bioactive drug molecules in the treatment of tuberculosis." *Critical Reviews™ in Therapeutic Drug Carrier Systems* 31 (1):49–88.

Kaur, Ranjot, Tarun Garg, Basant Malik, Umesh Datta Gupta, Pushpa Gupta, Goutam Rath, and Amit Kumar Goyal. 2016. "Development and characterization of spray-dried porous nanoaggregates for pulmonary delivery of anti-tubercular drugs." *Drug Delivery* 23 (3):872–877.

Kavaldzhiev, Mincho N, Jose E Perez, Rachid Sougrat, Ptissam Bergam, Timothy Ravasi, and Jürgen Kosel. 2018. "Inductively actuated micro needles for on-demand intracellular delivery." *Scientific Reports* 8:9918.

Khan, Nauman, Mohd S Harun, Asif Nawaz, Nurulaini Harjoh, and Tin W Wong. 2015. "Nanocarriers and their actions to improve skin permeability and transdermal drug delivery." *Current Pharmaceutical Design* 21 (20):2848–2866.

Kress, Hans G. 2009. "Clinical update on the pharmacology, efficacy and safety of transdermal buprenorphine." *European Journal of Pain* 13 (3):219–230.

Laffleur, Flavia, Benedikt Strasdat, Arshad Mahmood, Tobias Reichenberger, Melanie Gräber, and Kesinee Netsomboon. 2018. "Nasal patches containing naphazoline for management of nasal impairments." *Journal of Drug Delivery Science and Technology* 45: 54–59.

Lahiji, Shayan F, Manita Dangol, and Hyungil Jung. 2015. "A patchless dissolving microneedle delivery system enabling rapid and efficient transdermal drug delivery." *Scientific Reports* 5:7914.

Larraneta, Eneko, Rebecca EM Lutton, A David Woolfson, and Ryan F Donnelly. 2016. "Microneedle arrays as transdermal and intradermal drug delivery systems: Materials science, manufacture and commercial development." *Materials Science and Engineering: R: Reports* 104:1–32.

Luo, Zhimin, Wujin Sun, Jun Fang, KangJu Lee, Song Li, Zhen Gu, Mehmet R Dokmeci, and Ali Khademhosseini. 2019. "Biodegradable gelatin methacryloyl microneedles for transdermal drug delivery." *Advanced Healthcare Materials* 8 (3):1801054.

Luzuriaga, Michael A, Danielle R Berry, John C Reagan, Ronald A Smaldone, and Jeremiah J Gassensmith. 2018. "Biodegradable 3D printed polymer microneedles for transdermal drug delivery." *Lab on a Chip* 18 (8):1223–1230.

Ma, Hongdan, Dongyan Guo, Yu Fan, Jing Wang, Jiangxue Cheng, and Xiaofei Zhang. 2018. "Paeonol-loaded ethosomes as transdermal delivery carriers: design, preparation and evaluation." *Molecules* 23 (7):1756.

Mali, Audumbar Digambar. 2015. "An updated review on transdermal drug delivery systems." *International Journal of Advances in Scientific Research* 1 (06):244–254.

Malvey, Srilatha, J Venkateshwar Rao, and Kottai Muthu Arumugam. 2019. "Transdermal drug delivery system: A mini review." *The Pharma Innovation International Journal* 8 (1):181–197.

Marepally, Srujan, Cedar HA Boakye, Punit P Shah, Jagan Reddy Etukala, Adithi Vemuri, and Mandip Singh. 2013. "Design, synthesis of novel lipids as chemical permeation enhancers and development of nanoparticle system for transdermal drug delivery." *PloS one* 8 (12):e82581.

Marwah, Harneet, Tarun Garg, Amit K Goyal, and Goutam Rath. 2016. "Permeation enhancer strategies in transdermal drug delivery." *Drug Delivery* 23 (2):564–578.

Mathur, Vineet, Yamini Satrawala, and Mithun Singh Rajput. 2014. "Physical and chemical penetration enhancers in transdermal drug delivery system." *Asian Journal of Pharmaceutics (AJP)* 4 (3).

Menon, Gopinathan K, Gary W Cleary, and Majella E Lane. 2012. "The structure and function of the stratum corneum." *International Journal of Pharmaceutics* 435 (1):3–9.

Mezei, Michael, and Vijeyalakshmi Gulasekharam. 1982. "Liposomes—A selective drug delivery system for the topical route of administration: Gel dosage form." *Journal of Pharmacy and Pharmacology* 34 (7):473–474.

Michaels, AS, SK Chandrasekaran, and JE Shaw. 1975. "Drug permeation through human skin: theory and in vitro experimental measurement." *AIChE Journal* 21 (5):985–996.

Miller, MA, and E Pisani. 1999. "The cost of unsafe injections." *Bulletin of the World Health Organization* 77 (10):808.

Minghetti, Paola, Francesco Cilurzo, and Antonella Casiraghi. 2004. "Measuring adhesive performance in transdermal delivery systems." *American Journal of Drug Delivery* 2 (3):193–206.

Mitragotri, Samir. 2017. "Sonophoresis: Ultrasound-mediated transdermal drug delivery." In *Percutaneous Penetration Enhancers Physical Methods in Penetration Enhancement*. Springer:3–14.

Montenegro, Lucia, Francesco Lai, Alessia Offerta, Maria Grazia Sarpietro, Lucia Micicche, Anna Maria Maccioni, Donatella Valenti, and Anna Maria Fadda. 2016. "From nanoemulsions to nanostructured lipid carriers: A relevant development in dermal delivery of drugs and cosmetics." *Journal of Drug Delivery Science and Technology* 32:100–112.

Morrow, DIJ, PA McCarron, AD Woolfson, and RF Donnelly. 2007. "Innovative strategies for enhancing topical and transdermal drug delivery." *The Open Drug Delivery Journal* 1:36–59.

Nair, Rajesh Sreedharan, Tai Nyet Ling, Mohamed Saleem Abdul Shukkoor, and Balamurugan Manickam. 2013. "Matrix type transdermal patches of captopril: Ex vivo permeation studies through excised rat skin." *Journal of Pharmacy Research* 6 (7):774–779.

Narayanan, S Pradeep, and S Raghavan. 2018. "Fabrication and characterization of gold-coated solid silicon microneedles with improved biocompatibility." *The International Journal of Advanced Manufacturing Technology* 104(9–12):1–7.

Okumura, M, Y Nakamori, K Sugibayashi, and Y Morimoto. 1991. "Enhanced skin permeation of papaverine by a medium chain glyceride." *Drug Design and Delivery* 7 (2):147–157.

Otberg, Nina, Alexa Patzelt, Utkur Rasulev, Timo Hagemeister, Michael Linscheid, Ronald Sinkgraven, Wolfram Sterry, and Jürgen Lademann. 2008. "The role of hair follicles in the percutaneous absorption of caffeine." *British Journal of Clinical Pharmacology* 65 (4):488–492.

Pandey, Anushree, Ashu Mittal, Nitesh Chauhan, and Sanjar Alam. 2014. "Role of surfactants as penetration enhancer in transdermal drug delivery system." *Journal of Molecular Pharmaceutics & Organic Process Research* 2 (113):2–7.

Panzade, Prabhakar Satwaji. 2012. "Iontophoresis: A functional approach for enhancement of transdermal drug delivery." *Asian Journal of Biomedical and Pharmaceutical Sciences* 2 (11):1.

Pastore, Michael N, Yogeshvar N Kalia, Michael Horstmann, and Michael S Roberts. 2015. "Transdermal patches: History, development and pharmacology." *British Journal of Pharmacology* 172 (9):2179–2209.

Pathan, Inayat Bashir, and C Mallikarjuna Setty. 2009. "Chemical penetration enhancers for transdermal drug delivery systems." *Tropical Journal of Pharmaceutical Research* 8 (2).

Patil, Sunita, Parminder Singh, Christiane Szolar-Platzer, and Howard Maibach. 1996. "Epidermal enzymes as penetration enhancers in transdermal drug delivery?" *Journal of Pharmaceutical Sciences* 85 (3):249–252.

Peng, Hui, Ganggang Wei, Kanjun Sun, Guofu Ma, Enke Feng, Xue Yang, and Ziqiang Lei. 2018. "Integrated and heterostructured cobalt manganese sulfide nanoneedle arrays as advanced electrodes for high-performance supercapacitors." *New Journal of Chemistry* 42 (22):18328–18334.

Pentek, Tyler, Eric Newenhouse, Brennin O'Brien, and Abhay Chauhan. 2017. "Development of a topical resveratrol formulation for commercial applications using dendrimer nanotechnology." *Molecules* 22 (1):137.

Pichayakorn, Wiwat, Jirapornchai Suksaeree, Prapaporn Boonme, Thanaporn Amnuaikit, Wirach Taweepreda, and Garnpimol C Ritthidej. 2012. "Deproteinized natural rubber latex/hydroxypropylmethyl cellulose blending polymers for nicotine matrix films." *Industrial & Engineering Chemistry Research* 51 (25):8442–8452.

Pichayakorn, Wiwat, Jirapornchai Suksaeree, Prapaporn Boonme, Wirach Taweepreda, Thanaporn Amnuaikit, and Garnpimol C Ritthidej. 2013. "Deproteinised natural rubber used as a controlling layer membrane in reservoir-type nicotine transdermal patches." *Chemical Engineering Research and Design* 91 (3):520–529.

Pierre, Maria Bernadete Riemma, and Irina dos Santos Miranda Costa. 2011. "Liposomal systems as drug delivery vehicles for dermal and transdermal applications." *Archives of Dermatological Research* 303 (9):607.

Pîrvu, C Dinu, Cristina Hlevca, Alina Ortan, and Răzvan Prisada. 2010. "Elastic vesicles as drugs carriers through the skin." *Farmacia* 58 (2):128–135.

Polat, Baris E, Daniel Blankschtein, and Robert Langer. 2010. "Low-frequency sonophoresis: application to the transdermal delivery of macromolecules and hydrophilic drugs." *Expert Opinion on Drug Delivery* 7 (12):1415–1432.

Polat, Baris E, Douglas Hart, Robert Langer, and Daniel Blankschtein. 2011. "Ultrasound-mediated transdermal drug delivery: Mechanisms, scope, and emerging trends." *Journal of Controlled Release* 152 (3):330–348.

Prakash, Dev, Amrit Pal Singh, Nishant Singh Katiyar, Kamla Pathak, and D Pathak. 2016. "Penetration enhancers: Adjuvants in transdermal drug delivery system." *World Journal of Pharmacy and Pharmaceutical Sciences* 5 (5):353–376.

Prausnitz, Mark R, and Robert Langer. 2008. "Transdermal drug delivery." *Nature Biotechnology* 26 (11):1261.

Prausnitz, Mark R, Samir Mitragotri, and Robert Langer. 2004. "Current status and future potential of transdermal drug delivery." *Nature Reviews Drug Discovery* 3 (2):115.

Qiu, Yuqin, Yunhua Gao, Kejia Hu, and Fang Li. 2008. "Enhancement of skin permeation of docetaxel: a novel approach combining microneedle and elastic liposomes." *Journal of Controlled Release* 129 (2):144–150.

Quaroni, Gaia MG, Chiara GM Gennari, Francesco Cilurzo, Guylaine Ducouret, Costantino Creton, and Paola Minghetti. 2018. "Tuning the rheological properties of an ammonium methacrylate copolymer for the design of adhesives suitable for transdermal patches." *European Journal of Pharmaceutical Sciences* 111:238–246.

Rein, H. 1924. "Experimental electroendosmotic studies on living human skin." *Zeitschrift fur Biologie* 81:125–140.

Roberts, MS, Y Mohammed, MN Pastore, S Namjoshi, S Yousef, A Alinaghi, IN Haridass, E Abd, VR Leite-Silva, and HAE Benson. 2017. "Topical and cutaneous delivery using nanosystems." *Journal of Controlled Release* 247:86–105.

Ruan, Renquan, Ming Chen, Lili Zou, Pengfei Wei, Juanjuan Liu, Weiping Ding, and Longping Wen. 2016. "Recent advances in peptides for enhancing transdermal macromolecular drug delivery." *Therapeutic Delivery* 7 (2):89–100.

Saini, Sushila, Shikha Baghel, and SS Chauhan. 2014. "Recent development in penetration enhancers and techniques in transdermal drug delivery system." *Journal of Advanced Pharmacy Education & Research Jan-Mar* 4 (1).

Santos, Lúcia F, Ilídio J Correia, A Sofia Silva, and João F Mano. 2018. "Biomaterials for drug delivery patches." *European Journal of Pharmaceutical Sciences* 118:49–66.

Satas, Donatas. 1989. Handbook of Pressure Sensitive Adhesive Technology. Satas & Associates: Warwick, RI.

Scheuplein, Robert J. 1965. "Mechanism of percutaneous adsorption: I. Routes of penetration and the influence of solubility." *Journal of Investigative Dermatology* 45 (5):334–346.

Schoellhammer, Carl M, Daniel Blankschtein, and Robert Langer. 2014. "Skin permeabilization for transdermal drug delivery: Recent advances and future prospects." *Expert Opinion on Drug Delivery* 11 (3):393–407.

Shabbir, Maryam, Ali Sajid, Irfan Hamid, Ali Sharif, Muhammad Furqan Akhtar, Moosa Raza, Shoaib Ahmed, Sohaib Peerzada, and Muhammad Umair Amin. 2018. "Influence of different formulation variables on the performance of transdermal drug delivery system containing tizanidine hydrochloride: In vitro and ex vivo evaluations." *Brazilian Journal of Pharmaceutical Sciences* 54 (4).

Shetty, Pallavi Krishna, Jyothsna Manikkath, Karnaker Tupally, Ganesh Kokil, Aswathi R Hegde, Sushil Y Raut, Harendra S Parekh, and Srinivas Mutalik. 2017. "Skin delivery of EGCG and silibinin: Potential of peptide dendrimers for enhanced skin permeation and deposition." *AAPS PharmSciTech* 18 (6):2346–2357.

Sidat, Zainul, Thashree Marimuthu, Pradeep Kumar, Lisa C du Toit, Pierre PD Kondiah, Yahya E Choonara, and Viness Pillay. 2019. "Ionic liquids as potential and synergistic permeation enhancers for transdermal drug delivery." *Pharmaceutics* 11 (2):96.

Singh, Deependra, Madhulika Pradhan, Mukesh Nag, and Manju Rawat Singh. 2015. "Vesicular system: Versatile carrier for transdermal delivery of bioactives." *Artificial Cells, Nanomedicine, and Biotechnology* 43 (4):282–290.

Singh, Juhi, Pooja Mittal, Gunjan Vasant Bonde, Gufran Ajmal, and Brahmeshwar Mishra. 2018. "Design, optimization, characterization and in-vivo evaluation of Quercetin enveloped Soluplus®/P407 micelles in diabetes treatment." In: *Artificial Cells, Innanomedicine, and biotechnology* 46 (sup3):S546–S555.

Sinha, VR, and Maninder Pal Kaur. 2000. "Permeation enhancers for transdermal drug delivery." *Drug Development and industrial pharmacy* 26 (11):1131–1140.

Sivamani, Raja K, Dorian Liepmann, and Howard I Maibach. 2007. "Microneedles and transdermal applications." *Expert Opinion on Drug Yelivery* 4 (1):19–25.

Suksaeree, Jirapornchai, Jessada Prasomkij, Kamon Panrat, and Wiwat Pichayakorn. 2018. "Comparison of pectin layers for nicotine transdermal patch preparation." *Advanced Pharmaceutical Bulletin* 8 (3):401.

Sun, Mingjing, Aiping Fan, Zheng Wang, and Yanjun Zhao. 2012. "Dendrimer-mediated drug delivery to the skin." *Soft Matter* 8 (16):4301–4305.

Takeuchi, Issei, Yosuke Shimamura, Yuki Kakami, Tsunenori Kameda, Keitaro Hattori, Seiji Miura, Hiroyuki Shirai, Mutsuo Okumura, Toshio Inagi, and Hiroshi Terada. 2019. "Transdermal delivery of 40-nm silk fibroin nanoparticles." *Colloids and Surfaces B: Biointerfaces* 175:564–568.

Tiwari, Rohit, Manish Jaimini, Shailender Mohan, and Sanjay Sharma. 2013. "Transdermal Drug Delivery System: A Review."

Tsai, Jui-Chen, Richard H Guy, Carl R Thornfeldt, Wen Ni Gao, Kenneth R Feingold, and Peter M Elias. 1996. "Metabolic approaches to enhance transdermal drug delivery. 1. Effect of lipid synthesis inhibitors." *Journal of pharmaceutical sciences* 85 (6):643–648.

Uchechi, Okoro, John DN Ogbonna, and Anthony A Attama. 2014. "Nanoparticles for dermal and transdermal drug delivery." In Application of Nanotechnology in Drug Delivery. IntechOpen.

USFDA. Drugs@FDA: FDA approved drug products. accessed May 9, 2019. www.accessdata.fda.gov/scripts/cder/daf/.

van der Maaden, Koen, Jeroen Heuts, Marcel Camps, Maria Pontier, Anton Terwisscha van Scheltinga, Wim Jiskoot, Ferry Ossendorp, and Joke Bouwstra. 2018. "Hollow microneedle-mediated micro-injections of a liposomal HPV E7$_{43-63}$ synthetic long peptide vaccine for efficient induction of cytotoxic and T-helper responses." *Journal of Controlled Release* 269:347–354.

Van Gele, Mireille, Barbara Geusens, Lieve Brochez, Reinhart Speeckaert, and Jo Lambert. 2011. "Three-dimensional skin models as tools for transdermal drug delivery: Challenges and limitations." *Expert Opinion on Drug Delivery* 8 (6):705–720.

Vogt, Annika, Christian Wischke, Axel T Neffe, Nan Ma, Ulrike Alexiev, and Andreas Lendlein. 2016. "Nanocarriers for drug delivery into and through the skin—do existing technologies match clinical challenges?" *Journal of Controlled Release* 242:3–15.

Wang, Yatian, Boxin Zhao, Shengqi Wang, Qianying Liang, Yun Cai, Fuheng Yang, and Guofeng Li. 2016. "Formulation and evaluation of novel glycyrrhizic acid micelles for transdermal delivery of podophyllotoxin." *Drug Delivery* 23 (5):1623–1635.

Watkinson, Adam C, Mary-Carmel Kearney, Helen L Quinn, Aaron J Courtenay, and Ryan F Donnelly. 2016. "Future of the transdermal drug delivery market–have we barely touched the surface?" *Expert Opinion on Drug Delivery* 13 (4):523–532.

Weimann, Ludwig. 2018. Transdermal delivery of cannabidiol with other active moieties including cannabinoids. Google Patents.

Williams, Adrian C, and Brian W Barry. 2012. "Penetration enhancers." *Advanced Drug Delivery Reviews* 64:128–137.

Wokovich, Anna M, Suneela Prodduturi, William H Doub, Ajaz S Hussain, and Lucinda F Buhse. 2006. "Transdermal drug delivery system (TDDS) adhesion as a critical safety, efficacy and quality attribute." *European Journal of Pharmaceutics and Biopharmaceutics* 64 (1):1–8.

Wolff, Hans-Michael, Christoph Arth, Luc Quere, and Walter Müller. 2018. Polyvinylpyrrolidone for the stabilization of a solid dispersion of the non-crystalline form of rotigotine. Google Patents.

Wolff, HM. 2014. "Future of transdermal drug delivery systems (TDDS)." *American Pharmaceutical Review* 17 (4).

Wong, Tin Wui. 2014. "Electrical, magnetic, photomechanical and cavitational waves to overcome skin barrier for transdermal drug delivery." *Journal of Controlled Release* 193:257–269.

Wu, Ji, Kalpana S Paudel, Caroline Strasinger, Dana Hammell, Audra L Stinchcomb, and Bruce J Hinds. 2010. "Programmable transdermal drug delivery of nicotine using carbon nanotube membranes." *Proceedings of the National Academy of Sciences* 107 (26):11698–11702.

Yang, Guang, Yuqi Zhang, and Zhen Gu. 2018. "Punching and electroporation for enhanced transdermal drug delivery." *Theranostics* 8 (13):3688.

Yang, Yang, Jason Bugno, and Seungpyo Hong. 2013. "Nanoscale polymeric penetration enhancers in topical drug delivery." *Polymer Chemistry* 4 (9):2651–2657.

Yao, Wendong, Chenghao Tao, Jiafeng Zou, Hongyue Zheng, Jingjing Zhu, Zhihong Zhu, Jiazhen Zhu, Lin Liu, Fanzhu Li, and Xinli Song. 2019. "Flexible two-layer dissolving and safing Microneedle transdermal of Neurotoxin: A biocomfortable attempt to treat rheumatoid arthritis." *International Journal of Pharmaceutics* 563:91–100.

Ye, Yanqi, Jicheng Yu, Di Wen, Anna R Kahkoska, and Zhen Gu. 2018. "Polymeric microneedles for transdermal protein delivery." *Advanced Drug Delivery Reviews* 127:106–118.

Yu, Jicheng, Yuqi Zhang, Yanqi Ye, Rocco DiSanto, Wujin Sun, Davis Ranson, Frances S Ligler, John B Buse, and Zhen Gu. 2015. "Microneedle-array patches loaded with hypoxia-sensitive vesicles provide fast glucose-responsive insulin delivery." *Proceedings of the National Academy of Sciences* 112 (27):8260–8265.

Yue, Yaocun, Dandan Zhao, and Qiuwen Yin. 2018. "Hyaluronic acid modified nanostructured lipid carriers for transdermal bupivacaine delivery: In vitro and in vivo anesthesia evaluation." *Biomedicine & Pharmacotherapy* 98:813–820.

Zhan, Xiaoping, Guochun Tang, Sijing Chen, and Zhenmin Mao. 2006. "A new copolymer membrane controlling clonidine linear release in a transdermal drug delivery system." *International Journal of Pharmaceutics* 322 (1–2):1–5.

Zhang, Yongtai, Kai Zhang, Zhonghua Wu, Teng Guo, Beini Ye, Mingyun Lu, Jihui Zhao, Chunyun Zhu, and Nianping Feng. 2015. "Evaluation of transdermal salidroside delivery using niosomes via in vitro cellular uptake." *International Journal of Pharmaceutics* 478 (1):138–146.

Zhang, Yong-Tai, Li-Na Shen, Zhong-Hua Wu, Ji-Hui Zhao, and Nian-Ping Feng. 2014. "Comparison of ethosomes and liposomes for skin delivery of psoralen for psoriasis therapy." *International Journal of Pharmaceutics* 471 (1–2):449–452.

Zhao, Jian, Zhenjiang Li, Xiangcheng Yuan, Zhen Yang, Meng Zhang, Alan Meng, and Qingdang Li. 2018. "A high-energy density asymmetric supercapacitor based on Fe2O3 nanoneedle arrays and NiCo2O4/Ni (OH) 2 hybrid nanosheet arrays grown on SiC nanowire networks as free-standing advanced electrodes." *Advanced Energy Materials* 8 (12):1702787.

Zhao, Zhongfu, Peiying Liu, Chunqing Zhang, Xiuling Zhu, Wei Liu, Shiyun Li, Yandong Zhang, and Fanzhi Meng. 2019. "Hot-melt pressure-sensitive adhesives based on SIS-g-PB copolymer for transdermal delivery of hydrophilic drugs." *International Journal of Adhesion and Adhesives* 91:72–76.

Zhu, Dan Dan, Qi Lei Wang, Xu Bo Liu, and Xin Dong Guo. 2016. "Rapidly separating microneedles for transdermal drug delivery." *Acta Biomaterialia* 41:312–319.

Zhu, Xiaoyue, Muk Fung Yuen, Li Yan, Zhenyu Zhang, Fujin Ai, Yang Yang, Peter KN Yu, Guangyu Zhu, Wenjun Zhang, and Xianfeng Chen. 2016. "Diamond-nanoneedle-array-facilitated intracellular delivery and the potential Influence on cell physiology." *Advanced Healthcare Materials* 5 (10):1157–1168.

15 Mucoadhesive Chitosan-Based Nanoparticles for Oral Drug Delivery

Xin Zhang, Jian Guan, and Shirui Mao
Shenyang Pharmaceutical University

CONTENTS

15.1 INTRODUCTION

Oral drug delivery system is one of the preferred administration routes for patients due to excellent safety and patient compliance. Appropriate design of drug carrier is critical to increase the oral bioavailability of drugs. However, the complex gastrointestinal environment and mucus layer greatly affect oral delivery efficiency of drugs. Due to the faster secretion and clearance rate of mucus layer, most well-designed micro or nanopreparations cannot stay in the gastrointestinal tract for sufficiently long time, therefore with limited absorption by the intestinal epithelial cells.

The mucoadhesion and absorption enhancing properties of chitosan-based nanoparticles aid in increasing the residence time of drugs in the gastrointestinal tract and improving their bioavailability. Further modification of physical and chemical properties of chitosan or combination of other polymeric materials with chitosan further expands its application in drug delivery, making it not only suitable for small molecule water-soluble, poorly water-soluble drugs, but also for oral delivery of biomacromolecule drugs.

Thus, in this chapter, first of all, mucus structure, mucoadhesion mechanism, and mucoadhesion evaluation methods were introduced. Thereafter, properties of chitosan, synthesis of chitosan derivatives, and their biological properties were reviewed. Moreover, the application of chitosan in mucoadhesive nanoparticle delivery system and the fate of chitosan-based nanoparticles after oral administration were discussed.

15.2 FEATURES OF MUCUS AND MECHANISM OF MUCOADHESION

15.2.1 STRUCTURE OF MUCUS

The surface of the gastrointestinal tract is covered with a mucus layer. The multifunction of mucus including lubricating and selective permeation, which allows the body's required nutrients to enter the human body and blocks the harmful substances such as most bacteria and pathogens, is vital to the human body.

Mucus is mainly composed of mucin, salts, lipids, antibodies, bacteria, and cell debris. Apart from water which is 90%–95% of the mucus, mucin is the main component of mucus. The "PTS" region composed of proline, threonine, and serine can be found in the mucin structure. The threonine and serine could form a polysaccharide–protein complex with O-linked glycans. The carboxyl structure in polysaccharide makes mucin PTS region negatively charged. Partial cysteine-rich area formed by disulfide bonds also exists in the PTS regions. The mucin monomer ends with an N-linked sulfate group and connected by disulfide bond (Olmsted et al. 2001; Cone 2009). The scanning electron microscope (SEM)study showed that the spatial space between mucin fibers was about 100–500 nm (Saltzman et al. 1994), which allowed the nanoparticles less than that size to pass through.

Mucus layer undergoes a process of continuous secretion, shedding, digestion, and absorption, and ~10 L of mucus is secreted into the gastrointestinal tract and most of them are reabsorbed everyday (Ensign, Cone, and Hanes 2012). The mucus layer can be structurally divided into a loose layer and a dense layer, and the loose layer can flow with the chyme. The thickness of the intestinal mucus layer is about 15–450 μm varying with the location of the gastrointestinal tract, which is renewed according to mucus secretion rate and mucus degradation and shedding rate (Khanvilkar, Donovan, and Flanagan 2001). The mucus is non-Newtonian fluid in rheology with shear thinning characteristics. The viscosity of mucus is closely related to the content of mucin (Ensign, Cone, and Hanes 2012). The inevitable interaction between mucus and pharmaceutical formulations includes hydrophobic forces and electrostatic forces, and the complexity of the gastrointestinal environment further highlights the importance of mucus adhesion studies in oral drug delivery system.

15.2.2 MECHANISM OF MUCOADHESION

Different theories have been developed to explain the mucoadhesion mechanism of polymers. According to the molecular structure of polymers, different bonds could be involved in the interaction between mucoadhesive polymers and mucus, and the main mucoadhesion-related theories are listed in Table 15.1 (Andrews, Laverty, and Jones 2009). The bonds involved include ionic bonding, covalent bonding, hydrogen bonding, van der Waals force, and hydrophobic bonding.

TABLE 15.1

Theories of Mucoadhesion

Theories	Contents
The wetting theory	The spreading of liquid system on the mucus was the prerequisite for mucoadhesion. The contact angle reflects the interfacial tension of liquid and mucosa, and the lower contact angle indicated better spreadability
The electronic theory	Mucoadhesion is produced by attractive forces in electrical double layer due to electron transfer between polymer and mucus
The adsorption theory	Mucoadhesion is produced by the primary bonding: ionic, covalent, and metallic bonding and secondary bonding: hydrogen bonding and van der Waals' forces
The diffusion theory	Mucoadhesion is produced by interdiffusion of polymers and mucus layer
The mechanical theory	Mucoadhesion comes from the interlocking process between polymer and mucus
The fracture theory	The mucoadhesion bond between polymers and mucus is related to the required force for interphase separation

15.3 CHITOSAN AS A MUCOADHESIVE POLYMER

15.3.1 PROPERTIES OF CHITOSAN

Chitosan has been widely applied in oral drug delivery field because of its excellent mucoadhesive and biocompatible properties. Chitosan is a linear polysaccharide constituted of glucosamine and N-acetyl-D-glusoamine units linked by β-1, 4-bonds. In general, the deacetylation degree of chitosan is usually 40%–98% and its molecular weight ranges from 50 to 2,000 kDa (Mao, Sun, and Kissel 2010).

The primary amino group in chitosan is positively charged when the solution pH is lower than its pKa 6.5 (Pillai, Paul, and Sharma 2009). The positive charged nature of chitosan can interact with the negative charged mucus and exhibit good mucoadhesion. However, the low solubility of chitosan in neutral solution limits its application, which was also affected by its degree of deacetylation, distribution of acetyl groups, ionic strength, and molecular weight (Casettari et al. 2012). The physicochemical properties of chitosan can be further modified to satisfy the specific requirements by synthesizing chitosan derivatives.

15.3.2 CHITOSAN DERIVATIVES

To expand the application of chitosan, a series of chemical modification on C2 primary amine group and C6 hydroxyl groups of chitosan have been carried out to meet the requirements of drug delivery. The structure of chitosan and examples of chitosan derivatives are shown in Figure 15.1. The properties of chitosan derivatives can be conveniently adjusted by changing the degree of substitution and molecular structure of the modification group including carboxy group, alkyl group, carboxyalkyl group, sulfonic group, PEG group, and amino acid. Details can be found in the related book chapter (Tian et al. 2016).

Hydrophobic modification of chitosan is one of the most promising strategies to extend its application in drug delivery, which can be used as the carrier of micelles, stabilizers, and incorporation into liposome. Self-assemble properties of hydrophobic-modified chitosan derivatives depend on the hydrophobic interaction among molecules and can be evaluated by critical micelle concentration (CMC) and critical aggregation concentration (CAC). For example, in order to improve the bioavailability of 10-hydroxycamptothecin, hydrophobic glyceryl monooleate, which could inhibit P-gp expression, was grafted on the backbone of chitosan to form micelles by linking activated carboxyl

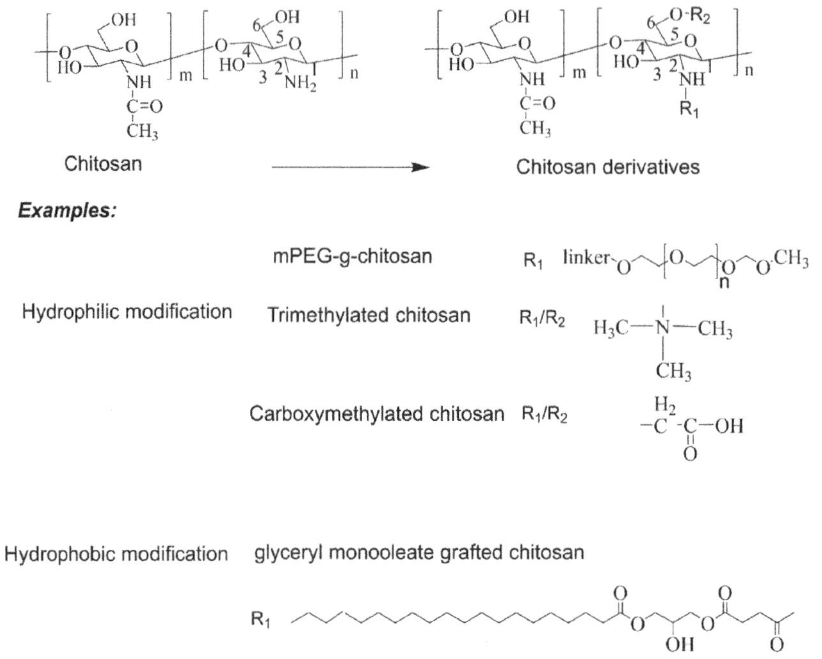

FIGURE 15.1 The structure of chitosan and examples of chitosan derivatives.

acid of glyceryl monooleate to amine groups of chitosan in the presence of carbodiimide(EDC) and N-Hydroxysuccinimide (NHS). 10-Hydroxycamptothecin was loaded in the micelles by pH adjustment method, and the particle size was about 340 nm with drug loading as high as 30%. The in vivo result demonstrated that the micelles prolonged drug circulation time in plasma for up to 96 h and exhibited comparable antitumor effects with the injection group (Tian et al. 2015b). In another study, glyceryl monocaprylate grafted chitosan was synthesized to prepare polyelectrolyte nanocomplexes with insulin, and hydrophobic modification was designed to increase the uptake of epithelial cells. The carboxyl groups of succinylated glyceryl monocaprylate was activated by NHS and EDC and then reacted with chitosan. The results showed that the hydrophobic modification of chitosan increased the mucoadhesion and prolonged the therapeutic effect of insulin (Liu et al. 2019b). In addition to hydrophobic component conjugation, based on the fact that hydrophobic cavity of cyclodextrins which was composed of 6–8 D-glucose units can be applied to load small molecular hydrophobic drugs, carboxymethyl β-cyclodextrin was grafted on hydroxypropyl chitosan to control the release rate of ketoprofen. The drug release rate was significantly reduced and the release behavior was pH dependent (Prabaharan and Mano 2005).

Hydrophilic modification of chitosan is an effective way to increase the solubility of chitosan in a broad pH range. Among different strategies, polyethylene glycol (PEG) modification is a popular one in pharmaceutical field, which can not only increase the hydrophilicity of the copolymer but also provide stealth or steric effect. For example, PEG modification can increase the water solubility of chitosan, prolong the circulation time of chitosan-based nanoparticles in the blood, and increase the mucus penetration ability. In a study, PEG-grafted chitosan was synthesized by PEG aldehyde in the presence of $NaCNBH_3$ and was then ionically crosslinked with tripolyphosphate and poly (glutamic acid) to form bovine serum albumin loaded nanoparticles with particle size of 150–600 nm. The influence of PEG chain length on drug release rate was studied. The results showed that higher molecular weight of PEG and high degree of substitution could increase the release rate of bovine serum albumin (Papadimitriou, Achilias, and Bikiaris 2012). In our previous study, in order to decrease the cytotoxicity of trimethyl chitosan, PEG-grafted trimethyl chitosan copolymers were synthesized and then applied to form nanocomplexes with insulin. The result showed that modification of trimethyl chitosan with PEG increased the half maximal inhibitory concentration (IC50) value of trimethyl chitosan against L929 cells from 100 to ~500 mg/mL (Mao et al. 2005).

Amino acid groups have also been introduced into chitosan to modify the solubility and mucoadhesion of chitosan and further improve delivery efficiency of nanoparticles. Inspired by nature, chitosan-modified L-Phe derivatives were synthesized to simulate the components of viral envelopes and then polyelectrolyte complexes (PECs) between CS-g-N-Phe copolymers and insulin were prepared to achieve both structure and composition simulation of virus envelope. It was demonstrated that both in vitro mucodiffusion and in vivo hypoglycemic effect were L-Phe graft ratio dependent, with CS-g-N-Phe 20.2%/insulin PECs presenting 2.0- to 2.2-fold higher relative pharmacological bioavailability than nonmodified CS/insulin PECs (Liu et al. 2019a). In another study, arginine-grafted chitosan and histidine-grafted chitosan were synthesized by adding the activated carboxyl groups of basic amino acid to chitosan solution. The synthesized amino acid based chitosan derivatives were further mixed with insulin to form polyelectrolyte nanocomplexes with particle size of 205–303 nm and surface charge of 14–27 mV. The uptake of insulin by Caco-2 cell was increased, and the pharmacological activity of insulin was about 2.29%–5.39% (Abbad et al. 2015).

15.3.3 BIOLOGICAL PROPERTIES OF CHITOSAN AND ITS DERIVATIVES

The anionic sialic acid, sulfonic acid groups, and hydrophobic structure in mucin provide the interaction site with mucoadhesive polymers such as chitosan and its derivatives. In general, electrostatic interaction, hydrophobic interaction, and hydrogen bonding contribute to the mucoadhesion properties of chitosan (Sogias, Williams, and Khutoryanskiy 2008). Among them, electrostatic interactions between cationic primary amino groups of chitosan and anionic mucin play a more important role. In order to further improve the mucoadhesive properties of chitosan, thiolated chitosan derivatives were synthesized (Kulkarni et al. 2017).

In addition to excellent mucoadhesion, chitosan is usually considered as a biocompatible, nontoxic, and safe polymeric excipient. It has been approved by regulatory authorities as food additives and excipients for wound dressing (Kean and Thanou 2010; Wedmore et al. 2006). Chitosan can be degraded into fragments by chemical or enzymatic biodegradation in vivo, such as acid-catalyzed degradation in stomach and enzyme degradation in the colon (Zhang and Neau 2002). Most chitosan derivatives also show good safety profile, which is greatly affected by the charge density of the structure (Kean and Thanou 2010). For example, trimethylation of chitosan could increase the toxicity of chitosan, and the cytotoxicity increased with the increase of degree of substitution (Thomas Kean, Roth, and Thanou 2005).

Another promising property of chitosan and its derivatives is that they could reversibly open the tight junction by rearrangement of tight junction correlated proteins to enhance the drug absorption by paracellular pathway (Lemmer and Hamman 2013). The mechanism of reversibly opening tight junction by chitosan was studied in Caco-2 cells. It is speculated that interaction between chitosan and epithelial cells would induce the redistribution and disruption of tight junction, and the function recovery was due to an increase in claudin-4 gene transcription (Yeh et al. 2011).

15.4 MUCOADHESION EVALUATION METHODS

In comparison with in vivo mucoadhesion evaluation methods, in vitro approaches were more convenient to be operated, and the variation of result is expected to be smaller. Various methods based on different mechanisms have been developed to evaluate the mucoadhesion of polymers or nanoparticles, which can be classified into mechanical force determination, rheology measurement, mucin particle interaction, particle tracking method (MPT), atomic force microscopy (AFM), and so on (Davidovich-Pinhas and Bianco-Peled 2010).

15.4.1 MECHANICAL FORCE DETERMINATION

In general, mucoadhesion characterization by mechanical force determination involves the measurement of tensile, shear, and peeling forces. Tensile force is obtained by measuring the detaching force of material from the mucus layer in an axial dimension. Among the methods for tensile measurement, texture analyzer and surface tensiometer are widely applied. During the measurement process by texture analyzer, the material or formulation is adhered to the probe and then interacted with mucosa or model gels with a defined force. After a period of time, the probe is moved up, and the detaching force is determined. According to the force–distance curve obtained by using texture analyzer, the maximum detachment force and total work of adhesion of material can be calculated (Hägerström and Edsman 2001). The parameters used during measurement including applied force, contact time, withdrawal speed, and temperature will affect the force–distance curve. If the withdrawal speed is faster, the curve will become narrower (Woertz et al. 2013).

Modified surface tensiometer can also be used to investigate the mucoadhesive properties of formulations. After the adhesive bond was formed between the formulation disc and mucosa, the formulation was detached from the mucosa with extremely low speed to break the bonds, and the force was recorded. Shear force was applied to evaluate the mucoadhesion by determining the interaction strength of materials and mucus layer under the applied shear forces. Many methods, such as flow method and rotating cylinder method, are used for measuring the shear force. Flow study can evaluate the binding strength of material to mucus tissue under a fixed shear force. As for the measurement procedure, the formulation or polymer coated glass sphere is first contacted with fresh mucus tissue to form stable adhesive bonds in a suitable environment. Thereafter, the mucus tissue is washed using phosphate buffer at a fixed flow rate. At a fixed time, the amount of formulation retained in the tissue is used to analyze the adhesive strength. The even flow rate is critical to ensure accuracy of the results. The rotating cylinder method is developed to measure the mucoadhesion by attaching the polymer tablets or granules to the mucosa, which is fixed on the surface of a stainless steel cylinder. The cylinder is then placed in the buffer solution and rotated with a certain speed to produce the shear force (Baloglu et al. 2011; Duggan et al. 2016).

15.4.2 RHEOLOGY MEASUREMENT

During the mucus adhesion process, the molecular interaction including electrostatic interaction, entanglement and molecular chain diffusion, or other bonds between chitosan and mucus will lead to a change of rheology. Therefore, rheology study provides a way to evaluate the mucosa adhesion of formulation and understand the molecular interaction mechanism. In general, the parameters of viscosity, storage modulus, and loss modulus are determined to evaluate the extent of mucoadhesion. The increase of viscosity due to interaction between formulations and mucus can be calculated (Hassan and Gallo 1990). In addition to viscosity, viscoelastic moduli which includes storage energy during elastic deformation (storage moduli, G') and loss of energy during plastic deformation (loss moduli, G'') can also be used to quantify the mucoadhesion (Rossi et al. 2018). However, the value of rheology parameters is greatly influenced by the mucus source. For commercial mucins, many characteristics of mucus will be lost during the extraction and purification process, although the results might show better reproducibility than that of the native mucus. In addition, the parameters used in rheology determination will also greatly influence the results. For example, according to mucin to chitosan ratio, the viscosity synergism of chitosan–mucin mixture might be observed or not (Rossi et al. 2001). The variation of rheology result under different determination conditions limits the comparability of mucoadhesion results measured in different studies.

15.4.3 MUCIN PARTICLE INTERACTION

Particle size and zeta potential measurement are important and convenient to analyze the properties of nanoparticles. In general, when the mucin–nanoparticle complex is formed, the particle size and zeta potential of nanoparticles will change. If the particle size of mucin solution is appropriate, the variance of nanoparticle properties due to adsorption of mucin can be directly measured. In order to obtain mucin nanoparticles with suitable size, ultrasonication and centrifugation treatment are usually applied. In addition to the simple determination process, the mucoadhesion difference between nanoparticles can be sensitively evaluated.

For example, the mucoadhesion of nanocomplex based on chitosan-grafted glyceryl monocaprylate, glyceryl monolaurate and glyceryl monostearate were compared by mucin particle interaction method. The particle size of mucin particles was controlled at 300 ± 20 nm, the mucin solution was incubated with a nanocomplex for 2 h at 37°C, and the increased particle size was used to evaluate mucoadhesion. The results showed that chitosan-grafted glyceryl monostearate owned the strongest mucoadhesion (Wang et al. 2014). However, this method also has certain limitations. While the property of mucin nanoparticles has been greatly changed in comparison with the native mucus, the results are mainly based on the adhesion interaction and ignore the influence of other factors. Another disadvantage of this method is that the aggregation of mucin nanoparticles may be formed depending on the stability of different nanoparticles, and this will cause misjudgment of mucus adhesion magnitude of different formulations.

15.4.4 ATOMIC FORCE MICROSCOPY

The AFM technology has been widely applied in the morphology study of materials on an atomic scale (Giessibl 2003). In addition, it has also been developed to understand the mucoadhesion process, both the morphology change of mucin and adhesive force of tested formulation to mucus can be obtained from AFM study. The formation of mucin–chitosan complex was observed by comparing images of mucin and mucin–chitosan mixture. In acetate buffer (pH 4.5), the conformation of pig gastric mucin and chitosan molecules has a linear structure. When pig gastric mucin was mixed with chitosan, the aggregation of molecules was observed, demonstrating the complex was formed (Deacon, McGurk, and Roberts 2000).

The adhesive force of polymer to mucus can also be measured by force–distance mode of AFM. In a study, the poly (lactic-co-glycolic acid) microsphere modified by chitosan was evenly attached to the probe and then interacted with the mucin film. The force between surface-modified probe and mucus was measured to analyze the mucoadhesion capacity, and the attractive force between chitosan and mucin was observed (Li et al. 2010).

Although AFM could directly determine the forces on molecular scale and observe the change of morphology due to mucoadhesion, limitations still exist. First, the preparation process is complicated, including the probe modification and preparation of mucus planar surface. In addition, the sampling speed, morphology of mucin layer, and contamination of probe will also affect the reproducibility of results (Cleary, Bromberg, and Magner 2004).

15.4.5 PARTICLE TRACKING METHOD

Limited understanding of real movement behavior of nanoparticles in the mucus hampers the advance of mucoadhesive formulation study. Therefore, in order to visually track the trajectories of nanoparticles, the real-time MPT methods have been extensively applied to evaluate the diffusion behavior of nanoparticles in mucus (Suh, Dawson, and Hanes 2005). Brownian movement of nanoparticles can be tracked by fluorescent microscopy technique, and the mobility of nanoparticles in mucus will be affected by their mucoadhesion ability. Thus, the mucoadhesion of nanoparticles can be calculated by analyzing the trajectories of nanoparticles. That is, the procedure of MPT methods involves the particle tracking process and data analysis. In order to track the nanoparticles, the nanoparticles are usually labeled with fluoresce, and high fluoresce intensity is critical to obtain high quality video of the movement process. The trajectories of tens of nanoparticles are further analyzed, mean-square displacement (MSD)-time scale and effective diffusivities-time scale are usually used as indicators of mobility. The adhesion of nanoparticles might lead to a decrease of MSD and effective diffusivities.

For example, the mobility of positively charged trimethyl chitosan coated nanoparticles in mucus was tracked by MPT method, and their trajectory was highly constrained, indicating the strong mucus adhesion of trimethyl chitosan (Liu et al. 2016). In another study, poly(lactic-co-glycolic acid) (PLGA) nanoparticles labeled by Coumarin 6 were used as probe, and chitosan was then coated on the surface via layer-by-layer method to study the influence of surface characteristics on the diffusion behavior of nanoparticles in mucus. The slowest diffusion rate of chitosan coated nanoparticles was observed due to the mucoadhesion of chitosan (Zhang et al. 2018). The MPT method could provide a new insight to determine the mucoadhesion of nanoparticles. However, the limited fluorescence intensity and small particle size of nanocarriers for drug delivery increase the difficulty to obtain high resolution trajectories of nanoparticles with appropriate video rate (15–30 frames/s). In addition, the analysis of nanoparticles is also time consuming, which reduces the efficiency of this method.

15.5 APPLICATION OF CHITOSAN-BASED MUCOADHESIVE DRUG DELIVERY SYSTEM

Because of mucoadhesive properties of chitosan and its derivatives, it has been widely applied in different oral delivery carriers, and the schematic representation of chitosan as carrier of micelles, stabilizer, matrix and coating material of nanosuspension, carrier of nanocomplex, coating material of liposomes, and matrix of nanoparticles is shown in Figure 15.2.

15.5.1 As the Carrier of Micelles

A series of problems were found in the clinical application of hydrophobic cancer drugs including the poor tumor targeting ability, low bioavailability, and toxic side effects. The micelles based on amphiphilic structure could effectively help to improve the oral bioavailability of anticancer drugs by increasing the membrane permeability, mucoadhesion, and receptor-mediated uptake (Gaucher et al. 2010; Tian and Mao 2012). Many polymeric materials can be used as the carrier of micelles, among them chitosan is most frequently used as the hydrophilic part. By introducing hydrophobic group in chitosan structure, chitosan-based micelles could be formed in aqueous solution by self-assembly, with a modifiable hydrophilic surface and hydrophobic core structure (Tian and Mao 2012). The hydrophilic surface could maintain stability of the micelles and provide modifiable site for multifunctional modification. The drug release behavior, drug loading efficiency, and the stability of micelles are greatly affected by the hydrophobic core structure. For example, benzyl group, naphthyl group, and octyl group were grafted on chitosan by reductive N-amination. Although all of the micelles exhibited similar spherical shape and low cytotoxicity, octyl group grafted chitosan showed the highest drug loading and best stability (Woraphatphadung et al. 2016). Thus, in order to design a more scientific and rational micellar structure, systemic understanding of the influence of hydrophobic group structure and substitution degree on the absorption of micelles is critical.

During the design of chitosan-based micelles, it should be noted that the compatibility of hydrophobic component with drug substance can influence the stability of micelles remarkably (Shi et al. 2016). For example, glyceryl monostearate, glyceryl monolaurate, and glyceryl monooleate were introduced to the chitosan backbone, and the compatibility between chitosan derivatives and

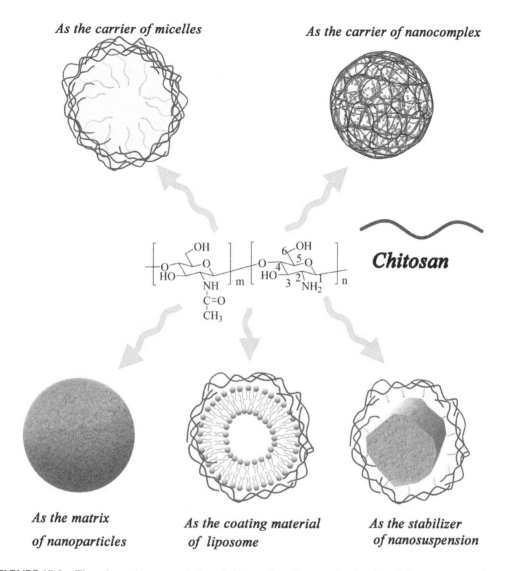

FIGURE 15.2   The schematic representation of chitosan-based mucoadhesive drug delivery systems.

hydroxycamptothecin was calculated by group contribution method and Flory–Huggins interaction parameter, respectively. It was demonstrated that good compatibility could increase the stability of the micelle, therefore the compatibility result can be applied to guide the design and screen of chitosan derivatives based micelles to achieve good stability and higher drug loading (Tian et al. 2015a).

15.5.2   As the Stabilizer, Matrix, and Coating Material of Nanosuspension

With an increase in the number of poorly water-soluble drugs, nanosuspension technology is becoming an effective strategy to overcome the poor bioavailability by improving the dissolution rate and solubility (Zhang, Li, and Mao 2014). According to Ostwald–Freundlich and Noyes–Whitney equations, the advantage of fast dissolution rate and increased solubility of nanosuspension mainly comes from the reduction of particle size and increase of surface area (Merisko-Liversidge and

Liversidge 2011). Therefore, appropriate stabilizers are crucial to obtain the nanosuspension with ideal particle size and good stability during storage. It has been demonstrated that polymeric stabilizers could adsorb on the surface of nanoparticles and provide steric stabilization effect to prevent the aggregation of nanosuspension (Ghosh et al. 2011). In comparison with the normal polymeric stabilizers, such as Hydroxypropyl methyl cellulose (HPMC), Hydroxypropyl cellulose (HPC), povidone, and polyvinyl alcohol, cationic charged chitosan can provide not only steric stabilization but also electrostatic stabilization, and moreover, making the nanosuspension own mucosal adhesion characteristics. In a previous study, chitosan and N-trimethyl chitosan were used as stabilizers of itraconazole nanosuspension, and it was found that their effectiveness was influenced by chitosan molecular weight, polymer charge density and environmental pH. Compared to 400 kDa chitosan, 50 kDa chitosan stabilized itraconazole nanosuspension showed smaller particle size, indicating steric stabilization effect provided by 50 kDa chitosan was enough to maintain stability of the nanosuspension and faster diffusion rate of low molecular weight chitosan contributed to the smaller particle size. The influence of charge density of chitosan and N-trimethyl chitosan in different pH environments was further compared. Nanosuspension stabilized by higher charged N-trimethyl chitosan showed smaller particle size, which provided a better stabilization effect (Sun et al. 2012).

Apart from stabilizers, chitosan and its derivatives can also be used as hydrogel matrix carrier and coating material of nanosuspension formulation. For example, buparvaquone nanosuspension stabilized by Poloxamer 188/PVA was prepared and was then incorporated into mucoadhesive chitosan hydrogels, with improved long-term stability (Müller and Jacobs 2002). The poor oral bioavailability and intestine stimulatory effect of diacerein greatly limit its application. In order to overcome these problems, chitosan coated nanosuspension was prepared by mixing chitosan solution with diacerein nanosuspension to enhance the mucoadhesive properties in the upper intestine. It was found that chitosan coating on diacerein nanosuspension increased its mucoadhesion by 16%. In the presence of mannitol, optimized chitosan coated nanosuspension also showed good stability during the lyophilization process (Allam, Hamdallah, and Abdallah 2017).

15.5.3 As the Carrier of Nanocomplex

As a promising drug carrier, nanocomplex can be prepared under mild condition, and it is especially suitable for the delivery of macromolecules. Due to its superior characteristics, chitosan is the most frequently used material to prepare nanocomplex for biological drug delivery, including insulin and genes (Mao et al. 2005). Chitosan-based nanocomplex could be prepared with oppositely charged polymers or drugs based on electrostatic interaction, and sometimes hydrogen bonds and hydrophobic interaction are also involved. Most of the negatively charged polysaccharides such as alginate, pectin, dextran sulfate, carboxymethyl chitosan, chondroitin sulfate, and poly glutamic acid can form nanocomplex with chitosan.

During the preparation of nanocomplex, because charge neutralization process of preparation may induce instability of the nanocomplex, the ratio of chitosan to anionic polymers should be therefore evaluated and an appropriate surface charge is usually required (Quiñones, Peniche, and Peniche 2018). In addition, both polymer molecular structure and preparation condition can affect the properties of nanocomplex. The electrostatic interaction strength between chitosan and anionic polymers is pH and ionic strength dependent, which will finally influence the particle size and stability. For example, the particle size of trimethyl chitosan–insulin nanocomplex prepared at pH 5.0 was 860 nm, and it was further decreased to 511 and 306 nm when the pH was increased to 6.8 and 7.4, respectively. As to the influence of ionic strength, when the concentration of sodium chloride solution was 15 mM, 60% of nanocomplex prepared at pH 5.0 was dissociated (Jintapattanakit et al. 2007). Chitosan modification degree can also influence the in vitro and in vivo behavior of the nanocomplex. For example, chitosan-grafted glyceryl monostearate copolymers with different substitution degrees were synthesized, their complex with enoxaparin was prepared, and the morphology, mucoadhesive properties, and in vivo absorption of enoxaparin loaded nanocomplex in fasted rats were compared. The results showed that the mucoadhesion and absorption of the chitosan derivatives based nanocomplex increased linearly with an increase of graft ratio when the graft ratio was below 11.1%. However, with the further increase of graft ratio, oral absorption of enoxaparin decreased. This may be due to the structure change of the nanocarrier, with the increase of substitution degree of hydrophobic group, instead of forming nanocomplex, a micelle-like structure might be formed due to a good hydrophile–lipophile balance achieved in the copolymer, with the hydrophobic group forming core therefore decreasing the surface distribution of hydrophobic chains (Wang et al. 2013).

The structure of hydrophobic components in modified chitosan copolymers can also influence the in vitro and in vivo behavior of the prepared nanocomplex. In a study, the influence of fatty glyceride chain length, including glyceryl monocaprylate, glyceryl monolaurate, and glyceryl monostearate in the modified chitosan copolymer on the oral absorption of enoxaparin after nanocomplex preparation was studied. The results showed that glyceryl monocaprylate-grafted chitosan exhibited better mucoadhesion and increased cell uptake via clathrin and caveolae dependent endocytosis mechanism (Wang et al. 2014).

In addition, during nanocomplex preparation, the synergistic effect of chitosan with other anionic polymers also provides promising properties for drug delivery. For example, taking advantage of CD 44 receptor targeting ability of hyaluronic acid, doxorubicin, and MicroRNA-34a coloaded in hyaluronic acid –chitosan (HA-CS)nanocomplex was successfully prepared, and the chemotherapy efficacy of DOX against triple negative breast cancer MDA-MB-231 was improved by overcoming drug resistance (Deng et al. 2014).

15.5.4 As the Coating Material of Nanoparticles

Chitosan coating on nanoparticles could offer a series of advantages to drug carrier including improving stability, controlling drug release rate, improving bioadhesion, and targeting colon segment. In general, chitosan coating layer could be directly formed during preparation process of nanoparticles or coated on the preformed nanoparticles by extra coating procedure. The electrostatic interaction between positive charged chitosan and negatively charged nanoparticles is usually utilized to form the coating layer. The chitosan coating layer on the surface of nanoparticles usually leads to an increase of particle size and a shift of zeta potential. For example, human serum albumin nanoparticles with particle size 241 nm and zeta potential -47 ± 3 mV was prepared by desolvation method. Chitosan was adsorbed on the surface by electrostatic interaction to form a coating layer, and particle size and zeta potential of nanoparticles after coating were increased to 261 nm and $+45 \pm 1$ mV, respectively (Piazzini et al. 2019).

Chitosan has been extensively explored for solid lipid nanoparticles (SLN) coating. Rapid drug release rate in the body, poor physical stability, and low drug loading due to chemical incompatibility are the bottlenecks for SLN development (Bugnicourt and Ladavière 2017). Chitosan coating showed a promising potential to address these issues and could additionally improve the mucoadhesion of SLNs. To obtain chitosan coated nanoparticles with ideal performance and maintain the stability of SLNs during coating, factors influencing the coating process including chitosan concentration, molecular weight, pH, and ionic strength of solution should be optimized. For example, after being coated by chitosan, the entrapment efficiency of indomethacin loaded SLNs increased from 81% to 92%. And compared to uncoated nanoparticles, the chitosan coating also increased the storage stability, and only a 15% increase in terms of particle size was found after storage at 40°C for 90 days (Balguri, Adelli, and Majumdar 2016). Similarly, for light-sensitive drug curcumin, chitosan coating layer not only improved the stability of curcumin loaded SLNs but also its oral bioavailability (Ramalingam, Yoo, and Ko 2016).

Chitosan can also be used for liposome coating. Liposomes are nanoparticles composed of self-assembled bilayer in an aqueous environment which can be used to encapsulate both hydrophilic and hydrophobic drugs. However, the molecular structure of liposome greatly limits its application in oral administration route, because the unstable membrane of liposome in the gastrointestinal environment including wide pH range, phospholipase enzymes, and bile salts would result in structure disruption and release of the entrapped drugs (Daeihamed, Dadashzadeh, and Akhlaghi 2016). Attempts to overcome these problems have developed a number of well-designed nanoparticle structures, among them surface coating of liposomes by chitosan showed promising application potential (Alavi, Haeri, and Dadashzadeh 2017). In a study, the stability of chitosan coated liposome in different pH and ionic strength environment was investigated. Without chitosan coating, the liposome was disrupted quickly in pH 2–3 solution and 10^{-2} to 10^{-3} M NaCl solution. In contrast, chitosan coating greatly enhanced the stability of liposomes in acidic solution and most of the nanoparticles were kept stable up to pH 1. Resistance of the liposome to high ionic strength environment was demonstrated and its structure was stable in 10^{-1} M NaCl concentration, although a higher ionic strength still led to aggregation of liposomes (Quemeneur et al. 2007). In addition, in order to understand the stability and integrity of chitosan coated liposomes in intestine, chitosan coating and liposome core were labeled by fluorescein isothiocyanate (FITC) and 1,1'-dioctadecyl-3,3,3',3'-tetramethylindocarbocyanine perchlorate (DiI), respectively. The mucoadhesion and penetration behavior of chitosan coated liposomes were observed by confocal laser scanning microscopy. The results showed that the chitosan coating layer was adsorbed on the surface, and the structure of chitosan coated liposome was maintained during the mucosa penetration process (Thongborisute et al. 2006). Similarly, calcitonin loaded mucoadhesive liposome was prepared by coating chitosan and carbopol, respectively. Intestine mucoadhesion study showed that positive charged chitosan coated liposome owned better mucoadhesive ability than that of carbopol coated liposome. The enhanced mucoadhesive properties, which showed prolonged retention time, also improved the oral delivery efficiency of calcitonin, and an in vivo study showing a reduction of calcium concentration in blood was significantly prolonged (Takeuchi et al. 2003).

In addition to enhanced mucoadhesion, chitosan coated nanoparticles can also be potentially applied for colon targeting drug delivery because chitosan can be degraded by colonic bacteria. In order to avoid the degradation of nanoparticles in the upper gastrointestinal tract, chitosan could be applied together with other insoluble polymers such as Eudragit® RS/RL to achieve the purpose of colon targeting (Gulbake and Jain 2012).

15.5.5 As the Matrix of Nanoparticles

Nanoparticles have many advantages in drug delivery, and chitosan is one of the most frequently used materials to prepare nanoparticles. Chitosan-based nanoparticles can be prepared using different methods, including precipitation, crosslinking, and electrospray methods (Naskar, Sharma, and Kuotsu 2019), depending on the properties of the active components to be encapsulated.

According to the solubility change of chitosan in different pH, chitosan nanoparticles can be prepared by precipitation method. For example, chitosan can be dissolved in the aqueous phase of emulsion. The evaporation and diffusion of methylene chloride/acetone oil phase into aqueous phase can reduce the solubility of chitosan and lead to formation of nanoparticles (El-Shabouri 2002). Chitosan solution with appropriate stabilizer can also be added to the dispersing phase which is miscible with water, and reduction of chitosan solubility would lead to formation of nanoparticles (Luque-Alcaraz et al. 2016).

Compared to precipitation method, crosslinking method is more widely applied to prepare chitosan nanoparticles for drug delivery. Crosslinkers such as glutaraldehyde, genipin, and tripolyphosphate can be used to prepare chitosan nanoparticles. The chemical aldimine condensation reaction can happen between the amine groups in chitosan structure and aldehyde groups to form chitosan nanoparticles. However, toxicity of the crosslinkers limits their applications in pharmaceutical area (Agnihotri, Mallikarjuna, and Aminabhavi 2004). Therefore, searching for crosslinkers with good safety profile is a good solution. Genipin is water-soluble crosslinker obtained from gademia. It can react with amino groups of chitosan to form a crosslinked hydrogel. The safety of genipin makes it a good substitute for glutaraldehyde (Muzzarelli 2009). Physical ionic crosslinking between anionic sodium tripolyphosphate (TPP) and cationic chitosan based on electrostatic interaction is also widely applied to prepare chitosan nanoparticles. Chitosan–TPP nanoparticles exhibited many promising advantages such as controllable particle size, excellent biocompatibility, and mild preparation environment. This makes it suitable to prepare biomacromolecules loaded nanoparticles and avoid denaturation of protein during crosslinking process (Hou et al. 2012). The properties of chitosan–TPP nanoparticles can be controlled by optimizing the preparation parameters including chitosan concentration, ratio of TPP to chitosan, pH and ionic strength of medium, stirring speed, and time. The chitosan–TPP nanoparticles with narrow size distributions could be prepared by changing the concentration of NaCl and particle size could be tuned from 100 to 900 nm. (Sawtarie, Cai, and Lapitsky 2017). Catechin loaded chitosan–TPP nanoparticles with a particle size of 130 ± 5 nm was prepared. The morphology study showed that the nanoparticles were spherical in shape with smooth surface, and 32% of catechin was released within 24 h. Mucoadhesion of FITC labeled nanoparticles was also studied using freshly excised porcine intestinal segment and 40% of catechin loaded nanoparticles was adhered to the mucosa (Dudhani and Kosaraju 2010).

In addition to precipitation and crosslinking methods, chitosan nanoparticles can also be directly prepared by electrospraying process. In comparison with traditional spray drying method, the particle size of droplets produced by electrospray dryer, which was atomized by coulomb repulsion, was much smaller (Hartman et al. 2000). The solution characteristics including viscosity, conductivity, and process parameters could affect properties of the formed nanoparticles. For example, the particles size of chitosan nanoparticle decreased with decreasing acetic acid concentration and chitosan concentration, and 124 nm nanoparticles could be obtained by optimizing the parameters (Zhang and Kawakami 2010).

15.6 THE IN VIVO FATE OF CHITOSAN-BASED NANOPARTICLES FOR ORAL DELIVERY

The convenience of oral route and excellent patient compliance make it the most popular administration route for nanoparticle delivery. Although the drug carrier based on nanotechnology has been extensively studied for years, the fate of nanoparticles in oral delivery process is still unclear, and related research and attempts are still scientifically challenging. The complexity of gastrointestinal tract including the digestive environment, protective mucus layer, and transport barrier of intestinal epithelium makes it hard to understand the whole fate of nanoparticles in oral administration process (Liu et al. 2018). In addition, the well-designed nanocarriers such as micelles, nanosuspensions, liposomes, and SLNs are composed of different structures and own different characteristics, and this will further increase the difficulty of analyzing and concluding the fate of nanoparticles in the gastrointestinal tract (Lagarce et al. 2010).

15.6.1 STABILITY AND INTEGRITY OF NANOPARTICLES

The stability and integrity of nanoparticles in gastrointestinal environment is the first factor that should be taken into consideration. The wide pH range (1.5–7), abundant digestive enzymes including trypsin, chymotrypsin, amylase, lipase, and surfactant will affect the stability of nanoparticles and lead to aggregation or disruption of nanoparticles. For example, the instability and burst release of SLNs in stomach limit their pharmaceutical application. In order to increase the stability of nanoparticles in acidic pH condition, N-trimethyl chitosan graft palmitic acid (TMC-g-PA) copolymer was synthesized and coated on the nanoparticles. The in vitro release study in simulated gastric fluid (SGF) showed that <10% of the drug was released from TMC-g-PA coated nanoparticles in 24 h. In contrast, more than 70% of the drugs was burst released from uncoated nanoparticles in 12 h.

The result indicated that chitosan derivatives improved the integrity of nanoparticles in stomach (Ramalingam and Ko 2016). Likewise, chitosan coating layer also improved the stability of liposome and slowed down drug release in the gastrointestinal environment. During 30 days of storage, 1.07-fold increase in particle size and 2.1% leakage ratio were found for 0.3% chitosan coated liposomes as compared to 1.37-fold and 9.4% for uncoated liposome, respectively. The drug burst release from uncoated liposomes in simulated intestinal fluid (SIF) may be due to the loss of structural integrity. With the increase of chitosan coating layer thickness, drug release from liposome in SGF and SIF decreased (Nguyen et al. 2014).

15.6.2   Mucus Adhesion and Penetration of Nanoparticles

For nanoparticles which could resist the gastrointestinal environment and maintain structure integrity, mucus layer is another barrier before being absorbed by intestinal epithelium. The protective mucus layer covered on epithelial surface forms an inevitable barrier for most nanoparticle drug delivery system. Taking advantage of mucoadhesive property of chitosan, chitosan-based nanoparticle drug delivery system could improve the bioavailability of drugs by prolonging drug residence time and increase the possibility of nanoparticles uptake by epithelium.

To improve the oral absorption of insulin, N-trimethyl chitosan was coated on the insulin loaded polylactide-co-glycoside nanoparticles with zeta potential of 45.2 ± 4.6 mV, which was expected to exhibit good mucoadhesion. Insulin was labeled with ^{125}I and the mucoadhesion of nanoparticles in intestinal segments was studied. Compared with PLGA nanoparticles, the movement speed of N-trimethyl chitosan-modified PLGA nanoparticles was greatly reduced and about 40% of nanoparticles was adhered to the small intestine after 3 h (Sheng et al. 2015).

In addition to enhancing mucoadhesion, chitosan was also applied in mucus penetration strategy to overcome the mucus diffusion barrier. Since the rapid mucus penetration ability of virus attracted researchers' attention (Cone 2009), many highly densely charged nanoparticles composed of chitosan and other anionic polymers were designed to mimic the surface characteristics of virus. In a study, chitosan–chondroitin sulfate nanocomplex with highly densely charged surface was designed, and their interaction with intestinal mucus and mucus diffusion ability of the nanocomplex was studied. The increase of particle size and reverse of zeta potential of positive charged nanoparticles in diluted mucus solution indicated the electrostatic interaction with mucus. Regardless of the slight difference in zeta potential, higher permeation ability of chitosan–chondroitin sulfate nanocomplex was found in comparison with hydrophilic reference nanoparticles (Pereira de Sousa et al. 2015).

Moreover, hydrophilic modification of chitosan can also be applied to increase the mucus penetration ability. For this objective, PEG-grafted chitosan was synthesized and applied to form polyelectrolyte nanocomplex with insulin. The result showed that PEG modification increased the hydrophilicity of nanocomplex and covered the charge of chitosan, which significantly reduced the interaction strength of the nanocomplex with mucin at lower PEG substitution degree. However, high degree of substitution (18%) of PEG enhanced the interaction between nanocomplex and mucus (Liu et al. 2019b).

15.6.3   Absorption Mechanism of Nanoparticles

The absorption mechanism of drugs in chitosan-based nanoparticles depends on the characteristics of nanoparticles and targeting site of administration. For local administration, the drug carriers can be disrupted in targeted site and release the drug for absorption. For systemic administration, chitosan-based nanoparticles can be uptaken by paracellular pathway, transcellular pathway, or M-cells pathway. Different mechanisms are involved in the transport process across the intestinal epithelium.

Intercellular space is linked by tight junctions which is composed of claudin-4 and correlated proteins, and the pathway for drug diffusion is estimated to be 0.3–1 nm which greatly limits the passage of nanocarriers (Nellans 1991). Cationic chitosan and its derivatives can reversibly open the tight junctions by reducing the concentration of calcium ion and redistribute transmembrane protein of tight junctions. In a study, different quaternized chitosan derivatives including trimethyl chitosan, dimethylethyl chitosan, diethylmethyl chitosan, and triethyl chitosan were synthesized, and their permeation enhancing ability by opening the tight junctions was compared. The transepithelial electrical resistance (TEER) value of Caco-2 cells was decreased in the presence of chitosan derivatives but it was reversible (Sadeghi et al. 2008). Although opening tight junctions could increase the opportunity of drugs to be absorbed via paracellular pathway, it is still difficult for intact nanocarriers to transport through. In general, it is presumed that the nanoparticles have to be disrupted first and then the released drug was being transported through the paracellular pathway (Lin et al. 2008). The TEER value can be measured to understand the paracellular permeation potential of nanocarriers (Sadeghi et al. 2008). For example, chitosan and poly (γ-glutamic acid) were used as the carrier to prepare pH-responsive nanoparticles based on their electrostatic interaction for oral delivery of insulin. Insulin, chitosan, and γ- polyglutamic acid (PGA) were labeled by Cy3, Cy5, and fluoresceinamine, respectively, to observe the transport process. It was found that the nanoparticles could open the tight junctions and thereafter the nanoparticles were disrupted and the released insulin was transported by paracellular pathway (Sung et al. 2012).

After intact nanoparticles penetrate through the mucus layer and reach the intestinal epithelial cells, they can be uptaken by intestinal epithelial cells including enterocytes and M cells by transcellular pathway. Compared to passive diffusion which is used to transport small, lipophilic drugs, nanoparticles are more likely being uptaken by energy-dependent active transport mechanism. The uptake mechanism can be studied by evaluating the nanoparticles uptake amount in cells pretreated with different inhibitors. For example, 5β-cholanic acid modified glycol chitosan was synthesized, self-assembled nanoparticles were prepared with a particle size of 359 nm and a zeta potential of 22 mV. The HeLa H2BGFP cells were incubated with chlorpromazine, filipin, and amiloride for 1 h at 37°C to inhibit clathrin-mediated endocytosis, caveolae-mediated endocytosis, and macropinocytosis, respectively. It was demonstrated that the uptake amount of nanoparticles was inhibited with different degrees, indicating all of the clathrin-mediated endocytosis, caveolae-mediated endocytosis, and macropinocytosis contributed to the uptake of 5β-cholanic acid modified glycol chitosan nanoparticles (Nam et al. 2009). In another study, insulin loaded chitosan–alginate nanocomplexes were prepared, and an endocytosis uptake mechanism in intestine was evaluated. The intestine was incubated with colchicine, chlorpromazine, and indomethacin to inhibit clathrin-mediated endocytosis, macropinocytosis, and caveolin-mediated endocytosis. The transport reduction of nanocomplex in intestine at 4°C was observed, indicating energy-dependent uptake process. Further study demonstrated that multiple endocytosis mechanisms were involved in the uptake process (Zhang et al. 2018).

Based on the specific requirement, chitosan-based nanoparticles can also be designed for M-cell targeting. It was reported that nanoparticles larger than 500 nm can be uptaken by M cells (Florence 2005). To enhance nanoparticles uptake by Peyer's patch, M cell-homing peptide CKSTHPLSC-grafted chitosan was synthesized, and it was demonstrated that binding affinity, uptake efficiency of chitosan-based nanoparticles by the M cells, was significantly improved, which can be used as a potentially M cell targeting carrier (Yoo et al. 2010). However, the limited number of M-cells (<1%) in intestinal epithelial cells reduced its contribution to the overall absorption of nanoparticles in the gastrointestinal tract (Brayden, Jepson, and Baird 2005).

After the nanoparticles were uptaken by intestinal epithelial cells, they may be transported through the cells and release the drug at the basolateral side. After dissociation of chitosan nanoparticle, chitosan will be degraded. The molecular weight and degree of acetylation of chitosan greatly affect its degradation rate. The enzymatic degradation of chitosan in the gastrointestinal tract may also be affected by chitosan's NH_2 availability (Kean and Thanou 2010).

15.7 CONCLUSIONS

The application of chitosan and its derivatives in nanoparticles oral drug delivery system has been extensively studied because of their excellent mucoadhesion, absorption enhancing ability, and biocompatibility. In addition to mucoadhesion, chitosan could also increase the stability of liposomes and SLNs in gastrointestinal tract, and the ability of reversibly opening tight junction potentially enhance the oral bioavailability of drugs, even for biomacromolecules. In summary, the modifiable properties of chitosan by introducing functional groups could further expand their application in mucoadhesive nanoparticles for oral drug delivery.

ACKNOWLEDGEMENT

This project is supported by the Natural Science Foundation of China (Grant No. 81273446, 31870987).

REFERENCES

Abbad, Sarra, Zhenhai Zhang, Ayman Y. Waddad, Were L. L. Munyendo, Huixia Lv, and Jianping Zhou. 2015. Chitosan-modified cationic amino acid nanoparticles as a novel oral delivery system for insulin. *Journal of Biomedical Nanotechnology* 11 (3): 486–99. doi: 10.1166/jbn.2015.1924.

Agnihotri, Sunil A., Nadagouda N. Mallikarjuna, and Tejraj M. Aminabhavi. 2004. Recent advances on chitosan-based micro- and nanoparticles in drug delivery. *Journal of Controlled Release* 100 (1): 5–28. doi: 10.1016/j.jconrel.2004.08.010.

Alavi, Sonia, Azadeh Haeri, and Simin Dadashzadeh. 2017. Utilization of chitosan-caged liposomes to push the boundaries of therapeutic delivery. *Carbohydrate Polymers* 157: 991–1012. Elsevier Ltd. doi: 10.1016/j.carbpol.2016.10.063.

Allam, Ahmed, Sherif Hamdallah, and Ossama Abdallah. 2017. Chitosan-coated diacerein nanosuspensions as a platform for enhancing bioavailability and lowering side effects: Preparation, characterization, and ex vivo/in vivo evaluation. *International Journal of Nanomedicine* 12 (July): 4733–45. doi: 10.2147/IJN.S139706.

Andrews, Gavin P., Thomas P. Laverty, and David S. Jones. 2009. Mucoadhesive polymeric platforms for controlled drug delivery. *European Journal of Pharmaceutics and Biopharmaceutics* 71 (3): 505–18. doi: 10.1016/j.ejpb.2008.09.028.

Balguri, Sai Prachetan, Goutham R. Adelli, and Soumyajit Majumdar. 2016. Topical ophthalmic lipid nanoparticle formulations (SLN, NLC) of indomethacin for delivery to the posterior segment ocular tissues. *European Journal of Pharmaceutics and Biopharmaceutics* 109 (December): 224–35. doi: 10.1016/j.ejpb.2016.10.015.

Baloglu, Esra, Zeynep Ay Senyıgıt, Sinem Yaprak Karavana, Anja Vetter, Dilek Yesim Metın, Suleyha Hilmioglu Polat, Tamer Guneri, and Andreas Bernkop-Schnurch. 2011. *In vitro* evaluation of mucoadhesive vaginal tablets of antifungal drugs prepared with thiolated polymer and development of a new dissolution technique for vaginal formulations. *Chemical and Pharmaceutical Bulletin* 59 (8): 952–58. doi: 10.1248/cpb.59.952.

Brayden, David J., Mark A. Jepson, and Alan W. Baird. 2005. Keynote review: Intestinal Peyer's patch M cells and oral vaccine targeting. *Drug Discovery Today* 10 (17): 1145–57. doi: 10.1016/S1359-6446(05)03536-1.

Bugnicourt, Loïc and Catherine Ladavière. 2017. A close collaboration of chitosan with lipid colloidal carriers for drug delivery applications. *Journal of Controlled Release* 256: 121–40. Elsevier B.V. doi: 10.1016/j.jconrel.2017.04.018.

Casettari, Luca, Driton Vllasaliu, Enzo Castagnino, Snjezana Stolnik, Steven Howdle, and Lisbeth Illum. 2012. PEGylated chitosan derivatives: Synthesis, characterizations and pharmaceutical applications. *Progress in Polymer Science* 37 (5): 659–85. Elsevier Ltd. doi: 10.1016/j.progpolymsci.2011.10.001.

Cleary, John, Lev Bromberg, and Edmond Magner. 2004. Adhesion of polyether-modified poly(acrylic acid) to mucin. *Langmuir* 20 (22): 9755–62. doi: 10.1021/la048993s.

Cone, Richard A. 2009. Barrier properties of mucus. *Advanced Drug Delivery Reviews* 61 (2): 75–85. Elsevier B.V. doi: 10.1016/j.addr.2008.09.008.

Daeihamed, Marjan, Simin Dadashzadeh, Azadeh Haeri, and Masoud Akhlaghi. 2016. Potential of liposomes for enhancement of oral drug absorption. *Current Drug Delivery* 13 (999): 1. doi: 10.2174/1567201813 666160115125756.

Davidovich-Pinhas, Maya and Havazelet Bianco-Peled. 2010. Mucoadhesion: A review of characterization techniques. *Expert Opinion on Drug Delivery* 7 (2): 259–71. doi: 10.1517/17425240903473134.

Deacon, Matthew P., Simon McGurk, and Clive J. Roberts. 2000. Atomic force microscopy of gastric mucin and chitosan mucoadhesive systems Matthew. *Biochemical Journal* 563: 557–63.

Deng, Xiongwei, Minjun Cao, Jiakun Zhang, Kelei Hu, Zhaoxia Yin, Zhixiang Zhou, and Xiangqian Xiao, et al. 2014. Hyaluronic acid-chitosan nanoparticles for co-delivery of MiR-34a and doxorubicin in therapy against triple negative breast cancer. *Biomaterials* 35 (14): 4333–44. Elsevier Ltd. doi: 10.1016/j. biomaterials.2014.02.006.

Dudhani, Anitha R. and Shantha L. Kosaraju. 2010. Bioadhesive chitosan nanoparticles: Preparation and characterization. *Carbohydrate Polymers* 81 (2): 243–51. Elsevier Ltd. doi: 10.1016/j.carbpol.2010.02.026.

Duggan, Sarah, Helen Hughes, Eleanor Owens, Elaine Duggan, Wayne Cummins, and Orla O' Donovan. 2016. Synthesis and characterisation of mucoadhesive thiolated polyallylamine. *International Journal of Pharmaceutics* 499 (1–2): 368–75. doi: 10.1016/j.ijpharm.2016.01.009.

El-Shabouri, Mohamed H. 2002. Positively charged nanoparticles for improving the oral bioavailability of cyclosporin-A. *International Journal of Pharmaceutics* 249 (1–2): 101–8. doi: 10.1016/ S0378-5173(02)00461-1.

Ensign, Laura M., Richard Cone, and Justin Hanes. 2012. Oral drug delivery with polymeric nanoparticles: The gastrointestinal mucus barriers. *Advanced Drug Delivery Reviews* 64 (6): 557–70. Elsevier B.V. doi:10.1016/j.addr.2011.12.009.

Florence, Alexander T. 2005. Nanoparticle uptake by the oral route: Fulfilling its potential? *Drug Discovery Today: Technologies* 2 (1): 75–81. doi: 10.1016/j.ddtec.2005.05.019.

Gaucher, Geneviève, Prashant Satturwar, Marie-Christine Jones, Alexandra Furtos, and Jean-Christophe Leroux. 2010. Polymeric micelles for oral drug delivery. *European Journal of Pharmaceutics and Biopharmaceutics* 76 (2): 147–58. doi: 10.1016/j.ejpb.2010.06.007.

Ghosh, Indrajit, Sonali Bose, Radha Vippagunta, and Ferris Harmon. 2011. Nanosuspension for improving the bioavailability of a poorly soluble drug and screening of stabilizing agents to inhibit crystal growth. *International Journal of Pharmaceutics* 409 (1–2): 260–68. Elsevier B.V. doi: 10.1016/j. ijpharm.2011.02.051.

Giessibl, Franz J. 2003. Advances in atomic force microscopy. *Reviews of Modern Physics* 75 (3): 949–83. doi: 10.1103/RevModPhys.75.949.

Gulbake, Arvind and Sanjay K. Jain. 2012. Chitosan: A potential polymer for colon-specific drug delivery system. *Expert Opinion on Drug Delivery* 9 (6): 713–29. doi: 10.1517/17425247.2012.682148.

Hägerström, Helene and Katarina Edsman. 2001. Interpretation of mucoadhesive properties of polymer gel preparations using a tensile strength method. *Journal of Pharmacy and Pharmacology* 53 (12): 1589–99. doi: 10.1211/0022357011778197.

Hartman, Ruppert P. A., D. J. Brunner, D. M. A. Camelot, Jan C. M. Marijnissen, and Brian. Scarlett. 2000. Jet break-up in electrohydrodynamic atomization in the cone-jet mode. *Journal of Aerosol Science* 31 (1): 65–95. doi: 10.1016/S0021-8502(99)00034-8.

Hassan, Emad Eldin and James M. Gallo. 1990. A simple rheological method for the in vitro assessment of mucin-polymer bioadhesive bond strength. *Pharmaceutical Research* 7 (5): 491–95. doi: 10.1023/A:1015812615635.

Hou, Yaping, Junli Hu, Hyejin Park, and Min Lee. 2012. Chitosan-based nanoparticles as a sustained protein release carrier for tissue engineering applications. *Journal of Biomedical Materials Research Part A* 100A (4): 939–47. doi: 10.1002/jbm.a.34031.

Jintapattanakit, Anchalee, Varaporn B. Junyaprasert, Shirui Mao, Johannes Sitterberg, Udo Bakowsky, and Thomas Kissel. 2007. Peroral delivery of insulin using chitosan derivatives: A comparative study of polyelectrolyte nanocomplexes and nanoparticles. *International Journal of Pharmaceutics* 342 (1–2): 240–49. doi: 10.1016/j.ijpharm.2007.05.015.

Kean, Thomas J. and Maya Thanou. 2010. Biodegradation, biodistribution and toxicity of chitosan. *Advanced Drug Delivery Reviews* 62 (1): 3–11. Elsevier B.V. doi: 10.1016/j.addr.2009.09.004.

Kean, Thomas, Susanne Roth, and Maya Thanou. 2005. Trimethylated chitosans as non-viral gene delivery vectors: Cytotoxicity and transfection efficiency. *Journal of Controlled Release* 103 (3): 643–53. doi: 10.1016/j.jconrel.2005.01.001.

Khanvilkar, Kavita, Maureen D. Donovan, and Douglas R. Flanagan. 2001. Drug transfer through mucus. *Advanced Drug Delivery Reviews* 48 (2–3): 173–93. doi: 10.1016/S0169-409X(01)00115-6.

Kulkarni, Abhijeet D., Harun M. Patel, Sanjay J. Surana, Yogesh H. Vanjari, Veena S. Belgamwar, and Chandrakantsing V. Pardeshi. 2017. N,N,N-trimethyl chitosan: An advanced polymer with myriad of opportunities in nanomedicine. *Carbohydrate Polymers* 157: 875–902. Elsevier Ltd. doi: 10.1016/j. carbpol.2016.10.041.

Lagarce, Frederic, Jean-Pierre Benoit, Emilie Roger, and Emmanuel Garcion. 2010. Biopharmaceutical parameters to consider in order to alter the fate of nanocarriers after oral delivery. *Nanomedicine* 5 (2): 287–306. doi: 10.2217/nnm.09.110.

Lemmer, Hendrik J. R. and Josias H. Hamman. 2013. Paracellular drug absorption enhancement through tight junction modulation. *Expert Opinion on Drug Delivery* 10 (1): 103–14. doi: 10.1517/17425247.2013.745509.

Li, Dong Xing, Hiromitsu Yamamoto, Hirofumi Takeuchi, and Yoshiaki Kawashima. 2010. A novel method for modifying AFM probe to investigate the interaction between biomaterial polymers (chitosan-coated PLGA) and mucin film. *European Journal of Pharmaceutics and Biopharmaceutics* 75 (2): 277–83. doi: 10.1016/j.ejpb.2010.02.013.

Lin, Yu Hsin, Kiran Sonaje, Kurt M. Lin, Jyuhn Huarng Juang, Fwu Long Mi, Han Wen Yang, and Hsing Wen Sung. 2008. Multi-ion-crosslinked nanoparticles with PH-responsive characteristics for oral delivery of protein drugs. *Journal of Controlled Release* 132 (2): 141–49. Elsevier B.V. doi: 10.1016/j. jconrel.2008.08.020.

Liu, Min, Jian Zhang, Xi Zhu, Wei Shan, Lian Li, Jiaju Zhong, Zhirong Zhang, and Yuan Huang. 2016. Efficient mucus permeation and tight junction opening by dissociable 'mucus-inert' agent coated tri- methyl chitosan nanoparticles for oral insulin delivery. *Journal of Controlled Release* 222: 67–77. Elsevier B.V. doi: 10.1016/j.jconrel.2015.12.008.

Liu, Chang, Yongqiang Kou, Xin Zhang, Hongbo Cheng, Xianzhi Chen, and Shirui Mao. 2018. Strategies and industrial perspectives to improve oral absorption of biological macromolecules. *Expert Opinion on Drug Delivery* 15(3): 223–233. doi: 10.1080/17425247.2017.1395853.

Liu, Chang, Huan Xu, Yian Sun, Xin Zhang, Hongbo Cheng, and Shirui Mao. 2019a. Design of virus- mimicking polyelectrolyte complexes for enhanced oral insulin delivery. *Journal of Pharmaceutical Sciences* 108: 3408–15. doi: 10.1016/j.xphs.

Liu, Chang, Yongqiang Kou, Xin Zhang, Wei Dong, Hongbo Cheng, and Shirui Mao. 2019b. Enhanced oral insulin delivery via surface hydrophilic modification of chitosan copolymer based self-assembly polyelectrolyte nanocomplex. *International Journal of Pharmaceutics* 554 (September 2018): 36–47. Elsevier. doi: 10.1016/j.ijpharm.2018.10.068.

Luque-Alcaraz, Ana Guadalupe, J. Lizardi-Mendoza, F. M. Goycoolea, I. Higuera-Ciapara, and W. Argüelles- Monal. 2016. Preparation of Chitosan Nanoparticles by Nanoprecipitation and Their Ability as a Drug Nanocarrier. *RSC Advances* 6 (64): 59250–56. doi:10.1039/C6RA06563E.

Mao, Shirui, Oliver Germershaus, Dagmar Fischer, Thomas Linn, Robert Schnepf, and Thomas Kissel. 2005. Uptake and transport of PEG-graft-trimethyl-chitosan copolymer-insulin nanocomplexes by epithelial cells. *Pharmaceutical Research* 22 (12): 2058–68. doi: 10.1007/s11095-005-8175-y.

Mao, Shirui, Wei Sun, and Thomas Kissel. 2010. Chitosan-based formulations for delivery of DNA and SiRNA. *Advanced Drug Delivery Reviews* 62 (1): 12–27. Elsevier B.V. doi: 10.1016/j.addr.2009.08.004.

Merisko-Liversidge, Elaine and Gary G. Liversidge. 2011. Nanosizing for oral and parenteral drug delivery: A perspective on formulating poorly-water soluble compounds using wet media milling technology. *Advanced Drug Delivery Reviews* 63 (6): 427–40. Elsevier B.V. doi: 10.1016/j.addr.2010.12.007.

Müller, Rainer Helmut and C. Jacobs. 2002. Buparvaquone mucoadhesive nanosuspension: Preparation, optimisation and long-term stability. *International Journal of Pharmaceutics* 237 (1–2): 151–61. doi: 10.1016/S0378-5173(02)00040-6.

Muzzarelli, Riccardo A. A. 2009. Genipin-crosslinked chitosan hydrogels as biomedical and pharmaceutical aids. *Carbohydrate Polymers* 77 (1): 1–9. doi: 10.1016/j.carbpol.2009.01.016.

Nam, Hae Yun, Seok Min Kwon, Hyunjin Chung, Seung-Young Lee, Seung-Hae Kwon, Hyesung Jeon, Yoonkyung Kim, et al. 2009. Cellular uptake mechanism and intracellular fate of hydrophobically modified glycol chitosan nanoparticles. *Journal of Controlled Release* 135 (3): 259–67. doi: 10.1016/j. jconrel.2009.01.018.

Naskar, Sweet, Suraj Sharma, and Ketousetuo Kuotsu. 2019. Chitosan-based nanoparticles: An overview of biomedical applications and its preparation. *Journal of Drug Delivery Science and Technology* 49 (October 2018): 66–81. Elsevier. doi: 10.1016/j.jddst.2018.10.022.

Nellans, Hugh N. 1991. (B) Mechanisms of peptide and protein absorption. *Advanced Drug Delivery Reviews* 7 (3): 339–64. doi: 10.1016/0169-409X(91)90013-3.

Nguyen, Thanh Xuan, Lin Huang, Li Liu, Ahmed Mohammed Elamin Abdalla, Mario Gauthier, and Guang Yang. 2014. Chitosan-coated nano-liposomes for the oral delivery of berberine hydrochloride. *Journal of Materials Chemistry B* 2 (41): 7149–59. Royal Society of Chemistry. doi: 10.1039/C4TB00876F.

Olmsted, Stuart S., Janet L. Padgett, Ashley I. Yudin, Kevin J. Whaley, Thomas R. Moench, and Richard A. Cone. 2001. Diffusion of macromolecules and virus-like particles in human cervical mucus. *Biophysical Journal* 81 (4): 1930–37. Elsevier. doi: 10.1016/S0006-3495(01)75844-4.

Papadimitriou, Sofia A., Dimitris S. Achilias, and Dimitrios N. Bikiaris. 2012. Chitosan-g-PEG nanoparticles ionically crosslinked with poly(glutamic acid) and tripolyphosphate as protein delivery systems. *International Journal of Pharmaceutics* 430 (1–2): 318–27. doi: 10.1016/j.ijpharm.2012.04.004.

Pereira de Sousa, Irene, Corinna Steiner, Matthias Schmutzler, Matthew D. Wilcox, Gert J. Veldhuis, Jeffrey P. Pearson, Christian W. Huck, Willi Salvenmoser, and Andreas Bernkop-Schnürch. 2015. Mucus permeating carriers: Formulation and characterization of highly densely charged nanoparticles. *European Journal of Pharmaceutics and Biopharmaceutics* 97 (November): 273–79. Elsevier B.V. doi: 10.1016/j.ejpb.2014.12.024.

Piazzini, Vieri, Elisa Landucci, Mario D'Ambrosio, Laura Tiozzo Fasiolo, Lorenzo Cinci, Gaia Colombo, Domenico E. Pellegrini-Giampietro, Anna Rita Bilia, Cristina Luceri, and Maria Camilla Bergonzi. 2019. Chitosan coated human serum albumin nanoparticles: A promising strategy for nose-to-brain drug delivery. *International Journal of Biological Macromolecules* 129 (May): 267–80. Elsevier B.V. doi: 10.1016/j.ijbiomac.2019.02.005.

Pillai, Chennakkattu K. S., Willi Paul, and Chandra P. Sharma. 2009. Chitin and chitosan polymers: Chemistry, solubility and fiber formation. *Progress in Polymer Science* 34 (7): 641–78. doi: 10.1016/j.progpolymsci.2009.04.001.

Prabaharan, Mani and João F. Mano. 2005. Hydroxypropyl chitosan bearing β-cyclodextrin cavities: Synthesis and slow release of its inclusion complex with a model hydrophobic drug. *Macromolecular Bioscience* 5 (10): 965–73. doi: 10.1002/mabi.200500087.

Quemeneur, Francois, Ayman Rammal, Marguerite Rinaudo, and Brigitte Pépin-Donat. 2007. Large and giant vesicles 'decorated' with chitosan: Effects of PH, salt or glucose stress, and surface adhesion. *Biomacromolecules* 8 (8): 2512–19. doi: 10.1021/bm061227a.

Quiñones, Javier Pérez, Hazel Peniche, and Carlos Peniche. 2018. Chitosan based self-assembled nanoparticles in drug delivery. *Polymers* 10 (3): 1–32. doi: 10.3390/polym10030235.

Ramalingam, Prakash and Young Tag Ko. 2016. Improved oral delivery of resveratrol from N-trimethyl chitosan-g-palmitic acid surface-modified solid lipid nanoparticles. *Colloids and Surfaces B: Biointerfaces* 139: 52–61. Elsevier B.V. doi: 10.1016/j.colsurfb.2015.11.050.

Ramalingam, Prakash, Sang Woo Yoo, and Young Tag Ko. 2016. Nanodelivery systems based on mucoadhesive polymer coated solid lipid nanoparticles to improve the oral intake of food curcumin. *Food Research International* 84: 113–19. Elsevier B.V. doi: 10.1016/j.foodres.2016.03.031.

Rossi, Silvia, Franca Ferrari, Maria Cristina Bonferoni, and Carla Caramella. 2001. Characterization of chitosan hydrochloride–Mucin rheological interaction: Influence of polymer concentration and polymer: Mucin weight ratio. *European Journal of Pharmaceutical Sciences* 12 (4): 479–85. doi: 10.1016/S0928-0987(00)00194-9.

Rossi, Silvia, Barbara Vigani, Maria Cristina Bonferoni, Giuseppina Sandri, Carla Caramella, and Franca Ferrari. 2018. Rheological analysis and mucoadhesion: A 30 year-old and still active combination. *Journal of Pharmaceutical and Biomedical Analysis* 156 (July): 232–38. Elsevier B.V. doi: 10.1016/j.jpba.2018.04.041.

Sadeghi, Assal Mir Mohamma, Farid A. Dorkoosh, Mohammad R. Avadi, Mirko Weinhold, Akbar Bayat, Florence Delie, Robert Gurny, Bagher Larijani, Morteza Rafiee-Tehrani, and Hans E. Junginger. 2008. Permeation enhancer effect of chitosan and chitosan derivatives: Comparison of formulations as soluble polymers and nanoparticulate systems on insulin absorption in caco-2 cells. *European Journal of Pharmaceutics and Biopharmaceutics* 70 (1): 270–78. doi: 10.1016/j.ejpb.2008.03.004.

Saltzman, William Mark, Michael L. Radomsky, Kevin J. Whaley, and Richard A. Cone. 1994. Antibody diffusion in human cervical mucus. *Biophysical Journal* 66 (2): 508–15. Elsevier. doi: 10.1016/S0006-3495(94)80802-1.

Sawtarie, Nader, Yuhang Cai, and Yakov Lapitsky. 2017. Preparation of chitosan/tripolyphosphate nanoparticles with highly tunable size and low polydispersity. *Colloids and Surfaces B: Biointerfaces* 157: 110–17. Elsevier B.V. doi: 10.1016/j.colsurfb.2017.05.055.

Sheng, Jianyong, Limei Han, Jing Qin, Ge Ru, Ruixiang Li, Lihong Wu, Dongqi Cui, Pei Yang, Yuwei He, and Jianxin Wang. 2015. N -trimethyl chitosan chloride-coated PLGA nanoparticles overcoming multiple barriers to oral insulin absorption. *ACS Applied Materials and Interfaces* 7 (28): 15430–41. doi: 10.1021/acsami.5b03555.

Shi, Chenjun, Yujiao Sun, Haiyang Wu, Chengyun Zhu, Guoguang Wei, Jinfeng Li, Tenglan Chan, Defang Ouyang, and Shirui Mao. 2016. Exploring the effect of hydrophilic and hydrophobic structure of grafted polymeric micelles on drug loading. *International Journal of Pharmaceutics* 512(1): 282–91. doi: 10.1016/j.ijpharm.2016.08.054.

Sogias, Ioannis A., Adrian C. Williams, and Vitaliy V. Khutoryanskiy. 2008. Why is chitosan mucoadhesive? *Biomacromolecules* 9 (7): 1837–42. doi: 10.1021/bm800276d.

Suh, Junghae, Michelle Dawson, and Justin Hanes. 2005. Real-time multiple-particle tracking: Applications to drug and gene delivery. *Advanced Drug Delivery Reviews* 57 (1 SPEC. ISS): 63–78. doi: 10.1016/j.addr.2004.06.001.

Sun, Wei, Wei Tian, Yuyang Zhang, Jianyong He, Shirui Mao, and Liang Fang. 2012. Effect of novel stabilizers-cationic polymers on the particle size and physical stability of poorly soluble drug nanocrystals. *Nanomedicine: Nanotechnology, Biology, and Medicine* 8 (4): 460–67. Elsevier Inc. doi: 10.1016/j.nano.2011.07.006.

Sung, Hsing-Wen, Kiran Sonaje, Zi-Xian Liao, Li-Wen Hsu, and Er-Yuan Chuang. 2012. PH-responsive nanoparticles shelled with chitosan for oral delivery of insulin: From mechanism to therapeutic applications. *Accounts of Chemical Research* 45 (4): 619–29. doi: 10.1021/ar200234q.

Takeuchi, Hirofiimi, Yuji Matsui, Hiromitsu Yamamoto, and Yoshiaki Kawashima. 2003. Mucoadhesive properties of carbopol or chitosan-coated liposomes and their effectiveness in the oral administration of calcitonin to rats. *Journal of Controlled Release* 86 (2–3): 235–42. doi: 10.1016/S0168-3659(02)00411-X.

Thongborisute, Jringjai, Hirofumi Takeuchi, H. Yamamoto, and Yuzuru Kawashima. 2006. Visualization of the penetrative and mucoadhesive properties of chitosan and chitosan-coated liposomes through the rat intestine. *Journal of Liposome Research* 16 (2): 127–41. doi: 10.1080/08982100600680816.

Tian, Ye and Shirui Mao. 2012. Amphiphilic polymeric micelles as the nanocarrier for peroral delivery of poorly soluble anticancer drugs. *Expert Opinion on Drug Delivery* 9 (6): 687–700. doi: 10.1517/174252 47.2012.681299.

Tian, Ye, Chenjun Shi, Yujiao Sun, Chengyun Zhu, Changquan Calvin Sun, and Shirui Mao. 2015a. Designing micellar nanocarriers with improved drug loading and stability based on solubility parameter. *Molecular Pharmaceutics* 12 (3): 816–25. doi: 10.1021/mp5006504.

Tian, Ye, Chenjun Shi, Xin Zhang, Yujiao Sun, Juan Wang, Yuyang Zhang, Jingyu Yang, Lihui Wang, Linlin Wang, and Shirui Mao. 2015b. Nanomicelle based peroral delivery system for enhanced absorption and sustained release of 10-hydrocamptothecin. *Journal of Biomedical Nanotechnology* 11 (2): 262–73. doi: 10.1166/jbn.2015.1909.

Tian, Ye, Yujiao Sun, Xiaodan Wang, Georgios Kasparis, and Shirui Mao. 2016. Chapter 15- Chitosan and its derivatives-based nano-formulations in drug delivery. In *Nanobiomaterials in Drug Delivery*, edited by Alexandru Mihai Grumezescu, 515–72. William Andrew Publishing. doi: 10.1016/B978-0-323-42866-8.00015-0.

Wang, Linlin, Liang Li, Yujiao Sun, Ye Tian, Ying Li, Conghao Li, Varaporn B. Junyaprasert, and Shirui Mao. 2013. Exploration of hydrophobic modification degree of chitosan-based nanocomplexes on the oral delivery of enoxaparin. *European Journal of Pharmaceutical Sciences* 50 (3–4): 263–71. Elsevier B.V. doi: 10.1016/j.ejps.2013.07.009.

Wang, Linlin, Yujiao Sun, Chenjun Shi, Liang Li, Jian Guan, Xin Zhang, Rui Ni, Xiaopin Duan, Yaping Li, and Shirui Mao. 2014. Uptake, transport and peroral absorption of fatty glyceride grafted chitosan copolymer-enoxaparin nanocomplexes: Influence of glyceride chain length. *Acta Biomaterialia* 10 (8): 3675–85. Acta Materialia Inc. doi: 10.1016/j.actbio.2014.05.003.

Wedmore, Ian, John G. McManus, Anthony E. Pusateri, and John B. Holcomb. 2006. A special report on the chitosan-based hemostatic dressing: Experience in current combat operations. *The Journal of Trauma: Injury, Infection, and Critical Care* 60 (3): 655–58. doi: 10.1097/01.ta.0000199392.91772.44.

Woertz, Christina, Maren Preis, Jörg Breitkreutz, and Peter Kleinebudde. 2013. Assessment of test methods evaluating mucoadhesive polymers and dosage forms: An overview. *European Journal of Pharmaceutics and Biopharmaceutics* 85 (3 PART B): 843–53. Elsevier B.V. doi: 10.1016/j.ejpb.2013.06.023.

Woraphatphadung, Thisirak, Warayuth Sajomsang, Pattarapond Gonil, Alongkot Treetong, Prasert Akkaramongkolporn, Tanasait Ngawhirunpat, and Praneet Opanasopit. 2016. PH-responsive polymeric micelles based on amphiphilic chitosan derivatives: Effect of hydrophobic cores on oral meloxicam delivery. *International Journal of Pharmaceutics* 497 (1–2): 150–60. doi: 10.1016/j.ijpharm.2015.12.009.

Yeh, Tzyy Harn, Li Wen Hsu, Michael T. Tseng, Pei Ling Lee, Kiran Sonjae, Yi Cheng Ho, and Hsing Wen Sung. 2011. Mechanism and Consequence of Chitosan-Mediated Reversible Epithelial Tight Junction Opening. *Biomaterials* 32 (26): 6164–73. doi:10.1016/j.biomaterials.2011.03.056.

Yoo, Mi Kyong, Sang Kee Kang, Jin Huk Choi, In Kyu Park, Hee Sam Na, Hyun Chul Lee, Eun Bae Kim, et al. 2010. Targeted delivery of chitosan nanoparticles to Peyer's patch using M cell-homing peptide selected by phage display technique. *Biomaterials* 31 (30): 7738–47. Elsevier Ltd. doi: 10.1016/j. biomaterials.2010.06.059.

Zhang, Hua and Steven H. Neau. 2002. In vitro degradation of chitosan by bacterial enzymes from rat cecal and colonic contents. *Biomaterials* 23 (13): 2761–66. doi: 10.1016/S0142-9612(02)00011-X.

Zhang, Shaoling and Kohsaku Kawakami. 2010. One-step preparation of chitosan solid nanoparticles by electrospray deposition. *International Journal of Pharmaceutics* 397 (1–2): 211–17. Elsevier B.V. doi: 10.1016/j.ijpharm.2010.07.007.

Zhang, Xin, Luk Li, and Shirui Mao. 2014. Nanosuspensions of poorly water soluble drugs prepared by top-down technologies. *Current Pharmaceutical Design* 20 (3): 388–407. doi: 10.2174/13816128113199990401.

Zhang, Xin, Hongbo Cheng, Wei Dong, Meixia Zhang, Qiaoyu Liu, Xiuhua Wang, Jian Guan, Haiyang Wu, and Shirui Mao. 2018. Design and intestinal mucus penetration mechanism of core-shell nanocomplex. *Journal of Controlled Release* 272 (December 2017): 29–38. Elsevier. doi: 10.1016/j.jconrel.2017.12.034.

16 Liposome-Based Delivery of Therapeutic Agents

Eneida de Paula, Juliana Damasceno Oliveira,
and Fernando Freitas de Lima
Institute of Biology, University of Campinas-UNICAMP

Lígia Nunes de Morais Ribeiro
Institute of Biology, University of Campinas-UNICAMP
Federal University of Uberlândia

CONTENTS

16.1 INTRODUCTION

Liposomes are micro, submicro, and nanometric vesicles that mimic cell membranes because of their overall structure: lipid bilayer(s) that involve inner aqueous core(s). They are spontaneously formed when specific lipids are exposed to water, under agitation. Indeed, due to the hydrophobic effect,[1] rod-shaped phospholipids, such as phosphatidylcholine (PC) in the presence of water tend to aggregate in concentric lamellae,[2] in which their acyl chains hide from water, leaving the polar head groups (inner and outer monolayers) exposed to it (Figure 16.1). Phospholipids are the major components of liposomes, followed by cholesterol (Chol) that inserts in-between the phospholipids, adjusting the fluidity of the bilayer in a biphasic mode that depends on the melting transition of the phospholipid.[3]

Liposomes can be classified by the number of concentric bilayers per vesicle (mono, oligo, or multivesicular), size (small, large, giant), surface charge (zwitterionic, anionic, and cationic)[1,3–7] The methods for liposome formation also deserve mention, going from the simple agitation in water, to sonication, extrusion, or phase inversion (solvent evaporation).[4,8] Finally, nonconventional liposomes can also be prepared, such as (i) elastic liposomes, that contain surface active compounds inside the bilayer to form deformable vesicles, suitable for dermal drug delivery[9]; (ii) ionic-gradient liposomes, in which pH or ion gradients allow the upload of higher drug amounts

---

[1] Notice that there are no positively charged natural lipids. Despite of that, and especially for gene-delivery purposes liposomes have been prepared with synthetic cationic lipids, such as DOTAP®, which electrostatically interact with nucleic acids.

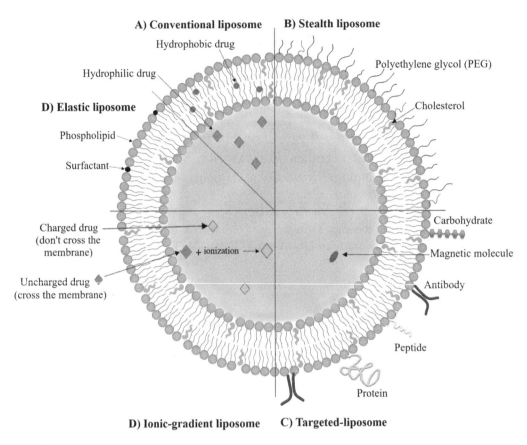

FIGURE 16.1 Schematic representation of different kinds of liposomes (A) conventional, B) stealth or PEGylated, C) targeted, D) ionic-gradient and E) elastic) in drug delivery, and their components.

into the inner aqueous core of the vesicles[10,11]; (iii) stealth liposomes, polyethylene glycol (PEG) ylated vesicles[2] that are able to evade the reticuloendothelial system (RES), remaining in circulation for longer periods,[13,14] and (iv) targeted-liposomes – loaded either with aptamers (proteins, peptides, antibodies, etc.) or magnetic molecules that, are able to target the vesicles to specific tissues[3,5,15] (Figure 16.1). Other assemblies involving lipid vesicles and adjuvants are also of interest as drug delivery systems (DDS), such as DepoFoam®[16] or either vesicles formed with nonionic surfactants, the niosomes.[17]

Although the original description of liposomes, by Bangham, was made in 1965,[18] and their clinical potential for enzyme replacement therapy in genetic deficiencies of lysosomal enzymes was reported in the 1970s.[4] The first liposomal-based drug delivery product for human use appeared in the 80s[3–4], containing doxorubicin (DOX), Doxyl® obtained regulatory approval in 1995.[13] Beyond advantages such as biocompatibility, biodegradability, and nonimmunogenicity, what distinguish liposomes from other drug delivery carriers is their ability to encapsulate both hydrophobic (partitioned in the lipid bilayer) and hydrophilic (dissolved in the inner aqueous core) drugs.[6,7]

Liposomes occupy a prominent position among DDS, having the largest number of products approved for human use.[19] Despite of that, technological drawbacks of liposomal systems include issues related to stability/vesicles size control during storage, scaling up production under sterile

---

[2] PEGylation consists in the attachment of polyethylene glycol polymer chains to a given molecule, e.g. PE in liposomes. PEGylation is a strategy to avoid opsonization of liposomes, by increasing the half-life and biological effect. It is also possible to functionalize PEG molecules with addition of aptamers, for targeting the vesicles to specific cells/tissues[12].

conditions, high price of pure lipids,[8,20] as well as concerns about the toxicity of liposomal formulations for anticancer agents,[21] or those prepared with cationic lipids.[22]

This chapter contains a systematic review of liposomal formulations in clinical and preclinical stages. The liposomal formulations were grouped into four categories: liposomes for the treatment of pain (including local anesthetics (LA), opioids, and anti-inflammatories), infections (antibiotics and antifungals), and cancer.

16.2 LIPOSOMAL FORMULATIONS FOR THE TREATMENT OF PAIN

Pain is one of the most frequent causes of medical demand, worldwide.[23-27] The pharmacological treatment is the most common approach to provide analgesia[28,29] using either LAs, opioids, or anti-inflammatory drugs.

LA are frequently used in surgical procedures and prevention of acute and chronic pain, relieving the symptom of syndromes such as diabetic neuropathy and advanced stage cancers, due to their capacity to inhibit the excitation of peripheral sensorial nerve fibers.[30-35] Liposomes have been used for the delivery of LAs since the end of 1970s with advantages such as the gradual LA release, prolongation of analgesia, and decrease of side effects.[36,37] Table 16.1 reviews studies in which formulations of LAs encapsulated in liposomes have been tested in human volunteers. Among them liposomal bupivacaine (Exparel®), launched in 2011, is the most known.[55]

Exparel® carries bupivacaine in multivesicular liposomes prepared by DepoFoam® technology. This system is described as honeycomb-like structures of vesicles, with average diameters of 10–30 μm, composed of phospholipids (dierucoyl and dipalmitoyl PC), Chol, and tricaprylin. Exparel® is able to release bupivacaine for ~72 h,[56,57] and a single-dose infiltration of Exparel® into surgical site through interscalene brachial plexus nerve block produces long-acting analgesia, decreasing the use of opioids.[46,58,59] Exparel® has been used in a variety of procedures, such as breast reconstruction after mastectomy and arthroplasty.[60-62]

Another example of successful encapsulation of LA in liposomes is LMX4®, a topical (liposomal lidocaine 4% cream) formulation. Taddio et al.[63] demonstrated its superior analgesia, shortening the onset of action with minimal vasoactive properties and minor dermal changes, when compared with other topical LA formulation such as lidocaine-prilocaine 5% cream (EMLA®) for intravenous cannulation in children.[63,64] Since there are many adverse effects related to EMLA, e.g. methemoglobinemia, vasoconstriction,[65-67] erythema, blanching, edema, and irritation,[68,69] encapsulation into liposomes was proposed to decrease them.[70]

Grant et al.[40] developed ionic gradient liposomes (IGL) for the encapsulation of bupivacaine (0.5%–2%). Large multivesicular vesicles (LMVV) of hydrogenated soybean PC (HSPC):Chol (2:1 mol%) with 250 mM ammonium sulfate were prepared. In ammonium sulfate IGL the anesthetic in its basic form crosses the bilayer of preformed liposomes prepared with high $(NH_4)_2SO_4$ in their internal aqueous core. The subsequent dissociation of ammonium ions ($NH_4^+ \leftrightarrow NH_3 + H^+$) and permeation of the resultant ammonia through the bilayer leaves protons that decrease the pH of the inner aqueous compartment of the liposomes. In such acidic medium protonation of the anesthetic takes place, and the low diffusion of the protonated LA species through the membrane keeps it inside the vesicles.[71,72] After intradermal injections in human volunteers, ultralong anesthesia (up to 19, 38 and 48 h for the IGL formulations containing 0.5%, 1.0%, and 2.0% bupivacaine, respectively) as achieved.

For the control of postoperative pain, opioids are the most important medicines, with morphine being the reference drug. DepoDur® is an extended-release liposome epidural morphine formulation, also prepared by DepoFoam® technology. It is able to promote analgesia for 48 h, preventing the administration of multiple doses of opioids for pain control.[73-75] There are several reports of significantly lower pain intensity scores and prolongation of analgesia after a single-dose DepoDur® (5–30 mg), in comparison to equivalent dose of plain morphine, for postoperative pain control.[76,77] In a study with 75 patients submitted to elective cesareans, the parturients received a single dose of

TABLE 16.1

Liposomal Systems for the Sustained Release of Local Anesthetics

Drug/Concentration	Liposome Type	Composition	Pharmacological Tests	Route	Biological Effect	Year	References
Tetracaine 0.5%	MLV	SPC:Chol in gel	Clinic, in human volunteers	Skin	Improvement and prolongation of the anesthetic effect.	1988	[38]
Bupivacaine 2%	Large unilamellar vesicle (LUV, 300 mM citrate-IGL)	DOPC:Chol (55:45 mol%)	Cutaneous wheal model, in guinea pigs	Intradermal	Sustained release (14 h)	1996	[39]
Mepivacaine 0.5; 1; 2%	LUV	EPC:Chol:α-tocopherol (4:3:0.07 mol%)	Paw withdraw test, mice	Sciatic nerve block	Prolongation of the anesthetic effect	2004	[28]
Bupivacaine 0.5; 1.0; 2.0%	LMVV	HSPC:Chol (2:1 mol%)	Clinic, in human volunteers	Intradermal	Prolongation of the anesthetic effect for more than 42 h	2004	[40]
Benzocaine 0.5; 1.0%	SUV/hydrogel	l-α-PC:Chol (1:1 mol%)	Conjunctival reflex test, in albino rabbits	Conjunctival sac	Sustained release and more intense anesthetic effect than the plain drug administration	2007	[41]
Ropivacaine 1%; 2%	LUV	EPC:Chol:α-tocopherol (4:3:0.07 mol%)	Clinic, in human volunteers	Oral mucosa	Improved duration of soft tissue anesthesia	2007, 2010	[42, 43]
Mepivacaine 2%; 3%	LUV	EPC:Chol:α-tocopherol (4:3:0.07 mol%)	Clinic, in human volunteers	Oral mucosa	Increased anesthetic effect.	2011	[44, 45]
Bupivacaine 0.5; 1.0; 2%	LMVV (127 mM ammonium sulfate-IGL)	HSPC:sphingomyelin:Chol (3:3:4 mol%) (Bupisome hydrogel)	Electrical stimulation testing, in mice	Intradermal	Sustained release (24 h)	2012	[46]
Benzocaine 10%	LUV	EPC:Chol:α-tocopherol (4:3:0.07 mol%)	Clinic, in human volunteers	Oral mucosa	Lower latency time compared to the commercial formulation	2013	[47]
Lidocaine 2.5; 5.0%	LUV	EPC:Chol:α-tocopherol (4:3:0.07 mol%)	Clinic, in human volunteers	Oral mucosa	Improvement of anesthetic permeability trough the mucosa	2015	[48]

(Continued)

TABLE 16.1 (*Continued*)
Liposomal Systems for the Sustained Release of Local Anesthetics

Drug/Concentration	Liposome Type	Composition	Pharmacological Tests	Route	Biological Effect	Year	References
Articaine 4%	LUV/LMV	EPC:Chol:α-tocopherol (4:3:0.07 mol%)	Inflamed hind paw model, in rats	Infiltrative	Anesthetic effect was not affected by inflammation.	2016	[49]
Butamben 10%	Elastic LUV/gel	EPC:Chol:α-tocopherol (4:3:0.07 mol%)	Tail-flick test, in rats	Sensory block into the base of the tail	Increased analgesic effect compared to plain drug.	2017	[50]
Ropivacaine 0.75: 2%	LMVV/LUV donor/acceptor (250 mM ammonium sulfate-IGL)	HSPC:Chol (2:1 mol%)	Von Frey test, in mice	Subcutaneous	Sustained release (*ca.* 7h).	2017	[51]
Ropivacaine 0.75: 2%	LMVV/LUV donor/acceptor (250 mM ammonium sulfate-IGL)	HSPC:Chol (2:1 mol%)	Pharmacokinetics evaluation, in white rabbits (New Zealand)	Sciatic nerve block	Reduced systemic exposure (low plasma LA concentration) and higher concentrations at the site of action.	2018	[52]
Dibucaine 0.012%	LMVV/LUV (250 mM ammonium sulfate-IGL)	HSPC:Chol (2:1 mol%)	Tail flick, in mice	Infiltrative	Sustained release (27 h) with a parenteral formulation of dibucaine.	2018	[53]
Lidocaine 2%	LUV	HSPC:Chol: mannitol (3:1:1.25 mol%)	Infraorbital blockage test, in rats	Infraorbital nerve	Prolonged duration of analgesia by more than 50% when compared with plain drug.	2019	[54]

liposomal morphine (5, 10, and 15 mg) or 5 mg of plain epidural morphine. Higher effectiveness of pain control 48 h postdose was observed with liposomal formulations (32%, 53%, and 74%, respectively) than with the control group (22%), although over 90% of parturients treated with morphine (liposomal or not) reported some adverse effects related to the opioid.[78]

Another opioid that has been encapsulated in liposomes is fentanyl. In 1995, Hung et al.[79] proposed a liposomal formulation for its pulmonary prolonged release, to be used in the control of postoperative pain. The results were satisfactory, although similar to a nonliposomal aerolized fentanyl formulation, and the authors concluded that the optimal liposome composition promoted sustained release. After that, a preparation of aerolized liposome-encapsulated fentanyl (AeroLEF®) was developed for the treatment of chronic and acute pain, resulting in rapid onset extended analgesia.[80–83]

Anti-inflammatory agents, such as nonsteroidal anti-inflammatory drugs (NSAIDs), are also widely used for pain control. However, adverse effects such as severe gastrointestinal tract damage are associated to the use of NSAIDs. To avoid that, the transdermal route may be an alternative, by decreasing the systemic effects, avoiding the first-pass effect and gastric degradation[84,85] Since the success of transdermal or topical delivery depends on the ability of the drug to cross the skin layers, liposomes were proposed to facilitate that passage for anti-inflammatory drugs.[86,87]

Gaur et al.[87] have tested different lipid compositions in the preparation of liposomes containing 1% ibuprofen, which were suspended in carbopol gel. Tested in Wistar rats such ibuprofen liposomal gel composed of PC:Chol:dicetylphosphate (7:3:1 mol%) significantly decreased the edema caused by carrageenan, in comparison to ibuprofen gel (control). Similar results were reported by Fetih et al.[88] with liposomes of HSPC:Chol at different molar ratios (7:3, 6:4, 5:5) containing 0.5% celecoxib and incorporated in different gels (hydroxyl ethyl cellulose, Pluronic F-127, Carbopol 934). When dispersed in carbopol, such liposomes were found effective in reducing paw edema compared with celecoxib gels, with sustained anti-inflammatory effects for more than 6 h.

The steroidal anti-inflammatory prednisolone, a glucocorticoid used in the therapy of rheumatoid arthritis and other inflammatory diseases, has also been tried in liposomal formulations: when tested in rats, there was remission of paw inflammation 2 days after treatment.[89] Nanocort® is a PEGylated liposomal formulation (in which lipid-bound PEG molecules produce sterically stabilized vesicles) of prednisolone phosphate for administration by intravenous infusion.[90,91] Nanocort® has been carried to phase I and II clinical trials in human volunteers with severe inflamed carotid or aortic atherosclerosis plaque but no conclusive results have been published so far.[92]

The potential of glucocorticoid prodrugs encapsulated in PEGylated liposomal formulation against several inflammatory diseases was examined by Turjeman and Barenholz[93] with promising results in relation to pharmacokinetics, bioavailability, and tolerability, when compared with free prodrugs tested for inflammation in six different animal models.

Despite the great number of researches related to liposomes for pain relief in the literature, and that dozens of formulations are published every year reporting the benefits of sustained release caused by pain-relief drugs encapsulation in liposomes, they somehow fail to reach clinical trials[37] since the only commercially available formulations so far are Exparel® and DepoDur®.

16.3 LIPOSOMES LOADED WITH ANTIBIOTICS AGENTS

Antibiotics are among the ten most important discoveries in the field of health, dramatically reducing mortality and morbidity caused by severe bacterial infections. Most medical procedures could not be safely performed without antimicrobial therapy. But the cell walls of Gram-negative and Gram-positive bacteria may significantly restrict or completely prevent the penetration of antibiotics therein.[94–96] Besides, the structural aspects of bacteria may limit the use of antibiotics. The emergence of multiresistant bacteria threatens public health and it is a global concern, since there are compelling evidences that the indiscriminate consumption of antibiotics induces multidrug resistance.[97,98]

Multiresistance of bacteria to conventional antimicrobial therapies has become one of the main factors that drive researchers towards new pharmaceutical approaches, including combination of therapies or encapsulation of antibiotics in DDS, including liposomes.[99–101] Liposomal systems can target antibiotics to specific cells or organs and help in the treatment of multiresistant bacterial infection, protect antibiotics from enzymatic degradation, potentiate and/or prolong their pharmacological action, and reduce toxic effects.[101–103]

Liposomes can fuse with bacterial membranes because of their unique lipid bilayer composition.[103,104] Phagocytes can also internalize liposomes in the blood (e.g. RES removal of liposomes larger than 100 nm from circulation), or at specific tissues.[103,105–108]

The development of liposomes loaded with antimicrobial drugs emerged in the 70s, but without *in vivo* application. In the 1990s a liposomal formulation containing 12.3 mg/mL amikacin (Mikasome®) was launched onto the market with effective results in the treatment of endocarditis caused by *Staphylococcus aureus*. However, the product was discontinued in 2000, when it was already in clinical trials.[109–112]

Nowadays a heterogeneity of antibiotics (amikacin, amoxicillin, ampicillin, ciprofloxacin, clofazimine, gentamicin, polymyxin B, rifampicin, and tobramycin) has been loaded in liposomes, mostly for the treatment of infections caused by Gram-negative bacteria. Table 16.2 depicts the main clinical and preclinical studies with antimicrobial agents encapsulated in liposomes, involving different classes of antibiotics and types of liposomes, since 1990.

Currently, there are three formulations in clinical trials: Arikace®, Lipoquin®, and Pulmaquin®. Arikace® allows targeting amikacin (280 or 560 mg) to the lungs, i.e. to the most common infection site for *Pseudomonas aeruginosa*. The results demonstrated good biological activity in cystic fibrosis patients infected by *P. aeruginosa* with only one daily administration and no unexpected adverse events. The product is currently undergoing phase III clinical trials and has been shown safe and well tolerated, without unexpected adverse effects.[13,136,137]

Aerosol forms of liposomal ciprofloxacin were also developed for the treatment of *P. aeruginosa* in noncystic fibrosis bronchiectasis and chronically infected patients. Lipoquin® (liposomal ciprofloxacin, 50 mg/mL) and Pulmaquin® (liposomal ciprofloxacin, 50 mg/mL, plus free ciprofloxacin 20 mg/mL) are already in clinical phase III. The results so far have shown no adverse effects and reduced bacterial density in the lungs, with benefits for patients with chronic *P. aeruginosa* lung infections with frequent exacerbations.[138–140]

16.4 ANTIFUNGAL LIPOSOMAL SYSTEMS

The rise of systemic fungal infections, in which diagnosis and therapeutic is not easy and leads to significant morbidity, is explained by the great number of immunocompromised patients. The number of cancerous, diabetic, and patients with AIDS under life-threatening presystemic and systemic fungal infections increased to alarming proportions in the last decades.[141] While a large number of fungi can cause topical mycoses, the most common fungal pathogens in neutropenic and bone marrow transplantation patients are *Candida* spp., *Aspergillus* spp., and *Cryptococcus neoformans*.[142]

The broadest spectrum agents of antifungal therapy worldwide in the last 50 years have been the polyene compounds (e.g. amphotericin, nystatin, hamycin, dermostatin, etc.). Amphotericin B (AMB) is the gold standard antifungal drug, but its use is still associated with severe adverse effects (mainly impairment of nephron function by cumulative doses, besides fever, chills, myalgia, and thrombophlebitis), low clinical response, and high mortality rates. Another class of antifungal, the azoles, include ketoconazole, fluconazole, and itraconazole (launched in the 80s), and later the second-generation triazoles voriconazole, ravuconazole, and posaconazole. Their good activity against molds brought some help to the antifungal therapy, although some of them are mostly used as topical agents. Allylamines, such as butenafine and naftifine, are the third class of antimycotic agents that are able to inhibit squalene epoxidase, restraining the synthesis of ergosterol.[143] In the beginning of the 21st century, another class of drugs, the echinocandins – noncompetitive inhibitors of β-1-3-glucan synthase, blocking the synthesis of the fungal cell wall – appeared as a promise for the candidiasis and aspergillosis treatment.[144,145]

TABLE 16.2

Liposomal Systems for the Sustained Release of Antibiotics, Classified According to Gram Stain

Drug/Concentration	Liposome Type	Composition	Pharmacological Tests	Route	Biological Effect	Year	References
			Gram-negative bacteria				
Gentamicin 20–80 mg/kg	LMV	EPC:EPG:Chol: α-tocopherol	In vivo test female mice (BALB/c)	Intravenous	Liposomal gentamicin directed antimicrobial agents to infected cells, increasing antimicrobial activity and decreasing toxicity (Salmonella dublin)	1990	[113]
Gentamicin 10 mg/kg	LMV	EPC (7.1 mol%)	In vivo test male mice (BALB/c)	Intravenous	Liposomal gentamicin greatly enhanced survival when given as a single dose, 1 or 2 days after infection, as well as up to 7 days before infection (Salmonella typhimurium)	1990	[114]
Ampicillin 50 mg/mL	LMV	SPC:Chol:PG (4:5:1 mol%)	In vivo test mice (C57BL/6)	Retro-orbital	Treatment with liposome-entrapped ampicillin reduced mortality (50%) compared with untreated controls or mice treated with nonloaded liposomes (Salmonella typhimurium)	1991	[115]
Gentamicin 25 mg/mL	LMV	EPC:Chol:SA (6:3:1 mol%)	In vivo test female mice (Swiss–Webster)	Intravenous	Cationic liposomes with gentamicin potentiated the therapeutic effect of the drug compared to free drug (Brucella abortus)	1997	[116]
Clofazimine 5–100 mg/mL	LMV	DMPC:DMPG (7:3 mol%)	In vivo test mice (BALB/c)	Intravenous	The treatment with liposomal clofazimine was efficient, with no recurrence, and bactericidal effect on liver and spleen (Mycobacterium tuberculosis)	1999	[117]
Gentamicin 50 mg/mL	pH-Sensitive Liposomes	DOPE:N-succinyl-DOPE (3.5:3 mol%)	In vivo test female mice (BALB/c)	Intravenous	pH-sensitive liposomes with gentamicin significantly reduced the presence of bacteria in spleen and liver (Salmonella enterica)	2000	[118]
Isoniazid 12 mg/kg; and Rifampicin 10 mg/kg	LMV	EPC:Chol:DPC: PEG-DSPE (2:1.5:0.2:0.2 mol%)	In vivo test mice (Mice (Laca strain)	Intravenous	Liposomal isoniazid reduced the number of Bacillus tuberculosis in lungs, liver, and spleen, improving patient compliance and reducing cost, dosage, and toxic effects of the therapy	2002	[119]

(Continued)

TABLE 16.2 (Continued)
Liposomal Systems for the Sustained Release of Antibiotics, Classified According to Gram Stain

Drug/Concentration	Liposome Type	Composition	Pharmacological Tests	Route	Biological Effect	Year	References
Polymyxin B 10 mg/mL	LUV	DPPC:Chol (2:1 mol%)	In vivo test male rats (Sprague-Dawley)	Intratracheal	The effectiveness of liposomal polymyxin B, administered intratracheally to the lungs of rats infected was confirmed in three consecutive treatment days (P. aeruginosa)	2002	[120]
Tobramycin 4.9 g/L	LUV	DPPC:DMPG (10:1 mol%)	In vivo test male rats (Sprague–Dawley)	Intratracheal	Liposomal tobramycin promoted drug retention in the lungs and therapeutic efficacy after multiple treatments (P. aeruginosa)	2003	[121]
Ciprofloxacin 22 mg/mL	SUV (ammonium sulfate -IGL)	EPC:Chol (1:1 mol%)	In vivo test female mice (BALB/c)	Aerosol inhalation	The aerosol form of liposomal ciprofloxacin, efficiently delivered the drug to the primary site of infection, increasing its efficacy (Francisella tularensis)	2003	[122]
Amikacin (Arikace™) 20–75 mg/kg	LUV	DPPC:Chol	In vivo test female rats (Sprague-Dawley)	Nebulization	Liposomal amikacin demonstrated efficacy with less toxicity, keeping most of the drug in the lung (P. aeruginosa)	2008	[123]
Amoxicillin 10 mg; and Ranitidine 10 mg	LMV LUV	PC:Chol:PE (7:3:0.5 mol%), PC:Chol:AS (7:3:0.2 mol%)	In vivo and in vitro tests albino rats	Oral via	The double liposomal system showed action on the gastric mucosa in Helicobacter pylori clearance. inhibition of bacterial growth was also shown by in vitro models	2012	[124]
Tobramycin 300 mg/L	LMV	PEG-DSPC: Chol (2:1 mol%)	In vivo test rats (Sprague-Dawley rats)	Intratracheal	Liposomal tobramycin effectively reduced the bacterial load in the lungs, compared with the free drug (P. aeruginosa)	2013	[125]
Polymyxin B 3 mg/kg	LUV	DPPC: Chol	In vivo test mice (Swiss Webster)	Intravenous	Liposomal Polymyxin B formulation demonstrated superior efficacy in the treatment of murine pneumonia (P. aeruginosa)	2013	[126]
Ciprofloxacin 50 mg/mL	SUV	---	In vivo test female mice (BALB/c)	Intranasal	Liposomal ciprofloxacin showed greater efficacy compared with the oral drug formulation (Francisella tularensis)	2014	[127]

(Continued)

TABLE 16.2 (*Continued*)
Liposomal Systems for the Sustained Release of Antibiotics, Classified According to Gram Stain

Drug/Concentration	Liposome Type	Composition	Pharmacological Tests	Route	Biological Effect	Year	References
Gram-positive bacteria							
Gentamicin 0.2–20 mg/kg	LMV	EPC	*In vivo* test beige mice (C57BL/6J-bg/bg)	Intravenous	The liposomal system showed a promising effect with bacterial decrease in the liver and spleen (*Mycobacterium Avium*)	1990	[128]
Ampicillin 50 mg/mL	LMV	SPC:Chol:PG (4:5:1)	*In vivo* test nude mice	Intravenous (tail vein)	Ampicillin-loaded liposomes showed greater effect on the bacterial count in the spleen (*Listeria monocytogenes*) of mice with induced chronic listeriosis	1991	[115]
Streptomycin 168 mg/mL	LUV	PG:PC:Chol (1:9:6.7 mol%) PEG-DSPE: DSPC: Chol (1:9:6.7 mol%)	*In vivo* test male beige mice (C57BL/6J-bg/bg)	Intravenous (tail vein)	Twice-weekly dosing of streptomycin encapsulated in the two kinds of liposomes reduced the level of infection (*Mycobacterium avium*)	1995	[129]
Clofazimine 5; 10; 25; 50 and 100 mg/kg	LMV	DMPC:DMPG (7:3 mol%)	*In vitro*	Macrophages peritoneal lavage of the mice	Liposomal clofazimine was more effective than equivalent doses of free drug, in reducing bacterial activity in the liver, spleen and kidney tissues (*Mycobacterium avium-M. intracellulare*)	1996	[130]
Amikacin (MiKasome®) plus Oxacillin (50 mg/kg)	SUV	HSPC:Chol: DSPG (2:1:0.1 mol%)	*In vivo* test white female rabbits (New Zealand)	Intravenous	The association of oxacillin and conventional amikacin (free or encapsulated in liposomes) promoted significant density reduction in all target tissues and were shown to protect the left ventricular function (*Staphylococcus aureus*)	1999	[111]
Ciprofloxacin 10 mg/kg and Vancomycin 15 mg/mL	LMV	EPC:SA:Chol (7:2:1 mol%)	*In vivo* test white rabbits (New Zealand)	Intravenous	The 14-day drug combination in cationic liposomes proved to be able to sterilize the bone marrow; a promising approach for the treatment of osteomyelitis (*S. aureus*)	2004	[131]

(Continued)

TABLE 16.2 (Continued)
Liposomal Systems for the Sustained Release of Antibiotics, Classified According to Gram Stain

Drug/Concentration	Liposome Type	Composition	Pharmacological Tests	Route	Biological Effect	Year	References
Amikacin 12 mg/kg	LUV	HEPC:Chol: PEG-DSPE (3.9:2:0.3 mol%)	*In vivo* test female mice (C57BL/6)	Intravenous (tail vein)	The liposomal formulation caused rapid decrease in mycobacterial load, followed by effective death (*Mycobacterium avium*)	2007	[132]
Vancomycin 50 mg/mL	LMV	DSPC:DCP:Chol (7:2:1 mol%)	*In vivo* test mice	Intravenous	Liposomes enhanced the antistaphylococcal efficacy of vancomycin (methicillin-resistant *S. aureus*)	2012	[133]
Daptomycin 20 mg/mL	SUV	SPC:sodium cholate (17:1 mol%)	*In vivo* test male mice (BALB/c)	Transdermal	Liposomes efficiently fused in the skin providing anti-infective and antibiofilm activities (methicillin-resistant *S. aureus*)	2013	[134]
Daptomycin 1.6 mg/kg Clarithromycin 51.8 mg/kg	SUV	HSPC:Chol: mPEG-DSPE (15:10:1)	*In vivo* test male and female mice (Kunming)	Intravenous (in tail vein)	Codelivery of daptomycin and clarithromycin by liposomes significantly prolonged the survival rate of infected animals (methicillin-resistant *S. aureus*)	2015	[135]

16.4.1 POLYENE ANTIMYCOTIC AGENTS

The mechanism of action of polyene agents and their specificity to fungi depends on their binding to ergosterol (the sterol of fungus) and the formation of transmembrane pores that not only change cell membrane permeability and cause death but also oxidative damage. To overcome the poor solubility of AMB, a colloidal suspension of AMB in deoxycholate salt was launched in the United States as Fungizone® in 1960. Other lipid-based carriers appeared later, such as a colloidal dispersion of AMB in cholesterol sulfate (Amphotec®, Amphocil®), AMB lipid complex (ABLC, a ribbon-like structure formed of L-α-dimyristoylphosphatidyl choline (DMPC) and L-α-dimyristoylphosphatidyl glycerol (DMPG) with AMB), AMB in 20% lipid emulsion (Intralipid) and L-AMB or AmBisome®, a true unilamellar liposome formulation.[146]

Liposomal antifungal formulations enhance the activity of the drug by enabling its entrapment in the RES and its delivery specifically to the site of infection. The small unilamellar vesicles (SUV) of L-AMB are composed of hydrogenated soy PC, 1,2-distearoyl-sn-glycero-3-phosphoglycerol (DSPG), Chol, and AMB in a 2:0.8:1:0.4 molar ratio. The small size (60–70 nm diameter) of the vesicles and the relative rigidity of the lipid bilayer, given by the higher transition temperature of its lipid components, provide longer circulation times to the formulation. L-AMB is considerably less nephrotoxic than AMB, and its LD_{50} after a single injection to mice and rats was also significantly higher (30–60 times) compared with that of conventional AMB.[142,147,148] Like all other lipid formulations and conventional AMB, it is unable to surpass the blood–brain barrier. Moreover, AMB-loaded liposomes penetrate the cell wall, have long half-life and retention in tissues, and show reduced toxicity at higher, more effective doses of AMB than the second most commonly used AmB product, Fungizone® or ABLC. Altogether, these features suggest that single or intermittent dosing regimens are feasible and should be of interest in clinical trials.[148] To highlight the prominence of L-AMB formulation, from 63 clinical trials involving fungal infection and liposomes at the National Institute of Health clinical trials site (https://clinicaltrials.gov/ct2/), 29 studied the performance of Ambisome®.

Recently, an antifungal immunoliposome formulation for AMB was reported. The authors employed commercial 100 nm size PEGylated liposomes (DSPC:Chol:PEG-DSPE, 53:47:5 mol%) to encapsulate 11% AMB. Then, Dectin-1 – a mammalian innate immune receptor present in the membrane of leukocytes that is able to bind beta-glucans of fungal cell walls – was covalently bound to PEG-DSPE and incorporated in the liposomes (1 mol%). Such modified liposomes were able to bind specifically to *Candida albicans* and *C. neoformans* cells, as revealed by fluorescence microscopy. The system has a great potential to improve even more benefits of liposomal AMB, when applied *in vivo*.[149]

Other polyene antifungals have also been entrapped in liposomes. A lyophilized DMPC:DMPS 7:3 multilamellar liposomes formulation (Nyotran®) has been proposed to overcome the low solubility of the polyene nystatin. When administered at doses of 0.25–4 mg/kg, the formulation decreased the toxicity and enabled systemic administration of nystatin, with good *in vivo* activity against candidiasis and aspergillosis.[147] Hamycin, another polyene antifungal which significant toxic side effects do not allow it to be parenterally administrated, has been formulated in multilamellar vesicle (MLV) composed of DMPC:DMPG (7:3 mol%) and different proportions (20–60 mol%) of Chol. Formulations with 30% Chol allowed systemic administration of hamycin, reduced its toxic effects, and increased its antifungal activity *in vitro* and *in vivo*.[141,150]

16.4.2 AZOLE ANTIFUNGAL AGENTS

Imidazole antifungal agents, such as miconazole and ketoconazole, have been used for treatment of various cutaneous and systemic mycoses. Liposomal formulations (MLV and SUV composed of soy and egg PC) for ketoconazole or miconazole have been reported[151]; *in vitro* such liposomes prolonged the antifungal action against *C. albicans*. Also for the topical treatment of candidiasis, elastic liposomes (160–180 nm) containing miconazole nitrate were described by Pandit et al.[152]

To produce the ultraflexible liposomes, surfactants (sodium deoxycholate, Span 80, Span 60, and Tween 80) were added to PC, improving the specificity of the antifungal liposomal formulation to the skin.

Le Conte et al.[153] reported the encapsulation of itraconazole in large (200 ± 230 nm) MLVs of 1,2-dipalmitoyl-sn-glycero-3-phosphocholine (DPPC), providing the first parenteral formulation for this azole antifungal. Its administration increased the tissue concentrations and antifungal efficacy, showing potential for the long-term treatment of immunocompromised patients. Later, SUV composed of soy PC:Chol:stearylamine (SA) (8:2:1 mol%) and itraconazole (1 mg/mL) for topical application showed better antifungal activity than the free drug in treatment of fungal keratitis in rats.[154]

Fluconazole was first encapsulated in MLV of DPPC:Chol:SA (5:3:1 mol%) and tested *in vitro*, being found onefold more active than free fluconazole against two strains of *C. albicans*.[155] PEGylated liposomes containing 2 mg/mL fluconazole were also described and used against keratitis in humans, leading to decreased instillation frequency and better healing from candidiasis.[156]

Voriconazole, a second-generation triazole derivative, has been incorporated in extruded liposomes (95.3 ± 1.27 nm) composed of PC:Chol: α-tocopherol (2:1:0.1 mol%) and voriconazole (2 mg/mL) for intravenous delivery against *C. albicans*. The formulation was compared to VFEND®, a commercially available formulation of voriconazole:sulfobutyl ether-β-cyclodextrin inclusion complex. The liposomal formulation improved tissue distribution and enhanced the antifungal activity of voriconazole.[157] Modified liposomes have also been reported for the delivery of voriconazole: ethosomes, prepared with HSPC and ethanol to enhance the permeation through the skin[158] and PEGylated liposomes designed to achieve longer circulation in the blood, by preventing liposome opsonization of the RES.[159] In both cases improved action of voriconazole was determined *in vitro*.

It is worth mentioning that different azole antifungal agents and AMB have also been formulated in niosomes, liposomes composed of nonionic surfactants, and Chol. Niosomal formulations seem to have a great potential for the treatment of topical fungal infections.[17] Finally, as for the other classes of fungicides, echinocandin and allyamines, there are no reports on liposomal formulations with clinical or preclinical studies reported so far.

16.5 LIPOSOMAL SYSTEMS FOR THE TREATMENT OF CANCER

Cancer is a multifactorial disease with higher mortality and morbidity rates. The World Health Organization registered ~9.6 million cancer-based deaths in 2018.[160] This progressive incidence can be related to the high heterogeneity of cancer cell proliferation, allied to the patient habits, physiological conditions, and environmental risks.[161–163] Traditional cancer therapies are often ineffective and aggressive to healthy tissues, recurrence being of common incidence for some types of cancer, after surgical, radio, or chemotherapy.[164]

The inexorable search for alternative cancer treatments has moving efforts from researches of several fields of knowledge, yielding thousands of published works in the last years.[165] Specially in the case of DDS, it is still a challenge to find effective systemic cancer therapies without causing severe side effects, but liposomes seem to be the most successful anticancer nanocarriers so far.[3,13,166] This can be evidenced by the high number of U.S. Food and Drug Administration (FDA) clinical approved formulations, as well as from the number of commercially available liposomal formulations (e.g. Doxil®, Onivyde®, Lipocurc® DaunoXome®, Myocet® MarqIbo®, DecpoCyt®). There are some mechanistic properties, intrinsic to liposomal formulations, that can be explored to efficiently target cancer cells, depending on the cancer type, localization, and stage. Generally, the success of liposomal formulations for cancer therapy is based on the enhanced permeability retention (EPR) effect on the tumor microenvironment. EPR allows liposomes (<200 nm) to penetrate and accumulate into the tumor by its porous blood capillaries and poor lymphatic drainage.[167] However, conventional liposomes have important disadvantages, such as physicochemical instability, renal clearance, and uptake by RES.[7] In order to overcome such limitations, functionalized and molecular planned liposomes had to be developed, as discussed below.

PEGylation of liposomes finds great application in cancer treatment. PEGylated (or stealth) liposomes have additional benefits in increasing the EPR effect and drug accumulation at the tumor site, compared to conventional liposomes.[168,169] A lot of researches and interesting reviews are available, that describe clinical trials of PEGylated liposomal antineoplastics for the treatment of breast, pancreas, ovarian, lung, prostate, and bladder cancers. PEGylation is certainly the most employed approach for the development of anticancer liposomal systems.[170–173]

DOX is the most studied anticancer drug in liposomal formulations. The first liposomal formulation for DOX (1980) was composed of egg PC and egg phosphatidylglycerol (EPC, EPG) and Chol, processed as oligolamellar liposomes. After some initial clinical trial failures, the formulation was redesigned to obtain lower particles sizes (80–90 nm), drug-load stability (high DOX concentration was required), and specific tumor cells recognition. Doxil®, with 20 mg/mL DOX in PEGylated liposomes composed of HSPC and Chol, was the first commercially available liposomal formulation for cancer treatment. It is claimed to increase the half-life of DOX while promoting specific release in the target tissue. Doxil® was first approved for Kaposi's sarcoma (1995), followed by breast (1999) and ovarian (2003) cancer treatments.[174] However, there are still reports of Doxil® undesirable side effects over healthy cells, similar to those observed with plain DOX.[175,176] Petersen et al.[177] conducted an important meta-analysis study to evaluate preclinical and clinical success of liposomal DOX. The authors selected several works (covering almost 3,000 patients) and evaluated the efficacy of liposomal and plain DOX for different cancer treatments. In general, liposomal DOX formulations showed a better preclinical performance than the plain drug, but these effects were not translated into increased anticancer efficacy in clinical trials. The authors argued that this incoherent performance between the *in vivo* (preclinical and clinical) studies reflects the need for standardization in the conduction of preclinical studies.

DOX has also been encapsulated in another nonconventional liposome formulation: Myocet® an ionic-gradient liposomal formulation formed by high concentrations of citrate in the internal aqueous compartments of the vesicles and indicated for ovarian cancer therapy.[10] Romeo et al. evaluated the efficacy and safety of Myocet® associated with carboplatin in comparison to the standard therapy based on carboplatin and PEGylated liposomal DOX, in a phase II trial. The results demonstrated a comparable performance of Myocet® and the standard therapy in terms of efficacy, and the authors concluded that Myocet® (50 mg/m^2) and carboplatin (5 g/min mL) administered each 4 weeks should contribute to improve the efficacy of cancer ovarian treatment. In general, the treatment was well tolerated, once almost of 80 % patients have received the initial planned six cycles application and the selected formulations were carried out to a phase III trial. However, undesirable side effects such as alopecia, nausea, fatigue, and neutropenia were observed in more than 50 % of patients that received Myocet® ($n = 84$).[178] Similarly, Myocet® plus paclitaxel and carboplatin were proposed as a neoadjuvant treatment in comparison with the traditional therapy based on epirubicin, paclitaxel, and cyclophosphamide, for breast cancer treatment. The study was conducted as a phase III trial and the traditional therapy was carried out in a daily dose-dense chemotherapeutics cycle, while Myocet® plus paclitaxel and carboplatin was weekly given to the patients ($n = 393$). The authors did not find statistical differences between the evaluated treatments. However, two deaths caused by pneumonia and cerebral embolism were recorded for patients under the neoadjuvant treatment.[179]

Other antineoplastic drugs have been successfully loaded in liposomes for the treatment of cancer. An important work proposed a final overall survival analysis for patients with metastatic pancreatic cancer, with more than 400 enrolled patients that were treated with liposomal tecan plus 5-fluoracil and leucovirin (n = 117), or 5-fluoracil and leucovirin (n = 149) for the first 4 of 6-week cycles. The treatment with liposomal irinotecan formulation plus 5-fluoracil nd leucovirin exhibited higher overall survival than the chemotherapeutics control (6.2 vs. 4.2 months, respectively). After 1 year, a total of 10 % patients under liposomal irinotecan therapy, 25 % in the irino-tecan liposomal plus 5-fluoracil and leucovirin therapy, and 13 % in the chemotherapeutics control have have survived.[180] In addition, Hubner et al.[181] monitored the quality of life of such patients, treated with liposomal irinotecan plus 5-fluorouracil and leucovorin in comparison to those treated only with the chemotherapeutics. In general, patients presented a combination of manageable and reversible symptoms, including diarrhea, vomits, and neutropenia, among others. The patients treated with the liposomal irinotecan formulation plus the chemotherapeutics presented lower pain score, but higher nausea, diarrhea, fatigue, and insomnia than the control. However, the patient compliance rate along the study severely decreased over time, majorly caused by the cancer final stage.

On the other hand, new anticancer drug candidates processed as nanodevices are required as innovator therapies. But clinical trials to prove their efficacy and safety are still scarce. That is the case of curcumin, whose antineoplastic activity *in vitro* is already well known. Lipocurc® is a liposomal curcumin formulation designed for intravenous administration, composed of dimyristoyl PC (DMPC):DMPG (9:1 mol %) plus curcumin (0.6 g %). Bolger et al. compared the pharmacokinetics of Lipocurc® as an adjuvant therapy in cancer patients and healthy individuals. The curcumin bloodstream levels in cancer patients showed lower distribution volume with shorter half-life when compared with healthy individuals. These factors probably occurred due to the nondisease conditions of control and the use of other drugs in cancer patients.[182] Eribulin-loaded liposomes were evaluated for the treatment of advanced solid tumors in a phase I clinical study ($n = 58$). Eribulin is a synthetic analog of halichondrin B, a natural product synthesized by marine sponges (*Halichondria okadai*) and approved as monotherapy for metastatic breast cancers, for patients previously exposed to a failed traditional therapy. Relevant clinical activity was observed in almost 10 % of treated patients, with desirable pharmacokinetic profile and tolerable side effects, in comparison with free drug.[183]

The clinical trial of liposomal formulations for cancer treatment is a crucial step for drugs to be approved. Unfortunately, clinical efficacy results are not as exciting as for *in vivo* studies, until now. Therefore, there are some important points to be addressed. In the trials, the efficacy and safety of liposomal antineoplastic formulations are misunderstood, once they are commonly administered in association with other drugs. In addition, liposomal formulations have not been the first choice for cancer treatment of the evaluated patients who usually show advanced metastatic conditions. It is also worth mentioning that the management of the life expectancy and life quality on the studied patients are essential parameters to be monitored, aspects still underexploited in most of clinical trials and case reports. The same is true for intratumor variability that has to be considered since it is directly related to the success of the treatment. Further clinical trials with other liposome-loaded chemotherapeutics are required, considering their particular interaction with each patient-based tumor variant cells.

Although embryonic, a personalized tumor treatment is a promising approach towards the cure of cancer, due to the high histopathological heterogeneity of the tumor cells, which is also proper to each person, site, and stage.[184] In that sense liposomes should be prepared with aptamers for active targeting the tumor. Thus, the formulations are designed under molecular and pharmacogenetics approaches, which is mandatory to a deep understanding of the individual tumor cell receptors.[185] Liposomes labeled with specific ligands should bind to tumor receptors, improving the therapeutic efficacy, without compromising the common physiological processes such as cellular uptake, intracellular trafficking, or immune response.[186,187] There is an exciting and long way to be explored therein. We hope that new personalized liposomal anticancer formulations may come to clinical trials in the near future.

16.6 CONCLUSIONS

Advances in liposome technology along the last 40 years allowed more efficient and less toxic therapeutic regimens for different classes of drugs, contributing to the World Public Health.

There is a wealth of research related to DDS for pain (acute and chronic) relief involving liposomes. Most studies report the benefits of sustained release and decrease of adverse effects caused by drug encapsulation in liposomes. However, so far, the only commercial formulations are

Exparel® and DepoDur®, for bupivacaine and morphine, respectively. Therefore, there is a wide field of research to be explored herein.

As considered before, encapsulation of antibiotics has reduced side effects and frequency of pharmacological administration, increased drug/bacteria cell interaction, the release time, and bactericidal activity. To the pharmaceutical industry, liposomal DDS offer a promising alternative to improve the bioavailability of antimicrobial drugs, rather than developing new drugs, especially for multiresistant bacteria.

As the population of immunocompromised patients continues to grow worldwide, fungal infections are on the rise. Antifungal agents are barely soluble in water, requiring strategies to improve their bioavailability. Liposomes have brought a new era to antifungal therapy since drug entrapped in liposomes could be specifically targeted to the RES cells, resulting in high concentration of therapeutic agents at the site of infection. AMB was the first antifungal agent to be entrapped in liposomes (Ambisome®), and up to now it is the most important liposomal antifungal medicine, with more than 20 clinical trials registered in the NIH. Conventional or modified (PEGylated, immuno and ethosomes) liposomal formulations have also been proposed for other polyene antifungals (nystatin, hamycin) and azoles (itraconazole, miconazole, ketoconazole, and voriconazole), in all cases achieving a decrease in drug toxicity.

Liposomal-based formulations are the most developed DDS aiming cancer therapy to reach the clinical trials. This is translated in thousand works published in the last years. PEGylated liposomes are the main strategy to enhance the half-life of antineoplastics, mainly in association with other drugs in the treatment of breast, prostate, pancreas, ovarian, lung, and bladder cancers. Despite the relevant advances reported, the perspective of successful cancer treatment is nowadays propelled by the development of personalized liposomal anticancer formulations (translational drug development), specific to each patient, that can be carried by liposomal systems.

ABBREVIATIONS

AMB:	amphothericin B
Chol:	Cholesterol
DMPC:	L-α-dimyristoylphosphatidyl choline
DMPG:	L-α-dimyristoylphosphatidyl glycerol
DOPC:	dioleoylphosphatidylcholine
DOPE:	dioleoylphosphatidylethanolamine
DOX:	doxorubicin
DPPC:	1,2-dipalmitoyl-sn-glycero-3-phosphocholine
DSPG:	1,2-distearoyl-sn-glycero-3-phosphoglycerol
EPC:	egg phosphatidylcholine
EPG:	egg phosphatidylglycerol
HEPC:	hydrogenated egg phosphatidylcholine
HSPC:	hydrogenated soybean phosphatidylcholine
IGL:	ionic-gradient liposomes
LMV:	large multilamellar vesicles
LMVV:	large multivesicular vesicles
LUV:	large unilamellar vesicles
MLV:	multilamellar vesicles
mPEG-2000-DSPE:	methylpolyethyleneglycol-1,2-distearyl-phosphatidylethanolamine conjugate
PEG-DSPC:	polyethyleneglycol-1,2-distearoyl-sn-glycero-3-phosphocholine
PEG-DSPE:	polyethyleneglycol 2000-distearylphosphatidyl-ethanolamine
PC:	phosphatidylcholine
PE:	phosphatidylethanolamine

PG: phosphatidylglycerol
SPC: soybean phosphatidylcholine
ST: stearylamine
SUV: small unilamellar vesicles

REFERENCES

1. Tanford, C. *The Hydrophobic Effect*, John Wiley and Sons, New York, 1980.
2. Lasic, D. D. Novel applications of liposomes. *Trends in Biotechnology*, 16(7), 307–321, 1998.
3. Allen, T. M.; Cullis, P. R. Liposomal drug delivery systems: From concept to clinical applications. *Advanced Drug Delivery Reviews* 2013, 65, 36–48.
4. Samad, A.; Sultana, Y.; Aqil, M. Liposomal drug delivery systems: An update review. *Current Drug Delivery* 2007, 4 297–305.
5. Torchilin, V. Liposomes in drug-delivery. Fundamentals and applications of controlled release. *Advances in Delivery Science and Technology* 2012, 1, 289–328.
6. Sercombe, L.; Veerati, T.; Moheimani, F.; Wu, S. I.; Sood, A. K.; Hua, S. Advances and challenges of liposome assisted drug delivery. *Frontiers in Pharmacology* 2015, 7, 1–13.
7. Bozzuto, G.; Molinari, A. Liposomes as nanomedical devices. *International Journal of Nanomedicine* 2015, 10, 975–999.
8. Patil, Y. P.; Jadhav, S. Novel methods for liposome preparation. *Chemistry and Physics of Lipids* 2014, 177, 8–18.
9. Chen, J.; Lu, W.-L.; Gu, W.; Lu, S.-S.; Chen, Z.-P.; Cai, B.-C. Skin permeation behavior of elastic liposomes: Role of formulation ingredients. *Expert Opinion in Drug Delivery* 2013, 10(6), 845–856.
10. Zucker, D.; Marcus, D.; Barenholz, Y.; Goldblum, A. Liposome drugs' loading efficiency: A working model based on loading conditions and drug's physicochemical properties. *Journal of Controlled Release* 2009, 139, 73–80.
11. Gubernator, J. Active methods of drug loading into liposomes: Recent strategies for stable drug entrapment and increased in vivo activity. *Expert Opinion on Drug Delivery* 2011, 8(5), 565–80.
12. Milani, D.; Athiyah, U.; Hariyadi, D. M.; Pathak, Y. V. Surface modifications of liposomes for drug targeting, Chapter 11. In: *Surface Modification of Nanoparticles for Targeted Drug Delivery*, Pathak, Y. (ed.), pp. 207–220, Springer, Berlin, Germany, 2019.
13. Immordino, M.; Dosio, F.; Cattel, L. Stealth liposomes: Review of the basic science, rationale, and clinical applications, existing and potential. *Intenational Journal of Nanomedicine* 2006, 1, 297–315.
14. Bulbake, U.; Doppalapudi, S.; Kommineni, N.; Khan, W. Liposomal formulations in clinical use: An updated review. *Pharmaceutics* 2017, 9(2), 1–33.
15. Gogoi, M.; Kuman, N.; Patra, S. Multifunctional magnetic liposomes for cancer imaging and therapeutic applications, Chapter 27. In: *Nanoarchitectonics for Smart Delivery and Drug Targeting*, Holban, A.-M.; Grumezescu, A. (eds), pp. 743–782. Elsevier, Amsterdam, 2016.
16. Mantripragada, S. A. Lipid based depot (DepoFoam® technology) for sustained release drug delivery. *Progress in Lipid Research* 2002, 41(5), 392–406.
17. Osanloo, M.; Assadpour, S.; Mehravaran, A.; Abastabar, M.; Akhtari, J. Niosome-loaded antifungal drugs as an effective nanocarrier system: A mini review. *Current Medical Mycology* 2018, 4(4), 31–36.
18. Bangham, A.; Standish, M.; Watkins, J. Diffusion of univalent ions across the lamellae of swollen phospholipids. *Journal of Molecular Biology* 1965, 13, 238–252.
19. Grewal, A.; Lather, V.; Sharma, N.; Singh, S.; Nrang, R. S.; Narang, J. K.; Pandita, D. Recent updates on nanomedicine based products: Current scenario and future opportunities. *Applied Clinical Research and Clinical Trials Regulatory Affairs* 2018, 5, 132–144.
20. Wagner, A; Vorauer-Uhl, A. Liposome technology for industrial purposes. *Journal of Drug Delivery* 2011, 2011, 591325.
21. He, K.; Tang, M. Safety of novel liposomal drugs for cancer treatment: Advances and prospects. *Chemical and Biological Interactions* 2018, 295, 13–19.
22. Knudsen, K. B.; Northeved, H.; Kumar, P. E.; Permin, A; Gjetting, T.; Andresen, T. L.; Larsen, S.; Wegener, K. M.; Lykkesfeldt, J.; Jantzen, K.; Loft, S.; Møller, P; Roursgaard, M. Nanomedicine: Nanotechnology, *Biology and Medicine* 2015, 11, 467–477.
23. Lynch, M. E.; Watson, C. P. N. The pharmacotherapy of chronic pain: A review. *Pain Research and Management* 2006, 11(1), 11–38.

24. Kroenke, K.; Krebs, E. E.; Bair, M. J. Pharmacotherapy of chronic pain: A synthesis of recommendations from systematic reviews. *General Hospital Psychiatry* 2009, 31(3), 206–219.

25. Harker, J.; Kleijnen, J.; Reid, K. J.; Bala, M. M.; Kellen, E.; Bekkering, G. E.; Truyers, C. Epidemiology of chronic non-cancer pain in Europe: Narrative review of prevalence, pain treatments and pain impact. *Current Medical Research and Opinion* 2011, 27(2), 449–462.

26. Giamberardino, M.A.; Evers, S.; Goebel, A; Svensson, P.; Treede, R.-D.; Rief, W.; Benoliel, R.; Vlaeyen, J. W. S.; Perrot, S.; Barke, A.; Nicholas, M.; Cohen, M.; Korwisi, B.; Aziz, Q.; Wang, S.-J. The IASP classification of chronic pain for ICD-11. *Pain* 2018, 160(1), 28–37.

27. Barke, A., Chronic pain has arrived in the ICD-11. International Association for the Study of Pain (IASP). Avaible from: www.iasp-pain.org/PublicationsNews/NewsDetail.aspx? ItemNumber=8340& navItemNumber=643. Acessed March 01, 2019.

28. de Araújo, D. R.; Cereda, C. M. S.; Brunetto, G. B.; Pinto, L. M.; Santana, M. H.; de Paula E. Encapsulation of mepivacaine prolongs the analgesia provided by sciatic nerve blockade in mice. *Canadian Journal of Anesthesia* 2004, 51(6), 566–572.

29. Gordon, S.; Mischenko, A. V.; Dionne, R. A. Long-acting local anesthetics and perioperative pain management. *Dental Clinics of North America* 2010, 54(4), 611–620.

30. Glazer, S.; Portenoy, R. K. Systemic local anesthetics in pain control. *Journal Pain Symptom Manage* 1991, 6(1), 30–39.

31. Chong, S. F.; Bretscher, M. E.; Mailliard, J.; Tschetter, L. K.; Kimmel, D. W.; Hatfield, A. K.; Loprinzi, C. L. Pilot study evaluating local anesthetics administered systemically for treatment of pain in patients with advanced cancer. *Journal of Pain Symptom Management* 1997, 13(2), 112–117.

32. Portenoy, R. K. Current pharmacotherapy of chronic pain. *Journal Pain Symptom Manage* 2000, 19(1), 16–20.

33. Bragagni, M.; Maestrelli, F.; Mennini, N.; Ghelardini, C.; Mura, P. Liposomal formulations of prilocaine: Effect of complexation with hydroxypropyl-ß-cyclodextrin on drug anesthetic efficacy. *Journal of Liposome Research* 2010, 20(4), 315–322.

34. Weinschenk, S. Neural therapy: A review of the therapeutic use of local anesthetics. *Acupuncture and Related Therapies* 2012, 1(1), 5–9.

35. Nagasaki, Y.; Mizukoshi, Y.; Gao, Z.; Feliciano, C. P.; Chang, K.; Sekiyama, H.; Kimura, H. Development of a local anesthetic lidocaine-loaded redox-active injectable gel for postoperative pain management. *Acta Biomaterialia* 2017, 57, 127–135.

36. Grant, G. J.; Barenholz, Y.; Piskoun, B.; Bansinath, M.; Turndorf, H.; Bolotin, E. M. DRV liposomal bupivacaine: Preparation, characterization, and in vivo evaluation in mice. *Pharmaceutical Research* 2001, 18(3), 336–343.

37. de Araújo, D. R.; Ribeiro, L. N. M.; de Paula, E. Lipid-based carriers for the delivery of local anesthetics. *Expert Opinion on Drug Delivery* 2019, 16(7), 701–714.

38. Gesztes, A.; Mezei, M. Topical anesthesia of the skin by liposome encapsulated tetracaine. *Anesthesia Analgesia* 1988, 67, 1079–1081.

39. Mowat, J. J.; Mok, M. J.; MacLeod, B. A. M. T. Liposomal bupivacaine. Extended duration nerve blockade using large unilamellar vesicles that exhibit a proton gradient. *Anesthesiology* 1996, 85(3), 635–643.

40. Grant, G. J.; Barenholz, Y.; Bolotin, E. M.; Bansinath, M.; Turndorf, H.; Piskoun, B.; Davidson, E. M. A novel liposomal bupivacaine formulation to produce ultralong-acting analgesia. *Anesthesiology* 2004, 101(1), 133–137.

41. Mura, P.; Maestrelli, F.; González-Rodríguez, M. L.; Michelacci, I.; Ghelardini, C.; Rabasco, A. M. Development, characterization and in vivo evaluation of benzocaine-loaded liposomes. *European Journal of Pharmaceutics and Biopharmaceutics* 2007, 67(1), 86–95.

42. Franz-Montan, M.; Silva, A. L. R.; Cogo, K.; Bergamaschi, C. D. C.; Volpato, M. C.; Ranali, J., de Paula, E.; Groppo, F. C. Liposome-encapsulated ropivacaine for topical anesthesia of human oral mucosa. *Anesthesia Analgesia* 2007, 104(6), 1528–1531.

43. Franz-Montan, M.; Silva, A. L. R.; Fraceto, L. F.; Volpato, M. C.; de Paula, E.; Ranali, J.; Groppo, F. C. Liposomal encapsulation improves the duration of soft tissue anesthesia but does not induce pulpal anesthesia. *Journal of Clinical Anesthesia* 2010, 22(5), 313–317.

44. Tofoli, G. R.; Cereda, C. M. S.; Groppo, F. C.; Volpato, M. C.; Franz-Montan, M.; Ranali, J.; de Araújo, D. R., de Paula, E. Efficacy of liposome-encapsulated mepivacaine for infiltrative anesthesia in volunteers. *Journal of Liposome Research* 2011, 21(1), 88–94.

45. Tofoli, G. R.; Cereda, C. M. S.; de Araújo, D. R.; Franz-Montan, M.; Groppo, F. C.; Quaglio, D.; Pedrazzoli Jr, E.; Calafatti, S. A.; Barros, F. A.; de Paula, E. Pharmacokinetic study of liposome-encapsulated and plain mepivacaine formulations injected intra-orally in volunteers. *Journal of Pharmacy and Pharmacology* 2011 64(3), 397–403.

46. Cohen, R.; Kanaan, H.; Grant, G. J.; Barenholz, Y. Prolonged analgesia from Bupisome and Bupigel formulations: From design and fabrication to improved stability. *Journal Control Release* 2012, 160(2), 346–352.

47. Franz-Montan, M.; Cereda, C. M.; Gaspari, A.; da Silva, C. M. G.; de Araújo, D. R.; Padula, C.; Santi, P.; Narvaes, E; Novaes, P. D.; Groppo, F. C.; de Paula, E. Liposomal-benzocaine gel formulation: Correlation between in vitro assays and in vivo topical anesthesia in volunteers. *Journal of Liposome Research* 2013, 23(1), 54–60.

48. Franz-Montan, M.; Baroni, D.; Brunetto, G.; Sobral, V. R. V.; Da Silva, C. M. G.; Venâncio, P.; Zago, P. W.; Cereda, C. M.; Volpato, M. C.; de Araújo, D. R.; de Paula, E.; Groppo, F. C. Liposomal lidocaine gel for topical use at the oral mucosa: Characterization, in vitro assays and in vivo anesthetic efficacy in humans. *Journal of Liposome Research* 2015, 25(1), 11–19.

49. da Silva, C. B.; Groppo, F. C.; dos Santos, C. P.; Serpe, L.; Franz-Montan, M.; Paula, Ed; Ranali, J., Volpato, M. C. Anaesthetic efficacy of unilamellar and multilamellar liposomal formulations of articaine in inflamed and uninflamed tissue. *British Journal of Oral and Maxillofacial Surgery* 2016, 54(3), 295–300.

50. Cereda, C. M. S.; Guilherme, V. A.; Alkschbirs, M. I.; de Brito Junior, R. B.; Tofoli, G. R.; Franz-Montan, M.; de Araújo, D. R.; de Paula, E. Liposomal butamben gel formulations: Toxicity assays and topical anesthesia in an animal model. *Journal of Liposome Research* 2017, 27(1), 74–82.

51. da Silva, C. M. G; Franz-Montan, M.; Limia, C. E. G.; Ribeiro, L. N. M.; Braga, M. A.; Guilherme, V. A.; Silva, C. B.; Casadei, B. R.; Cereda, C. M. S.; de Paula, E. Encapsulation of ropivacaine in a combined (donor-acceptor, ionic-gradient) liposomal system promotes extended anesthesia time. *PLoS One* 2017, 12(10), 1–16.

52. Rennó, C. C.; Cereda, C. M. S.; Martinez, E.; de Paula, E.; Papini, J. Z. B.; Calafatti, S. A.; Tófoli, G. R. Preclinical evaluation of ropivacaine in 2 liposomal modified systems. *Anesthesia and Analgesia* 2019, 129(2), 387–396.

53. Couto, V. M.; Prieto, M. J.; Igartúa, D. E.; Feas, D. A.; Ribeiro, L. N. M.; Silva, C. M. G.; Castro, S. R.; Guilherme, V. A.; Dantzger, D. D.; Machado, D.; Alonso, S. D. V.; de Paula, E. Dibucaine in ionic-gradient liposomes: Biophysical, toxicological, and activity characterization. *Journal of Pharmaceutical Sciences* 2018, 107(9), 2411–2419.

54. Almeida, A. C. P.; Pinto, L. M. A.; Alves, G. P.; Ribeiro, L. N. M.; Santana, M. H. A.; Cereda, C. M. S.; Fraceto, L. F.; de Paula, E. Liposomal-based lidocaine formulation for the improvement of infiltrative buccal anaesthesia. *Journal of Liposome Research* 2019, 29(1), 66–72.

55. Ilfeld, B. M.; Viscusi, E. R.; Hadzic, A.; Minkowitz, H. S.; Morren, M. D.; Lookabaugh, J.; Joshi, G. P. Safety and side effect profile of liposome Bupivacaine (Exparel) in Peripheral Nerve Blocks. *Regional Anesthesia and Pain Medicine* 2015, 40(5), 572–582.

56. Chahar, P.; Cummings III, K. Liposomal bupivacaine: A review of a new bupivacaine formulation. *Journal of Pain Research*, 2012, 5, 257.

57. Baxter, R.; Bramlett, K.; Onel, E.; Daniels, S. Impact of local administration of liposome bupivacaine for postsurgical analgesia on wound healing: A review of data from ten prospective, controlled clinical studies. *Clinical Therapeutics* 2013, 35(3), 312–320.

58. Vogel, J. Liposome bupivacaine (exparel) for extended pain relief in patients undergoing ileostomy reversal at a single institution with a fast-track discharge protocol: An improve phase IV health economics trial. *Journal Pain Research* 2013, 6, 605–610.

59. Mont, M. A.; Beaver, W. B.; Dysart, S. H.; Barrington, J. W.; Del Gaizo, D. J. Local infiltration analgesia with liposomal bupivacaine improves pain scores and reduces opioid use after total knee arthroplasty: Results of a randomized controlled trial. *Journal Arthroplasty* 2018, 33(1), 90–96.

60. Butz, D. R.; Shenaq, D. S.; Rundell, V. L. M.; Kepler, B.; Liederbach, E.; Thiel, J.; Pesce, C.; Murphy, G. S.; Sisco, M.; Howard, M. A. Postoperative pain and length of stay lowered by use of exparel in immediate, implant-based breast reconstruction. *Plastic and Reconstructive Surgery: Global Open* 2015, 3(5), 1–5.

61. Surdam, J. W.; Licini, D. J.; Baynes, N. T.; Arce, B. R. The use of exparel (liposomal bupivacaine) to manage postoperative pain in unilateral total knee arthroplasty patients. *Journal Arthroplasty* 2015, 30(2), 325–329.

62. Vyas, K. S.; Rajendran, S.; Morrison, S. D.; Shakir, A.; Mardini, S.; Lemaine, V.; Nahabedian, M. Y.; Baker, S. B.; Rinker, B. D.; Vasconez, H. C. Systematic review of liposomal bupivacaine (exparel) for postoperative analgesia. *Plastic and Reconstructive Surgery* 2016, 138(4), 748–756.

63. Taddio, A.; Soin, H. K.; Schuh, S.; Koren, G.; Scolnik, D. Liposomal lidocaine to improve procedural success rates and reduce procedural pain among children: A randomized controlled trial. *Canadian Medical Association Journal* 2005, 172(13), 1691–1695.

64. Lehr, V. T.; Taddio, A. Topical anesthesia in neonates: Clinical practices and practical considerations. *Seminars in Perinatology* 2007, 31(5), 323–329.

65. Bahruth, A. J. Peripherally inserted central catheter insertion problems associated with topical anesthesia. *Journal of Infusion Nursing* 1996, 19(1), 32–34.

66. Hahn, I. H.; Hoffman, R. S.; Nelson, L. S. EMLA-induced methemoglobinemia and systemic topical anesthetic toxicity. *Journal of Emergency Medicine* 2004, 26, 85–88.

67. Raso, S. M.; Fernandez, J. B.; Beobide, E. A.; Landaluce, A. F. Methemoglobinemia and CNS toxicity after topical application of EMLA to a 4-year-old girl with molluscum contagiosum. *Pediatric Dermatology* 2006, 23, 592–593.

68. Chen, B. K.; Cunningham, B. B. Topical anesthetics in children: Agents and techniques that equally comfort patients, parents, and clinicians. *Current Opinion in Pediatrics* 2001, 13, 324–330.

69. Parker, J. F.; Vats, A.; Bauer, G. EMLA toxicity after application for allergy skin testing. *Pediatrics* 2004, 113, 410–411.

70. Young, K. D. What's new in topical anesthesia. *Clinical Pediatric Emergency Medicine* 2007, 8(4), 232–239.

71. Barenholz, Y.; Haran, G. Method of amphiphaticdrug loading in lposomes by ammonum ion gradent. US Patent 5,316,771, 1994.

72. Oliveira, J. D.; Ribeiro, L. N. M.; Da Silva, G. H. R.; Casadei, B. R.; Couto, V. M.; Martinez, E. F.; de Paula, E. Sustained release from ionic-gradient liposomes significantly decreases ETIDOCAINE cytotoxicity. *Pharmaceutical Research* 2018, 35, 229.

73. Hartrick, C. T.; Martin, G.; Kantor, G.; Koncelik, J.; Manvelian, G. Evaluation of a single-dose, extended-release epidural morphine formulation for pain after knee arthroplasty. *The Journal of Bone and Joint Surgery* 2006, 88(2), 273–281.

74. Nagle, P. C.; Gerancher, J. C. DepoDur® (extended-release epidural morphine): A review of an old drug in a new vehicle. *Techniques in Regional Anesthesia and Pain Management* 2007, 11(1), 9–18.

75. Hartrick, C. T.; Hartrick, K. A. Extended-release epidural morphine (DepoDur): Review and safety analysis. *Expert Review of Neurotherapeutics* 2008, 8(11), 1641–1648.

76. Viscusi, E. R.; Kopacz, D.; Hartrick, C.; Martin, G.; Manvelian, G. Single-dose extended-release epidural morphine for pain following hip arthroplasty. *American Journal of Therapeutics* 2006, 13(5), 423–431.

77. Carvalho, B.; Roland, L. M.; Chu, L. F.; Campitelli, V. A.; Riley, E. T. Single-dose, extended-release epidural morphine (DepoDur™) compared to conventional epidural morphine for post-cesarean pain. *Anesthesia and Analgesia* 2007, 105(1), 176–183.

78. Carvalho, B.; Riley, E.; Cohen, S. E.; Gambling, D.; Palmer, C.; Huffnagle, H. J.; Polley, L.; Muir, H.; Segal, S.; Lihou, C.; Manvelian, G. Single-dose, sustained-release epidural morphine in the management of postoperative pain after elective cesarean delivery: Results of a multicenter randomized controlled study. *Anesthesia and Analgesia* 2005, 100(4), 1150–1158.

79. Hung, O. R.; Whynot, S. C.; Varvel, J. R.; Shafer, S. L.; Mezei, M. Pharmacokinetics of inhaled liposome-encapsulated fentanyl. *Anesthesiology* 1995, 83, 277–284.

80. Hung, O. R.; Sellers, E. M.; Kaplan, H. L.; Romach, M. K. Phase Ib clinical trial of aerosolized liposome encapsulated fentanyl (AeroLEF™). *Clinical Pharmacology and Therapeutics* 2004, 75(2), P4.

81. Hung, O.; Pliura, D. Comparative phase I PK study of aerosolized free and liposome-encapsulated fentanyl (AeroLEF) demonstrates rapid and extended plasma fentanyl concentrations following inhalation. *The Journal of Pain* 2008, 9(4), 36.

82. Clark, A.; Rossiter-Rooney, M.; Valle-Leutri, F. Aerosolized liposome-encapsulated fentanyl (AeroLEF) via pulmonary administration allows patients with moderate to severe post-surgical acute pain to self-titrate to effective analgesia. *The Journal of Pain* 2008, 9(4), 42.

83. Brull, R.; Chan, V. A. Randomized controlled trial demonstrates the efficacy, safety and tolerability of aerosolized free and liposome-encapsulated fentanyl (AeroLEF) via pulmonary administration. *The Journal of Pain* 2008, 9(4), 42.

84. Chen, J.; Gao, Y. Strategies for meloxicam delivery to and across the skin: A review. *Drug Delivery* 2016, 23(8), 3146–3156.

85. Jain, S.; Jain, N.; Bhadra, D.; Tiwary, A.; Jain, N. Transdermal delivery of an analgesic agent using elastic liposomes: Preparation, characterization and performance evaluation. *Current Drug Delivery* 2005, 2(3), 223–333.

86. Ashtikar, M.; Nagarsekar, K.; Fahr, A. Transdermal delivery from liposomal formulations: Evolution of the technology over the last three decades. *Journal of Controlled Release* 2016, 242, 126–140.

87. Gaur, P. K.; Bajpai, M.; Mishra, S.; Verma, A. Development of ibuprofen nanoliposome for transdermal delivery: Physical characterization, in vitro/in vivo studies, and anti-inflammatory activity. *Artificial Cells, Nanomedicine and Biotechnology* 2016, 44(1), 370–375.

88. Fetih, G.; Fathalla, D.; El-Badry, M., Liposomal gels for site-specific, sustained delivery of celecoxib: In vitro and in vivo evaluation. *Drug Development Research* 2014, 75(4), 257–266.

89. Metselaar, J. M.; Wauben, M. H.; Wagenaar-Hilbers, J. P.; Boerman, O. C.; Storm, G. Complete remission of experimental arthritis by joint targeting of glucocorticoids with long-circulating liposomes. *Arthritis and Rheumatology* 2003, 48(7), 2059–2066.

90. Schiffelers, R. M.; Banciu, M.; Metselaar, J. M.; Storm, G. Therapeutic application of long-circulating liposomal glucocorticoids in auto-immune diseases and cancer. *Journal of Liposome Research* 2006, 16(3), 185–194.

91. Van Tomme, S. R.; Metselaar, J. M.; Schiffelers, R. M.; Storm, G. Therapeutic nanomedicine: Liposomal corticosteroid as targeted antiinflammatory nanomedicine. *European Journal Nanomedicine* 2008, 1(1), 15–19.

92. Stroes, E. S. G. Silencing inflammatory activity by injecting nanocort in patients at risk for atherosclerotic disease (SILENCE). ClinicalTrials gov Identifier:NCT01601106, 2012.

93. Turjeman, K.; Barenholz, Y. Liposomal nano-drugs based on amphipathic weak acid steroid prodrugs for treatment of inflammatory diseases. *Journal of Drug Targeting* 2016, 24(9), 805–820.

94. Nikaido, H. Prevention of drug access to bacterial targets: Permeability barriers and active efflux. *Science* 1994, 264(5157), 382–388.

95. Silhavy, T. J.; Kahne, D.; Walker, S. The bacterial cell envelope. *Cold Spring Harbor Perspectives in Biology* 2010, 2(5), a000414.

96. Santos, R. S.; Figueiredo, C.; Azevedo, N. F.; Braeckmans, K.; De Smedt, S. C. Nanomaterials and molecular transporters to overcome the bacterial envelope barrier: Towards advanced delivery of antibiotics. *Advanced Drug Delivery Reviews* 2018, 136, 28–48.

97. Leibovici, L.; Paul, M.; Garner, P.; Sinclair, D. J.; Afshari, A.; Pace, N. L.; Cullum, N.; Williams, H. C.; Smyth, A.; Skoetz, N.; Del Mar, C. Addressing resistance to antibiotics in systematic reviews of antibiotic interventions. *Journal of Antimicrobial Chemotherapy* 2016, 71(9), 2367–2369.

98. Inoue, H.; Minghui, R. Antimicrobial resistance: Translating political commitment into national action. *Bulletin of the World Health Organization* 2017, 95(4), 242.

99. Segatore, B.; Bellio, P.; Setacci, D.; Brisdelli, F.; Piovano, M.; Garbarino, J. A.; Nicoletti, M.; Amicosante, G.; Perilli, M.; Celenza, G. *In vitro* interaction of usnic acid in combination with antimicrobial agents against methicillin-resistant *Staphylococcus aureus* clinical isolates determined by FICI and ΔE model methods. *Phytomedicine* 2012, 19(3–4), 341–347.

100. Pumerantz, A.; Betageri, G.; Wang, J. J. U.S. Patent No. 9,566,238. Washington, DC: U.S. Patent and Trademark Office, 2017.

101. Cavalcanti, I. M. F.; Menezes, T. G. C.; Campos, L. A. D. A.; Ferraz, M. S.; Maciel, M. A. V.; Caetano, M. N. P.; Santos-Magalhães, N. S. Interaction study between vancomycin and liposomes containing natural compounds against methicillin-resistant *Staphylococcus aureus* clinical isolates. *Brazilian Journal of Pharmaceutical Sciences* 2018, 54(2), 1–8.

102. Abed, N.; Couvreur, P. Nanocarriers for antibiotics: A promising solution to treat intracellular bacterial infections. *International Journal of Antimicrobial Agents* 2014, 43(6), 485–496.

103. Rukavina, Z.; Vanić, Ž. Current trends in development of liposomes for targeting bacterial biofilms. *Pharmaceutics* 2016, 8(2), 18.

104. Rukavina, Z.; Klarić, M. Š.; Filipović-Grčić, J.; Lovrić, J.; Vanić, Ž. Azithromycin-loaded liposomes for enhanced topical treatment of methicillin-resistant *Staphyloccocus aureus* (MRSA) infections. *International Journal of Pharmaceutics* 2018, 553(1–2), 109–119.

105. Raz, A.; Bucana, C.; Fogler, W. E.; Poste, G.; Fidler, I. J. Biochemical, morphological, and ultrastructural studies on the uptake of liposomes by murine macrophages. *Cancer Research* 1981, 41(2), 487–494.

106. Allen, T. M.; Austin, G. A.; Chonn, A.; Lin, L.; Lee, K. C. Uptake of liposomes by cultured mouse bone marrow macrophages: Influence of liposome composition and size. *Biochimica et Biophysica Acta (BBA): Biomembranes* 1991, 1061(1), 56–64.

107. Drulis-Kawa, Z.; Dorotkiewicz-Jach, A. Liposomes as delivery systems for antibiotics. *International Journal of Pharmaceutics* 2010, 387(1–2), 187–198.

108. Muppidi, K.; Wang, J.; Betageri, G.; Pumerantz, A. S. PEGylated liposome encapsulation increases the lung tissue concentration of vancomycin. *Antimicrobial Agents and Chemotherapy* 2011, 55(10), 4537–4542.

109. Duzgunes, N.; Perumal, V. K.; Kesavalu, L.; Goldstein, J. A.; Debs, R. J.; Gangadharam, P. R. Enhanced effect of liposome-encapsulated amikacin on *Mycobacterium avium*-M. intracellulare complex infection in beige mice. *Antimicrobial Agents and Chemotherapy* 1988, 32, 1404–1411.

110. Leitzke, S.; Bucke, W.; Borner, K.; Muller, R.; Hahn, H.; Ehlers, S. Rationale for and efficacy of prolonged-interval treatment using liposome-encapsulated amikacin in experimental *Mycobacterium avium* infection. *Antimicrobial Agents and Chemotherapy* 1998, 42, 459–461.

111. Xiong, Y. Q.; Kupferwasser, L. I.; Zack, P. M.; Bayer, A. S. Comparative efficacies of liposomal amikacin (MiKasome) plus oxacillin versus conventional amikacin plus oxacillin in experimental endocarditis induced by *Staphylococcus aureus*: Microbiological and echocardiographic analyses. *Antimicrobial Agents and Chemotherapy* 1999, 43(7), 1737–1742.

112. Schiffelers, R.; Storm, G.; Bakker-Woudenberg, I. Liposome-encapsulated aminoglycosides in pre-clinical and clinical studies. *Journal of Antimicrobial Chemotherapy* 2001, 48, 333–344.

113. Fierer, J. O.; Hatlen, L.; Lin, J. P.; Estrella, D.; Mihalko, P.; Yau-Young, A. Successful treatment using gentamicin liposomes of *Salmonella dublin* infections in mice. *Antimicrobial Agents and Chemotherapy* 1990, 34(2), 343–348.

114. Swenson, C. E.; Stewart, K. A.; Hammett, J. L.; Fitzsimmons, W. E.; Ginsberg, R. S. Pharmacokinetics and *in vivo* activity of liposome-encapsulated gentamicin. *Antimicrobial Agents and Chemotherapy* 1990, 34(2), 235–240.

115. Fattal, E.; Rojas, J.; Youssef, M.; Couvreur, P.; Andremont, A. Liposome-entrapped ampicillin in the treatment of experimental murine listeriosis and salmonellosis. *Antimicrobial Agents and Chemotherapy* 1991, 35(4), 770–772.

116. Vitas, A. I.; Díaz, R.; Gamazo, C. Protective effect of liposomal gentamicin against systemic acute murine brucellosis. *Chemotherapy* 1997, 43(3), 204–210.

117. Adams, L. B.; Sinha, I.; Franzblau, S. G.; Krahenbuhl, J. L; Mehta, R. T. Effective treatment of acute and chronic murine tuberculosis with liposome-encapsulated clofazimine. *Antimicrobial Agents and Chemotherapy* 1999, 43(7), 1638–1643.

118. Cordeiro, C.; Wiseman, D. J.; Lutwyche, P.; Uh, M.; Evans, J. C.; Finlay, B. B.; Webb, M. S. Antibacterial efficacy of gentamicin encapsulated in pH-sensitive liposomes against an *in vivo Salmonella enterica* serovar typhimurium intracellular infection model. *Antimicrobial Agents and Chemotherapy* 2000, 44(3), 533–539.

119. Labana, S.; Pandey, R.; Sharma, S.; Khuller, G. K. Chemotherapeutic activity against murine tuberculosis of once weekly administered drugs (isoniazid and rifampicin) encapsulated in liposomes. *International Journal of Antimicrobial Agents* 2002, 20(4), 301–304.

120. Omri, A.; Suntres, Z. E.; Shek, P. N. Enhanced activity of liposomal polymyxin B against *Pseudomonas aeruginosa* in a rat model of lung infection. *Biochemical Pharmacology* 2002, 64(9), 1407–1413.

121. Marier, J. F.; Brazier, J. L.; Lavigne, J.; Ducharme, M. P. Liposomal tobramycin against pulmonary infections of *Pseudomonas aeruginosa*: A pharmacokinetic and efficacy study following single and multiple intratracheal administrations in rats. *Journal of Antimicrobial Chemotherapy* 2003, 52(2), 247–252.

122. Wong, J. P.; Yang, H.; Blasetti, K. L.; Schnell, G.; Conley, J.; Schofield, L. N. Liposome delivery of ciprofloxacin against intracellular *Francisella tularensis* infection. *Journal of Controlled Release* 2003, 92(3), 265–273.

123. Meers, P.; Neville, M.; Malinin, V.; Scotto, A. W.; Sardaryan G.; Kurumunda, R.; Mackinson, C.; James, G.; Fisher, S.; Perkins, W. R. Biofilm penetration, triggered release and *in vivo* activity of inhaled liposomal amikacin in chronic *Pseudomonas aeruginosa* lung infections. *Journal of Antimicrobial Chemotherapy* 2008, 61(4), 859–868.

124. Jain, A. K.; Agarwal, A.; Agrawal, H.; Agrawal, G. P. Double-liposome–based dual-drug delivery system as vectors for effective management of peptic ulcer. *Journal of Liposome Research* 2012, 22(3), 205–214.

125. Alhariri, M.; Omri, A. Efficacy of liposomal bismuth-ethanedithiol-loaded tobramycin after intratracheal administration in rats with pulmonary *Pseudomonas aeruginosa* infection. *Antimicrobial Agents and Chemotherapy* 2013, 57(1), 569–578.

126. He, J.; Abdelraouf, K.; Ledesma, K. R.; Chow, D. S.; Tam, V. H. Pharmacokinetics and efficacy of liposomal polymyxin B in a murine pneumonia model. *International Journal of Antimicrobial Agents* 2013, 42(6), 559–564.

127. Hamblin, K. A., Armstrong, S. J.; Barnes, K. B.; Davies, C.; Wong, J. P.; Blanchard, J. D.; Harding, S. V.; Simpson, A. J.; Atkins, H. S. Liposome encapsulation of ciprofloxacin improves protection against highly virulent *Francisella tularensis* strain Schu S4. *Antimicrobial Agents and Chemotherapy*, 2014, 58(6), 3053–3059.

128. Klemens, S. P.; Cynamon, M. H.; Swenson, C. E.; Ginsberg, R. S. Liposome-encapsulated-gentamicin therapy of *Mycobacterium avium* complex infection in beige mice. *Antimicrobial Agents and Chemotherapy* 1990, 34(6), 967–970.

129. Gangadharam, P. R.; Ashtekar, D. R.; Flasher, D. L.; Düzgüneş, N. Therapy of *Mycobacterium avium* complex infections in beige mice with streptomycin encapsulated in sterically stabilized liposomes. *Antimicrobial Agents and Chemotherapy* 1995, 39(3), 725–730.

130. Mehta, R. T. Liposome encapsulation of clofazimine reduces toxicity in vitro and in vivo and improves therapeutic efficacy in the beige mouse model of disseminated *Mycobacterium avium-M. intracellulare* complex infection. *Antimicrobial Agents and Chemotherapy* 1996, 40(8), 1893–1902.

131. Kadry, A. A.; Al-Suwayeh, S. A.; Abd-Allah, A. R. A.; Bayomi, M. A. Treatment of experimental osteomyelitis by liposomal antibiotics. *Journal of Antimicrobial Chemotherapy* 2004, 54, 1103–1108.

132. Steenwinkel, J. E.; Van Vianen, W.; Ten Kate, M. T.; Verbrugh, H. A.; Van Agtmael, M. A.; Schiffelers, R. M.; Bakker-Woudenberg, I. A. Targeted drug delivery to enhance efficacy and shorten treatment duration in disseminated *Mycobacterium avium* infection in mice. *Journal of Antimicrobial Chemotherapy* 2007, 60(5), 1064–1073.

133. Sande, L.; Sanchez, M.; Montes, J.; Wolf, A. J.; Morgan, M. A.; Omri, A.; Liu, G. Y. Liposomal encapsulation of vancomycin improves killing of methicillin-resistant *Staphylococcus aureus* in a murine infection model. *Journal of Antimicrobial Chemotherapy* 2012, 67(9), 2191–2194.

134. Li, C.; Zhang, X.; Huang, X.; Wang, X.; Liao, G.; Chen, Z. Preparation and characterization of flexible nanoliposomes loaded with daptomycin, a novel antibiotic, for topical skin therapy. *International Journal of Nanomedicine* 2013, 8, 1285–1292.

135. Li, Y.; Su, T.; Zhang, Y.; Huang, X.; Li, J.; Li, C. Liposomal co-delivery of daptomycin and clarithromycin at an optimized ratio for treatment of methicillin-resistant *Staphylococcus aureus* infection. *Drug Delivery* 2015, 22(5), 627–637.

136. Clancy, J. P.; Dupont, L.; Konstan, M. W.; Billings, J.; Fustik, S.; Goss, C. H.; Lymp, J.; Minic, P.; Quittner, A. L.; Rubenstein, R. C.; Young, K. R. Phase II studies of nebulised Arikace in CF patients with Pseudomonas aeruginosa infection. *Thorax* 2013, 68(9), 818–825.

137. Bilton, D.; Pressler, T.; Fajac, I.; Clancy, J. P.; Sands, D.; Minic, P.; Cipolli, M.; LaRosa, M.; Galeva, I.; Sole, A. A.; Staab D. Phase 3 efficacy and safety data from randomized, multicenter study of liposomal amikacin for inhalation (ARIKACE) compared with TOBI in cystic fibrosis patients with chronic infection due to *Pseudomonas Aeruginosa*. *Pediatric Pulmonology* 2013, 48(S36), 207–453.

138. Cipolla, D.; Blanchard, J.; Gonda, I. Development of liposomal ciprofloxacin to treat lung infections. *Pharmaceutics* 2016, 8(1), 1–6.

139. Haworth, C.; Wanner, A.; Froehlich, J.; O'Neal, T.; Davis, A.; Gonda, I.; O'Donnell, A. Inhaled liposomal ciprofloxacin in patients with bronchiectasis and chronic *Pseudomonas aeruginosa* infection: Results from two parallel phase III trials (ORBIT-3 and-4). *B14. Clinical Trials Across Pulmonary Disease* 2017, 195, A7604–A7604.

140. Haworth, C.; Bilton, D.; Chalmers, J. D.; Davis, A. M.; Froehlich, J.; Gonda, I; Thompson, B.; Wanner, A.; O'Donnell A. E. Two randomised controlled trials of inhaled liposomal ciprofloxacin (ARD-3150) in patients with non-cystic fibrosis bronchiectasis and chronic lung infection with *Pseudomonas Aeruginosa*. *The Lancet Respiratory Medicine* 2018 7(3): 213–226.

141. Ng, A. W.; Wasan, K. M.; Lopez-Berestein, G. G. Development of liposomal polyene antibiotics: An historical perspective. *Journal of Pharmaceutical Sciences* 2003 6(1), 67–83.

142. Arikan, S.; Rex, J. H. Lipid-based antifungal agents current status. *Current Pharmaceutical Design* 2001, 7(5), 395–417.

143. Birnbaum, J. E. Pharmacology of the allylamines. *Journal of the American Academy of Dermatology* 1990, 23(4), 782–785.

144. Maertens, J. A. History of the development of azole derivatives. *Clinical Microbiology and Infection* 2004, 10(1), 1–10.

145. Larkin, E. L., Dharmaiah, S.; Ghannoum, M. A. Biofilms and beyond: Expanding echinocandin utility. *Journal of Antimicrobial Chemotherapy* 2018, 73(1), i73–i81.

146. Clemons, K. V., Stevens, D. A. Comparative efficacies of four amphotericin B formulations: fungizone, amphotec (amphocil), AmBisome, and abelcet: Against systemic murine aspergillosis. *Antimicrob Agents Chemother* 2004, 48(3), 1047–1050.

147. Lopez-Berestein, G. Liposomes as carriers of antifungal. *Drugs Antimicrobial Agents and Chemotherapy* 1987, 31(5), 675–678.

148. Stone, N. R. H.; Bicanic, T.; Salim, R.; Hope, W. Liposomal amphotericin B (AmBisome®): A review of the pharmacokinetics, pharmacodynamics, clinical experience and future directions. *Drugs* 2016, 76(4), 485–500.

149. Ambati, S.; Ferarro, A. R.; Earl Khang, S.; Lin, J.; Lin, X.; Momany, M.; Lewis, Z.; Meagher, R. B. Dectin-1-targeted antifungal liposomes exhibit enhanced efficacy. *mSphere* 2019, 4, e00025-19.

150. Mehta, R. T.; McQueen, T. J.; Keyhani, A.; Lopez-Berestein, G. Liposomal hamycin: Reduced toxicity and improved antifungal efficacy in vitro and in vivo. *Journal of Infectious Diseases* 1991, 164(5), 1003–1006.

151. de Logu, A.; Fadda, A. M.; Anchisi, C.; Maccioni, A. M.; Sinico, C.; Schivo, M. L.; Alhaique, F. Effects of in-vitro activity of miconazole and ketoconazole in phospholipid formulations. *Journal of Antimicrobial Chemotherapy* 1997, 40(6), 889–893.

152. Pandit, J., Garg, M.; Jain, N. K. Miconazole nitrate bearing ultraflexible liposomes for the treatment of fungal infection. *Journal of Liposome Research* 2014, 24(2), 163–169.

153. Le Conte, P.; Joly, V.; Saint-Julien, L., Gillardin, J.-M., Carbon, C., Yeni, P. Tissue distribution and anti-fungal effect of liposomal itraconazole in experimental cryptococcosis and pulmonary aspergillosis. *American Reviews in Respiratory Disease* 1992, 145(2), 424–429.

154. Leal, A. F.; Leite, M. C.; Medeiros, C. S.; Cavalcanti, I. M.; Wanderley, A.G.; Magalhães, N. S.; Neves, R. P. Antifungal activity of a liposomal itraconazole formulation in experimental Aspergillus flavus keratitis with endophthalmitis. *Mycopathologia* 2015, 179(3–4), 225–229.

155. Singh, M.; Maiti, S. N.; Gandhi, A.; Atwal, H. Preparation of liposomal fluconazole and their in vitro antifungal activity. *Journal of Microencapsulation* 1993, 10(2), 229–236.

156. Abdel-Rhaman, M. S.; Soliman, W., Habib, F.; Fathalla, D. A new long-acting liposomal topical antifungal formula: Human clinical study. *Cornea* 2011, 31(2), 126–129.

157. Veloso, D. F. M. C.; Benedetti, N. I. G. M.; Ávila, R. I.; Bastos, T. S. A.; Silva, T. C.; Silva, M. R. R.; Batista, A. C.; Valadares, M. C.; Lima, E. M. Intravenous delivery of a liposomal formulation of voriconazole improves drug pharmacokinetics, tissue distribution, and enhances antifungal activity. *Drug Delivery* 2018, 25(1), 1585–1594.

158. Hamdan, A. M. Design, formulation and characterization of liposomal preparation of voriconazole (VRC). *Journal of Pharmaceutical and Biomedical Sciences* 2015, 5(10), 822–827.

159. Patel, A. T.; Modiya, P. R.; Shinde, G.; Patel, R. Formulation and characterization of long circulating liposomes of antifungal drug. *International Journal of Pharmacy Research and Technology* 2018, 2, 32–42.

160. Kohi, T. W.; von Essen, L.; Masika, G. M.; Gottvall, M.; Dol, J. Cancer-related concerns and needs among young adults and children on cancer treatment in Tanzania: A qualitative study. *BMC Cancer* 2019, 9, 82–90.

161. White, M. C.; Holman, D. M.; Boehm, J. E.; Peipins, L. A.; Grossman, M.; Henley, S. J., Age and cancer risk: A potentially modifiable relationship. *American Journal of Preventive Medicine* 2014, 46, S7–S15.

162. Rayyan-Assi, H.; Ziv, A.; Dankner, R. The metabolic syndrome and its components are differentially associated with chronic diseases in a high-risk population of 350,000 adults: A cross-sectional study. *Diabetes/Metabolism Research and Reviews* 2019, 35, e3121.

163. Sontheimer-Phelps, A.; Hassell, B. A.; Ingber, D. E. Modelling cancer in microfluidic human organs-on-chips. *Nature Reviews Cancer* 2019, 19, 65–81.

164. Samstein, R. M.; Lee, C. H.; Shoushtari, A. N.; Hellmann, M. D.; Shen, R.; Janjigian, Y. Y.; Barron, D. A.; Zehir, A.; Jordan, E. J.; Omuro, A.; Kaley, T. J.; Kendall, S. M.; Motzer, R. J.; Hakimi, A. A.; Voss, M. H.; Russo, P.; Rosenberg, J.; Iyer, G.; Bochner, B. H.; Bajorin, D. F.; Al-Ahmadie, H. A.; Chaft, J. E.; Rudin, C. M.; Riely, G. J.; Baxi, S.; Ho, A. L.; Wong, R. J.; Pfister, D. G.; Wolchok, J. D.; Barker, C. A.; Gutin, P. H.; Brennan, C. W.; Tabar, V.; Mellinghoff, I. K.; DeAngelis, L. M.; Ariyan, C. E.; Lee, N.; Tap, W. D.; Gounder, M. M.; D'Angelo, S. P.; Saltz, L.; Stadler, Z. K.; Scher, H. I.; Baselga, J.; Razavi, P.; Klebanoff, C. A.; Yaeger, R.; Segal, N. H.; Ku, G. Y.; DeMatteo, R. P.; Ladanyi, M.; Rizvi, N. A.; Berger, M. F.; Riaz, N.; Solit, D. B.; Chan, T. A.; Morris, H. G. T. Tumor mutational load predicts survival after immunotherapy across multiple cancer types. *Nature Genetics* 2019, 51, 202–206.

165. Chen, H.; Zhang, W.; Zhu, G.; Xie, J.; Chen, X. Rethinking cancer nanotheranostics. *Nature Reviews Materials* 2017, 2, 17024.

166. Chang, H. I.; Yeh, M. K. Clinical development of liposome-based drugs: Formulation, characterization, and therapeutic efficacy. *International Journal of Nanomedicine* 2012, 7, 49–60.

167. Maiolo, D.; Del Pino, P.; Metrangolo, P.; Parak, W. J.; Bombelli, F. B. Nanomedicine delivery: Does protein corona route to the target or off road? *Nanomedicine*, 2015, 10, 3231–3247.

168. Mishra, P.; Nayak, B.; Dey, R. K. PEGylation in anti-cancer therapy: An overview. *Asian Journal of Pharmaceutical Sciences* 2016, 11, 337–348.

169. Riaz, M.; Riaz, M. A.; Zhang, X.; Lin, C.; Wong, K. H.; Chen, X.; Zhang, G.; Lu, A.; Yang, Z. Surface functionalization and targeting strategies of liposomes in solid tumor therapy: A review. *International Journal of Molecular Sciences* 2018, 19(1), E195.

170. Blake, E. A.; Bradley, C. A.; Mostofizadeh, S.; Muggia, F. M.; Garcia, A. A.; Roman, L. D.; Matsuo, K. Efficacy of pegylated liposomal doxorubicin maintenance therapy in platinum-sensitive recurrent epithelial ovarian cancer: A retrospective study. *Archives of Gynecology and Obstetrics* 2019, 299, 1641–1649.

171. Landrum, L. M.; Brady, W. E.; Armstrong, D. K.; Moore, K. N.; Di Silvestro, P. A.; O'Malley, D. M.; Tenney, M. E.; Rose, P. G.; Fracasso, P. M. A phase I trial of pegylated liposomal doxorubicin (PLD), carboplatin, bevacizumab and veliparib in recurrent, platinum-sensitive ovarian, primary peritoneal, and fallopian tube cancer: An NRG Oncology/Gynecologic Oncology Group study. *Gynecologic Oncology* 2016, 140, 204–209.

172. Mahner, S.; Meier, W.; du Bois, A.; Brown, C.; Lorusso, D.; Dell'Anna, T.; Cretin, J.; Havsteen, H.; Bessette, P.; Zeimet, A. G.; Vergote, I.; Vasey, P.; Pujade-Lauraine, E.; Gladieff, L.; Ferrero, A. Carboplatin and pegylated liposomal doxorubicin versus carboplatin and paclitaxel in very platinum-sensitive ovarian cancer patients: Results from a subset analysis of the CALYPSO phase III trial. *European Journal of Cancer* 2015, 51, 352–358.

173. Marth, C.; Vergote, I.; Scambia, G.; Oberaigner, W.; Clamp, A.; Berger, R.; Kurzeder, C.; Colombo, N.; Vuylsteke, P.; Lorusso, D.; Hall, M.; Renard, V.; Pignata, S.; Kristeleit, R.; Altintas, S.; Rustin, G.; Wenham, R. M.; Mirza, M. R.; Fong, P. C.; Oza, A.; Monk, B. J.; Ma, H.; Vogl, F. D.; Bach, B. A. ENGOT-ov-6/TRINOVA-2: Randomised, double-blind, phase 3 study of pegylated liposomal doxorubicin plus trebananib or placebo in women with recurrent partially platinum-sensitive or resistant ovarian cancer. *European Journal of Cancer* 2017, 70, 111–121.

174. Barenholz, Y. C. Doxil®: The first FDA-approved nano-drug: Lessons learned. *Journal of Controlled Release* 2012, 160, 117–134.

175. Rahman, A. M.; Yusuf, S. W.; Ewer, M. S. Anthracycline-induced cardiotoxicity and the cardiac sparing effect of liposomal formulation. *International Journal of Nanomedicine* 2007, 2, 567–583.

176. O'Brian, M. E.; Wigler, N.; Inbar, M.; Rosso, R.; Grischke, E.; Santoro, A.; Catane, R.; Kieback, D. G.; Tomczak, P.; Ackland, S. P.; Orlandi, F.; Mellars, L.; Alland, L.; Tendler, C. Reduced cardiotoxicity and comparable efficacy in a phase III trial of pegylated liposomal doxorubicin HCl (Caelyx/Doxil) versus conventional doxorubicin for first-line treatment of metastatic breast cancer. *Annals of Oncology* 2004, 15, 440–449.

177. Petersen, G. H.; Alzghari, S. K.; Chee, W.; Sankari, S. S.; NinhM, L. B. Meta-analysis of clinical and preclinical studies comparing the anticancer efficacy of liposomal versus conventional non-liposomal doxorubicin. *Journal of Controlled Release* 2016, 232, 255–264.

178. Romeo, R.; Joly, F.; Ray-Coquard, I.; El Kouri, C.; Mercier-Blas, A.; Berton-Rigaud, D.; Kalbacher, E.; Cojocarasu, O.; Fabbro, M.; Cretin, J.; Zannetti, A.; Abadie-Lacourtoisie, S.; Mollon, D.; Hardy-Bessard, A.; Provansal, M.; Blot, E.; Delbaldo, C.; Lesoi, A.; Freyer, G.; You, B. Non-pegylated liposomal doxorubicin (NPLD, Myocet®)+carboplatin in patients with platinum sensitive ovarian cancers: A ARCAGYGINECO phase IB-II trial. *Gynecologic Oncology* 2019, 152, 68–75.

179. Schneeweiss, A.; Möbus, V.; Tesch, H.; Hanusch, C.; Denkert, C.; Lübbe, K.; Huober, J.; Klare, P.; Kümmel, S.; Untch, M.; Kast, K.; Jackisch, C.; Thomalla, J.; Ingold-Heppner, B.; Blohmer, J.; Rezai, M.; Frank, M.; Engels, K.; Rhiem, K.; Fasching, P. A.; Nekljudova, V.; von Minckwitz, G.; Loibl, S. Intense dose-dense epirubicin, paclitaxel, cyclophosphamide versus weekly paclitaxel, liposomal doxorubicin (plus carboplatin in triple-negative breast cancer) for neoadjuvant treatment of high-risk early breast cancer (GeparOctodGBG 84): A randomized phase III trial. *European Journal of Cancer* 2019, 106, 181–192.

180. Wang-Gillam, A.; Hubner, R. A.; Siveke, J. T.; Von Hoff, D. D.; Belanger, B.; de Jong, F. A.; Mirakhur, B.; Chen, L. NAPOLI-1 phase 3 study of liposomal irinotecan in metastatic pancreatic cancer: Final overall survival analysis and characteristics of long-term survivors. *European Journal of Cancer* 2019, 108, 78–87.

181. Hubner, R. A.; Cubillo, A.; Blanc, J. F.; Melisi, D.; Von Hoff, D. D.; Wang-Gillam, A.; Chen, L. T.; Becker, C.; Mamlouk, K.; Belanger, B.; Yang, Y.; de Jong, F. A.; Siveke, J. T. Quality of life in metastatic pancreatic cancer patients receiving liposomal irinotecan plus 5-fluorouracil and leucovorin. *European Journal of Cancer* 2019, 106, 24–33.

182. Bolger, G. T.; Licollari, A.; Tan, A.; Greil, R.; Vcelar, B.; Greil-Ressler, S.; Weiss, L.; Schönlieb, C.; Magnes, T.; Radl, B.; Majeed, M.; Sordillo, P. P. Pharmacokinetics of liposomal curcumin (Lipocurc™) infusion: Effect of co-medication in cancer patients and comparison with healthy individuals. *Cancer Chemotherapy and Pharmacology* 2019, 83, 265–275.

183. Evans, T. R. J.; Dean, E.; Molife, L. R.; Lopez, J.; Ranson, M.; El-Khouly, F.; Zubairi, I.; Savulsky, C.; Reyderman, L.; Jia, Y.; Sweeting, L.; Greystoke, A.; Barriuso, J.; Kristeleit, R. Phase 1 dose-finding and pharmacokinetic study of eribulin liposomal formulation in patients with solid tumours. *British Journal of Cancer* 2019, 120, 379–386.

184. Colapicchioni, V.; Tilio, M.; Digiacomo, L.; Gambini, V.; Palchetti, S.; Marchini, C.; Pozzi, D.; Occhipinti, S.; Amici, A.; Caracciolo, G. Personalized liposome–protein corona in the blood of breast, gastricand pancreatic cancer patients. *The International Journal of Biochemistry and Cell Biology* 2016, 75, 180–187.

185. Guo, P.; Yang, J.; Liu, D.; Huang, L.; Fell, G.; Huang, J.; Moses, M. A.; Auguste, D. T. Dual complementary liposomes inhibit triple-negative breast tumor progression and metastasis. *Science Advances* 2019, 5, eaav5010.

186. Caracciolo, G. Clinically approved liposomal nanomedicines: Lessons learned from the biomolecular corona. *Nanoscale* 2018, 10, 4167–4172.

187. Papi, M.; Caputo, D.; Palmieri, V.; Coppola, R.; Palchetti, S; Bugli, F.; Martini, C.; Digiacomo, L.; Pozzi, D.; Caracciolo, G. Clinically approved PEGylated nanoparticles are covered by a protein corona that boosts uptake by cancer cells. *Nanoscale* 2017, 9, 10327–10334.

17 Targeted Intestinal Delivery of Probiotics

Kevin Enck and Emmanuel Opara
Virginia Tech-Wake Forest School of Biomedical Engineering and
Sciences (SBES), Wake Forest Institute for Regenerative Medicine

Alec Jost
Wake Forest School of Medicine

CONTENTS

17.1   INTRODUCTION

Probiotics are, by definition, live microorganisms which when administered in adequate amounts confer a health benefit to the host. This is the characterization given by the Food and Agriculture Association of the United Nations (FAO) and World Health Organization (WHO).[1] Within our gastrointestinal tract (GIT) we have ~10^{14} microbes that make up an ecosystem of both beneficial and harmful functions that is known as the microbiome or microbiota.[2,3] This is an order of magnitude higher than the number of cells that make up the human body (~10^{13}), which illustrates the scale and complexity of the microbiome. Researchers are just now beginning to understand how these bacteria function and the role they play in diseases such as obesity, diabetes, cancer, and others. This review will discuss this role and show how probiotics may work to treat or prevent these diseases, as well as current barriers to successful use of probiotics, in addition to approaches to overcome those barriers, and lastly we will describe innovation technologies that may improve the targeted delivery for these probiotics.

There are four main functions of the gut microbiota: (i) nutrient absorption, (ii) energy metabolism, (iii) intestinal barrier integrity maintenance, and (iv) expression of genes involved in immunity.[4,5] Dysbiosis is known as a shift in composition of intestinal microbiota, and this change leads to a disruption in these four functions, which can eventually lead to a diseased state.[4,6] For example in a study following patients who received bariatric surgery, investigators found significant changes to patients' gut microbiota, specifically *Faecalibacterium prausnitzii*.[6,7] Following the surgery, the patients had a significant increase in *F. prausnitzii* which has been shown to be anti-inflammatory.[8–11] Obesity, type 2 diabetes (T2D), and insulin sensitivity are all now known to be associated with systemic and adipose tissue inflammation,[2,6,12–15] and a lack of bacteria such as *F. prausnitzii* is believed to be part of the problem.

17.1.1   "Leaky" Gut

While there are trillions of bacteria providing a symbiotic relationship with the gut, their presence in the peripheral tissue triggers an immense immune response because the body perceives the microbes as foreign invaders. The concept of a "leaky" gut due to dysbiosis has gained traction in the scientific community and is used to explain a potential cause or contributor to metabolic diseases such as obesity and T2D, as well as cancer,[2,16–18] and even autoimmune diseases.[3,19–22] The barrier that separates bacteria from the peripheral tissue is a single layer of highly absorptive epithelium. This layer is protected by the mucosal layer, defensins, and antibacterial lectins which make up the mucosal immune system.[23] The exact mechanisms for how the barrier becomes compromised is still not fully known, but eventually the tight junctions that create the barrier are damaged or destroyed leading to increased permeability and eventual translocation of bacteria into the periphery. This triggers a cascade of inflammatory responses as mentioned earlier. Because the system is so complex, there is even some evidence to support the notion that the inflammatory response occurs first and that is what causes the damage to the epithelium barrier[24] (Figure 17.1).

17.1.2   Obesity, T2D, and Insulin Sensitivity

T2D is a metabolic disease that is caused by decreased sensitivity to insulin, which creates a higher demand for insulin production by pancreatic β cells. These cells are thus required to overproduce insulin and are eventually destroyed because of this burden.[2] What T2D patients have in common with obese people is a measured increase in T_{cells}[25,26] and mast cells,[27] which are both proinflammatory, as well as a decrease in T_{reg} cells.[6,28] All of these changes lead to adipose tissue inflammation and are thought to be a contributor to the pathogenesis of obesity and T2D. T_{reg} cells are well studied and known for their inflammation suppressive capabilities. This mechanism of action is through expression of inhibitory cytokines like Interleukin-10 (IL-10), Tumor Growth Factor-β (TGF-β),

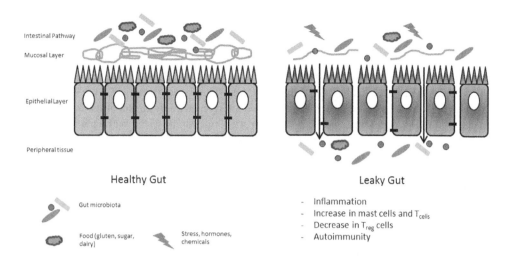

FIGURE 17.1 Illustration of a healthy gut lining (left) and a leaky gut (right). The mucosal layer and tight junctions of the epithelial cells protect the peripheral tissue from the contents of the intestinal pathway. In a leaky gut, these contents are able to pass through to the peripheral tissue where they trigger many inflammatory pathways and, over extended periods of time, pathogenesis of certain diseases.

and IL-35 as well as disruption of cellular metabolism through expression of IL-2 receptors. They also have been shown to target the maturation of dendritic cells through cell surface expression of certain molecules.[29] Probiotics such as *Lactobacillus casei* and *Bifidobacteria longum* have been shown to modulate the T_{reg} cell response[29] and significantly decrease their numbers in obese and T2D patients. Another possible contributor to the pathogenesis of the disease is lipopolysaccharides, which are a microbe-derived inflammatory molecule. While harmless in the gut, when they are transported through the "leaky" gut barrier and into peripheral tissue they cause adipose tissue inflammation.[6,30] Plasma lipopolysaccharide levels are elevated in obese and T2D patients further supporting this theory. In obese humans and mice, adipose tissue is infiltrated with large numbers of macrophages.[12,31,32] These macrophages secrete cytokines such as TNF-α and IL-1β due to highly activated proinflammatory pathways most likely from lipolysaccharides.[2,12,15,33] In healthy patients, these macrophages and microbes in the periphery are minimal to non-existent.

These proinflammatory molecules and highly activated proinflammatory pathways are believed to cause obesity and insulin resistance.[32–35] From this evidence, it would make sense that a reversal of the dysbiosis could prevent further damage or treat the disease all together. An established successful treatment for obesity and T2D, bariatric surgery, mentioned earlier illustrates this reversal. While it has been shown to be effective, the surgery is expensive, extensive, and exclusive. Patients need to have serious weight-related health problems and all other weight loss efforts would have been unsuccessful among other qualifications for the surgery. For this reason, other treatment options should be investigated to help treat patients before they reach that level of disease state. Fecal microbiota transplantation (FMT) is another clinically approved procedure that has been shown to help in the treatment of many gastrointestinal diseases.[36–38] In FMT, strains of bacteria from a healthy donor are transplanted into the gut of a patient in order to prevent or treat a disease. When performed on males with insulin resistance, beneficial metabolic effects were observed including improved peripheral insulin sensitivity.[39,40] Not every treatment option requires a medical procedure either; diet alone has been shown to alter the gut microbiota towards a healthier state.[6,41] By reintroducing therapeutic bacteria into the GIT, through any of the methods mentioned above, intestinal barrier integrity and intestinal immunity are improved, and inflammation has been shown to be reduced.[4,42]

17.1.3   IBD: Crohn's and UC

Inflammatory Bowel Disease (IBD) is a gastrointestinal disorder that affects 100–200 patients per 100,000 people in North America and Northern Europe.[43] As the name suggests, IBD involves a chronic inflammatory response in gut that can lead to diarrhea, ulceration, intestinal obstruction, and even perforation of the GIT. Two of the most common phenotypes are Crohn's Disease (CD) and Ulcerative Colitis (UC) and both have been characterized with dysbiosis of the microbiota.[2,44,45] While these are two unique diseases that affect patients differently, the pathogenesis and how it relates to the microbiome is believed to be fairly similar. It is well established that environmental factors play a role in rapid progression of IBD as the rate of development is different for industrialized western nations compared with their Asian or less developed counterparts.[46] The relevant factors are still being determined, but a reduction in complexity of the gut microbiome appears to be the result. With a reduction in immune modulating and anti-inflammatory bacteria such as *F. prausnitzii* and *Butyricoccus pullicaecorum* and an increase in proinflammatory strains such as *Escherichia coli*, there is an inflammatory response that proliferates throughout the gut.[46] An example of this response starts with *E. coli* stimulating the release of proinflammatory cytokines such as Interferon-γ (IFN-γ) and IL-6 which activates Matrix Metallopeptidase (MMPs) that trigger matrix degradation, epithelial cell detachment, and ulceration.[46,47] There is evidence that demonstrates that the reintroduction of bacteria such as *F. prausnitzii*[8] and *B. pullicaecorum*[44] back into the gut attenuates some of the inflammation and has led to extended remission periods in patients. Both oral delivery of specific probiotics and FMT have been used with varying degrees of success to repopulate the microbiome of patients with IBD.[36,38]

17.1.4   *Clostridium difficile* Infection

One of the first disorders treated with FMT was *Clostridium difficile* infection. *C. diff* is a bacterium that is known to cause serious infections following antibiotic therapy. The strain is extremely resilient and commonly occurs in long-term care facilities such as hospitals.[48] A healthy individual's gut microbiome can resist colonization by *C. diff*, but the microbiome of a patient who has received antibiotics can be depleted of those same protective microbes. This leads to colonization and release of toxins that can cause inflammation and mucosal damage. FMT is used to repopulate the gut microbiome in order to resist the spreading and damage caused by *C. diff* and has been shown to be around 90% effective.[36,38,49]

17.1.5   Cancer

The association of infectious agents and inflammation with cancer has been well known for decades.[50,51] Inflammation caused by dysbiosis and infection is associated with an increased regenerative response. When this inflammation goes from acute to chronic, the risk of developing an oncogenic mutation is increased. Improvements in cell proteomics and genomics have led to a better understanding of this relationship and helped define the actual pathways for tumorogenesis. As with the other diseases mentioned above, dysbiosis is seen as a main contributor to the development of cancerous growth.[52] A mouse model of gastric cancer has demonstrated that gastric infection caused by *Helicobacter felis* is associated with an "aberrant regenerative response that may account for the development of this type of cancer."[16] Many environmental factors, including obesity and diet, are indicated as contributing to the carcinogenic cell pathways,[52] and these factors are directly tied to the gut microbiome as we have discussed above. The therapeutic use of probiotics for cancer treatment is limited as there is no evidence of bacteria being able to reverse the oncogenic mutations caused by the repeat injury to the tissue. However, it can be used preventatively as a way to rebalance the microbiome and downregulate some of the key proinflammatory cytokines and chemokines that are produced by the harmful bacteria.

17.1.6 PARKINSON'S AND ALZHEIMER'S

There is a complex grouping of neurons known as the enteric nervous system (ENS) located in the intestines, and there is direct communication between it and the central nervous system (CNS).[19] This communication influences brain activity, behavior, as well as neurotransmitters and neuro-trophic factors.[3,53–57] Neurological disorders such as Parkinson's (PD) and Alzheimer's Disease (AD) are now beginning to be linked to the overall gut health, and researchers are studying how dysbiosis plays a role in their pathogenesis. Both PD and AD are affected by oxidative damage and neurodegeneration that is caused by chronic inflammation.[58] While the pathways are still not fully understood, researchers of PD believe ENS neurodegeneration is tied to the synucelinopathy that defines the disease.[3] Gut microbiota directly influences the activity of enteric neurons, which could possibly affect cellular α-synuclein deposition in the brain and gut. Some of the microbiome changes involved in the dysbiosis are an increased presence of *Enterobacteriaceae* and *H. pylori*, which are proinflammatory, and a decrease in *Prevotellacae* and *Faecalibacterium* which are known anti-inflammatory microbes.[22] Almost all (80%) of the patients with PD suffer from consti-pation, which is associated with α-synuclein accumulation in the gut, and recently a clinical study found that regular intake of fermented milk containing *L. casei* improved constipation and bowel movements in patients with PD.[59]

The oxidative damage that is caused by a compromised immune system is particularly impact-ful in AD.[58] This neurodegeneration is brought typically with age, and there is evidence that shows how the microbiome diversity decreases over time, especially in patients with AD.[58,60] This disease has also been tied to T2D as AD pathogenesis involves impaired glucose metabolism and insulin signaling as well as chronic inflammation.[21] Conversely, centenarians typically have major differences in their microbiota compared with other seniors, indicating a possible corre-lation between gut health and a long, healthy life.[61] Similar to cancer, probiotics have not been shown to reverse the symptoms of AD, but administering them prophylactically could result in a decreased risk.

17.1.7 TYPE 1 DIABETES

Type 1 Diabetes (T1D) is an autoimmune disorder that results from improper self-destruction of pancreatic β-cells by the immune system. This is notably different from T2D where the β-cells are destroyed because of metabolic stress and overproduction of insulin due to decreased insulin sensitivity. There is growing evidence that the pathogenesis of T1D could originate from the gut. In addition to genetic and possible environmental factors, a compromised gut microbiome could lead to a permeable gut barrier. In a diabetic rat model, increased gut permeability has been observed before the onset of the disease. This leaky gut leads to an improper activation of T_{cells} which may lead to pancreatic islet inflammation and destruction of pancreatic β-cells.[62–64] It has been shown in a Non-obese Diabetic (NOD) mouse model that delivery of certain probiotics can prevent spontaneous autoimmune diabetes, which helps support the case for the gut microbiota having a major impact on autoimmune disease development[65] (Table 17.1).

17.2 BARRIERS TO SUCCESSFUL USE OF PROBIOTICS IN DISEASE TREATMENT/PREVENTION

A major commonality among the various diseases discussed above is the therapeutic benefit of rein-troducing beneficial bacteria into the GIT. Different strains of probiotics provide different effects for protecting the gut, and there is enough evidence to suggest a strong correlation between gut health and disease pathogenesis.[4,42,69] There are many challenges to successfully providing the ther-apeutic effect of probiotics to the host.

TABLE 17.1

List of Some Diseases and Currently Accepted Probiotics Used for Treatment

Disease	Bacteria Strain	Outcome of Treatment	Reference
Rotavirus diarrhea	*Lactobacillus rhamnosus* GG	Reduction of symptoms	[66]
C. difficile infection	*Bifidobacterium lactis*	Prevention of diarrhea	[67]
	FMT (multiple species)	Prevention of spreading and further damage	[36,38,49]
IBD	*Faecalibacterium prasnitzii*	Attenuation of inflammation and extended remission	[8]
	Butyricoccus pullicaecorum	Attenuation of inflammation and extended remission	[44]
	Saccharomyces boulardii	Extended remission or decrease in clinical signs	[68]
PD	*L. casei*	Improved bowel movements	[59]
Obesity and T2D	*Bifidobacterium longum* & *L. casei*	Modulate Tcell response	[29]
	FMT (multiple species)	Improved insulin sensitivity	[49]
	Faecalibacterium prasnitzii	Reduction of inflammation	[6,7]

17.2.1 DESTRUCTION OF PROBIOTICS IN THE STOMACH

The first and most relevant is the difficulty in delivering probiotics orally. Bacteria are easily destroyed by the harsh stomach acid before they can even get to the gut.[70,71] Gastric emptying time ranges from 5 minutes up to 2 hours and is different for every patient, which has made it difficult to design effective drug delivery vehicles.[71] This has been the main reason for the continued use of FMT for therapeutic bacteria delivery as it avoids the stomach all together. FMT is not ideal for diseases that require daily drug therapy for a long period of time such as IBD, diabetes, as well as any prophylactic treatment, as it requires trained medical personnel to administer the therapy.

17.2.2 IMPROVED PRECISION OF PROBIOTIC STRAIN USAGE

Another challenge is the use of probiotic preparations composed of multiple species.[72–74] FMT transplants hundreds if not thousands of different strains of bacteria of a healthy donor into a patient in what is known as a "shotgun" approach. Doctors know that only a few of the strains will provide the desired therapeutic effect while others will provide no benefit at all. For any other cell therapy, this same approach would never be approved by regulators, but FMT has been proven effective and the gut is much more resilient than most other tissues. That being said, more research needs to be done to understand the mechanism and effect of each strain so that precise probiotic "cocktails" can be prescribed to patients for maximized therapeutic benefit.

17.2.3 DRYING AND PROCESSING PROBIOTICS REDUCES VIABILITY

Manufacturing processes also need to be improved as they have been shown to decrease cell viability, thus lowering therapeutic efficacy. Drying of probiotics is a popular processing method as it improves handling and long-term storage, but it is known to be damaging to the bacteria.[71] Cook et al. have described many of these processes and the advantages and disadvantages to each of them such as fluid bed drying, vacuum oven drying, and freeze drying.[71] All of them result in a loss of viability, but some are more damaging than others. Other properties such as clustering, cost, and time contribute to which processes are used as well.

17.2.4 IMPROVEMENT OF CLINICAL TRIALS TO SHOW PROOF OF PROBIOTIC EFFICACY

As the probiotic field grows, clinical trial design will need to improve to better understand how these microbes are functioning. Sanders et al. have made a compelling argument for difficulties with trial design based on both internal and external factors.[52] Internally, there has yet to be explicit causality and reversal of a disease from probiotics as most evidence has shown strong correlations at best. By designing experiments in a way that isolates the effect of probiotics alongside improved genomic and proteomic sequencing, causality should be improved, and probiotics use would be much more effective. Externally, there is increased pressure by regulators in Europe and USA to substantiate claims as stating improved or "maintained" health is difficult to prove due to the complexity of the cellular and molecular pathways involved.[52] Also, if probiotics are deemed to help treat or prevent a disease, they are considered a drug and would be regulated as such. This makes it more difficult to incorporate them into food products, which fall under a different and less complex regulatory pathway.

17.2.5 PUBLIC OPINION

Lastly, public opinion of probiotics is starting to grow and is susceptible to negative or incorrect discussion that could hinder their applications and development. An area that has not yet been addressed in this review is the bioengineering of probiotics to be more resilient or more potent. These fall under the classification of genetically modified organisms (GMOs) which is highly scrutinized by the public. Being described as such may be enough to discourage funding or potential buyers even if the product is extremely effective.[72] On the other end of the spectrum is the high praise for probiotics and their "cure-all" capabilities. While researchers are finding new uses for them constantly, the term "probiotics" may be oversaturating the market and overpromising its benefits, similar to the term "organic". If regulators allow the term to be used without proper justification, general disbelief of ineffectiveness may grow when some of the products may not even fall under the umbrella of probiotics in the first place.[75]

There are many barriers to successful use of probiotics and not all can be overcome through proper research alone. Outside of designing better methods of delivering the microbes to the gut, there needs to be improved communication and coordination between scientists, regulators, and the general public. Within the realm of scientific research, we will further discuss how these challenges have been approached and improved upon.

17.3 APPROACHES TO OVERCOME THE BARRIERS

17.3.1 MANUFACTURING PROCESSES

Manufacturers and researchers have begun to focus on three areas to develop improved probiotic use: delivery, survival, and efficacy.[72,76] Delivery applies to what occurs before the probiotics are ingested. First, discovering better ways to store, package, and deliver probiotics as a product is extremely important. This involves proper scaling drying methods from clinical to manufacturing scale so that the loss in cell viability is minimized. Once the products are packaged, storing them in consistent conditions ensures that they will not die or become activated before being ingested. One approach has been to develop mutant strains of bacteria that are more resistant to the stress from manufacturing processes.[72] Survival has to do with improved competitiveness and durability in the GIT. Researchers are currently looking at designing the probiotics to express host-specific survival factors in order to better survive the acidic environment as well as compete for space in the intestines.[76] Lastly, efficacy is about improving the therapeutic effect of probiotics. The catchy term is "designer probiotics," and these strains are engineered to produce specific molecules in order to prevent and/or treat specific diseases.[77,78] These approaches look at improving probiotics directly, but there are other strategies for protecting the bacteria from the stomach acid and delivering them to the desired therapeutic location in the gut.

17.3.2 Incorporation with Food

The first paper that described probiotics was published in 1906 and discussed the benefits of fermented milk and how it could displace pathogens and increase longevity.[79] Since then, probiotics have been closely associated with food and food manufacturing. While some foods, such as milk and yogurt are known to contain some probiotics, others are being supplemented with them to provide some of the beneficial effects described. Evidence shows that incorporating probiotics with food protects them from the stomach acid better than if the bacteria were ingested on their own.[80] Following a meal, the pH can be raised as high as 5, which increases the ability of the bacteria to survive until they reach the gut.[70,80] There are some challenges with adding bioactive ingredients to foods though. When adding bioactive ingredients to food, it is critical to ensure that there are no undesirable interactions between the food and the bacteria.[81,82] Champagne et al. have performed an extensive review on the addition of probiotics to food sources and how to best approach the problems that are present.[81] Some of the major points to consider are the viability in storage, the activity level based on the food source, and the identification of strain-food compatibilities. If the amount of colony forming units (CFU) is different from what is described, it could lead to an ineffective or even overly toxic effect depending on the patient's health and microbiota. As mentioned previously, adding probiotics to food and claiming that they can treat or prevent disease may prolong or even halt their approval with regulators since they could be classified as a drug. This may not be desirable or profitable for food companies, which is why encapsulation has become another platform for probiotic administration.

17.3.3 Microencapsulation

Microencapsulation of probiotics for oral drug delivery has been researched for many years now.[71,82,83] By surrounding the bacteria with a protective matrix, the acidic stomach environment is less effective at destroying the microbes before they reach the GIT. Once they reach the gut, it is important that they release their payload into the intestines. This is the goal for any oral drug delivery vehicle, not just for probiotics[84–87] but since probiotics are much larger than drug molecules, the capsules need to degrade to release them into the gut. Alginate has been the most used biomaterial for the purpose of bacteria encapsulation for reasons that include the following: (i) alginate is nontoxic and approved as an accepted food additive,[88,89] (ii) it is not antimicrobial and provides good protection from acid,[71,88] and (iii) eventually dissolves in the gut after about 8–10 hours due to swelling caused by the intestinal fluids.[84,90,91] Xanthan gum is a biomaterial that is very similar to alginate in that it crosslinks with divalent cations and has comparable protective effects in acidic environments.[92] While alginate is still used more frequently, Xanthan gum is a good alternative. Pectin is another biomaterial that has been used in drug delivery as it is broken down by colonic microflora which can be useful for drug delivery that is specifically targeted for the colon.[93] Since alginate remains the most commonly used biomaterial for probiotic encapsulation, we will explore the various ways it has been used in the field as well as how it can be improved to better address the problems associated with oral delivery of probiotics.

17.3.3.1 Alginate

The two most popular methods for alginate-based encapsulation are extrusion[88,94,95] and emulsion.[96–99] Extrusion entails pushing alginate through a junction that separates it into small droplets which are collected and crosslinked with divalent cations such as Ca^{2+}. Emulsion methods combine alginate with large volumes of hydrophobic compounds, typically oil, and spin them at high speeds. This forms droplets due to alginate being immiscible in oil. The droplets are subsequently crosslinked by addition of a crosslinking solution to the mixture. The advantage of the extrusion method is the precision and control over which the microbeads are created. Beads can range from 10 μm to a few mm in diameter depending on the device being used,[100–102] but the size is typically fairly monodisperse.[100,103,104] A disadvantage of the extrusion method is the speed and scale at which it can be done. As much as a few 100 capsules can be produced per second, while the emulsion method's limitation is based solely on the scale of equipment being used. A large manufacturing facility measures the amount of alginate beads they produce in pounds instead of number of beads, which shows the vast difference in production rate.[82,105] The alginate beads can also be produced as small as the nanoscale, depending on the speed at which the solution is spun. The downside of the emulsion method is the lack of control over bead size. Since the beads are formed based on immiscibility, the distribution of bead size is quite large. This is not ideal for encapsulation of single cell clusters such as pancreatic islets[106–109] as well as precise concentrations of single cell types such as mesenchymal stem cells.[110–112] For that reason, the extrusion method is typically employed when a lower number of beads and high precision is necessary for drug delivery. That being said, both methods are still frequently used when it comes to probiotic encapsulation and determining which method to use is based on the needs of the researchers/manufacturers.

17.4 INNOVATIONS FOR IMPROVED TARGETED DELIVERY

Current innovation strategies for improving the delivery of probiotics to the gut are focused around either chemical or physical modifications of the delivery vehicle. These modifications are intended to either improve the protection of probiotics in the acidic stomach or improve the release rate in the gut. The microbiome changes with the regions of the GIT, therefore having a vehicle with a targeted release property would improve treatment efficacy.[113] In order to have a delivery vehicle that can target a specific site, there needs to be a stimulus that causes change in the material properties. The most common stimuli used, regardless of application, are: temperature, pH, light, electric field, ultrasound, and mechanical stress.[114] For oral drug delivery, pH is the most commonly used stimuli due to the large difference between gastric and intestinal pHs. Once the vehicle material comes in contact with the stimulus, it would swell or degrade in order to release the therapeutic payload rapidly. This strategy works well for all soluble drugs, but is not always effective for probiotics since they are much larger and cannot diffusive easily through the hydrogels. Therefore, some modifications that have shown efficacy in oral chemical drug delivery studies may not be pertinent for probiotic delivery and will not be discussed in this chapter.

17.4.1 PHYSICAL MODIFICATIONS

There is evidence that suggests increasing the size of the beads better protects the probiotics from the gastric environment.[88,96,98] By decreasing the surface area-to-volume ratio, larger beads expose their payload to less surrounding fluids. This is an advantage for protection of probiotics but a disadvantage for dissolution of the beads in the gut. Another common physical modification is to form biomaterial complexes in order to take advantage of the compound material properties. Some of the most popular complexes are alginate–chitosan[115–121] and xanthan–chitosan.[122,123] Chitosan is cationic and can supplement Ca^{2+} as a crosslinking agent. On its own, it can deliver drugs in a sustained manner at neutral pH, but a major limitation is its ease of dissolution at low pH in the stomach.[118] By combining alginate or xanthan gum with chitosan, the stability of the hydrogel is greatly improved, which may be useful for delayed release of probiotics in the large intestine or colon.[123] Chitosan can also be used to coat the outer layer of alginate which has been shown to increase the survival of B. breve in simulated gastric fluid (SGF).[121] Other biomaterials such as dextran[124] and gelatin[125] provide a similar effect of increasing the durability of the hydrogel when combined with alginate. While this approach can be useful for both gastric protection and delayed release of probiotics, neither is useful if rapid release is desired. For this reason, chemical modifications have been explored.

17.4.2 Chemical Modifications

By chemically modifying a hydrogel biomaterial, most of the advantageous properties of the material are preserved while gaining an additional benefit depending on what is chemically attached to the material. All pH-sensitive polymers have acidic or basic groups that can either accept or donate a proton based on the pH environment. With this proton donation, relatively large structural changes can occur that allow for either bead shrinking or swelling. For targeted release, bead swelling is desired as this leads to degradation and eventual release of the therapeutic. The addition of carboxylic groups has been shown to cause bead swelling and expansion as the chain becomes ionized at pH of 4.4 or greater.[126,127] El-Sherbiny et al. combined both physical and chemical modifications by adding alginate to a chitosan modified with a carboxymethyl group in order to provide protection in gastric fluid and targeted release in the gut.[128] Another group added an alginate-protamine outer layer to their alginate capsules, which increased viability in gastric fluid due to the closing of alginate pores with protamine molecules as well as increased release of bacteria in the intestines due to protamine positively interacting with trypsin in the gut.[129] Our lab has chemically oxidized the vicinal dialcohol backbone of the alginate polymer as a way to increase pH sensitivity.[130] We also showed that by varying the degree of modification, the degradation rate could be controlled, which expands the use of the hydrogel for oral drug delivery since it can be used to target different sections of GIT (Figure 17.2).

17.4.3 Assessment of Targeted Delivery

From research lab to manufacturing product development, the properties of the desired drug delivery vehicle need to be assessed and adapted for scaling up production. This involves testing of the material and the probiotics encapsulated within it. For the material, encapsulation efficiency, size,

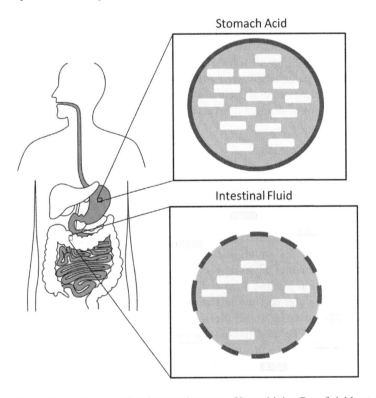

FIGURE 17.2 Chemical modification of alginate to increase pH sensitivity. Beneficial bacteria (light gray) encapsulated in alginate (dark gray) is protected from the harsh stomach acid while degrading in the neutral intestinal fluid and releasing the bacteria.

degradation rate, and drug release kinetics are important characteristics to control and monitor throughout the process. For the bacteria, the critical characteristics are viability in gastric fluid, viability following manufacturing processes such as storage and drying, as well as the therapeutic effect once the bacteria have reached the desired location.

17.4.3.1 *In Vitro* Assessment

Throughout the entirety of the development process, *in vitro* assessment can be used to quickly and inexpensively understand the material and product properties listed above. Capsules containing bacteria can be placed in SGF or simulated intestinal fluid (SIF) to study the pharmacokinetics between capsules and body-like conditions. To replicate the motility in the GIT, a United States Pharmacopeia (USP) Dissolution Apparatus is typically used at physiological temperature for most drug delivery studies. Once the capsules have been recovered, the probiotics release can be quantified with UV spectrophotometry and their viability can be determined via culturing on agar plates. These quantities can be used to determine loading efficiency, release rate, and bacteria viability, while size can be determined using standard microscopy or Scanning Electron Microscope (SEM) imaging. The effectiveness of the bacteria would be more difficult to determine and is typically reserved for *in vivo* studies.

17.4.3.2 *In Vivo* Assessment

While it is more difficult to determine release rate and bacteria viability *in vivo* compared with the *in vitro* assays, the advantages of delivering the bacteria in a physiological system outweighs the challenge. Animal models include but are not limited to rats, mice, rabbits, and dogs.[84] Each model typically correlates to a specific disease state or demographic, and extensive literary research should be done to determine what animal model best suits the disease being investigated. Regardless of the model, therapeutic efficacy can be measured in a number of ways. Reversal of symptoms is one of the more apparent methods to determine efficacy, but is often difficult to troubleshoot as a lack of treatment does not necessarily correlate to an ineffective product. To better understand if, how, and where the bacteria is releasing into the gut, histological samples can be taken after euthanasia. Many of the potential inflammatory factors, epithelial cell integrity, and therapeutic molecules can be detected by staining tissue samples of the GIT. The difficulty with histopathological assessment is that the samples are taken posthumously which may limit the design of experiments.

Another effective method is to measure bacteria diversity in stool samples. This has the advantage of permitting multiple measurements throughout an experiment, but not the sensitivity or precision of histological samples. These methods are not mutually exclusive as they are often done in conjunction to improve the output of the experiment. While these *in vivo* animal experiments can demonstrate the therapeutic effect of the bacteria, they do not guarantee the same effect when administered to humans. Clincal trials, as described above, have the difficult challenge of proving the direct benefit of probiotics based on the complex pathways of the GIT. Stool samples and patient health are the output measurements used during clinical trials since histological samples of gut are rarely possible.[131,132] When the trials are successful, scaling up the production is the next obstacle and this is generally outsourced owing to the complexity and variation of challenges.

17.4.3.3 Manufacturing and Production Assessment

The goal of the scaling up process is to produce the same product but on a larger scale. Most research labs perfect the product on a small scale and get it to work under specific conditions. To reduce cost, these settings are exchanged for more industrial environments where the processes are automated, speed up, and/or increased in scale, which introduces errors and challenges that were not present in the labs.[71,72,75,82,83,133] The first concern is that the upscaling process changes the material properties. The encapsulation polymer needs to perform as it did in the previous assessments in order for it to have a similar therapeutic effect. This is a common concern for all products and the solution involves having feedback and communication between manufacturers and researchers so that any change in material properties can be better understood and alleviated. For example, if the encapsulation polymer degrades slower than expected, researchers can study the manufactured material, detect the change, and come up with a solution to have the material perform as expected. As we discussed earlier, encapsulated probiotics are dried via various methods, which can greatly reduce the viability of the cells due to the harsh conditions in which they occur. The drying techniques give the product an extended shelf-life, which is critical for successful marketing and use.

Other concerns are the storage and widespread distribution of the products to stores. Heat and moisture are what typically activate the bacteria from their dried state, which would both occur following ingestion. The challenge is preventing both of those two conditions during shipment and storage. This requires proper packaging and labeling for both shipment and receiving, which are both not controlled by the manufacturers, to properly handle them before being sold. Manufacturing is an important and overlooked process by researchers and requires communication between all parties that are involved in product development in order to provide consumers with a viable product.

17.5 CONCLUSION

Symbiosis of bacteria with the human gut has been known to be beneficial to our health for over 100 years.[79] These "good bacteria" are already present in our GIT, but a change in the microbiota composition, dysbiosis, has been shown to contribute to a whole host of diseases. Patients with metabolic diseases such as obesity and T2D, as well as IBD all have increased proinflammatory cytokines and/or decreased immune regulating bacteria present in their gut or peripheral tissue.[13,21,33,34,40,41] The same correlation is seen in patients with autoimmune disorders such as T1D, as well as neurodegenerative diseases including AD and PD.[3,19,20,22,23,134] This increased presence of proinflammatory factors is believed to trigger some of the improper cellular pathways such as destruction of pancreatic beta cells or deposition of α-synuclein. As this inflammation turns into a chronic condition, the likelihood of oncogenic mutation is greatly increased, which is why cancers such as colorectal cancer have been closely linked to dysbiosis as well.[2,16,17,50]

Evidence shows that by reintroducing the beneficial bacterial strains back into the GIT early enough in the pathogenesis, many of these diseases can be prevented, or sometimes, even treated.[52,69,135] In this chapter, we have discussed some of the major barriers that impair successful use of probiotics for disease treatment/prevention. These include limited success in delivery of the bacteria as well as inadequate understanding of what strains should be used for specific diseases and why. This burden of proof has been difficult as disease states are complicated. There are hundreds of different strains in our gut, and each person has a slightly different microbiome, akin to a fingerprint. Regardless of strain, researchers have tried to administer probiotics through oral delivery for many years now. It is much less intensive and can be prescribed frequently unlike the FMT.[36,37]

Encapsulation in polymers, such as alginate, has become a popular method of delivery as it is nontoxic to both the body and the bacteria, and the capsules provide protection from the acidic gastric fluid. Herein we have described modifications to some of the polymers to allow for better protection and/or improved targeted delivery. Since the microbiome changes at different parts of the GIT, targeting the release of the encapsulated probiotics to specific sites where they are typically found is critical for treatment efficacy.[113] Lastly, we have detailed how researchers have assessed the material properties to determine degradation rate and released bacterial potency. Overall, the field of probiotics and gut health is rapidly growing as we use cutting-edge genomics and proteomics to better understand how important and versatile our microbiome is. While there are many different ways to deliver probiotics, encapsulation appears to be a popular choice as it provides protection and opportunity for targeted release. While these bacterial strains are being improved and better studied for biological effects, so too are the materials being used to deliver these microbes.

ACKNOWLEDGEMENT

Our foray into probiotics delivery research has been made possible by a Collaborative Pilot Grant from Office of Research & Sponsored Programs of Wake Forest University and another Pilot Grant from the Center on Diabetes, Obesity, and Metabolism of the Wake Forest School of Medicine. In addition, we acknowledge the support of NIH Pre-doctoral Training Program: Studies in Translational Regenerative Medicine (T32 NIBIB Grant #1T32EB014836-01A1, A. Atala, PI) for Kevin Enck.

REFERENCES

1. WHO/FAO. Evaluation of health and nutritional properties of powder milk and live lactic acid bacteria. *Food and Agriculture Organization of the United Nations and World Health Organization Expert Consultation Report* 2001, 1–34.
2. Karin, M.; Lawrence, T.; Nizet, V., Innate immunity gone awry: Linking microbial infections to chronic inflammation and cancer. *Cell* **2006**, *124* (4), 823–835.
3. Scheperjans, F.; Aho, V.; Pereira, P. A.; Koskinen, K.; Paulin, L.; Pekkonen, E.; Haapaniemi, E.; Kaakkola, S.; Eerola-Rautio, J.; Pohja, M., Gut microbiota are related to Parkinson's disease and clinical phenotype. *Movement Disorders* **2015**, *30* (3), 350–358.
4. Hemarajata, P.; Versalovic, J., Effects of probiotics on gut microbiota: Mechanisms of intestinal immunomodulation and neuromodulation. *Therapeutic Advances in Gastroenterology* **2013**, *6* (1), 39–51.
5. Larsson, E.; Tremaroli, V.; Lee, Y. S.; Koren, O.; Nookaew, I.; Fricker, A.; Nielsen, J.; Ley, R. E.; Bäckhed, F., Analysis of gut microbial regulation of host gene expression along the length of the gut and regulation of gut microbial ecology through MyD88. *Gut* **2012**, *61* (8), 1124–1131.
6. Tremaroli, V.; Bäckhed, F., Functional interactions between the gut microbiota and host metabolism. *Nature* **2012**, *489*, 242.
7. Furet, J.-P.; Kong, L.-C.; Tap, J.; Poitou, C.; Basdevant, A.; Bouillot, J.-L.; Mariat, D.; Corthier, G.; Doré, J.; Henegar, C., Differential adaptation of human gut microbiota to bariatric surgery–induced weight loss: Links with metabolic and low-grade inflammation markers. *Diabetes* **2010**, *59* (12), 3049–3057.
8. Sokol, H.; Pigneur, B.; Watterlot, L.; Lakhdari, O.; Bermúdez-Humarán, L. G.; Gratadoux, J.-J.; Blugeon, S.; Bridonneau, C.; Furet, J.-P.; Corthier, G., Faecalibacterium prausnitzii is an anti-inflammatory commensal bacterium identified by gut microbiota analysis of Crohn disease patients. *Proceedings of the National Academy of Sciences* **2008**, *105* (43), 16731–16736.
9. Fanning, S.; Hall, L. J.; Cronin, M.; Zomer, A.; MacSharry, J.; Goulding, D.; Motherway, M. O. C.; Shanahan, F.; Nally, K.; Dougan, G., Bifidobacterial surface-exopolysaccharide facilitates commensal-host interaction through immune modulation and pathogen protection. *Proceedings of the National Academy of Sciences* **2012**, *109* (6), 2108–2113.
10. Tsilingiri, K.; Barbosa, T.; Penna, G.; Caprioli, F.; Sonzogni, A.; Viale, G.; Rescigno, M., Probiotic and postbiotic activity in health and disease: Comparison on a novel polarised ex-vivo organ culture model. *Gut* **2012**, *61* (7), 1007–1015.
11. von Schillde, M.-A.; Hörmannsperger, G.; Weiher, M.; Alpert, C.-A.; Hahne, H.; Bäuerl, C.; van Huynegem, K.; Steidler, L.; Hrncir, T.; Pérez-Martínez, G., Lactocepin secreted by Lactobacillus exerts anti-inflammatory effects by selectively degrading proinflammatory chemokines. *Cell Host & Microbe* **2012**, *11* (4), 387–396.
12. Osborn, O.; Olefsky, J. M., The cellular and signaling networks linking the immune system and metabolism in disease. *Nature Medicine* **2012**, *18* (3), 363.
13. Oliver, E.; McGillicuddy, F.; Phillips, C.; Toomey, S.; Roche, H. M., The role of inflammation and macrophage accumulation in the development of obesity-induced type 2 diabetes mellitus and the possible therapeutic effects of long-chain n-3 PUFA. *Proceedings of the Nutrition Society* **2010**, *69* (2), 232–243.
14. Kanda, H.; Tateya, S.; Tamori, Y.; Kotani, K.; Hiasa, K.-I.; Kitazawa, R.; Kitazawa, S.; Miyachi, H.; Maeda, S.; Egashira, K., MCP-1 contributes to macrophage infiltration into adipose tissue, insulin resistance, and hepatic steatosis in obesity. *The Journal of Clinical Investigation* **2006**, *116* (6), 1494–1505.
15. Schenk, S.; Saberi, M.; Olefsky, J. M., Insulin sensitivity: Modulation by nutrients and inflammation. *The Journal of Clinical Investigation* **2008**, *118* (9), 2992–3002.

16. Houghton, J.; Stoicov, C.; Nomura, S.; Rogers, A. B.; Carlson, J.; Li, H.; Cai, X.; Fox, J. G.; Goldenring, J. R.; Wang, T. C., Gastric cancer originating from bone marrow-derived cells. *Science* **2004**, *306* (5701), 1568–1571.

17. Karin, M.; Greten, F. R., NF-κB: Linking inflammation and immunity to cancer development and progression. *Nature Reviews Immunology* **2005**, *5* (10), 749.

18. Sears, C. L.; Pardoll, D. M., Perspective: Alpha-bugs, their microbial partners, and the link to colon cancer. *Journal of Infectious Diseases* **2011**, *203* (3), 306–311.

19. Hu, X.; Wang, T.; Jin, F., Alzheimer's disease and gut microbiota. *Science China Life Sciences* **2016**, *59* (10), 1006–1023.

20. Jiang, C.; Li, G.; Huang, P.; Liu, Z.; Zhao, B., The gut microbiota and Alzheimer's disease. *Journal of Alzheimer's Disease* **2017**, *58* (1), 1–15.

21. I Naseer, M.; Bibi, F.; H Alqahtani, M.; G Chaudhary, A.; I Azhar, E.; A Kamal, M.; Yasir, M., Role of gut microbiota in obesity, type 2 diabetes and Alzheimer's disease. *CNS & Neurological Disorders-Drug Targets (Formerly Current Drug Targets-CNS & Neurological Disorders)* **2014**, *13* (2), 305–311.

22. Parashar, A.; Udayabanu, M., Gut microbiota: Implications in Parkinson's disease. *Parkinsonism & Related Disorders* **2017**, *38*, 1–7.

23. Anders, H.-J.; Andersen, K.; Stecher, B., The intestinal microbiota, a leaky gut, and abnormal immunity in kidney disease. *Kidney International* **2013**, *83* (6), 1010–1016.

24. Andersson, H.; Van den Berg, A., Microfluidic devices for cellomics: A review. *Sensors and Actuators B: Chemical* **2003**, *92* (3), 315–325.

25. Nishimura, S.; Manabe, I.; Nagasaki, M.; Eto, K.; Yamashita, H.; Ohsugi, M.; Otsu, M.; Hara, K.; Ueki, K.; Sugiura, S., CD8+ effector T cells contribute to macrophage recruitment and adipose tissue inflammation in obesity. *Nature Medicine* **2009**, *15* (8), 914.

26. Winer, S.; Chan, Y.; Paltser, G.; Truong, D.; Tsui, H.; Bahrami, J.; Dorfman, R.; Wang, Y.; Zielenski, J.; Mastronardi, F., Normalization of obesity-associated insulin resistance through immunotherapy. *Nature Medicine* **2009**, *15* (8), 921.

27. Liu, J.; Divoux, A.; Sun, J.; Zhang, J.; Clément, K.; Glickman, J. N.; Sukhova, G. K.; Wolters, P. J.; Du, J.; Gorgun, C. Z., Genetic deficiency and pharmacological stabilization of mast cells reduce diet-induced obesity and diabetes in mice. *Nature Medicine* **2009**, *15* (8), 940.

28. Feuerer, M.; Herrero, L.; Cipolletta, D.; Naaz, A.; Wong, J.; Nayer, A.; Lee, J.; Goldfine, A. B.; Benoist, C.; Shoelson, S., Lean, but not obese, fat is enriched for a unique population of regulatory T cells that affect metabolic parameters. *Nature Medicine* **2009**, *15* (8), 930.

29. Round, J. L.; Mazmanian, S. K., The gut microbiota shapes intestinal immune responses during health and disease. *Nature Reviews Immunology* **2009**, *9* (5), 313.

30. Creely, S. J.; McTernan, P. G.; Kusminski, C. M.; Fisher, F. M.; Da Silva, N.; Khanolkar, M.; Evans, M.; Harte, A.; Kumar, S., Lipopolysaccharide activates an innate immune system response in human adipose tissue in obesity and type 2 diabetes. *American Journal of Physiology-Endocrinology and Metabolism* **2007**, *292* (3), E740–E747.

31. Weisberg, S. P.; McCann, D.; Desai, M.; Rosenbaum, M.; Leibel, R. L.; Ferrante, A. W., Obesity is associated with macrophage accumulation in adipose tissue. *The Journal of Clinical Investigation* **2003**, *112* (12), 1796–1808.

32. Xu, H.; Barnes, G. T.; Yang, Q.; Tan, G.; Yang, D.; Chou, C. J.; Sole, J.; Nichols, A.; Ross, J. S.; Tartaglia, L. A., Chronic inflammation in fat plays a crucial role in the development of obesity-related insulin resistance. *The Journal of Clinical Investigation* **2003**, *112* (12), 1821–1830.

33. Olefsky, J. M.; Glass, C. K., Macrophages, inflammation, and insulin resistance. *Annual Review of Physiology* **2010**, *72* (1), 219–246.

34. Heilbronn, L. K.; Campbell, L. V., Adipose tissue macrophages, low grade inflammation and insulin resistance in human obesity. *Current Pharmaceutical Design* **2008**, *14* (12), 1225–1230.

35. Cani, P. D.; Amar, J.; Iglesias, M. A.; Poggi, M.; Knauf, C.; Bastelica, D.; Neyrinck, A. M.; Fava, F.; Tuohy, K. M.; Chabo, C., Metabolic endotoxemia initiates obesity and insulin resistance. *Diabetes* **2007**, *56* (7), 1761–1772.

36. Borody, T. J.; Khoruts, A., Fecal microbiota transplantation and emerging applications. *Nature Reviews Gastroenterology & Hepatology* **2012**, *9* (2), 88.

37. Vrieze, A.; de Groot, P. F.; Kootte, R. S.; Knaapen, M.; Van Nood, E.; Nieuwdorp, M., Fecal transplant: A safe and sustainable clinical therapy for restoring intestinal microbial balance in human disease? *Best Practice & Research Clinical Gastroenterology* **2013**, *27* (1), 127–137.

38. Bakken, J. S.; Borody, T.; Brandt, L. J.; Brill, J. V.; Demarco, D. C.; Franzos, M. A.; Kelly, C.; Khoruts, A.; Louie, T.; Martinelli, L. P., Treating Clostridium difficile infection with fecal microbiota transplantation. *Clinical Gastroenterology and Hepatology* **2011**, *9* (12), 1044–1049.

39. Vrieze, A.; Van Nood, E.; Holleman, F.; Salojärvi, J.; Kootte, R. S.; Bartelsman, J. F.; Dallinga–Thie, G. M.; Ackermans, M. T.; Serlie, M. J.; Oozeer, R., Transfer of intestinal microbiota from lean donors increases insulin sensitivity in individuals with metabolic syndrome. *Gastroenterology* **2012**, *143* (4), 913–916. e7.

40. Hartstra, A. V.; Bouter, K. E.; Bäckhed, F.; Nieuwdorp, M., Insights into the role of the microbiome in obesity and type 2 diabetes. *Diabetes Care* **2015**, *38* (1), 159–165.

41. Ley, R. E.; Turnbaugh, P. J.; Klein, S.; Gordon, J. I., Microbial ecology: Human gut microbes associated with obesity. *Nature* **2006**, *444* (7122), 1022.

42. O'Toole, P. W.; Cooney, J. C., Probiotic bacteria influence the composition and function of the intestinal microbiota. *Interdisciplinary Perspectives on Infectious Diseases* **2008**, *2008*, 1–9.

43. Cho, J. H., The genetics and immunopathogenesis of inflammatory bowel disease. *Nature Reviews Immunology* **2008**, *8* (6), 458.

44. Eeckhaut, V.; Machiels, K.; Perrier, C.; Romero, C.; Maes, S.; Flahou, B.; Steppe, M.; Haesebrouck, F.; Sas, B.; Ducatelle, R., Butyricicoccus pullicaecorum in inflammatory bowel disease. *Gut* **2013**, *62* (12), 1745–1752.

45. Manichanh, C.; Rigottier-Gois, L.; Bonnaud, E.; Gloux, K.; Pelletier, E.; Frangeul, L.; Nalin, R.; Jarrin, C.; Chardon, P.; Marteau, P., Reduced diversity of faecal microbiota in Crohn's disease revealed by a metagenomic approach. *Gut* **2006**, *55* (2), 205–211.

46. Manichanh, C.; Borruel, N.; Casellas, F.; Guarner, F., The gut microbiota in IBD. *Nature Reviews Gastroenterology & Hepatology* **2012**, *9* (10), 599.

47. Pender, S. L., Do metalloproteinases contribute to tissue destruction or remodeling in the inflamed gut? *Inflammatory Bowel Diseases* **2008**, *14* (suppl_2), S136–S137.

48. Kelly, C. P.; Pothoulakis, C.; LaMont, J. T., Clostridium difficile colitis. *New England Journal of Medicine* **1994**, *330* (4), 257–262.

49. Kim, B.-S.; Jeon, Y.-S.; Chun, J., Current status and future promise of the human microbiome. *Pediatric Gastroenterology, Hepatology & Nutrition* **2013**, *16* (2), 71–79.

50. Marchesi, J. R.; Dutilh, B. E.; Hall, N.; Peters, W. H. M.; Roelofs, R.; Boleij, A.; Tjalsma, H., Towards the human colorectal cancer microbiome. *PloS one* **2011**, *6* (5), e20447.

51. Parkin, D. M., The global health burden of infection-associated cancers in the year 2002. *International Journal of Cancer* **2006**, *118* (12), 3030–3044.

52. Sanders, M. E.; Guarner, F.; Guerrant, R.; Holt, P. R.; Quigley, E. M.; Sartor, R. B.; Sherman, P. M.; Mayer, E. A., An update on the use and investigation of probiotics in health and disease. *Gut* **2013**, *62* (5), 787–796.

53. Bercik, P.; Denou, E.; Collins, J.; Jackson, W.; Lu, J.; Jury, J.; Deng, Y.; Blennerhassett, P.; Macri, J.; McCoy, K. D., The intestinal microbiota affect central levels of brain-derived neurotropic factor and behavior in mice. *Gastroenterology* **2011**, *141* (2), 599–609. e3.

54. Forsythe, P.; Kunze, W. A., Voices from within: Gut microbes and the CNS. *Cellular and Molecular Life Sciences* **2013**, *70* (1), 55–69.

55. Heijtz, R. D.; Wang, S.; Anuar, F.; Qian, Y.; Björkholm, B.; Samuelsson, A.; Hibberd, M. L.; Forssberg, H.; Pettersson, S., Normal gut microbiota modulates brain development and behavior. *Proceedings of the National Academy of Sciences* **2011**, *108* (7), 3047–3052.

56. Tillisch, K.; Labus, J.; Kilpatrick, L.; Jiang, Z.; Stains, J.; Ebrat, B.; Guyonnet, D.; Legrain–Raspaud, S.; Trotin, B.; Naliboff, B., Consumption of fermented milk product with probiotic modulates brain activity. *Gastroenterology* **2013**, *144* (7), 1394–1401. e4.

57. Cryan, J. F.; Dinan, T. G., Mind-altering microorganisms: The impact of the gut microbiota on brain and behaviour. *Nature Reviews Neuroscience* **2012**, *13* (10), 701.

58. Westfall, S.; Lomis, N.; Kahouli, I.; Dia, S. Y.; Singh, S. P.; Prakash, S., Microbiome, probiotics and neurodegenerative diseases: Deciphering the gut brain axis. *Cellular and Molecular Life Sciences* **2017**, *74* (20), 3769–3787.

59. Cassani, E.; Privitera, G.; Pezzoli, G.; Pusani, C.; Madio, C.; Iorio, L.; Barichella, M., Use of probiotics for the treatment of constipation in Parkinson's disease patients. *Minerva gastroenterologica e dietologica* **2011**, *57* (2), 117–121.

60. Cheng, J.; Palva, A. M.; de Vos, W. M.; Satokari, R., Contribution of the intestinal microbiota to human health: From birth to 100 years of age. In *Between Pathogenicity and Commensalism. Current Topics in Microbiology and Immunology*, Dobrindt, U., Hacker, J., Svanborg, C., Eds. vol. 358, Springer, Berlin, Heidelberg, **2011**; pp. 323–346.

61. Biagi, E.; Nylund, L.; Candela, M.; Ostan, R.; Bucci, L.; Pini, E.; Nikkïla, J.; Monti, D.; Satokari, R.; Franceschi, C., Through ageing, and beyond: Gut microbiota and inflammatory status in seniors and centenarians. *PloS one* **2010**, *5* (5), e10667.

62. Vaarala, O.; Atkinson, M. A.; Neu, J., The "perfect storm" for type 1 diabetes: The complex interplay between intestinal microbiota, gut permeability, and mucosal immunity. *Diabetes* **2008**, *57* (10), 2555–2562.

63. Kostic, A. D.; Gevers, D.; Siljander, H.; Vatanen, T.; Hyötyläinen, T.; Hämäläinen, A.-M.; Peet, A.; Tillmann, V.; Pöhö, P.; Mattila, I., The dynamics of the human infant gut microbiome in development and in progression toward type 1 diabetes. *Cell Host & Microbe* **2015**, *17* (2), 260–273.

64. Zheng, P.; Li, Z.; Zhou, Z., Gut microbiome in type 1 diabetes: A comprehensive review. *Diabetes/Metabolism Research and Reviews* **2018**, e3043.

65. Calcinaro, F.; Dionisi, S.; Marinaro, M.; Candeloro, P.; Bonato, V.; Marzotti, S.; Corneli, R.; Ferretti, E.; Gulino, A.; Grasso, F., Oral probiotic administration induces interleukin-10 production and prevents spontaneous autoimmune diabetes in the non-obese diabetic mouse. *Diabetologia* **2005**, *48* (8), 1565–1575.

66. Szajewska, H.; Wanke, M.; Patro, B., Meta-analysis: The effects of Lactobacillus rhamnosus GG supplementation for the prevention of healthcare-associated diarrhoea in children. *Alimentary Pharmacology & Therapeutics* **2011**, *34* (9), 1079–1087.

67. Goldenberg, J. Z.; Yap, C.; Lytvyn, L.; Lo, C. K. F.; Beardsley, J.; Mertz, D.; Johnston, B. C., Probiotics for the prevention of Clostridium difficile-associated diarrhea in adults and children. *Cochrane Database of Systematic Reviews* **2017**, *12*, CD006095.

68. Meijer, B. J.; Dieleman, L. A., Probiotics in the treatment of human inflammatory bowel diseases: Update 2011. *Journal of Clinical Gastroenterology* **2011**, *45*, S139–S144.

69. Sánchez, B.; Delgado, S.; Blanco-Míguez, A.; Lourenço, A.; Gueimonde, M.; Margolles, A., Probiotics, gut microbiota, and their influence on host health and disease. *Molecular Nutrition & Food Research* **2017**, *61* (1), 1600240.

70. Abuhelwa, A. Y.; Foster, D. J.; Upton, R. N., A quantitative review and meta-models of the variability and factors affecting oral drug absorption—part I: Gastrointestinal pH. *The AAPS Journal* **2016**, *18* (5), 1309–1321.

71. Cook, M. T.; Tzortzis, G.; Charalampopoulos, D.; Khutoryanskiy, V. V., Microencapsulation of probiotics for gastrointestinal delivery. *Journal of Controlled Release* **2012**, *162* (1), 56–67.

72. Foligné, B.; Daniel, C.; Pot, B., Probiotics from research to market: The possibilities, risks and challenges. *Current Opinion in Microbiology* **2013**, *16* (3), 284–292.

73. Petrof, E.; Claud, E.; Gloor, G.; Allen-Vercoe, E., Microbial ecosystems therapeutics: A new paradigm in medicine? *Beneficial Microbes* **2012**, *4* (1), 53–65.

74. Lemon, K. P.; Armitage, G. C.; Relman, D. A.; Fischbach, M. A., Microbiota-targeted therapies: An ecological perspective. *Science Translational Medicine* **2012**, *4* (137), 137rv5–137rv5.

75. Reid, G., Probiotics and prebiotics – Progress and challenges. *International Dairy Journal* **2008**, *18* (10), 969–975.

76. Bron, P. A.; Van Baarlen, P.; Kleerebezem, M., Emerging molecular insights into the interaction between probiotics and the host intestinal mucosa. *Nature Reviews Microbiology* **2012**, *10* (1), 66.

77. Wells, J., Mucosal vaccination and therapy with genetically modified lactic acid bacteria. *Annual Review of Food Science and Technology* **2011**, *2*, 423–445.

78. Daniel, C.; Roussel, Y.; Kleerebezem, M.; Pot, B., Recombinant lactic acid bacteria as mucosal biotherapeutic agents. *Trends in Biotechnology* **2011**, *29* (10), 499–508.

79. Metchnikoff, I. I.; Mitchell, P., *Prolongation of Life: Optimistic Studies*. Springer Publishing Company: New York, United States, **2004**.

80. Saxelin, M.; Korpela, R.; Mäyrä-Mäkinen, A., Introduction: Classifying functional dairy products. In *Woodhead Publishing Series in Food Science, Technology and Nutrition, Functional Dairy Products Functional Dairy Products*, Mattila-Sandholm, T., Saarela, M. Elsevier, **2003**; pp. 1–16.

81. Champagne, C. P.; Gardner, N. J.; Roy, D., Challenges in the addition of probiotic cultures to foods. *Critical Reviews in Food Science and Nutrition* **2005**, *45* (1), 61–84.

82. Champagne, C. P.; Fustier, P., Microencapsulation for the improved delivery of bioactive compounds into foods. *Current Opinion in Biotechnology* **2007**, *18* (2), 184–190.

83. Krasaekoopt, W.; Bhandari, B.; Deeth, H., Evaluation of encapsulation techniques of probiotics for yoghurt. *International Dairy Journal* **2003**, *13* (1), 3–13.

84. Agüero, L.; Zaldivar-Silva, D.; Peña, L.; Dias, M. L., Alginate microparticles as oral colon drug delivery device: A review. *Carbohydrate Polymers* **2017**, *168*, 32–43.

85. Sosnik, A. Alginate particles as platform for drug delivery by the oral route: State-of-the-art. *ISRN Pharmaceutics* **2014**, *2014*, 1–17.

86. Sastry, S. V.; Nyshadham, J. R.; Fix, J. A., Recent technological advances in oral drug delivery–A review. *Pharmaceutical Science & Technology Today* **2000**, *3* (4), 138–145.

87. Sharpe, L. A.; Daily, A. M.; Horava, S. D.; Peppas, N. A., Therapeutic applications of hydrogels in oral drug delivery. *Expert Opinion on Drug Delivery* **2014**, *11* (6), 901–915.

88. Chandramouli, V.; Kailasapathy, K.; Peiris, P.; Jones, M., An improved method of microencapsulation and its evaluation to protect Lactobacillus spp. in simulated gastric conditions. *Journal of Microbiological Methods* **2004**, *56* (1), 27–35.

89. Prevost, H.; Divies, C., Cream fermentation by a mixed culture of lactococci entrapped in two-layer calcium alginate gel beads. *Biotechnology Letters* **1992**, *14* (7), 583–588.

90. Tønnesen, H. H.; Karlsen, J., Alginate in drug delivery systems. *Drug Development and Industrial Pharmacy* **2002**, *28* (6), 621–630.

91. Lee, K. Y.; Mooney, D. J., Alginate: Properties and biomedical applications. *Progress in Polymer Science* **2012**, *37* (1), 106–126.

92. Ding, W.; Shah, N. P., Effect of various encapsulating materials on the stability of probiotic bacteria. *Journal of Food Science* **2009**, *74* (2), M100–M107.

93. Chourasia, M.; Jain, S., Pharmaceutical approaches to colon targeted drug delivery systems. *Journal of Pharmacy and Pharmaceutical Sciences* **2003**, *6* (1), 33–66.

94. Graff, S.; Hussain, S.; Chaumeil, J.-C.; Charrueau, C., Increased intestinal delivery of viable Saccharomyces boulardii by encapsulation in microspheres. *Pharmaceutical Research* **2008**, *25* (6), 1290–1296.

95. Albertini, B.; Vitali, B.; Passerini, N.; Cruciani, F.; Di Sabatino, M.; Rodriguez, L.; Brigidi, P., Development of microparticulate systems for intestinal delivery of Lactobacillus acidophilus and Bifidobacterium lactis. *European Journal of Pharmaceutical Sciences* **2010**, *40* (4), 359–366.

96. Sabikhi, L.; Babu, R.; Thompkinson, D. K.; Kapila, S., Resistance of microencapsulated Lactobacillus acidophilus LA1 to processing treatments and simulated gut conditions. *Food and Bioprocess Technology* **2010**, *3* (4), 586–593.

97. Mandal, S.; Puniya, A.; Singh, K., Effect of alginate concentrations on survival of microencapsulated Lactobacillus casei NCDC-298. *International Dairy Journal* **2006**, *16* (10), 1190–1195.

98. Hansen, L. T.; Allan-Wojtas, P.; Jin, Y.-L.; Paulson, A., Survival of Ca-alginate microencapsulated Bifidobacterium spp. in milk and simulated gastrointestinal conditions. *Food Microbiology* **2002**, *19* (1), 35–45.

99. Sultana, K.; Godward, G.; Reynolds, N.; Arumugaswamy, R.; Peiris, P.; Kailasapathy, K., Encapsulation of probiotic bacteria with alginate–starch and evaluation of survival in simulated gastrointestinal conditions and in yoghurt. *International Journal of Food Microbiology* **2000**, *62* (1–2), 47–55.

100. Choi, C.-H.; Jung, J.-H.; Rhee, Y. W.; Kim, D.-P.; Shim, S.-E.; Lee, C.-S., Generation of monodisperse alginate microbeads and in situ encapsulation of cell in microfluidic device. *Biomedical Microdevices* **2007**, *9* (6), 855–862.

101. McQuilling, J.; Arenas-Herrera, J.; Childers, C.; Pareta, R.; Khanna, O.; Jiang, B.; Brey, E.; Farney, A.; Opara, E. New alginate microcapsule system for angiogenic protein delivery and immunoisolation of islets for transplantation in the rat omentum pouch. In *Transplantation Proceedings*, Elsevier, **2011**; pp. 3262–3264.

102. Tendulkar, S.; McQuilling, J.; Childers, C.; Pareta, R.; Opara, E.; Ramasubramanian, M. A scalable microfluidic device for the mass production of microencapsulated islets. In *Transplantation Proceedings*, Elsevier, **2011**; pp. 3184–3187.

103. Utech, S.; Prodanovic, R.; Mao, A. S.; Ostafe, R.; Mooney, D. J.; Weitz, D. A., Microfluidic generation of monodisperse, structurally homogeneous alginate microgels for cell encapsulation and 3D cell culture. *Advanced Healthcare Materials* **2015**, *4* (11), 1628–1633.

104. Tan, W. H.; Takeuchi, S., Monodisperse alginate hydrogel microbeads for cell encapsulation. *Advanced Materials* **2007**, *19* (18), 2696–2701.

105. Gibbs, B. F., Kermasha, S., Alli, I., Mulligan, C. N., Encapsulation in the food industry: A review. *International Journal of Food Sciences and Nutrition* **1999**, *50* (3), 213–224.

106. Calafiore, R.; Basta, G., Alginate/poly-L-ornithine microcapsules for pancreatic islet cell immunoprotection. In *Cell Encapsulation Technology and Therapeutics*, Springer: **1999**; pp. 138–150.

107. De Vos, P.; De Haan, B.; Wolters, G.; Strubbe, J.; Van Schilfgaarde, R., Improved biocompatibility but limited graft survival after purification of alginate for microencapsulation of pancreatic islets. *Diabetologia* **1997**, *40* (3), 262–270.

108. Weir, G., Islet encapsulation: Advances and obstacles. *Diabetologia* **2013**, *56* (7), 1458–1461.

109. Opara, E. C.; McQuilling, J. P.; Farney, A. C., Microencapsulation of pancreatic islets for use in a bioartificial pancreas. In *Organ Regeneration: Methods and Protocols*, Basu, J.; Ludlow, J. W., Eds. Humana Press: Totowa, NJ, **2013**; pp. 261–266.

110. Krishnan, R.; Alexander, M.; Robles, L.; Foster 3rd, C. E.; Lakey, J. R., Islet and stem cell encapsulation for clinical transplantation. *The Review of Diabetic Studies: RDS* **2014**, *11* (1), 84.

111. Shintaku, H.; Kuwabara, T.; Kawano, S.; Suzuki, T.; Kanno, I.; Kotera, H., Micro cell encapsulation and its hydrogel-beads production using microfluidic device. *Microsystem Technologies* **2007**, *13* (8–10), 951–958.

112. Collins, D. J.; Neild, A.; deMello, A.; Liu, A.-Q.; Ai, Y., The Poisson distribution and beyond: Methods for microfluidic droplet production and single cell encapsulation. *Lab on a Chip* **2015**, *15* (17), 3439–3459.

113. Hillman, E. T.; Lu, H.; Yao, T.; Nakatsu, C. H., Microbial ecology along the gastrointestinal tract. *Microbes and Environments* **2017**, *32* (4), 300–313.

114. Priya James, H.; John, R.; Alex, A.; Anoop, K. R., Smart polymers for the controlled delivery of drugs – A concise overview. *Acta Pharmaceutica Sinica B* **2014**, *4* (2), 120–127.

115. Chen, S.-C.; Wu, Y.-C.; Mi, F.-L.; Lin, Y.-H.; Yu, L.-C.; Sung, H.-W., A novel pH-sensitive hydrogel composed of N, O-carboxymethyl chitosan and alginate cross-linked by genipin for protein drug delivery. *Journal of Controlled Release* **2004**, *96* (2), 285–300.

116. Chung, T. W.; Yang, J.; Akaike, T.; Cho, K. Y.; Nah, J. W.; Kim, S. I.; Cho, C. S., Preparation of alginate/galactosylated chitosan scaffold for hepatocyte attachment. *Biomaterials* **2002**, *23* (14), 2827–2834.

117. Florczyk, S. J.; Kievit, F. M.; Wang, K.; Erickson, A. E.; Ellenbogen, R. G.; Zhang, M., 3D porous chitosan–alginate scaffolds promote proliferation and enrichment of cancer stem-like cells. *Journal of Materials Chemistry B* **2016**, *4* (38), 6326–6334.

118. George, M.; Abraham, T. E., Polyionic hydrocolloids for the intestinal delivery of protein drugs: Alginate and chitosan — A review. *Journal of Controlled Release* **2006**, *114* (1), 1–14.

119. Ramdas, M.; Dileep, K.; Anitha, Y.; Paul, W.; Sharma, C. P., Alginate encapsulated bioadhesive chitosan microspheres for intestinal drug delivery. *Journal of Biomaterials Applications* **1999**, *13* (4), 290–296.

120. Yang, J.; Chen, J.; Pan, D.; Wan, Y.; Wang, Z., pH-sensitive interpenetrating network hydrogels based on chitosan derivatives and alginate for oral drug delivery. *Carbohydrate Polymers* **2013**, *92* (1), 719–725.

121. Cook, M. T.; Tzortzis, G.; Charalampopoulos, D.; Khutoryanskiy, V. V., Production and evaluation of dry alginate-chitosan microcapsules as an enteric delivery vehicle for probiotic bacteria. *Biomacromolecules* **2011**, *12* (7), 2834–2840.

122. Argin, S. Microencapsulation of probiotic bacteria in xanthan-chitosan polyelectrolyte complex gels. **2007**.

123. Argin, S.; Kofinas, P.; Lo, Y. M., The cell release kinetics and the swelling behavior of physically cross-linked xanthan–chitosan hydrogels in simulated gastrointestinal conditions. *Food Hydrocolloids* **2014**, *40*, 138–144.

124. Huguet, M. L.; Neufeld, R. J.; Dellacherie, E., Calcium-alginate beads coated with polycationic polymers: Comparison of chitosan and DEAE-dextran. *Process Biochemistry* **1996**, *31* (4), 347–353.

125. Ferreira Almeida, P.; Almeida, A. J., Cross-linked alginate–gelatine beads: A new matrix for controlled release of pindolol. *Journal of Controlled Release* **2004**, *97* (3), 431–439.

126. Alvarez-Lorenzo, C.; Blanco-Fernandez, B.; Puga, A. M.; Concheiro, A., Crosslinked ionic polysaccharides for stimuli-sensitive drug delivery. *Advanced Drug Delivery Reviews* **2013**, *65* (9), 1148–1171.

127. Agüero, L.; Zaldivar, D.; Peña, L.; Solís, Y.; Ramón, J.; Dias, M. L., Preparation and characterization of pH-sensitive microparticles based on polyelectrolyte complexes for antibiotic delivery. *Polymer Engineering & Science* **2015**, *55* (5), 981–987.

128. El-Sherbiny, I. M., Enhanced pH-responsive carrier system based on alginate and chemically modified carboxymethyl chitosan for oral delivery of protein drugs: Preparation and in-vitro assessment. *Carbohydrate Polymers* **2010**, *80* (4), 1125–1136.

129. Mei, L.; He, F.; Zhou, R.-Q.; Wu, C.-D.; Liang, R.; Xie, R.; Ju, X.-J.; Wang, W.; Chu, L.-Y., Novel intestinal-targeted Ca-alginate-based carrier for pH-responsive protection and release of lactic acid bacteria. *ACS Applied Materials & Interfaces* **2014**, *6* (8), 5962–5970.

130. Banks, S. R.; Enck, K.; Wright, M. W.; Opara, E. C.; Welker, M. E., Chemical modification of alginate for controlled oral drug delivery. *Journal of Agricultural and Food Chemistry* **2019**, *67* (37), 10481–10488.

131. Dutta, P.; Mitra, U.; Dutta, S.; Rajendran, K.; Saha, T. K.; Chatterjee, M. K., Randomised controlled clinical trial of Lactobacillus sporogenes (Bacillus coagulans), used as probiotic in clinical practice, on acute watery diarrhoea in children. *Tropical Medicine & International Health* **2011**, *16* (5), 555–561.

132. Manabe, N.; Haruma, K.; Ito, M.; Takahashi, N.; Takasugi, H.; Wada, Y.; Nakata, H.; Katoh, T.; Miyamoto, M.; Tanaka, S., Efficacy of adding sodium alginate to omeprazole in patients with nonerosive reflux disease: A randomized clinical trial. *Diseases of the Esophagus* **2012**, *25* (5), 373–380.

133. de Vos, P.; Faas, M. M.; Spasojevic, M.; Sikkema, J., Encapsulation for preservation of functionality and targeted delivery of bioactive food components. *International Dairy Journal* **2010**, *20* (4), 292–302.

134. Ljungberg, M.; Korpela, R.; Ilonen, J.; Ludvigsson, J.; Vaarala, O., Probiotics for the prevention of beta cell autoimmunity in children at genetic risk of type 1 diabetes—the PRODIA study. *Annals of the New York Academy of Sciences* **2006**, *1079* (1), 360–364.

135. Amara, A.; Shibl, A., Role of probiotics in health improvement, infection control and disease treatment and management. *Saudi Pharmaceutical Journal* **2015**, *23* (2), 107–114.

Index